Geropsychiatric and Mental Health Nursing

Edited by

Karen Devereaux Melillo

PhD, APRN, BC, FAANP
Professor, Department of Nursing
School of Health and Environment
University of Massachusetts Lowell
Lowell, MA

Susan Crocker Houde

PhD, APRN, BC
Associate Professor and
Director of Master's Program in Nursing
University of Massachusetts Lowell
Lowell, MA

JONES AND BARTLETT PUBLISHERS

Sudbury, Massachusetts

BOSTON   TORONTO   LONDON   SINGAPORE

World Headquarters
Jones and Bartlett Publishers
40 Tall Pine Drive
Sudbury, MA 01776
978-443-5000
info@jbpub.com
www.jbpub.com

Jones and Bartlett Publishers
Canada
6339 Ormindale Way
Mississauga, ON L5V 1J2
CANADA

Jones and Bartlett Publishers
International
Barb House, Barb Mews
London W6 7PA
UK

Jones and Bartlett's books and products are available through most bookstores and online booksellers. To contact Jones and Bartlett Publishers directly, call 800-832-0034, fax 978-443-8000, or visit our website www.jbpub.com.

Substantial discounts on bulk quantities of Jones and Bartlett's publications are available to corporations, professional associations, and other qualified organizations. For details and specific discount information, contact the special sales department at Jones and Bartlett via the above contact information or send an email to specialsales@jbpub.com.

Copyright © 2005 by Jones and Bartlett Publishers, Inc.

ISBN-13: 978-0-7637-3272-1
ISBN-10: 0-7637-3272-9

Library of Congress Cataloging-in-Publication Data
Geropsychiatric and mental health nursing / [edited by] Karen Devereaux Melillo, Susan Crocker Houde.
    p. ; cm.
   Includes bibliographical references and index.
   ISBN 0-7637-3272-9 (pbk.)
   1. Geriatric psychiatry.   2. Geriatric nursing.   3. Psychiatric nursing.
I. Milillo, Karen Devereaux.   II. Houde, Susan Crocker.
   [DNLM: 1. Geriatric Nursing—methods.   2. Geriatric Psychiatry—methods.   3. Mental Disorders—nursing—Aged.
WY 152 G37774 2005]RC451.4.A5G479 2005
   618.97'689--dc22

                                                              2004025831

Production Credits
Acquisitions Editor: Kevin Sullivan
Production Director: Amy Rose
Associate Editor: Amy Sibley
Production Assistant: Kate Hennessy
Marketing Manager: Emily Ekle

Manufacturing and Inventory Coordinator: Amy Bacus
Composition: Bookwrights
Cover Design: Timothy Dziewit
Printing and Binding: Malloy, Inc.
Cover Printing: Malloy, Inc.

6048

Printed in the United States of America
10 09 08   10 9 8 7 6 5 4 3

Contents

Contributors

Julia K. Bail, MS, APRN, BC
Geriatric Nurse Practitioner and Clinical Nurse Specialist
West Los Angeles Veterans Administration
Los Angeles, CA

Charles E. Blair, PhD, RN, CS, LNFA
Director, Nursing Education and Research
The University of Texas Health Center at Tyler
Tyler, TX
John A. Hartford Foundation Institute for Geriatric Nursing Scholar

Marguarette M. Bolton, BA
Division of Nursing
The Steinhardt School of Education
New York University
New York, NY

Lisa A. Brown, MS, APRN, BC
Psychiatric Mental Health Nurse Practitioner
Health and Education Services, Inc.
Lawrence, MA

Kathleen C. Buckwalter, PhD, RN, FAAN
Distinguished Professor of Nursing
Co-Director, National Health Law and Policy Resource Center
The University of Iowa
Iowa City, IA

Eve Heemann Byrd, MSN, MPH, RN, FNP
Associate Director
Fuqua Center for Late-Life Depression
Wesley Woods Center of Emory University
Atlanta, GA

Jane Cloutterbuck, PhD, RN
Associate Professor
College of Nursing and Health Sciences
University of Massachusetts Boston
Boston, MA

Karen Dick, PhD, APRN, BC, FAANP
Assistant Professor
College of Nursing and Health Sciences
University of Massachusetts Boston
Boston, MA
John A. Hartford Foundation Institute for Geriatric Nursing Scholar

Michelle Doran, MS, APRN, BC, ANP, GNP, PCM
Palliative Care Consult Team
Hospice of the North Shore
Danvers, MA

Priscilla Ebersole, RN, PhD, FAAN
Professor Emerita
San Francisco State University
San Francisco, CA

Barbara J. Edlund, RN, PhD, ANP-BC
Associate Professor and Gerontological Track Coordinator
College of Nursing
Medical University of South Carolina
Charleston, SC

Kathy J. Fabiszewski, PhD, APRN, BC
Assistant Professor
School of Nursing
Salem State College
Salem, MA
and
Gerontological Nurse Practitioner
Family Doctors
Swampscott, MA

Terry Fulmer, PhD, RN, FAAN
The Erline Perkins McGriff Professor and Head, Division of Nursing
New York University
New York, NY
John A. Hartford Foundation Institute for Geriatric Nursing

May Futrell, PhD, RN, FAAN, FGSA
Professor and Chair
Department of Nursing
University of Massachusetts Lowell
Lowell, MA

Karyn Geary, MS, APRN, BC, ANP, GNP, PCM
Palliative Care Consult Team
Hospice of the North Shore
Danvers, MA

Linda A. Gerdner, PhD, RN
Assistant Professor
University of Minnesota
School of Nursing
Minneapolis, MN

Lisa Guadagno, MPA
Project Director
The Steinhardt School of Education
Division of Nursing
New York University
New York, NY

Lee Ann Hoff, PhD, MSN, MA
Author, "People in Crisis"
International Consultant: "Violence, Crisis, and Gender Issues"
Boston, MA

Susan Crocker Houde, PhD, APRN, BC
Associate Professor and Director of Master's Program in Nursing
University of Massachusetts Lowell
Lowell, MA
John A. Hartford Foundation Institute for Geriatric Nursing Scholar

Martha A. Huff, MS, APRN, BC
*Psychiatric/Mental Health Nurse Practitionaer, Gerontological Nurse Practitioner,
    Behavioral Health Fellow*
Harvard Vanguard Medical Associates
Chelmsford, MA

Madelyn Iris, PhD
Clinical Associate Professor
Buehler Center on Aging
The Feinberg School of Medicine
Northwestern University
Evanston, IL

Cindy H. Sullivan Kerber, PhD, APN, CS
Post-doctoral Fellow
College of Nursing
University of Iowa
Iowa City, IA
Assistant Professor
School of Nursing
Illinois Wesleyan University
Bloomington, IL

Diane Feeney Mahoney, PhD, APRN, BC
Director of Enhanced Family Caregiving Through Technology Program and Senior Research Scientist
Research and Training Institute
Hebrew Rehabilitation Center for Aged
Boston, MA

Geoffry McEnany, PhD, APRN, BC
Associate Professor
Department of Nursing
University of Massachusetts Lowell
Lowell, MA

Karen Devereaux Melillo, PhD, APRN, BC, FAANP
Professor
Department of Nursing
School of Health and Environment
University of Massachusetts Lowell
Lowell, MA

Janet C. Mentes, PhD, APRN, BC
Assistant Professor
School of Nursing
University of California Los Angeles
Los Angeles, CA
John A. Hartford Foundation Building Academic Geriatric Nursing Capacity Postdoctoral Fellow

Catherine R. Morency, MS, APRN, BC
Health Care Coordinator
Society of Jesus of New England
Boston, MA

Betty D. Morgan, PhD, APRN, BC
Assistant Professor
Coordinator, Adult Psychiatric and Mental Health Nursing Program
Department of Nursing
University of Massachusetts Lowell
Lowell, MA

Ruth Remington, PhD, APRN, BC
Assistant Professor
Department of Nursing
School of Health and Environment
University of Massachusetts Lowell
Lowell, MA

Barbara Resnick, PhD, CRNP, FAAN, FAANP
Associate Professor
University of Maryland School of Nursing
Baltimore, MD

Marianne Shaughnessy, PhD, CRNP
Assistant Professor
University of Maryland School of Nursing
Baltimore, MD

Kathleen Sherrell, RN, PsyD
Research Associate
Buehler Center on Aging
Associate Professor Emeritus
The Feinberg School of Medicine
Department of Psychiatry and Behavioral Sciences
Northwestern University
Evanston, IL

Marjorie Simpson, MS, CRNP
Doctoral Student
University of Maryland School of Nursing
Baltimore, MD

Marianne Smith, MS, ARNP, CS
Research Associate
The University of Iowa College of Nursing
Iowa City, IA
John A. Hartford Foundation Building Academic Geriatric Nursing Capacity
    Scholar

James Sterrett, BS, PharmD, CDE
Adjunct Clinical Assistant Professor
College of Pharmacy
Medical University of South Carolina
Pharmacist
Walgreens Pharmacy
Charleston, SC

Ann X. Wallace, MSN, RN, APRN, BC, NP-C
Capiton Medical Clinic
Taunton State Hospital
Taunton, MA

Donna McCarten White, RN, PhD, CADAC-II, LADC-I
Addiction Specialist
Lemuel Shattuck Hospital
Jamaica Plain, MA

Lin Zhan, PhD, RN, FAAN
Professor, Director of Nursing PhD Program
School of Health and Environment
University of Massachusetts Lowell
Lowell, MA

Acknowledgments

This book became a reality thanks to the dedicated and knowledgeable contributors who devoted their time and expertise to advance the important field of geropsychiatric and mental health nursing. I am amazed and humbled by the contributions of these nationally recognized gerontological and psychiatric and mental health nursing leaders. The Scholars Program at The John A. Hartford Institute for Geriatric Nursing at New York University was instrumental in our search for knowledgeable experts, and the behind-the-scenes mentorship and guidance provided to a number of the contributors by Dr. Kitty Buckwalter was most appreciated.

I have been fortunate to be mentored by Dr. May Futrell whose role modeling has been instrumental in many of the professional choices I have made. Most notable among these was my decision to pursue graduate education in gerontological nursing as a gerontological nurse practitioner at the University of Massachusetts Lowell in 1977; my decision to return five years later in a nurse practitioner faculty role; and my pursuit of doctoral education at Brandeis University, where May Futrell herself was among one of the first nurse graduates of the PhD in Social Policy Program. Many years of professional colleagueship with Dr. Futrell have resulted in opportunities to collaborate in countless teaching, research, and scholarship activities. Now, as Dr. Futrell plans for her retirement after 47 years of teaching, I find I am again indebted to her mentorship as I assume the role of department chair that she will vacate in June 2005. Her visionary leadership has been a beacon of light in all I have done, and I know it will continue to shine.

For the past and present gerontological nurse practitioner students with whom I have had the pleasure to teach, I thank you. Your enthusiasm, commitment, and motivation toward quality care for older adults have been a source of immense satisfaction. Our opportunity to work together in enabling you to reach your educational goals, in combination with the quality nursing care provided to the older adults entrusted to our care, has been a gift to me. For the first class of Geropsychiatric and Mental Health Nursing Certificate students enrolled in the core course, I wish to thank you for taking the journey with us, the faculty, in this course: Eileen Allosso, Wendy Arena, Bridget Langa, Irene Laventure, Sharon

Lefebvre, Brenda Lorrey, and Mary Jane (Dee Dee) Powers. For my faculty colleagues in this course, Drs. Betty Morgan and Carol Picard, thank you for sharing your expertise and for demonstrating how gerontological nursing and adult psychiatric mental health nursing does, indeed, blend into the needed geropsychiatric and mental health nursing specialty.

For my co-editor, Susan Crocker Houde, I have been truly blessed to work with a professional colleague and friend whose knowledge, work ethic, attention to detail, perseverance, support, and conscientiousness are traits unrivaled by anyone with whom I have worked. From the initiation of the project, throughout its development, and into its submission stage, Susan has stood out as a colleague that every professional should have the chance to work alongside. Long before this project, Susan was my first nurse practitioner instructor and was instrumental in encouraging me to apply for her position when she had made a decision to leave academia for the practice arena. Her continued involvement as a part-time instructor with the Master's Degree Nursing Program at the University of Massachusetts Lowell during her doctoral studies was pivotal to its success. Returning to the university seven years ago and now as an associate professor, Dr. Susan Crocker Houde has been an outstanding asset to the university, school, and department, and to the many students she has so positively influenced.

And, finally, my family deserves recognition for their support and encouragement throughout this process. To Bob, my husband of 31 years, this likely seemed like just another project, but he remained positive and encouraging despite the workload and hours required. For each of my four children—Michael, Marc, Eric, and Kara—you offered your own unique perspectives and laughter when it was needed, and always helped to ground me in this endeavor. To my parents, Bob and Helen Devereaux, and to your parenting formula that raised five self-reliant, highly independent, hard-working daughters, thank you. You have been my inspiration in both my professional and personal life.

To Jones and Bartlett Publishers who undertook this project, to Kevin Sullivan, the Acquisitions Editor who approached us about the project, to Amy Sibley who helped to assure the manuscript was prepared for launching, and to Kate Hennessy and the copyediting staff, thank you.

Karen Devereaux Melillo, co-editor

There are a number of people to whom I would like to express my sincere thanks for their assistance and support during the last two years of co-editing this book. First and foremost, I would like to express my appreciation to Karen Devereaux Melillo, whose hard work, organizing skills, keen mind for detail, dedication, and friendship have made working on this book such a pleasure. It is rare, I believe, to find someone with such outstanding qualities with whom to share your career.

I would like to thank Jones and Bartlett Publishers for recognizing that this book needed to be written, and to express appreciation for the assistance and support of Kevin Sullivan and Amy Sibley with the publication of this manuscript.

I would also like to recognize the assistance provided by Mathy Mezey and Amy Berman at The John A. Hartford Foundation Institute of Geriatric Nursing at New York University. They were instrumental in helping us to identify several contributors for the book who are leading experts in the field of geropsychiatric and mental health nursing. The efforts of the Hartford Institute have done so much to improve the nursing care of older adults and to educate nurses about the value of gerontological nursing as a specialty area.

Words cannot express my gratitude for the contributions of Kitty Buckwalter, who provided suggestions for the selection of contributors as well as editorial assistance to contributors, who reviewed the original book proposal and offered suggestions in its early stages of development, and who contributed to the text. We are indeed fortunate to have such leaders in the field of geropsychiatric and mental health nursing to guide us on our way.

How can one thank the contributors to this text? They are professionals who were willing to share their knowledge and expertise in this important specialty area, and who were willing to do this with little reward other than the knowledge and satisfaction that they were helping to prepare the geropsychiatric and mental health nurses of tomorrow.

To my lifetime mentor in the field of gerontological nursing, Dr. May Futrell, I express my gratitude for the support and guidance provided to me all these years. I have indeed been fortunate to have been tucked under the wing of such a pioneer and leader in this evolving specialty so many years ago.

Geoffry McEnany, my thanks for the lack of hesitation in agreeing to review a section of the book at a time when other work demands must have been overwhelming.

The support of colleagues and the administration at the University of Massachusetts Lowell has helped to make this text a reality. My students, thank you, for the inquisitive questions that keep me searching for answers in the important specialty of gerontological nursing. This book has been written for you.

I would like to express my appreciation to my family—Chuck, Courtney, and Katelyn—for tolerating my distraction and long hours at the computer during the co-editing of this text. Your presence and understanding help me to keep a healthy perspective in my life.

I would also like to thank Ram R. Gautam for his support and encouragement throughout the past year. He has taught me that anything is possible, that one should set high goals and strive for success. It is my hope that this text will help you, the readers, to achieve your professional goals in the specialty area of geropsychiatric and mental health nursing!

Susan Crocker Houde, co-editor

SECTION I

Overview of Aging and Mental Health Issues

CHAPTER 1

Introduction and Overview of Aging and Older Adulthood

Karen Devereaux Melillo, PhD, APRN, BC, FAANP

INTRODUCTION

The impetus for the development of this textbook is the projected change in the demographics of aging. Nationally, persons 65 years or older represent 12.3% of the US population. Demographic projections are that 20% of the population will be 65 and older by 2030, with phenomenal growth anticipated for older minority populations, from 16.4% of the elderly population in 2000 to 26.4% in the year 2030 (Administration on Aging [AOA], 2003). This growth will enlarge the population experiencing mental health issues and psychiatric disorders. For the gerontological nurse, this will require increasing knowledge and skills. In fact, *Mental Health: A Report of the Surgeon General* (Dept. of Health and Human Services [DHHS], 1999) notes "disability due to mental illness in individuals over 65 years old will become a major public health problem in the near future. . . . In particular, dementia, depression, and schizophrenia, among other conditions, will all present special problems in this age group" (p. 85). Furthermore, the American Psychiatric Association (APA, 1994) estimates that 15–25% of older adults suffer from symptoms of mental illness, with depression being considered the most common mental disorder, affecting up to 20% of those 65 and older.

MENTAL HEALTH AND OLDER ADULTS

The promotion of mental health in older adults is of critical importance. "Mental health is a state of well-being in which the individual realizes his or her own abilities, can cope with the normal stresses of life, can work productively and fruitfully, and is able to make a contribution to his or her community" (World Health Organization [WHO] Fact Sheet, 2001). Mental health promotion includes encouragement in the use of both individual and family resources and skills. It reflects a social ecology model of health and health promotion, recognizing that improvements in the socioeconomic environment are key.

This social ecology model of health promotion, including mental health, suggests the need for individually oriented behavior-change strategies in the care and treatment of mental health and psychiatric disorders, and proposes health promotion activities that emphasize a social causation of disease requiring changes in both physical and social environments (McLeroy, Bibeau, Steckler, & Glanz, 1988). The ecological perspective implies a reciprocal relationship between the individual and the environment. The five levels of analysis in an ecological model for mental health promotion include:

- Intrapersonal factors (psychological, values, personality, skills, knowledge, attitudes, behavior, self-concept, self-efficacy, self-esteem, and developmental history of the individual)

- Interpersonal processes and primary groups (formal and informal social networks, social support, family, work group, friendship networks, peers, and neighbors)

- Institutional and organizational factors (social institutions, schools, work settings, with organizational characteristics or culture, management styles, organization structure, communication networks, and rules and regulations)

- Community factors (relationships among organizations, institutions, churches, voluntary associations, neighborhoods, area economics, community resources, social and health services, governmental structures, formal and informal leadership, and folk practices)

- Public policy (local, state, and national laws; taxes; regulatory agencies and policies; political parties; citizen participation; and bureaucracies) (McLeroy, et al., 1988; McLeroy, Steckler, Goodman & Burdine, 1992).

Each of these social–ecological levels must be considered when addressing mental health promotion for older adults. Gerontological nurses can be key in defining the impact of each level on behavior when assessing and providing care for older adults.

Globally, WHO has emphasized that national mental health policies should enhance public awareness of mental illness while also addressing those broader issues that affect the mental health of all sectors of society. A mental health promotion policy must include the social integration of severely marginalized groups, including refugees, disaster victims, the socially alienated, the mentally disabled, the very old and infirm, abused children and women, and the poor (WHO, 1999).

The US Surgeon General's *Report on Mental Health* summarized themes that are important to consider when promoting mental health in the older adult:

- Important life tasks remain for individuals as they age. Older individuals continue to learn and contribute to society, in spite of physiologic changes due to aging and increasing health problems;

- Continued intellectual, social, and physical activity throughout the life cycle are important for the maintenance of mental health in late life;

- Stressful life events, such as declining health and/or the loss of mates, family members, or friends often increase with age. However, persistent bereavement or serious depression is not 'normal' and should be treated;

- Normal aging is not characterized by mental or cognitive disorders. Mental or substance-use disorders that present alone or co-occur should be recognized and treated as illnesses;

- Disability due to mental illness in individuals over 65 years old will become a major public health problem in the near future because of demographic changes. In particular . . .

  ○ Dementia produces significant dependency and is a leading contributor to the need for costly long-term care in the last years of life.

  ○ Depression contributes to the high rates of suicide among males in this population.

  ○ Schizophrenia continues to be disabling in spite of recovery of function by some individuals in mid to late life.

- There are effective interventions for most mental disorders experienced by older persons (for example, depression and anxiety), and many mental health problems, such as bereavement;
- Older individuals can benefit from the advances in psychotherapy, medication, and other treatment interventions for mental disorders enjoyed by younger adults, when these interventions are modified for age and health status;
- Treating older adults with mental disorders accrues other benefits to overall health by improving the interest and ability of individuals to care for themselves and follow their primary care provider's directions and advice, particularly about taking medications;
- Primary care practitioners are a critical link in identifying and addressing mental disorders in older adults. Opportunities are missed to improve mental health and general medical outcomes when mental illness is underrecognized and undertreated in primary care settings; and,
- Barriers to access exist in the organizing and financing of services for aging citizens. There are specific problems with Medicare, Medicaid, nursing homes, and managed care (US Surgeon General, 1999, p. 381).

Nurses should be vigilant in assessing how older adults respond to life events, transitions, and challenges to their physical and mental well-being in order to initiate appropriate interventions in a timely manner (DHHS 2001).

■ INTRODUCTION TO MENTAL HEALTH ISSUES AND DISORDERS

Overall, only one third of Americans of all ages with mental illness or mental health problems get care. This figure is likely higher among older adults (US Surgeon General, 1999). Butler, Lewis and Sunderland (1998)

suggest that stigma and embarrassment may be largely responsible, along with too few health care workers prepared to assess and treat this special population.

There is often a lack of clear terminology to define the experiences of those suffering from mental disorders. A mental disorder is "conceptualized as a clinically significant behavioral or psychological syndrome or pattern that occurs in an individual and that is associated with present distress (e.g., a painful symptom) or disability (i.e., impairment in one or more important areas of functioning) or with a significantly increased risk of suffering death, pain, disability or with an important loss of freedom. In addition, this syndrome or pattern must not be merely an expectable and culturally sanctioned response to a particular event, for example, the death of a loved one" (APA, 2000, p. xxxi).

Nearly 20% of the population 55 and older experience specific mental disorders that are not part of normal aging (AOA, 2001; US Surgeon General, 1999), including "depression, Alzheimer's disease, alcohol and drug misuse and abuse, anxiety, late-life schizophrenia, and other conditions" (US Surgeon General, 1999, para. 3). The National Institute of Mental Health (NIMH, 2001) has reported that four of the 10 leading causes of disability in the United States and other developed countries are mental disorders—major depression, bipolar disorder, schizophrenia, and obsessive–compulsive disorder.

The National Council on the Aging (Cutler, Whitelaw, & Beattie, 2002), reported on interviews conducted by telephone with a nationally representative sample of 3048 community-residing older adults. On the topic of health and aging, 11% of respondents reported being diagnosed with depression. As expected, there was disparity in those reporting depression by age, gender, education, and race. For the 65–74-year-old age group, 12% reported being diagnosed with depression, while 10% of those over 75 reported depression. A recent doctoral dissertation similarly reported depression to be greatest in the 65–74-year-old age group versus oldest-old adults, suggesting that resilience and coping of advanced-age survivors may be a factor in ameliorating the effects of depressive symptomatology for some (Butler, 2003).

Cutler et al. (2002) found that females more frequently reported depression (13%) versus males (8%). High school graduates reported depression less frequently than those who did not graduate from high school (10% compared to 14%). Blacks reported depression more (14%) than white respondents (10%). Overall, depression ranked ninth in the number of diseases or medical problems diagnosed (following high blood pressure, arthritis, prostate problems, heart disease, diabetes, respiratory problems, cancer, and osteoporosis) (Cutler et al.). These findings underscore the prevalence and impact of depressive disorders among older adults.

Relationship of Functional Status and Mobility Impairments to Mental Health

For gerontological nurses, the notion that the mind and body cannot be separated is widely recognized. Nurses have long viewed people in terms of wholeness of mind, body, and spirit, noting the interdependence of affective, behavioral, cognitive, social, and spiritual factors on physical well-being and vice versa (Edmands, Hoff, Kaylor, Mower, & Sorrell, 1999). Chronic health problems are more common in older adults than in younger adults, and functional impairments often occur as a result. Because of this, older adults may be experiencing mental health issues and problems in combination with the burden of chronic disease and functional disability or impairment. Consideration of these combined issues is essential in providing effective nursing care for older adults.

In the United States, approximately 80% of all persons 65 years and older have at least one chronic condition, and 50% have at least two. These chronic conditions often translate into limitations of activities, either instrumental or daily, and this becomes increasingly so with age (Figure 1-1). In 2001, 26.1% of those 65–74 years old reported a limitation, compared to 45.1% of those 75 years and over (AOA, 2003). For those 80+, almost three fourths (73.6%) report at least one disability. There is a strong relationship between disability status and

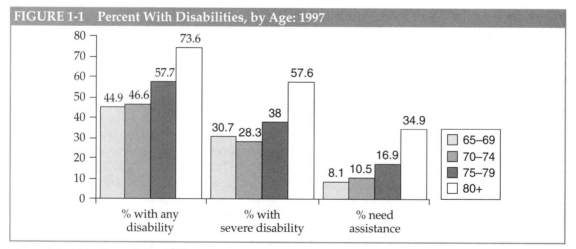

FIGURE 1-1   Percent With Disabilities, by Age: 1997

Source: Administration on Aging, 2003, p. 13.

reported health status such that 68% of those 65+ with a severe disability reported fair or poor health status (AOA). Severe disability presence is also associated with both lower income and lower educational attainment. Campbell, Crews, Moriarty, Zack, and Blackman (1999) examined data representing individuals 65 and older regarding activity limitations and sensory impairments for 1994 and health-related quality of life for 1993–97. They found that 6.2% of respondents 65 years and older had related that during the preceding 30 days their physical or mental health was "not good" (Campbell et al.). There appears to be a strong relationship between mental health and physical health and perceived health status in the older adult population.

Functional impairment with activity limitation is a common problem in the older adult population. Over 50% of the older population reported having at least one disability of some type (including both physical and nonphysical) (AOA, 2003). The presence of a disability can have a major impact on mental health. Research by Manton and Gu (2001) has identified a decline in recent disability rates using statistics from the National Long-Term Care Survey of the American population. In fact, the age-standardized prevalence of those with disability fell from 26.2% to 19.7%, between 1982 and 1999. The current emphasis on health promotion by the American public and health professionals may be responsible for this improvement.

▰▰ VULNERABLE POPULATIONS

Certain populations of older adults are at particular risk for mental health disorders and psychiatric illnesses. The following highlights some of these populations.

Chronically and Persistently Mentally Ill

Severe and persistent mental illness refers to the experience of an individual who has a psychiatric disorder that persists over time with remissions and recurrence of severe and disabling symptoms (Scholler-Jaquish, 2004). The most common psychiatric diagnoses responsible for chronic and persistent mental illness include schizophrenia, mood disorders, delusional disorders, dementia, amnesia, and other cognitive or psychotic disorders (APA, 2000). Gurland and Toner (1991) have suggested the following quality of life criteria in identifying chronicity of mental illness:

(a) Impairments of functional status in the performance of the basic and instrumental activities of daily life, and in such areas as social relationships, morale and life satisfaction, intellectual processes, communication skills, work, use of leisure time, initiative, and access to environmental and material resources

(b) Severity levels of symptomatic distress, or behaviors which are dangerous or disturbing to others because of the mental condition

(c) The extent to which current impairments of the sufferer's functional status are the basis for planning and decisions respecting the future

(d) The extent to which major options affecting quality of life, such as location of residence and degree of independence, have been predicated on the illness effects (Gurland & Toner, p. 5).

Some older adults with severe and persistent mental illness have had mental illness for decades while others may have been diagnosed later in life. In either case, the geropsychiatric nurse can play an important role. He/she can assist older adults by working with other multidisciplinary mental health team members in fostering access to coordinated care services and treatment programs that are geriatric-specific and by referring to agencies that can assist in assuring appropriate care.

Older Adults with Mental Retardation/ Developmental Disabilities and Their Aging Family Caregivers

Older adults, individuals over age 60, with lifelong intellectual and developmental disabilities (I/DD) numbered 641,000 in the United States in 2000. By 2030, these numbers are expected to double to 1,242,800 (Heller, Janicki, Hammel, & Factor, 2002). The life expectancy of persons with intellectual disabilities was 66 years in 1993, up from 19 years in the 1930s and 59 years in the 1970s. For individuals with Down's syndrome, the life expectancy in 1993 was 56 years, compared to the average age at death in the 1920s of nine years. Despite these significant demographic increases, few nurses have been educated to anticipate the needs or provide care for this unique population. Additionally, families are the primary providers of care for over two-thirds of adults with I/DD who live at home, and 25% of these caregivers are themselves over age 60 (Heller et al.). Expanding life expectancy has created significant demands for residential services where advocates note thousands on such waiting lists.

A report has been generated with recommendations for new directions in research in policy that addresses: (1) promoting healthy aging, (2) supporting families, and (3) creating age-friendly communities for those aging with developmental disabilities. The recommendations included:

- Assess and conduct public health surveillance of the health status of adults aging with I/DD and track their health care experiences.
- Conduct research on the reciprocal relationships between mental and emotional status, physical health, and environmental factors, including poverty, abusive, and stressful situations.
- Identify factors contributing to obesity and malnutrition, including nutritional status, medication use, and physical activ-

ity for persons with varying conditions and syndromes through longitudinal studies.

- Develop and evaluate health promotion programs encompassing health behavior education, nutrition, and physical activity, including analyses of differential effects for different syndromes and diagnostic groups, the impact on nontraditional exercise methods (e.g., tai chi), and methods of increasing exercise adherence (Heller, et al., 2002, p. 10).

Nursing has developed its own *Scope and Standards for the Nurse who Specializes in Developmental Disabilities and/or Mental Retardation* (American Nurses Association [ANA] 1998). However, few nurses have had any clinical experience in the care of this population, and nursing curricula do not adequately address this mental health area in the educational preparation of their graduates. This growing need, as evidenced by the demographic trends toward increasing life expectancy and community-based care settings, should be the basis for expanding model programs using nurses as pivotal care providers to adults and, more importantly, their caregivers.

The Homeless

Researchers have noted that homeless individuals at age 50 look and act like those 10 to 20 years older; thus, the *older homeless* population often refers to those age 50 and over (Cohen, 1999; Cohen, Teresi, Holmes, & Roth, 1988). Estimates of the proportion of individuals 50 and older in the homeless population range from 15–28% in shelter samples and up to 50% in street samples (DeMallie, North & Smith, 1997). Obviously, locating and recruiting any homeless population for study can be quite difficult, and, as a result, older homeless people are especially neglected in the research literature.

Unfortunately, many people with serious mental illness are among the homeless. "At least 30% of homeless persons suffer from some type of mental disorder" (Hogstel, 1995, p. 314). In fact, five to six times as many people who are homeless suffer from serious mental illnesses compared to the US population (Substance Abuse and Mental Health Services Administration [SAMHSA], 2003). Reporting on the mental illnesses experienced by the homeless population, SAMHSA notes that as many as 50% have had a diagnosable substance abuse disorder at some point during their lives, and up to 50% have had both substance use disorders and co-occurring mental illnesses, such as depression, bipolar disorder, schizophrenia, and severe personality disorders.

In one large study of homeless individuals, 13% of the 600 men and 3% of the 300 women were in the older age group of 50 years or more, with a mean age of 57.1 ± 6.9, and a range of 50–82 (DeMallie, North, & Smith, 1997). The study, designed to identify differences in psychiatric disorders between older and younger homeless subgroups, indicated that older subjects were more likely to be male and white, had lower incomes than their younger counterparts, and complained of worse health. Substance abuse history was present in nine out of 10 older men with a psychiatric disorder. More than one third of the older population suffered from the following: schizophrenia, bipolar disorder, major depression, generalized anxiety disorder, panic disorder, posttraumatic stress disorder, organic mental disorder, antisocial personality disorder, and conduct disorder (DeMallie et al. 1997).

Older women are the least frequently studied group of homeless individuals, and are estimated to be 20% of the older homeless population (Cohen, Ramirez, Teresi, Gallagher, & Sokolovsky, 1997). Unlike males, older women seem to have the best potential for finding housing, according to the interviews conducted with 237 women. Using the SHORT-CARE instrument, 40% of the women sampled evidenced psychotic

symptoms, including hallucinations, delusions, or disorganized thinking, 27% admitted to prior psychiatric hospitalizations, and 8% were moderate, heavy, or spree drinkers (Cohen, et al., 1997). Not surprisingly, older participants who found housing were significantly less likely to exhibit psychotic symptoms. This research suggests that, for older homeless women, both individual risk factors and systemic factors related to the availability of low-cost housing contribute to the etiology of homelessness.

The National Resource Center on Homelessness and Mental Illness (1999) serves as a clearinghouse of information and has published an annotated bibliography on homelessness and mental illness among older Americans. It is available at http://www.nrchmi.com. In one such referenced document, the challenges and opportunities in applying a population health approach to mental health services are described by the University of British Columbia's Institute of Health Promotion Research for the Health Systems Section of Health Canada (1999). This document emphasizes that forces and factors beyond the health care system strongly influence health, and that programs and policies that emphasize personal lifestyle and behavioral factors ("victim blaming") will overlook the broader determinants of health, and especially mental health. Some of the determinants are biological (genetics, age, gender, and race/ethnicity) while others, termed "distal determinants of health" (Frankish, Bishop & Steeves, 1999), include education, employment, income, housing, social support, and health-promoting behaviors. The population health approach to identifying and addressing the needs of older persons with mental illness in general, and homeless older persons in particular, is in keeping with the social ecology model of health promotion described earlier in this chapter.

▆ SUMMARY OF MENTAL HEALTH PROBLEMS EXPERIENCED BY OLDER ADULTS

The US Administration on Aging has reported on the following about mental health issues and older adults:

- **Age**—While suicide rates for persons 65 and older are higher than for any other age group, the suicide rate for persons 85+ is the highest of all—nearly twice the overall national rate.

- **Gender**—Women on average live seven years longer than men and are much more likely than older men to be widowed, to live alone, to be institutionalized, to receive a lower retirement income from all sources, and to suffer disproportionately from chronic disabilities and disorders. However, white men 85+ have the highest suicide rate among older adults.

- **Older Gay Men and Lesbians**—Social support, an important element of mental health for all older people, may be especially critical for older people who are gay, lesbian, or bisexual and who may have been exposed to prejudice, stigmatization, and antigay violence.

- **Marital Status**—Emotional and economic well-being of older Americans is strongly linked to their marital status.

- **Minority Status**—Minority populations, now representing 16% of the elderly population, are expected to represent 25% by 2030. Minorities face additional stressors such as higher rates of poverty and greater health problems. In the mental health arena, it is important to note that Westernized mental health treatment emphasizes verbal inquiry, interaction, and response, which may not be compatible with minority cultural beliefs and practices.

- **Income**—Poverty may be a risk factor associated with mental illness. Among older adults, women, African-Americans, persons living alone, very old persons, those living in rural areas, or those with a combination of these characteristics tend to be at greater risk for poverty.

- **Living Arrangements**—Only a small percentage (4.2% or 1.43 million) of older persons live in nursing homes, but this percentage increases dramatically with age. The majority of nursing home residents have mental health disorders, including dementia, depression or schizophrenia.

- **Physical Health**—Most older persons have at least one chronic condition, and many have multiple problems. These chronic problems can result in functional limitations in the ability to carry out activities of daily living (bathing, eating, transfer) or instrumental activities of daily living (shopping, managing money, housework, taking medications). Functional limitations can contribute to mental health difficulties (AOA, 2001).

Many have suggested that underreporting of mental health problems in older adults is likely. Estimates that 8–20% of older adults in the community, and up to 37% of those who receive primary care, experience symptoms of depression have been reported (Hoyert, Kochanke, & Murphy, 1999). For nursing home residents, approximately two-thirds suffer from mental disorders (Butler, Lewis, & Sunderland, 1998).

While some older adults with mental health disorders have suffered from serious and persistent mental illness most of their lives, a substantial number of elders may experience a mental health problem for the first time in late adulthood. The morbidity from mental health problems can range from problematic to disabling to fatal. Assessment and diagnosis can be difficult with older adults as many present with different symptoms than younger people—emphasizing somatic complaints rather than psychological troubles (US Surgeon General, 1999).

It is reported in *The State of Aging and Health in America* (Merck Institute of Aging & Health and the Gerontological Society of America [GSA], 2003) that of the 20% of older adults who experience mental disorders, many are never screened for or diagnosed with these illnesses, so they do not receive treatment. In fact, while constituting nearly 13% of the US population, older adults use a disproportionately lower share of inpatient and outpatient mental health services, accounting for 7% of all inpatient mental health services, 6% of community-based mental health services, and 9% of private psychiatric care (Merck Institute & GSA). Barriers to this care seeking include the mistaken belief that mental health problems are a normal part of aging and the stigma this cohort associates with seeking help for mental illness.

Provider barriers are also apparent, in which many primary care physicians and other health care providers associate depression with aging or believe that treatment with older adults is not effective. The often-cited statistic that many older adults who committed suicide had visited a primary care provider very close to the time of the suicide—20% on the same day; 40% within one week; and 70% within one month of the suicide (Merck Institute & GSA, 2003—should be impetus for including training in mental health assessment as part of gerontological assessment and nursing care.

▰ INTRODUCTION TO GERONTOLOGY

Demographics/Population Characteristics

The United States is not the only country experiencing a demographic shift toward an aging society. Globalization of aging is apparent. The World Health Organization (1999) reports a demographic revolution under way throughout the world. In fact, the proportion of people age 60 and over is growing faster than any other age group. Both longer lives and declining birthrates contribute to this aging phenomenon. The projections of rapid population aging will require health care systems to provide the care required for this aging world. As the WHO notes, "Aging is a privilege and a societal achievement. It is also a challenge, which will impact on all aspects of 21st century society. It is a challenge that cannot be addressed by the public or private sectors in isolation; it requires joint approaches and strategies" (WHO, *Towards Policy*, n.d., para 4).

Facts About World Aging (WHO, n.d.)

- People aged 60 and over: about 600 million in 2000, 1.2 billion in 2025, and 2 billion in 2050

- Currently about two-thirds of all older persons are living in the developing world; by 2025 that will rise to 75%

- In the developed world, the very old (age 80+) is the fastest growing population group.

- Women outlive men in virtually all societies; consequently in very old age the ratio of women:men is 2:1 (para 5).

In the United States, the Administration on Aging releases its *Profile of Older Adults* annually. The highlights of the 2003 profile are summarized in Table 1-1 (AOA, 2004). The information is an important resource for the gerontological nurse to understand the current implications of the statistics for nursing practice.

Older Americans today represent about one of every eight Americans; this number has increased by 3.3 million or 10.2% since 1992, and the number of Americans 45–64 (the "baby boomers"), who will reach 65 over the next two decades, increased by 38% during this period (AOA, 2004). Clearly women

TABLE 1-1   A Profile of Older Americans: 2003 Highlights*

- The older population (65+) numbered 35.6 million in 2002 (the most recent year for which data are available), an increase of 3.3 million or 10.2% since 1992.
- The number of Americans aged 45–64—the "baby boomers" who will reach 65 over the next two decades—increased by 38% during this decade.
- About one in every eight, or 12%, of the population is an older American.
- Over 2 million persons celebrated their 65th birthday in 2002.
- Persons reaching age 65 have an average life expectancy of an additional 18.1 years (19.4 years for females and 16.4 years for males).
- Older women outnumber older men at 20.8 million older women to 14.8 million older men.
- About 31% (10.5 million) noninstitutionalized older persons live alone (7.9 million women, 2.6 million men).
- Half of older women age 75+ live alone.
- Almost 400,000 grandparents aged 65 or more had the primary responsibility for their grandchildren who lived with them.
- By the year 2030, the older population will more than double to about 71.5 million.
- The 85+ population is projected to increase from 4.6 million in 2002 to 9.6 million in 2030.
- Members of minority groups are projected to represent 26.4% of the older population in 2030, up from 16.4% in 2000.
- The median income of older persons in 2002 was $19,436 for males and $11,406 for females. Median money income of all households headed by older people (after adjusting for inflation) fell by 1.4% for older people from 2001 to 2002; however, the difference was not statistically significant.
- The Social Security Administration reported that the major sources of income for older people were:
  Social Security (reported by 91% of older persons)
  Income from assets (reported by 58%)
  Public and private pensions (reported by 40%)
  Earnings (reported by 22%)
- About 3.6 million older persons lived below the poverty level in 2002. The poverty rate for older persons was 10.4% in 2002, which is not statistically different from the rate in 2001. Another 2.2 million or 6.4% were classified as "near poor" (income between poverty level and 125% of this level).

*The profile incorporates the latest data available but not all items are updated on an annual basis.
Sources: US Bureau of the Census, the National Center on Health Statistics, and the Bureau of Labor Statistics.

outnumber men with the ratio of women to men increasing with each passing decade. The ratio in 2000 was 143 women for every 100 men over the age of 65, but the ratio increased to 245 women per 100 men for persons 85 and over (AOA, 2003).

Life expectancy varies by gender. In 2000, women reaching age 65 had an average life expectancy of an additional 19.2 years (84.2)

while men's life expectancy had an average of 16.3 years (81.3). There were 50,545 persons aged 100 or more in 2000 (0.02% of the total population)—a 35% increase from 1990 (AOA, 2003). Life expectancy at birth for a child born in 2000 was 76.9 years, 29 years longer than a child born in 1900. Interestingly, Hayflick (2000) reported that the dramatic changes in life expectancy occurred in the first 70 years of the 20th century, with only a six-year increase in life expectancy from 1970–97, suggesting an important but neglected area of "aging" research.

Patterns of future growth of the older adult population suggest the largest growth will be among minorities, which, in 2030, are projected to represent 25.4% of the elderly population, up from 16.4% in 2000. "Between 1999 and 2030, the white [excludes persons of Hispanic origin] population 65+ is projected to increase by 81% compared with 219% for older minorities, including Hispanics (328%), African-Americans (131%), American Indians, Eskimos and Aleuts (147%), and Asians and Pacific Islanders (285%)" (AOA, 2003). Implications of these projections for the gerontological nurse include the need to tailor assessments and nursing interventions that are culturally competent.

Poverty statistics vary for different segments of the older adult population. In 2001, about 3.4 million elderly persons (10.1%) were below the poverty level. "Poverty statistics are based on definitions originally developed by the Social Security Administration. These include a set of money income thresholds that vary by family size and composition. These thresholds are updated annually by the US Census Bureau to reflect changes in the Consumer Price Index for all urban consumers" (Federal Interagency Forum on Aging-Related Statistics, 2000, p. 114). The 2004 US Department of Health and Human Services Poverty Guidelines (used for determining financial eligibility for certain federal programs) for a family unit of one was $9310; for a family unit of two, $12,490 (DHHS, 2004). Another 2.2 million or 6.5% of older adults were classified as "near poor," meaning that their income was between the poverty level and 125% of this level. Near poor older adults are challenged to meet their economic needs but may not be eligible for needs-based programs and services as a result of the definition of poverty.

Examination by race, ethnicity, and gender highlights the disparity in poverty among older adults. For elderly whites, 8.9% were poor in 2001, compared to 21.9% of elderly African-Americans and 21.8% of elderly Hispanics. Furthermore, older women had a higher poverty rate (12.4%) than older men (7.0%) in 2000. Those living alone or with nonrelatives were much more likely to be poor (19.7%) than were older persons living with families (5.5%) (AOA, 2003).

Poverty rates also vary by where older adults live. Compared with overall poverty rates of 10.1% for the 65+ population in general, persons who lived in central cities had poverty rates of 12.8%, while those living in rural areas had rates of 12.2% and those in the South, 12.4%. The highest poverty rates were experienced by older Hispanic women who lived alone or with nonrelatives, according to the Administration on Aging 2000 statistics (AOA, 2003).

The gerontological nurse recognizes that economic well-being is an essential component of overall quality of life for older adults. Without financial means, accessing needed resources for mental health and general well-being may be severely limited. Additionally, a lifetime exposure to financial hardships can add additional stress and burden in coping with age-related changes and access to health care for physical and mental health problems.

Theories of Aging

Gerontology is the multidisciplinary study of aging and older adults. Disciplines representing biology, psychology, and sociology were among the first to propose theories of aging based on research findings. These theories are an attempt to understand the phenomenon of aging as experienced by, and occurring within, older adults themselves and to enable professionals to adequately assess, plan, implement, and evaluate care, services, and policies that affect older adults. While most nurses are familiar with a number of nursing models and theories, few have been exposed to gerontology as a formal course and thus would be unfamiliar with how sociologists, psychologists, and biologists have viewed the structure and function of aging. An introduction to the most commonly cited theories of aging will be presented. This is not an exhaustive treatment of the subject, but an overview that will frame the issues and concerns for the nurse in understanding and providing individualized geropsychiatric and mental health nursing care.

Biological Theories of Aging   The biological theories of aging attempt to explain the complex factors related to how and why aging occurs. These theories fall into two main groups—one emphasizing internal programmed biological clocks, and the other external error or environmental forces that damage cells and organs until they can no longer function adequately (National Institute on Aging (NIA), n.d.). The programmed theories view aging as a predetermined, time phenomenon. One of the first programmed theories, cellular aging, proposed by internationally recognized cellular biology researcher Leonard Hayflick (2000), described normal human cells as having a finite capacity for reproduction (approximately 50 doublings) and then dying. Other examples of the programmed theories of aging include programmed senescence (where aging is the result of sequential switching on and off of certain genes, with senescence being defined as the time when age-associated deficits are manifested), endocrine theory (with biological clocks acting through hormones to control the pace of aging), and immunological theory (programmed decline in immune system functions leading to an increased vulnerability to infectious disease and thus aging and death) (NIA).

Error theories, on the other hand, are thought to be randomly occurring events that accumulate over time. Among these theories are the wear and tear theory (where cells and tissues have vital parts that wear out), crosslinking (accumulation of cross-linked proteins damages cells and tissues, slowing down bodily processes), and free radicals (where accumulated damage caused by oxygen radicals causes cells—and eventually organs—to stop functioning) (NIA, n.d.). Antioxidant use in the form of vitamins E and C, beta-carotene, and selenium, represents the public's interest in attempting to reverse the damaging effects of free radicals on the aging process.

Another emerging error theory is caloric restriction. This theory, termed rate of living or metabolic theory of aging, proposes that the greater an organism's rate of oxygen basal metabolism, the shorter its life span. The implications of this long-known phenomenon in laboratory animals are now being investigated for its effect on human aging (Hadley et al., 2001).

With the mapping of the human genome, research is also underway to examine the relationship of DNA and the aging process. In a study by Puca et al. (2001), a genome-wide scan for linkage to human exceptional longevity identified a locus on chromosome 4. The authors propose that this might exert a substantial influence on the ability to achieve exceptional old age. This knowledge could lead to important insights on cellular pathways important to the aging process (Puca et al.). A second development is the discovery of telomeres, arms located at the ends of chromosomes that may function as the cells' biological clocks (Hayflick, 1998). The field of biological aging continues to evolve.

However, even with the knowledge of these biological aging theories, we continue to be perplexed by the social and psychological responses and processes that occur in the context of aging for individuals and society. Psychological and social theories of aging offer an important glimpse into these processes. This knowledge can enable the nurse to assist older adults in achieving their self-defined "successful aging." For some, successful aging may be the ability to maintain the three key characteristics described by Rowe and Kahn (1998, p. 38): "low risk of disease and disease-related disability, high mental and physical function, and active engagement with life" (p. 38). Others have suggested that positive spirituality is a fourth dimension that intersects with Rowe and Kahn's three key behaviors for successful aging (Crowther, Parker, Achenbaum, Larimore, & Koenig, 2002).

Psychological Theories of Aging Psychological theories address how a person responds to the developmental tasks of his or her age (Madison, 2000). These theories recognize that both biology and sociology influence psychological responses. Examples of these psychological theories include Maslow's hierarchy of human needs, Jung's theory of individualism, Erikson's eight stages of life, and Peck's expansion on Erikson's theory.

Maslow's pyramid of human needs posits that basic physiologic needs for air, food, elimination, sleep, activity, and comfort must be met before advancing to higher orders on the pyramid. While illnesses and life crises may periodically require individuals to move up or down on the pyramid, the ultimate achievement for all humans is that of self-actualization. This can only be achieved when all basic needs for physiologic integrity, safety and security, love and belonging, and ego strength and self-esteem are met. As a psychological theory for understanding aging and older adults, Maslow's top rung of self-actualization can be compared to Rowe and Kahn's successful aging.

Jung's theory of individualism suggests that human aging is accompanied by transcendence from the inner self to an emphasis on the external world and the need to contribute to the good of the larger society (Hooyman & Kiyak, 2002). Jung also noted

that the psychological characteristics of anima/animus tend to be displayed in aging men and women. These characteristics enable older adults to psychologically adapt to aging and cope with age-related changes.

Erik Erikson proposed eight stages of human development (Erikson, 1963). Achievement of each stage is required before higher order stages can be met. Failure to achieve a stage renders the individual on the negative side of that stage's proposed dichotomy. In midlife, for example, if an individual cannot realize generativity in his/her chosen work, social roles, or life circumstances, then stagnation rather than generativity would prevail. For older adults who achieve the midlife developmental stage of generativity, Erikson proposes the final stage of ego-integrity versus despair. For those who are able to review their life with a sense of inner peace, having made various life choices that, upon reflection, were made with the best intentions and ability at the time, ego integrity can be achieved. Failing to see positives and suffering regrets over life decisions and outcomes would render the older adult with despair. Various psychosocial and psychotherapeutic therapies can enable older adults to gain insight into these negative perceptions and thus offer hope and provide opportunity for achieving ego integrity. Ego integrity is akin to Maslow's self-actualization—a psychological goal sought by all.

Peck expanded Erikson's original theory and divided the eighth stage—ego integrity versus despair—into additional stages occurring during middle age and older adulthood. The middle age stages consist of valuing wisdom versus valuing physical powers, socializing versus sexualizing in human relationships (redefining men and women as individuals versus sexual objects), cathectic flexibility versus cathectic impoverishment (suggesting emotional flexibility in being able to reinvest emotions in other people and pursuits is necessary for emotional health), and mental flexibility versus mental rigidity (openness to new experiences versus reliance on fixed rules of behavior from prior experience). In older adults, Peck's theory includes ego differentiation versus work-role preoccupation (shift in value system from vocational roles to broader range of role activities), body transcendence versus body preoccupation (transcending physical decline and discomforts and enjoying social and mental sources of pleasure), and ego transcendence versus ego preoccupation (inner contentment through children, contributions to the culture, and through friendships as enduring signs of self-perpetuation after death). Peck suggests that stages in late life may be far less predictable in terms of chronological age than is true of the childhood stages proposed by Erikson (Peck, 1968).

Sociological Theories of Aging   Early sociological theories focused on the social role losses as problems experienced by older adults and how individuals and society respond. Examples of these early theories, termed *first generation theories* by some (Bengtson, Burgess, & Parrott, 1997), include disengagement theory (Cumming & Henry, 1961), activity theory (Neugarten, Havighurst, & Tobin, 1968), and subculture theory of aging. These reflect theories published between 1949 and 1969.

The controversial disengagement theory proposed that "social equilibrium is achieved by a mutually beneficial process of reciprocal withdrawal between society and older people" (Miller, 2004, p. 51). This theory places society's needs over individual needs, but also suggests that older adults desire this withdrawal and are satisfied with the disengagement process. Among the limitations of this proposed theory are that successfully aging individuals do not benefit by disengaging and withdrawing from social roles.

The essence of the activity theory of aging, on the other hand, suggests there is a positive

relationship between activity and life satisfaction. Havighurst (1963, 1968) proposed the importance of social role participation for positive adjustment in old age. Other researchers examined activity in general, and interpersonal activity in particular, and noted that activity offers channels for acquiring role supports that sustain one's self-concept (Lemon, Bengtson, & Peterson, 1972). Thus, replacing roles lost would be essential for maintaining life satisfaction in old age.

The subculture of aging theory suggests that there is a benefit derived for older adults who maintain involvement and activities with their similarly aged cohort. This cohort shares similar norms, expectations, beliefs, and habits, and thus integrates better among themselves, as compared with people from other age groups (Miller, 2004). This formation of a subculture is primarily a response of the loss of status resulting from old age in American society and the strength that can result from membership in a peer group.

In the second period of theory development, 1970–85, new theoretical perspectives emerged that either built on or rejected these early theories (Bengtson, Burgess, & Parrott, 1997). Among these sociologic theories were continuity theory (Atchley, 1972; Neugarten, Havighurst, & Tobin, 1968), exchange theory, life course, age stratification, person-environment fit, and political economy of aging.

Neugarten et al. (1968) advanced the continuity theory because neither the activity nor the disengagement theory adequately explained successful aging. They proposed that personality characteristics, in place long before reaching older adulthood, continue. Thus, those coping strategies employed to adjust to changes throughout life will also be used to adjust to aging. Their research demonstrated that personality type (identified as integrated, armored–defended, passive–dependent, and unintegrated–disorganized), extent of social role activity, and degree of life satisfaction more accurately reflect patterns of aging. Thus, the person's lifelong experience creates in him/her certain predispositions that will be maintained if at all possible.

Social exchange theories proposed that those who maintain an active contribution to and engagement with society, whether through paid or unpaid employment, volunteering, or community involvement, will adapt most readily to aging.

Age stratification theory was first proposed by Riley and colleagues in 1972 and "addresses the interdependencies between age as an element of the social structure and the aging of people and cohorts as a social process" (Miller, 2004, p. 52). This theory notes that aging people and society are constantly influencing one another. Societal expectations for each age strata differ from one another based on stage of life and historical events that have characterized that group's life.

The person–environment fit theory, put forth by Lawton (1982), considers the interrelationships between personal competence and the environment. Personal competence "involves ego strength, motor skills, biologic health, cognitive capacity, and sensory–perceptual capacity" (Miller, 2004, p. 53). The individual interacts with an environment, which is viewed as having the potential for eliciting a behavioral response from the person. Lawton asserts that for each level of competence, there is a corresponding level of environmental demand, or environmental press, that can best enable that person to function effectively. Those with lower-level competence can tolerate only lower levels of environmental press; those with higher levels of competence can respond well to higher levels of environmental press.

Political economy of aging theory would suggest that power is in the hands of those who control the means of production or can influence the economy. Thus, in a social system where older adults are encouraged to retire, their power base is minimized. Estes (1979) pointed out that the "aging enterprise" in America benefits providers and practitioners more than older adults themselves—dispersing power among the owners of the capital versus the elders whom these programs, services, and agencies are intended to serve. Empowering older adults would change the balance of power; organizations such as AARP are intended to address this imbalance.

Theories described since the late 1980s could be said to be refinements of earlier proposed theories as well as the development of new theories. Reflecting the multidisciplinary scope in gerontology, these theories represent the disciplines of sociology, psychology, history, and economics. Many of these theories encompass both individual and social structures as influencing behaviors or experiences of older adults. Included among these newer third generation theories are social constructionist, feminist theories of aging, phenomenological, and critical gerontology.

Summary of Theories of Aging The biological/physiological, psychological/developmental, and social/gerontological theories of aging continue to evolve and shape our thinking about gerontology. These varied theoretical perspectives make comparisons about theories of aging difficult, in part because many view the process and outcomes of aging from their own discipline-specific lens. Biologists, for example, are interested in predicting length of life or the viability of organ systems while psychologists examine changes in a wide range of behavioral capacities, including learning, perception, and memory. Social scientists address theory as it relates to social status, life satisfaction, and adjustment to role changes associated with age, and include such concepts as culture, family, and cohort effects. As a result, there is no one integrated overall theory for examining and evaluating the complexities of aging and the aged. Instead, the value of an eclectic approach to the heterogeneous older adult population should be emphasized.

Each person ages in ways that are impacted by biological, psychological, and sociological factors. An understanding of the ways in which each of these factors affects individuals' and society's response to aging can be influential in the nurse's approach to geropsychiatric and mental health care. Ultimately, the goal of enhancing older adult well-being, quality of life, life satisfaction, and, what some have termed "successful aging," can be fostered when nursing assessments and interventions for older adults consider these factors. In fact, knowledge of these theories in the practice of geropsychiatric and mental health nursing care can be helpful in enabling older adults to achieve the WHO definition of mental health.

Growth and Development in Old Age

As the various psychological and social theories of aging suggest, older adulthood is a dynamic period, and older adults themselves represent an extremely heterogeneous group of individuals. Research and clinical practice have long recognized that development and adaptation occur throughout life. Development, defined as learning to live with oneself as one changes, and adaptation, learning to live in a particular way according to a particular set of values as one or as one's culture changes (Clark & Anderson, 1967; Matteson, McConnell, & Linton, 1997, p. 591), are necessary components in the quest for successful aging. Successful aging is possible for those experiencing chronic disease and/or functional limitations.

Rowe and Kahn's (1998, p. 39) model of successful aging includes "absence of disease and disability, maintaining high cognitive and physical function, and active engagement with life." Strawbridge, Wallhagen, and Cohen (2002) evaluated this model in their study of 867 Alameda County Study participants aged 65–99 and found that 50.3% of the participants self-rated themselves as aging successfully compared to 18.8% when using

the Rowe and Kahn criteria exclusively. The major differentiating factor in their study seemed to be that older adults with chronic conditions and functional difficulties still perceive their aging as successful. Thus, the high prevalence of chronic disease and functional limitations experienced by older adults need not be an obstacle toward the goal of successful aging and optimal mental wellness.

Other researchers have reexamined the Rowe and Kahn model and suggested the addition of a fourth factor to capture successful aging—positive spirituality. Incorporation of spirituality in interactions with older adults could strengthen efforts of health care providers and gerontological specialists to promote well-being in older adults (Crowther, Parker, Achenbaum, Larimore, & Koenig, 2002). The results of this research lend support for gerontological and psychiatric mental health nurses to incorporate positive spirituality in their assessment and interventions with older adults.

Holstein and Minkler (2003) have offered a critical perspective on aging that challenges the Rowe and Kahn view of successful aging. "If how we live determines how we age, and if how we live is shaped by many factors beyond individual choice, then success is far harder to come by for some than for others" (Holstein & Minkler, p. 791). These authors suggest that the avoidance of disease and disability and the maintenance of high physical and functional capacity, as representing successful aging, are not inevitably under individual control. An elder who is disabled (either due to a physical or mental illness or condition) is not so simply because he or she failed to try harder to make different health-promoting choices and decisions. As suggested earlier by the social–ecological model of health and mental health promotion, contextual factors, including economic conditions, physical and social environments, improvements in health and health care access, most certainly shape the conditions of individual "choice" and must be foremost in the mind of the gerontological nurse as an instrument of change/change agent/ advocate.

Cognitive Changes with Age

"All of the following processes are basic to much of our mental life and behavior, and they are all encompassed under the term cognition: intelligence, perception, attention, learning, memory, thought, and communication" (NIMH, 2000, para 1). Nurses adept at conducting mental status evaluations with older adults will be familiar with the testing and instruments needed to assess these dimensions of cognition.

- **Intelligence**—The theoretical limit of an individual's performance (Hooyman & Kiyak, 2002); the capacity to comprehend relationships, to think, to solve problems and to adjust to new situations (Tabers, 1989)

- **Attention**—"The power of concentration, the ability to focus on one specific thing without being distracted by many environmental stimuli" (Jarvis, 2004, p. 106)

- **Learning**—"The process by which new information (verbal and nonverbal) or skills are encoded, or put into one's memory" (Hooyman & Kiyak, 2002, p. 158)

- **Memory**—"The process of retrieving or recalling the information stored in the brain when needed; *memory* also refers to skills learned throughout a person's lifetime (i.e., how to ride a bicycle)." (Hooyman & Kiyak, 2002, p. 158)

Three types of memory:

1. Sensory—Information received through the sense organs and passed on to primary or secondary memory; it is only stored for a few 10ths of a second

   a. Iconic (visual memory, i.e., remembering faces)

   b. Echoic (auditory memory, i.e., sound of ocean)

2. Primary memory—Temporary stage for holding and organizing information, and does not necessarily refer to a storage area in the brain; i.e., most adults recall seven plus or minus two pieces of information for 60 seconds or less (local seven-digit phone numbers); working memory that decides what information to be attended to or ignored

3. Secondary (long-term) memory—To retain information in our permanent memory, it must be rehearsed or processed actively; requires cues to retrieve stored information (Hooyman & Kiyak, 2002)

Thus, true learning implies that the material we have acquired through our sensory and primary memories has been stored in "secondary memory" and can be retrieved. *Recall* is the process of searching through secondary memory in response to a specific external cue (Hooyman & Kiyak, 2002).

Research has demonstrated the following age-related changes in cognition that are important to consider in caring for older adults. Intelligence is one aspect of cognition where there is controversy as to whether age-associated changes occur. For one thing, it is well known that standardized testing and the time pressures associated with test-taking are more detrimental to older than younger persons. With these caveats in mind, certain age-associated changes have been identified. First, testing of fluid intelligence does demonstrate that older adults perform significantly worse on performance scales (Hooyman & Kiyak, 2002). Fluid intelligence consists of skills that are biologically determined, independent of experience or learning, and may be similar to what is called "native intelligence." It includes spatial orientation, abstract reasoning, and perceptual speed. *Crystallized intelligence,* on the other hand, refers to knowledge and abilities that the individual acquires through education and lifelong experiences. As measured with the verbal scales of the WAIS-R, crystallized intelligence remains stable (Hooyman & Kiyak). These cognitive changes in intelligence, known as the *classic aging pattern,* do hold up in both cross-sectional and longitudinal studies, with major changes generally not evident until the mid-70s.

Cohort effects may play a part in the results of these age-associated intelligence tests, including such factors as educational attainment, involvement in complex versus mechanistic work, cardiovascular disease, hypertension, sensory deficits, cognitive engagement (that is, involvement in intellectual pursuits), nutritional deficiencies, and depression (Hooyman & Kiyak, 2002). Also reported in the literature is the rapid decline in cognitive function within five years of death, known as the "terminal drop," whereby test scores that are low may not be so much a function of age at testing as proximity to death (Kleemeier, 1962).

Age-related changes in memory are a source of significant concern for many older adults who fear this may be the onset of Alzheimer's or a related dementia. "Normal aging does not result in significant declines in intelligence, memory, and learning ability" (Hooyman & Kiyak, 2002, p. 199). However, recently released American Academy of Neurology (AAN) guidelines have documented that mild cognitive impairment (MCI) is important to identify and monitor for progression to Alzheimer's disease (AD) (Table 1-2). "MCI is a classification of persons with memory impairment who are not demented (normal general cognitive function; intact activities of daily living)" (Peterson et al., 2001, p. 2). Other literature uses the terms *age-associated memory impairment* and *age-associated cognitive decline* to refer to the concept of

TABLE 1-2	Mild Cognitive Impairment Criteria
Memory complaint, preferably corroborated by an informant
Objective memory impairment
Normal general cognitive function
Intact activities of daily living
Not demented

Reproduced with permission of the American Academy of Neurology (2001). *Mild cognitive impairment.* Retrieved July 16, 2003, from http://www.aan.com

increasing memory impairment with age compared to memory function in younger normal adult subjects.

According to the American Academy of Neurology, "between 6% and 25% of MCI patients progress to dementia or AD each year. Therefore, older adults with MCI should be evaluated regularly for progression to AD" (Peterson et al., 2001, p. 2). The National Institute on Aging and the National Institutes of Health reported that in certain studies, about 40% of individuals with MCI develop AD within three years while others have not progressed to AD, even after eight years (NIA, NIH, 2002).

The National Institute on Aging and the National Institutes of Health's (2002) Progress Report on Alzheimer's Disease 2001-2002, reported on a study that examined 404 people who had either mild memory loss (classified as MCI) or no memory problems. The 227 people with MCI were placed in one of three categories that reflected the researchers' degree of confidence that subtle signs of memory loss might indicate the onset of AD (fairly confident, suspicious, uncertain) with volunteers being reassessed annually for up to 9.5 years. By the end of 9.5 years, all the volunteers with the most severe form of MCI had developed the clinical symptoms of AD. The findings were interpreted to mean that MCI is an early stage of AD (NIA, NIMH, 2002)

The American Psychiatric Association (APA, 2000, p. 741) lists Age-Related Cognitive Decline (780.9) under other conditions that may be a focus of clinical assessment. According to the DSM-IV-TR (APA), this category is used when there is an "objectively identified decline in cognitive functioning consequent to the aging process that is within normal limits given the person's age. Individuals with this condition may report problems remembering names or appointments or may experience difficulty in solving complex problems" (APA, p. 741). It is assumed that a specific mental disorder or neurological condition has been ruled out as a cause for the cognitive impairment.

In contrast, dementia is described as "the development of multiple cognitive deficits that include memory impairment and at least one of the following cognitive disturbances: aphasia, apraxia, agnosia, or a disturbance in executive functioning. The cognitive deficits must be sufficiently severe to cause impairment in occupational and social functioning and must represent a decline from a previously higher level of functioning. A diagnosis of a dementia should not be made if the cognitive deficits occur exclusively during the course of a delirium" (APA, 2000, p. 148).

While research continues to determine the significance and impact of mild cognitive impairment on older adults, the gerontological nurse must recognize that the concerns and fears of older adults and their family members regarding any cognitive changes must be carefully assessed and support provided during the diagnostic processes.

SUMMARY

This chapter has introduced the field of aging and older adulthood. Current demographics of the aging population, and those projected for the future, certainly portray that society's needs for mental health and psychiatric care of older adults will continue to grow. There continue to be too many older adults who experience mental health issues and psychiatric disorders that go underdiagnosed and undertreated, in part because they fail to access needed services or are not seen as suffering by health care providers who dismiss the client's complaints as being caused by normal aging. Knowledge about particularly vulnerable populations, including the developmentally disabled, the chronically and persistently mentally ill, and the homeless, is essential for the gerontological nurse to adequately address their mental health care needs.

While this chapter was not intended to be a comprehensive review of the field of gerontology, basic concepts to assist in the understanding of the lifespan perspective of aging and older adults have been introduced. An introduction to the biological, social, and psychological theories of aging has been presented as an overview for the geropsychiatric nurse. Growth and development in old age, and the concept of successful aging, have been presented. A review of the cognitive changes occurring with age and their implications for the aged and the geropsychiatric nurse, have also been included in an effort to provide the context for the assessment and treatment of mental health issues and psychiatric disorders that follows.

REFERENCES

Administration on Aging (2001). *Older adults and mental health 2001: Issues and opportunities.* Retrieved June 24, 2004, from http://www.protectassets.ccm/ssa/Older-AdultsandMH2001.pdf

Administration on Aging (2003). *A profile of older Americans: 2002.* Retrieved June 24, 2004, from http://www.aoa.dhhs.gov/prof/Statistics/profile/profiles2002.asp

Administration on Aging (2004). *A profile of older Americans: 2003.* Retrieved June 24, 2004, from http://www.aoa.dhhs.gov/prof/statistics/profile/profiles.asp

American Academy of Neurology (2001). Mild cognitive impairment. Retrieved July 16, 2003, from http://www.aan.com

American Nurses Association (1998). *Scope and standards for the nurse who specializes in developmental disabilities and/or mental retardation.* Washington, DC: Author.

American Psychiatric Association (1994). *Diagnostic and statistical manual of mental disorders.* (4th ed.). Washington, DC: Author.

American Psychiatric Association (2000). *Diagnostic and statistical manual of mental disorders. DSM-IV-TR* (text revison). Washington, DC: Author.

Atchley, R. C. (1972). *The social forces in later life.* Belmont, CA: Wadsworth.

Bengtson, V. L., Burgess, E. O., & Parrott, T. M. (1997). Theory, explanation, and a third generation of theoretical development in social gerontology. *Journal of Gerontology: Social Sciences, 52B*(2), S72–S88.

Butler, H. A. (2003). *Motivation: The role in diabetes self-management in older adults.* Unpublished doctoral dissertation, University of Massachusetts Lowell.

Butler, R. N., Lewis, M. I., & Sunderland, T. (1998). *Aging and mental health: Positive psychosocial and biomedical approaches* (5th ed.). Boston: Allyn and Bacon.

Campbell, V. A., Crews, J. E., Moriarty, D. G., Zack, M. M., & Blackman, D. K. (1999). Surveillance for sensory impairment, activity limitation, and health-related quality of life among older adults: United State, 1993-1997. *Surveillance Summaries, 48*(SS08), 131–156. Retrieved August 15, 2003, from http://www.cdc.gov/mmwr/preview/mmwrhtml/ss4808a6.htm

Clark, M., & Anderson, P. B. (1967). *Culture and aging.* Springfield, IL: Charles C. Thomas.

Cohen, C. I. (1999). Aging and homelessness. *The Gerontologist 39*(1), 5–14.

Cohen, C. I., Ramirez, M., Teresi, J., Gallagher, M., & Sokolovsky, J. (1997). Predictors of becoming redomiciled among older homeless women. *The Gerontologist, 37,* 67–74.

Cohen, C. I., Teresi, J. A., Holmes, D., & Roth. E. (1988). Survival strategies of older homeless men. *The Gerontologist, 28,* 58–65.

Crowther, M. R., Parker, M. W., Achenbaum, W. A., Larimore, W. L., & Koenig, H. G. (2002). Rowe and Kahn's model of successful aging revisited: Positive spirituality—the forgotten factor. *The Gerontologist, 42*(5), 613–620.

Cumming, E., & Henry, W. E. (1961). *Growing old.* New York: Basic Books.

Cutler, N. E., Whitelaw, N. A. & Beattie, B. L. (2002). *2002 American perspectives of aging in the 21st century: A myths and realities of aging chartbook.* Washington, DC: The National Council on the Aging.

DeMallie, D. A., North, C. A., & Smith, E. M. (1997). Psychiatric disorders among the homeless: A comparison of older and younger groups. *The Gerontologist, 37*(1), 61–66.

Department of Health and Human Services (1999). *Mental health: A report of the Surgeon General.* Rockville, MD: U.S. Department of Health and Human Services, Substance Abuse and Mental Health Services Administration, Center for Mental Health Services, National Institutes of Health, National Institute of Mental Health. Retrieved June 22, 2004, from http://www.surgeongeneral.gov/library/mentalhealth

Department of Health and Human Services (2001). *National strategy for suicide prevention: Goals and objectives for action.* Rockville, MD; Author.

Department of Health and Human Services (2004). *Poverty guidelines.* Retrieved June 22, 2004, from http://aspe.hhs.gov/poverty/04poverty.htm

Edmands, M. S., Hoff, L. A., Kaylor, L., Mower, L., & Sorrell, S. (1999). Bridging gaps between mind, body, spirit: Healing the whole person. *Journal of Psychosocial Nursing, 37*(10), 35–42.

Erikson, E. H. (1963). *Childhood and society* (2nd ed.). New York: W.W. Norton.

Estes, C. L. (1979). *The aging enterprise.* San Francisco: Jossey-Bass.

Federal Interagency Forum on Aging-Related Statistics (as of 2000) (2002). *Older Americans 2000:*

Key indicators of well-being. Hyattsville, MD: Author.

Frankish, C. J., Bishop, A., & Steeves, M. (1999). *Challenges and opportunities in applying a population health approach to mental health services: A discussion paper*. Institute of Health Promotion Research. University of British Columbia for the Health Systems Section of Health Canada. Retrieved August 4, 2003, from: www.ihpc. ubc.ca/pdfs/mentalhealthdraft.pdf

Gurland, B., & Toner, J. A. (1991). The chronically mentally ill elderly: Epidemiological perspectives on the nature of the population. In E. Light & B. D. Levowitz (Eds.). *The elderly with chronic mental illness* (Ch. 1). New York: Springer.

Hadley, E. C., Dutta, C., Finkelstein, J., Harris, T. B., Lane, M. A., Roth, G. S., Sherman, S. S., & Starke-Reed, P. E. (2001). Human implications of caloric restriction's effects on aging in laboratory animals: An overview of opportunities for research. *Journals of Gerontology: Biological Sciences and Medical Sciences, 56*, 5–6.

Havighurst, R. J. (1963). Successful aging. In R. Williams, C. Tibbits, & W. Donahue (Eds.). *Processes of aging* (Vol. 1). New York: Atherton Press.

Havighurst, R. J. (1968). Personality and patterns of aging. *The Gerontologist, 38*, 20–23.

Hayflick, L. (1998). How and why we age. *Experimental Gerontology, 33*(7–8), 639–653.

Hayflick, L. (2000). The nature of aging. *Nature, 408*, 267–269.

Heller, T., Janicki, M., Hammel, J., & Factor, A. (2002). *Promoting healthy aging, family support, and age-friendly communities for persons with developmental disabilities: Report of the 2001 Invitational Research Symposium on Aging with Developmental Disabilities*. Chicago: The Rehabilitation Research and Training Center on Aging with Developmental Disabilities, Department of Disability and Human Development, University of Illinois at Chicago.

Hogstel, M. O. (1995). *Geropsychiatric nursing*. St. Louis, MO: C.V. Mosby.

Holstein, M. B., & Minkler, M. (2003). Self, society, and the "new gerontology," *The Gerontologist, 43*(6), 787–796.

Hooyman, N. R., & Kiyak, H. A. (2002). *Social gerontology: A multidisciplinary perspective*. Boston: Allyn and Bacon.

Hoyert, D. L., Kochanke, K. D., & Murphy, S. L. (1999). Deaths: Final data for 1997. *National Vital Statistics Reports, 47*(9). Hyattsville, MD: National Center for Health Statistics.

Jarvis, C. (2004). *Physical examination & health assessment* (4th ed.). St. Louis, MO: Saunders.

Kleemeier, R. W. (1962). Intellectual changes in senium. Proceedings of the Social Statistics Section of the American Statistical Association, 1, 290–295.

Lawton, M. P. (1982). Competence, environmental press, and the adaptation of older people. In M. P. Lawton, P. G. Windley, & T. O. Byerts (Eds.). *Aging and the environment: Theoretical approaches* (pp. 33–59). New York: Springer.

Lemon, B., Bengston, V. L., & Peterson, J. A. (1972). An exploration of the activity theory of aging: Activity types and life satisfaction among in-movers to a retirement community. *Journal of Gerontology, 27*, 511–523.

Madison, H. E. (2000). Theories of aging. In A. G. Lueckenotte, *Gerontologic nursing* (2nd ed., p. 21). St. Louis, MO: C.V. Mosby.

Manton, K. G., & Gu, X. L. (2001). Dramatic decline in disability continues for older Americans. In *Proceedings of the National Academy of Sciences* (May 8, 2001). National Institutes of Health, National Institute on Aging, NIH News Release. Retrieved July 2, 2003, from http://www.nia. nih.gov/news/pr/2001/0507.htm

Matteson, M. A., McConnell, E. S., & Linton, A. D. (1997). *Gerontological nursing: Concepts and practice*. (2nd ed.). Philadelphia: W.B. Saunders.

McLeroy, K. R., Bibeau, D., Steckler, A., & Glanz, K. (1988). An ecological perspective on health promotion programs. *Health Education Quarterly, 15*(4), 351–377.

McLeroy, K. R., Steckler, A., Goodman, R., & Burdine, J. N. (1992). Health education research, theory and practice: Future directions. *Health Education Research: Theory and Practice, 7*(1), 1–8.

Merck Institute of Aging & Health and The Gerontological Society of America (2003). *The state of aging and health in America*. Washington, DC: Authors.

Miller, C. A. (2004). *Nursing for wellness in older adults. Theory and practice* (4th ed.). Philadelphia: Lippincott, Williams & Wilkins.

National Institute on Aging and the National Institutes of Health (2002). *Progress report on Alzheimer's disease, 2001–2002.* Washington, DC: Author. Retrieved November 15, 2004, from *http://www.alzheimers.org/pr01-02/fulltext.htm*

National Institute on Aging (n.d.). *Secrets of aging.* Retrieved July 1, 2003, from http://www.nia.nih.gov/health/pubs/secrets-of-aging/p1.htm

National Institute of Mental Health (2000). *Cognitive research at the National Institute of Mental Health.* Retrieved November 15, 2004, from http://www.nimh.nih.gov/publicat/NIMHcognitiveresfact.cfm

National Institute of Mental Health (2001). *The numbers count: Mental disorders in America.* Retrieved June 24, 2004, from http://www.nimh.nih.gov/publicat/numbers/cfm

National Resource Center on Homelessness and Mental Illness (1999). *Annotated bibliography on homelessness and mental illness among older Americans.* Retrieved August 4, 2003, from http://www.ihpr.ubc.ca/pdfs/mentalhealthdraft.pdf

Neugarten, B., Havighurst, R. J., & Tobin, S. S. (1968). Personality and patterns of aging. In B. L. Neugarten (Ed.). *Middle age and aging.* Chicago: University of Chicago Press.

Peck, R. (1968). Psychological determinants in the second half of life. In B. L. Neugarten (Ed.). *Middle age and aging.* Chicago: University of Chicago Press.

Peterson, R. C., Stevens, J. C., Ganguli, M., Tangalos, E. G., Cummings, J. L., & DeKosky, S. T. (2001). Practice parameter: Early detection of dementia: Mild cognitive impairment (an evidence-based review). Report of the Quality Standards Subcommittee of the American Academy of Neurology. *Neurology, 56,* 1133–1142. Retrieved June 22, 2004, from http://www.neurology.org/cgi/reprint/56/9/1133.pdf

Puca, A. A., Daly, M. J., Brewster, S. J., Matsie, T. C., Barrett, J., Shea-Drinkwater, M., Kang, S., Joyce, E., Nicoli, J., Benson, E., Kunkel, L. M., & Perls, T. (2001). A genome-wide scan for linkage to human exceptional longevity identifies a locus on chromosome 4. *Proceedings of the National Academy of Sciences, 98*(18), 10505–10508.

Riley, M. W., Johnson, J., & Foner, A. (1972). *Aging and society: A sociology of age stratification* (Vol. 3). New York: Russell Sage Foundation.

Rowe, J. W., & Kahn, R. L. (1998). *Successful aging.* New York: Pantheon Books.

Scholler-Jaquish, A. (2004). Persons with severe and persistent mental illness. In K. M. Fortinash & P. A. Holoday Worret, *Psychiatric mental health nursing* (3rd ed., pp. 617–644). St. Louis, MO: C. V. Mosby.

Strawbridge, W. J., Wallhagen, M. I., & Cohen, R. D. (2002). Successful aging and well-being: Self-rated compared with Rowe and Kahn. *The Gerontologist, 42*(6), 727–733.

Substance Abuse and Mental Health Services Administration (SAMHSA), The Center for Mental Health Services (2003). *Blueprint for change: Ending chronic homelessness for persons with serious mental illnesses and/or co-occurring substance use disorders.* Rockville, MD: Author. Retrieved August 27, 2004, from http://www.nrchmi.samhsa.gov/publications/default.asp

Taber's cyclopedia medical dictionary (17th ed.) (1989). Philadelphia: F.A. Davis.

The John A. Hartford Institute for Geriatric Nursing (n.d.). *Fast facts: Emphasis needed on geriatric nursing.* Retrieved June 27, 2003, from http://www.hartfordign.org/resources/policy/fastfacts.html

University of British Columbia (1999). *Institute of Health Promotion Research: Mental health draft for the Health Systems Section of Health Canada.* Retrieved August 4, 2003, from http://www.ippc.umc.ca/pdfs/mentalhealthdraft.pdf

World Health Organization (1999). *Report of the Secretary General. Highlights of an expert consultation on developing a policy framework for a society for all ages.* Retrieved February 9, 2003, from http://www.un.org/esa/socdev/ageing/agepfram.htm

World Health Organization (2001). *Mental health: Strengthening mental health promotion. Fact sheet 220. Revised November 2001.* Retrieved

June 25, 2004, from http://www.who/int/mediacentre/factsheets/fs220/en/

World Health Organization (n.d.). *Towards policy for health and ageing.* Retrieved June 25, 2003, from http://www.who.int

World Health Organization (n.d.). *About ageing and lifecourse.* Retrieved November 15, 2004, from http://www.who.int/hpr/ageing

ACKNOWLEDGMENT

The author wishes to acknowledge the helpful critique of an earlier draft of this chapter provided by Judith Conahan, RN, MS, PhD(c).

CHAPTER 2

Geropsychiatric Nursing as a Subspecialty

Karen Devereaux Melillo, PhD, APRN, BC, FAANP
Lee Ann Hoff, PhD, MSN, MA
Martha A. Huff, MS, APRN, BC

GEROPSYCHIATRIC MENTAL HEALTH NURSING— INTRODUCTION

There is inadequate geropsychiatric and mental health training and preparation for all health care professionals, including nurses. This fact can negatively affect individuals and families experiencing geropsychiatric and mental health issues. In the *Consensus Statement on the Upcoming Crisis in Geriatric Mental Health,* authors Jeste et al. (1999) acknowledge that a national crisis in geriatric mental health care is emerging. A myriad of factors are cited: inadequate research infrastructure, inadequate health care financing, lack of adequately trained mental health care personnel, and fragmented mental health care delivery systems that cannot meet the challenges posed by the explosion in the numbers of older adults, and of older adults needing psychiatric care. Consensus statement authors suggest that urgent action is needed now.

Currently, only 5–6% of an estimated 70,000–80,000 advanced practice nurses have been certified in gerontological nursing (American Academy of Nursing, 2002). Mezey and Fulmer (2002) reported that only 63 programs nationwide prepare advanced geronto-

logical nurses, and these programs graduate a mean of three students annually, making few available for the gerontological nursing care needed in health care settings. As reported by M. Smolensky, executive director of the American Nurses Credentialing Center (personal communication, January 2002, as cited in Mezey & Fulmer, 2002), there are only 3400 gerontological nurse practitioners and 800 gerontological clinical nurse specialists currently certified.

Basic preparation in gerontology is also lacking for many practicing nurses and current nursing students. An online review of *Peterson's Guide,* which provides detailed profiles of more than 2100 colleges and universities in the U.S. and Canada, revealed only 86 two- or four-year schools offering any gerontology coursework (Peterson's Guide, 2003). This suggests that today few college graduates in any major are equipped to understand the unique aspects of aging and older adults. This group of ill-prepared graduates includes nursing professionals. Nurses are often educated without the benefit of even a basic introductory undergraduate gerontology course. Even fewer have completed a nursing course dedicated to the unique health care and nursing needs required for older adults. As for most nurses practicing today, whose average age is 46 years, even fewer have had the opportunity to take a required course in geriatric/gerontological nursing.

In fact, one study noted only 23% of baccalaureate nursing programs have a required geriatric/gerontological nursing course (Rosenfeld, Bottrell, Fulmer, & Mezey, 1999). Clearly, gerontology content is "woefully lacking in medical schools and nursing programs, and primary care and specialty health care professionals, who are likely to care for large numbers of older patients, continue to receive inadequate training" (Kovner, Mezey, & Harrington, 2002, para. 7). Kovner et al. report that

> Only 4% of more than 670 baccalaureate nursing programs met all criteria for exemplary geriatrics education (defined as a stand-alone geriatrics course, two or more clinical placement sites in geriatrics, and at least one FT faculty member nationally certified in geriatrics). Only 23% of baccalaureate nursing programs required and 14% had as an elective a stand-alone geriatrics course. At the same time, 58% of the programs reported no FT faculty certified in geriatric nursing (2002, para. 14).

In fact, the Hartford Institute notes that "older people represent 60% of all adult primary care visits, 80% of home care visits, 46% of all hospital days and 85% of residents in nursing homes," and yet geriatric nursing is underrepresented at all levels of nursing practice and nursing education (John A. Hartford Institute, Fast Facts, n.d.).

Within the specialty field of gerontological nursing, there are unique mental health problems and specialized approaches needed to understand and care for older adult clients that educational programs have not fully addressed. To address this need, nursing professionals with additional specialized knowledge are needed.

Nurses are educationally prepared at the basic level for psychiatric mental health nursing. According to the American Psychiatric Nurses Association (APNA), basic level clinical practice of psychiatric mental health nursing includes registered nurses who "work with individuals, families, groups, and communities, assessing mental health needs, developing a nursing diagnosis and a plan of nursing care, implementing the plan, and finally evaluating the nursing care. Basic level practice is characterized by interventions that promote and foster health and mental health, assist clients to regain or improve their coping skills or abilities, and prevent further disability" (APNA, n.d.). The assessment, diagnosis, treatment, and evaluation of older adults with geropsychiatric and mental health problems is seldom the primary focus of the educational preparation in generic baccalaureate nursing programs, however.

Unlike basic-level psychiatric mental health nursing, geropsychiatric nursing is a master's-level subspecialty within the adult psychiatric mental health nursing field. Sub-specialization in a particular area of practice, according to Burgess (1997) "occurs during master's and doctoral preparation in nursing and/or through continuing professional education. Subspecialization is focused on the development of additional knowledge and skills for providing services to a population. Subspecializations within psychiatric mental health nursing are based on current and anticipated societal needs for various specialty nursing services. This subspecialization may be categorized according to:

- A developmental period (e.g., child and adolescent, adult, geriatric)

- A specific mental/emotional disorder (e.g., addiction, depression, chronic mental illness)

- A particular practice focus (e.g., community, group, couple, family, individuals), and/or

- A specific role or function (e.g., forensic nursing, psychiatric consultation/liaison) (Burgess, 1997, p. 21).

Currently, no certification examination for this specialty is offered by the American Nurses Credentialing Center (ANCC) (Kovner et al., 2002). In fact, Deirdre Thornlow, director of the Gerontology Project with the American Association of Colleges of Nursing, reports knowing of only five programs that offer an MS Geropsychiatric CNS/NP degree, and among them are the University of Arkansas, University of Michigan, and Case Western (D. Thornlow, personal communication, July 28, 2003). However, increasingly universities offer the needed continuing professional education for this specialty. The University of Massachusetts Lowell, for example, offers a 12-credit post-baccalaureate certificate in Geropsychiatric and Mental Health Nursing, and several other such programs are developing nationwide.

Fortunately, national specialty nursing groups and organizations are spearheading efforts to foster improved mental health promotion and psychiatric care for older adults. The National Conference of Gerontological Nurse Practitioners identified, among its 2002–03 Health Affairs Agenda, the need to "Advocate for improving the quality of mental health for elders, especially those who reside in nursing homes" (National Conference of Gerontological Nurse Practitioners, 2003). The Hartford Foundation's Institute for Geriatric Nursing has likewise identified strategies and tactics for the years 2001–06. These include "important nursing education initiatives to assure that all advanced practice and baccalaureate nursing graduates are competent in geriatrics, to imbue best practice nursing care of older adults and their families across the continuum of care settings, to foster innovative clinical geriatric nursing research, and to shape the national agenda to improve nursing care to older adults" (Hartford Institute, Fast Facts, n.d.).

The International Society for Education and Research in Psychiatric–Mental Health Nursing (SERPN) has established an Adult and Geropsychiatric–Mental Health Nurses Division to "identify, disseminate, and grow the unique body of knowledge that constitutes the scientific foundation for advanced practice psychiatric/mental health nurses who provide mental health care for adults, the elderly, their families, and communities" (SERPN, n.d., para 1). Among the goals identified for the division are to promote appropriate educational preparation for the undergraduate and graduate-level education of adult and geropsychiatric nurses (SERPN).

The American Psychiatric Nurses Association (APNA) describes itself as a professional organization representing the specialty practice of psychiatric–mental health nursing. It has more than 4000 members and is the largest national association of psychiatric nurses (www.apna.org). Among its initiatives is the receipt of a geropsychiatric grant awarded from the Atlantic Philanthropies by the American Nurses Foundation in partnership with the Hartford Institute for Geriatric Nursing to address Geriatric Competence of Specialty Nurses. The goal for APNA is to develop a web-based geropsychiatric education program consisting of five short courses/lectures designed to fill the gap for nurses in the area of geropsychiatry. As pointed out by APNA, few formal programs exist to provide education in this subspecialty. The need is critical to fill this knowledge gap (APNA, 2003). Key to addressing older adults' mental health care will be the preparation of nurses with geropsychiatric and mental health nursing knowledge and skills.

REVIEW OF STANDARDS

Geropsychiatric and mental health nursing is guided by a number of professional standards, beginning with the *ANA Standards of Clinical Nursing Practice* (1998a), the *ANA Code of Ethics for Nurses with Interpretive Statements* (2001), and the *ANA Social Policy Statement* (1996). Standards serve as criteria against which to measure one's nursing practice (Table 2-1). The American Nurses Association notes

TABLE 2-1	Standards of Care Comparing the Gerontological Nurse, Psychiatric Mental Health Nurse, and Nurse Who Specializes in Care of Developmentally Disabled Adults		
Standard	**Gerontological Nurse**	**Psychiatric-MH Nurse**	**Nurse Specializing in Care of Developmentally Disabled Adults**
Assessment	The gerontological nurse collects patient health data.	The psychiatric-mental health nurse collects patient health data.	The nurse who specializes in DD and/or MR collects data relevant to persons with DD and/or MR.
Diagnosis	The gerontological nurse analyzes the assessment data in determining the diagnosis.	The psychiatric-mental health nurse analyzes the assessment data in determining diagnoses.	The nurse who specializes in DD and/or MR analyzes assessment data in determining nursing diagnoses.
Outcome identification	The gerontological nurse identifies expected outcomes individualized to the older adult.	The psychiatric-mental health nurse identifies expected outcomes individualized to the patient.	The nurse who specializes in DD and/or MR assists the client in identifying expected outcomes individualized to the client, family, or community.
Planning	The gerontological nurse develops a plan of care that prescribes interventions to attain expected outcomes.	The psychiatric-mental health nurse develops a plan of care that is negotiated among the patient, nurse, family, and health care team and prescribes evidence-based interventions to attain expected outcomes.	The nurse who specializes in DD and/or MR develops a plan that prescribes interventions to attain expected outcomes.
Implementation	The gerontological nurse implements the interventions identified in the plan of care.	The psychiatric-mental health nurse implements the interventions identified in the plan of care (includes counseling, milieu therapy, promotion of self-care, psychobiological interventions, health teaching, case management, health promotion, and health maintenance).	The nurse who specializes in DD and/or MR implements interventions identified in the plan of care.
Evaluation	The gerontological nurse evaluates the older adult's progress toward attainment of expected outcomes.	The psychiatric-mental health nurse evaluates the patient's progress in attaining expected outcomes.	The nurse who specializes in DD and/or MR evaluates the client's, family's, and community's progress toward attainment of outcomes.

Sources: American Nurses Association (1998). *Scope and standards for the nurse who specializes in developmental disabilities and/or mental retardation.* Washington, DC: Author.

American Nurses Association (2001). *Scope and standards of gerontological nursing practice.* (2nd ed.). Washington, DC: Author.

American Nurses Association (2000). *Scope and standards of psychiatric-mental health nursing practice.* Washington, DC: Author.

Reproduced with permission from ANA.

"psychogeriatric nursing practice is a rapidly developing [sub-]specialty that addresses the mental health needs of older adults" (ANA, 2001, p. 7). The practice of geropsychiatric and mental health nursing is also guided by two sets of practice guidelines: *Scope and Standards of Gerontological Nursing Practice* (ANA, 2001) and *Scope and Standards of Psychiatric Mental Health Nursing Practice* (ANA, 2000).

The ANA has also published the *Scope and Standards for the Nurse who Specializes in Developmental Disabilities and/or Mental Retardation* (ANA, 1998b), an important field in caring for older adults with disabilities. Nurses caring for older adults will likely be providing care to those with mental retardation and other developmental disabilities (e.g., cerebral palsy) and their family members. Current estimates by the American Association on Mental Retardation suggest the numbers of adults age 60 and older with mental retardation will double to 1,065,000 by 2030 when the last of the "baby boom" generation reaches its 60s (AAMR, Fact Sheet, 2002).

According to the American Association on Mental Retardation, mental retardation is not a medical disorder nor a mental disorder. Rather, mental retardation is an important subcategory of developmental disabilities. Mental retardation, which originates before age 18, is defined as "a disability characterized by significant limitations both in intellectual functioning and adaptive behavior as expressed in conceptual, social, and practice adaptive skills" (AAMR, Definition of Mental Retardation, 2002).

In its Statement on the Scope of Practice (ANA, 1998b), the American Nurses Association recognizes that persons with developmental disabilities and/or mental retardation are living longer. There is a need for both the nurse generalist and the advanced practice nurse to provide safe and effective care for this population using the Standards of Professional Performance, which reflect the role functions of nursing, and Standards of Care, which reflect many of the components of the nursing process (ANA, 1998a). Both are described in the Statement on the *Scope and Standards for the Nurse Who Specializes in Developmental Disabilities and/or Mental Retardation.*

■ THEORETICAL FOUNDATIONS FOR GEROPSYCHIATRIC AND MENTAL HEALTH NURSING

Gerontological nursing is a highly complex specialty, which has borrowed theories of aging from several disciplines, including psychology, biology, and sociology. Gerontological nursing has adapted these theories to the person, health, nursing, and environment paradigm in nursing. Eliopoulos has offered her interpretation of the information system needed by the gerontological nurse (Figure 2-1) (Eliopoulos, 1997, p. 12).

In addition to theories of aging, geropsychiatric nursing borrows from the interdisciplinary foundations of psychiatric/mental health nursing. The complexity of care for many older adults with psychiatric/mental health problems requires an interdisciplinary team approach. Similarly, geropsychiatric nursing draws upon the theories and concepts of many disciplines. These include nursing, psychiatry, social and behavioral sciences, and the humanities. Following is an overview and critique of several disciplines' contribution to geropsychiatric nursing. The section concludes with a case example illustrating the theoretical underpinnings of geropsychiatric care in the nursing paradigm.

Psychoanalytic and Personality Theories

In the 1800s and the early 1900s, Sigmund Freud was a pioneer in the study of human behavior. His psychoanalytic theory focused on the behavior of disturbed individuals. It acknowledges and emphasizes the role of early childhood conflicts in the development of neurotic symptoms in later life. This approach is termed determinism, and is widely criticized today (Greenspan, 1983;

FIGURE 2-1   Information System of the Gerontological Nurse

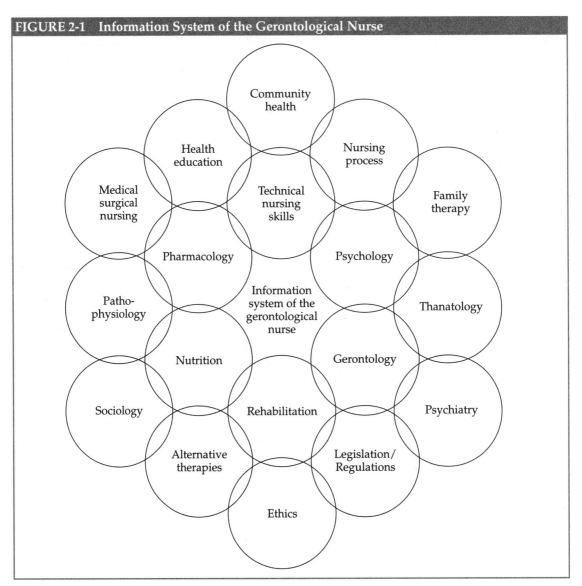

From Eliopoulos, C. 1997. *Gerontological nursing,* (4th ed.). Philadelphia: J. B. Lippincott, p. 12. Reproduced with permission from Lippincott, Williams, & Wilkins.

Rieker & Carmen, 1984; Walsh, 1987). Nevertheless, many psychiatric nurses and others in psychotherapy roles routinely inquire about a client's childhood experiences, perhaps as a result of Freud's work.

Freud was the first to propose an unconscious level of mental functioning and the three-part system of personality—id, ego, and superego. He believed that one must maintain a balance (equilibrium) among the three parts to avoid psychopathology. Freud's psychoanalytic technique of listening is the mainstay of the modern therapeutic relationship. His insight into human behavior marked the beginning of modern psychiatry, and he has influenced the contemporary writings of theorists in the social and behavioral sciences.

Harry Stack Sullivan (1947) and Erik Erikson (1963) modified Freud's ideas into less deterministic, more developmental theories for explaining human behavior. Sullivan, heavily influenced by sociology, focused on the social, interpersonal aspects of personality and one's cognitive representations of self and others, which he called personifications. He believed that personality continues to develop well into adulthood, but he did not directly address the development in older adults.

Erikson's *Theory of Psychosocial Development* is the first theory to identify a stage of personality development in older adulthood, although his early work omitted the oldest-old. His theory has also been critiqued for its support of traditional family structures that produce increased stress for women who bear the burden of disproportionate caretaking roles over the lifespan (Buss, 1979). Despite these limitations, Erikson's theory offers valuable insights to our understanding of human development.

The theory describes eight stages of development, each with two possible outcomes. The successful completion of each stage results in healthy personality development. As longevity becomes the norm, Erikson's ideas regarding "middle adulthood," (whose successful completion results in generativity) may apply to individuals in their early retirement years. *Ego Integrity vs. Despair*, the final stage, acknowledges the need for older adults to feel that they have led productive lives and that they have met their life goals. Unsuccessful completion of this stage results in depression and despair. Interventions such as intergenerational programs at nursing homes and senior centers, life review and reminiscence groups promote the development of ego integrity in the older adult.

Abraham Maslow's (1970) five-leveled *Hierarchy of Needs* has been widely used as a model to explain human behavior. Basically, Maslow stated that some needs take precedence over others. Individuals must meet the needs of one level before moving onto the next, higher level of need. However, Maslow suggested that individuals with extreme problems at a particular level may become "fixated" on those needs for the rest of their life. Regression to a lower level of needs may occur in response to life stress.

Existential Stress and Social Learning Theories

Viktor Frankl's book, *Man's Search for Meaning* (1963), was in part a reaction to the reductionism of both medicine and psychology, demonstrated by their biological, mechanistic explanations of the mind and of human behavior. Frankl sought a balance between physiology and humanity/spirituality. He emphasized the responsibility that an individual has for being human, and that one cannot be given meaning in life. Meaning must be a lived experience. However, a therapist can assist people in their search for meaning. Frankl's writings about the existential search for meaning have relevance for psychiatric nursing in general, and in particular for geropsychiatric nurses.

In the existential framework, theories of the classical stress response (Selye, 1956) are expanded to include values and meanings of people coping with life stressors. Hans Selye is the founder of the concept of stress. He believes that failure to cope with stressors (whether positive or negative) can result in "diseases of adaptation," or can affect the body's capacity to respond to injury and disease.

Developed by Albert Bandura (1977, 1997), the theory of social learning and self-efficacy views individuals as self-organizing, proactive, self-reflecting and self-regulating rather than as reactive organisms shaped by environmental forces or driven by unconscious impulses. From this theoretical perspective, human behavior is seen as the product of personal, behavioral, and environmental influences.

Antonovsky's (1980, 1987) research with concentration camp survivors and women in menopause led to his concept of "resistance resources"—including social support and a concept of "Sense of Coherence (SOC)"—to explain differential responses to stressful situations. SOC includes the person's perception of events as comprehensible, manageable, and meaningful. Applied to stress response, a person with a strong SOC will define social stressors as social rather than assuming blame for trouble that did not originate from oneself. One's resistance resources can make the difference between positive or negative responses to developmental transitions or to extreme stress (which a clinician might define as "crisis"), such as an older person's loss of spouse and major source of support. Research with abused women (Hoff, 1990) supports these views and the interaction between stress, crisis, and illness—physical, emotional, and mental (Hoff, 2001).

One model, the Progressively Lowered Stress Threshold (PLST) (Hall & Buckwalter, 1987) has been offered as a conceptual foundation for the effects of stress on persons with Alzheimer's disease and related disorders. "The model is adapted from psychologic theories of stress, adaptation, and coping—in addition to behavioral and physiologic research of Alzheimer's disease" (Hall & Laloudakis, 1999, para 6). Dysfunctional behaviors are a direct result of four groups of symptom clusters: (1) the cognitive or intellectual losses, (2) affective or personality changes, (3) conative or planning losses that cause a predictable decline in ADL abilities, and (4) the loss of stress threshold (Hall & Laloudakis, 1999). When any of six common triggers occurs (fatigue; change in environment, routine, or caregiver; misleading stimuli or inappropriate stimulus levels; affective responses to perceptions of loss; internal or external demands that exceed functional capacity; and physical stressors, such as pain, discomfort, infection, acute illness, comorbid conditions), the patient's stress threshold is exceeded and dysfunctional behavior (problematic behaviors that may be upsetting for family members) or catastrophic events can occur (Hall & Laloudakis, 1999).

The PLST has been used in the design and evaluation of experimental interventions to assist caregivers in understanding and planning care for behavioral problems exhibited by patients (Gerdner, Buckwalter, & Reed, 2002) and in a caregiver training protocol for dementia management (Gerdner, Hall, & Buckwalter, 1996). PLST has been cited in an evidence-based protocol on wandering (Futrell & Melillo, 2002), using expert opinion to offer this model as a basis for physical and psychosocial interventions to decrease wandering by eliminating stressors from the environment, including cold at night, changes in daily routines, and extra people at holidays (Hall & Laloudakis, 1999). This model is a useful framework in applying theory to practice for geropsychiatric and mental health nursing.

Crisis Theory, Public Health, and Preventive Psychiatry

The unique contribution of crisis theory, public health, and preventive psychiatry is the focus on identification and early intervention with vulnerable populations. Typically, the growing number of seniors require more rather than fewer resources to maintain health and safety in chosen locales. Of particular note for older persons is Lindemann's (1944) classic work on loss, grief, and early support through mourning that is pivotal in avoiding the hazards of depression.

Lindemann's (1944) study of bereavement following the disastrous Cocoanut Grove fire in Boston defined the grieving process people went through after sudden death of a relative. Lindemann found that survivors of this disaster who developed serious psychopathologies had failed to go through the normal process of grieving. His findings are particularly relevant in the care of older people who typically have suffered many losses, but who often lack the assistance and social approval necessary for grief work following loss and instead may be offered only medication (Hoff, 2001). Grief work consists of the process of mourning one's loss, experiencing the pain of such loss, and eventually accepting the reality of loss and adjusting to life without the loved person or object. Encouraging and supporting people to experience normal grieving can prevent depression and other negative outcomes of crises due to loss.

Among all the pioneers in crisis theory and preventive psychiatry, perhaps none is more outstanding than Gerald Caplan. In 1964 he developed a conceptual framework for understanding the process of crisis development. Caplan also emphasized a community-wide—i.e., public health—approach to crisis intervention. Public health includes education programs and consultation with various caretakers such as geriatric care managers and community-based nurses in preventing destructive outcomes of crises such as suicide or abuse of others. In his classic work *Principles of Preventive Psychiatry* (1964), Caplan's focus is on prevention, mastery, and the importance of social, cultural, and material "supplies" necessary to avoid crisis arising from stressful life events. This public health framework resonates with a current emphasis on human rights and the intrinsic connection between health and socioeconomic security and social justice for disadvantaged groups such as older persons who are poor and/or homeless (Rodriguez-Garcia & Akhter, 2000).

Although Caplan's contribution to the development of crisis theory and practice is widely accepted, his conceptual framework is grounded in disease rather than health concepts (Brandt & Gardner, 2000; Hoff, 1990, 2001), including some of the mechanistic concepts set forth by Freud—e.g., equilibrium between id, ego, and superego psychic func-

tions. The static concept of homeostasis and maintaining equilibrium shortchanges the dynamic processes of growth, development, and creative integration of life experience that are so important during late stages of the life cycle. This limitation is offset, however, by Caplan's emphasis on prevention. A more dynamic interpretation of stressful events and the crisis experience corresponds with ego psychology and developmental theory, which emphasize one's potential for growth and change through all stages of the life cycle (Erikson, 1963).

Crisis Care and Psychiatric Stabilization

Similar to the growing emphasis on primary health care is the integration of crisis approaches on behalf of those suffering from acute psychotic episodes. Typically, such persons are seen in the crisis unit of community mental health centers or in the emergency service of general hospitals, where the emphasis is on triage and rapid disposition. Psychopharmacologic agents are often used to stabilize distressed people. The strong medical orientation in such units warrants greater caution than usual by providers, particularly with older adults. The aim is to assure that chemical stabilization is not used as a substitute for crisis intervention techniques to restore acutely upset persons to a state of "equilibrium" or homeostasis.

For older people under stress or in acute crisis, overreliance on stabilization with psychotropic drugs is particularly hazardous. Chemical tranquilization practiced without humanistic crisis intervention is related to iatrogenesis (illness induced by physicians and other health providers) (McKinlay, 1990). Among some older persons with multiple social stressors and physical ailments or disabilities, it is all too easy to compound these problems by overmedication, failure to identify and prevent interactive side effects, and insufficient attention to contextual factors such as economic status, social support, secure housing, and 24-hour access to help when needed—a pivotal element of comprehensive community mental health.

Community Mental Health

Caplan's concepts about crisis emerged during the same period in which the community mental health movement was born. An important influence on preventive intervention and crisis care during this era was the 1961 Report of the Joint Commission on Mental Illness and Health in the United States, *Action for Mental Health* (1961). This work documented through five years of study the crucial fact that people were not getting the help they needed, when they needed it, and where they needed it—close to their natural social setting. It underscores a key facet of healthy aging and the desires of older people needing mental health care: Aging in place and receiving care at home or close to a familiar community and trusted social network, and coordinating such care with skilled medical and nursing interventions.

However, despite federal legislation and funding, the ideals of community-based mental health care are yet to be realized in the nationwide struggle for universal access, cost control, and insurance parity for mental health service (Hoff & Adamowski, 1998). Such service includes integration of mental health basics in primary care settings where most people are first seen, whether the presenting problem is medical or psychosocial. But even among those that include holistic approaches, emergency and other services are often far from ideal. In these settings the growing percentages of clients are age 65 or older, while the majority of primary care providers have minimal preparation in gerontology and geropsychiatric care.

Political and fiscal policies in recent decades resulted in further departures from community mental health ideals worldwide (Hoff, 1993; Marks & Scott, 1990). In the United States, this can be traced in part to

several historic themes: (1) the mind–body split in health practice (Edmands, Hoff, Kaylor, Mower, & Sorrell, 1999); (2) an individualistic vs. population-based focus in health service delivery (Fee & Brown, 2000); and (3) continuing bias against and disparity in health insurance coverage for those with mental or emotional illness (Ustun, 1999).

Reform movements in Canada, Italy, and the United States—with support from WHO—have attempted to reverse this course and alleviate the global burden of mental illness (Kaseje & Sempebwa, 1989; Mosher & Burti, 1989; Rachlis & Kushner, 1994; Scheper-Hughes & Lovell, 1986; Ustun, 1999; US Department of Health and Human Services, 2001). Progress toward reform, cost-saving, and a community mental health ideal to replace the current patchwork system leads to consideration of sociocultural and feminist factors influencing geropsychiatric care.

Sociocultural and Feminist Influences

Discussion of theory influencing geropsychiatric nursing practice thus far suggests that the momentum has come largely from psychological, psychiatric, or community sources. Yet sociology, anthropology, and feminist scholars offer invaluable insights into our understanding and practice of geropsychiatry. We are conceived, born, grow and develop, and die in a social context. We experience distress, illness, and crisis in our social milieu. People near us—friends, family, the community—help or hinder us during stressful life events. And death, even for those who die alone and abandoned, demands some response from the society left behind.

Multidisciplinary research has supported a shifting emphasis from individual to social approaches in helping distressed people (e.g., Antonovsky, 1980, 1987; Boissevain, 1970; Hoff, 1990; Mitchell, 1969). Despite the prevalence of individual intervention techniques, overwhelming evidence now shows that social networks and support are primary factors in a person's susceptibility to disease, the process of becoming ill and seeking help, the treatment process, and the outcome of illness, whether that be rehabilitation and recovery or death (e.g., Berkman & Syme, 1979; Loustau-nau & Sobo, 1997; Robinson, 1971; Sarason & Sarason, 1985). The work of clinicians during the golden age of social psychiatry supports the prolific social science literature on social approaches to distressed people (Hoff, 2001). Among earlier writers, psychiatrist Hansell (1976), building on Caplan's (1964) work, has done the most to stress social influences on preventive intervention with persons in distress and avoiding destructive outcomes of crisis, with particular application to the seriously and persistently mentally ill. His social-psychological approach to mental health theory and practice resonates with cross-cultural influences in the field.

Cross-Cultural and Diversity Influences

Political, social, and technological developments have contributed to more permeable national boundaries, and at the same time have sharpened cultural awareness, unique ethnic identities, and sensitivity to diversity issues. These observations have implications for cross-cultural and diversity issues in the experience of crisis, as well as variance in response to older people in chronic or acute distress. The rich data on rites of passage marking human transition states in traditional societies are another significant contribution of cultural and social anthropology to the understanding of vulnerable populations in transition. These insights from other cultures are particularly relevant to older people who typically face the challenge of successfully navigating several transitions together or in rapid succession; for example: a change in status from healthy to disabled, or a diagnosis of life-threatening illness; a move from home to institution; role change from spouse to widowed; and the final transition from life to death. Sadly, many older adults lack the sup-

port they need and deserve during these life-altering transitions (Hoff, 2001).

Attention to and competency in caring for persons from diverse cultural groups is challenging for many providers as they face a multitude of languages and belief systems among their clients. Of central importance here is recognizing the wisdom and clinical relevance of a key principle in working with anyone different from ourselves: Whatever our ethnic or cultural identity, we should never assume that—even with extensive study and exposure—we will ever be fully knowledgeable about a culture other than our own.

Rather, a helpful way of conveying respect for another's values and meaning system is to focus on a set of eight questions developed by medical anthropologist Arthur Kleinman and applied by Fadiman (1997, p. 260–261) to a Hmong family's serious culture clash with medical practitioners in California who treated their daughter's seizures:

1. What do you call the problem?
2. What do you think has caused the problem?
3. Why do you think it started when it did?
4. What do you think the sickness does? How does it work?
5. How severe is the sickness? Will it have a short or long course?
6. What kind of treatment do you think the patient should receive? What are the most important results you hope are received from this treatment?
7. What are the chief problems the sickness has caused?
8. What do you fear most about the sickness?

To Kleinman's eight questions, we add: How do you think we [at this agency, clinic, or hospital] can best help you with this problem?

These generic questions can be adapted to any treatment situation or concern in which successful outcomes depend heavily on the nurse's attempt to understand the other's point of view—no matter how different from one's own or deviant from treatment protocols entirely foreign to the client. Such an approach embodies the essence of respect, which is fundamental to the interpersonal process of effective nursing care.

Complementing sociocultural influences, feminist theory offers important insights on the mental health status of older adults and a gender-sensitive response to their needs by geropsychiatric providers. By feminist influences we mean taking gender into account in respect to theory, research, and geropsychiatric nursing practice with individuals and families. For example, burden falls disproportionately on women in caregiving roles, despite some progress in gender equality and egalitarian relationships; marriage patterns result in more companionless women than men in old age; traditional gender roles often leave widowed men at greater risk of depression and suicide than women; gender bias in paid and unpaid work roles typically leaves women with insufficient time for self-care and health-promoting leisure activity; and gender bias also results in women's greater risk of poverty and institutionalization in old age (Estes, 1995).

Nursing Theories

Geropsychiatric nursing practice has benefited greatly from the nursing theories developed by Dorothea E. Orem and Hildegarde E. Peplau, who began their careers in the early 1930s. Both nursing theorists continued to develop their concepts over many years. Orem's sixth edition of *Nursing: Concepts of Practice* was published in 2001. Peplau's original work, *Interpersonal Relations in Nursing* (1952/1991), is required reading in many nursing schools. Her psychodynamic nursing theory is particularly useful for psychiatric nurses.

Orem's *Self-Care Deficit Nursing Theory (SCDNT)* (1980) establishes nursing as a practical science having a focus that is distinct

from other disciplines. Orem's SCDNT is actually a model that encompasses three theories: self-care, self-care deficits, and nursing systems. Self-care is a human regulatory function that people either perform for themselves or have performed for them to maintain life, health, development, and well-being. The abstract term *self-care deficit* refers to the relationship between a person's capabilities and his or her need for care. Nursing is an intentional human action and includes operations of diagnosis, prescription, and regulation (Taylor et. al, 1998). *SCDNT* provides a framework for understanding the nursing process in general, but it is particularly helpful when thinking of older clients who may be experiencing "deficits" as part of the normal aging process.

Hildegarde Peplau's Psychodynamic Nursing Theory was influenced by Freud, Maslow, and especially by H. S. Sullivan, with whom she studied. The functions of psychodynamic nursing are "Being able to understand one's own behavior to help others identify felt difficulties, and to apply principles of human relations to the problems that arise at all levels of experience" (Peplau, 1991, p. xi). Peplau emphasized the importance of the nurse–patient relationship and identified four phases of that relationship: orientation, identification, exploitation, and resolution. During the relationship, both the patient and the nurse experience growth through experiences. Peplau stated that illness brings up feelings derived from prior experiences, and that the nurse–patient relationship is an opportunity for nurses to assist clients to finish developmental tasks.

Geropsychiatric nurses can use Peplau's phases of the interpersonal relationship to track their progress in guiding clients (whether individuals or communities) toward mutually agreed-upon goals. Additionally, they can promote the positive resolution of the later developmental tasks.

Peplau's writings encouraged nursing to become self-directed, rather than responsive to the direction of medicine. In the early 1950s she was encouraging nurses to promote "a new view of the *nurse as associate with other professional workers*" (Peplau, 1991, p. 45). She was truly a pioneer in terms of nursing theory and leadership.

THE NURSING PARADIGM APPLIED TO GEROPSYCHIATRIC NURSING

Our overview of multidisciplinary theories and concepts underpinning gerontology and geropsychiatric nursing offers a rich source for bridging gaps between theory and practice. In the everyday demands of nursing practice, a firm grasp of theory and confidence in its application is sometimes shortchanged. When that happens, desired outcomes of nursing interventions may also be compromised. This section aims to bridge the divide between theory and practice.

In Figure 2-2, the nursing paradigm is presented with its key interrelated concepts: person/family, environment; health, and nurse/provider. Each of the paradigm's key concepts depicts the interdisciplinary theoretical underpinnings of the particular concept with reference to geropsychiatric nursing practice.

The figure is adapted from an educational program for preparing health professionals on violence issues (Hoff, 1994). It illustrates the following theories and concepts encompassed in the nursing paradigm applied to geropsychiatric nursing from beginning to expert levels of learning and practice.

1. Person/Family
   a. Developmental, life-cycle theories
   b. Gender and role theories
   c. Personality theory
   d. Existential theory
2. Environmental
   a. Social stress
   b. Community mental health
   c. Sociocultural, feminist influences
   d. Socioeconomic theory
3. Health
   a. Psychoanalytic theory
   b. Crisis, public health theories
   c. Emotional stress
   d. Orem's Self-Care Deficit theory
   e. Social support and preventive psychiatry
4. Nurse/Provider
   a. Peplau's Interpersonal Relationship theory
   b. Attitudes, knowledge and skills in caring for older adults

The following case example illustrates the application and integration of the nursing paradigm's four concepts.

Case Study

Frank Kelly, a 72-year-old widowed Caucasian male, presents at the emergency room of a community hospital complaining of chest pain. His daughter Kate, the youngest of three children, encouraged him to seek treatment and is with him. His cardiac workup is negative, but during the assessment he is tearful and says that he wishes he were dead so that he could be with his wife. She died two years ago, and since then, weekly visits from his children, who all live close by, have been Frank's only social support. "I think about killing myself all the time, but I was raised Irish Catholic and I don't want to go to hell." He admits feeling depressed most of his life, but never sought help, saying "Who would I have asked?" Kate states that Frank's sister is treated with Celexa for depression.

continues

Case Study *(continued)*

Frank and his wife sold their house five years ago and bought a condo unit in a complex for seniors. He never developed friendships with neighbors because he focused on his wife during her last two years. Since then he has remained isolated, and his only distraction is watching TV. He has no hobbies, but used to like hunting and has several guns. Frank smiles briefly and expresses pride in his career as a pipe fitter, which enabled him to provide a comfortable lifestyle for his wife and children. His pension and Social Security income cover his living expenses now, but he is worried about escalating costs of his Medicare Part B coverage.

Frank admits that he has not seen his primary care physician since just after his wife died. At that time his physician suggested that he join a widowers support group, but he did not want to share his feelings at that point. Frank takes ASA 81 mg and hydrochlorothiazide daily for hypertension, but has called the office for refills without further evaluation. He has pain from osteoarthritis that is "pretty bad most days," but does not take any medication for this. About every four months his right great toe swells and is tender— "one time a doctor said it was gout."

Frank has never smoked and quit drinking 20 years ago because his wife objected to it. However, six months ago he started drinking beer again. He currently has five to seven beers a day, three to four times a week. He drinks alone at home and notes, "It sort of dulls the arthritis pain, so I can sleep better. I nod off in front of the TV." Frank estimates that he sleeps a total of seven to 10 hours a day, with many naps. He reports a fair appetite, but Kate thinks he has lost about 15 pounds in the last two years.

Application of Theory

Using the nursing paradigm, the nurse notes that Frank Kelly, "Person," is an older widowed white male who has not adjusted to his retired status or his role as widower. The nurse remembers that older white males as a group have the highest rate of suicide. Frank's difficulty in adjusting is interpreted considering developmental, life-cycle, gen-

der, and role theories. Additionally, existential theory relates to Frank's lack of meaning apart from his traditional, gender-specific role as a worker/provider. Accepting assistance from his children, members of the "Sandwich Generation" (the generation caring for both children and parents), may threaten his self-esteem.

Environmental factors particular to this case include social isolation, unresolved grief with inappropriate coping (alcohol), ethnic/religious influences, financial concerns, and the general absence of community mental health services given current priorities in health care. Sociocultural and socioeconomic theories, as well as the concepts of social stress and community mental health must be considered as the nurse assesses Frank's environment.

Evaluation of Frank's health is informed by psychoanalytic, crisis, and public health theories, as well as the concept of emotional stress. A suicide risk assessment would note that he has access to a lethal means of killing himself, and that his drinking (which increases impulsive behavior) increases his risk further. Orem's Self-Care Deficit Theory, social support, and concepts of preventive psychiatry should be considered as the nurse notes Frank's depression and weight loss, his arthritic pain and his self-medication with alcohol. Assessment of his ability to live independently should include an assessment of social support. Current support (his children) may be inadequate to meet his present needs, as he attempts to cope with the loss of his wife. The nurse can provide Frank with information about accessing medical and mental health care.

The nurse/provider uses the Interpersonal Relationship (Peplau) as a therapeutic tool in working with Frank. Nurses must become aware of their own attitudes toward older adults (ageism), and should develop interpersonal skills best suited for this population. Physical assessment is guided by the nurse's knowledge of normal changes associated with aging. Finally, application of mind–body concepts allows the nurse to integrate all data obtained, so as to provide holistic care.

FIGURE 2-2   Nursing Paradigm

This model illustrates the centrality of the four **key/anchor** concepts in the nursing paradigm: **nurse/provider, person/family, health, environment.** A few supporting concepts (especially those pertaining to geropsychiatric nursing) are illustrated as well; e.g. threat to safety, vulnerability, social isolation, coping (healthy and unhealthy).

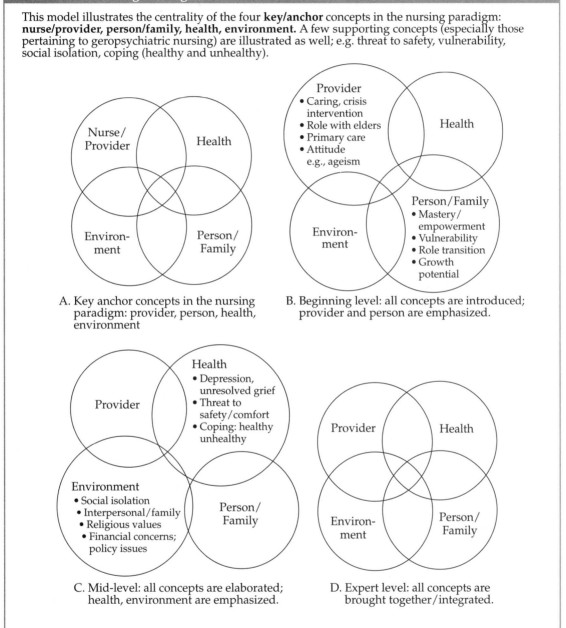

A. Key anchor concepts in the nursing paradigm: provider, person, health, environment

B. Beginning level: all concepts are introduced; provider and person are emphasized.

C. Mid-level: all concepts are elaborated; health, environment are emphasized.

D. Expert level: all concepts are brought together/integrated.

Source: *Violence issues: An interdisciplinary curriculum guide for health professionals.* Mental Health Division, Health Services Directorate, Health Canada. Reproduced with permission from: *Violence issues: An interdisciplinary curriculum guide for health professionals.* National Clearinghouse on Family Violence, Health Canada (1994) & reproduced with the permission of the Minister of Public Works and Government Services Canada, 2004.

REFERENCES

American Academy of Nursing (2002). New initiative on geriatric nursing education issues formal report outlining goals and strategies. (Press release) Retrieved February 22, 2002, from http://www.nursingworld.org/pressrel/2002/pr0204a.htm

American Association on Mental Retardation (2002). Fact sheet: Aging, older adults and their caregivers. Retrieved August 29, 2003, from http://www.aamr.org/Policies/faq_aging.shtml

American Association on Mental Retardation (2002). Definition of mental retardation. Retrieved August 29, 2003, from http://www.aamr.org/Policies/faq_mental_retardation.shtml

American Nurses Association (2001). *Code of ethics for nurses with interpretive statements.* Washington, DC: Author.

American Nurses Association (1998b). *Scope and standards for the nurse who specializes in developmental disabilities and/or mental retardation.* Washington, DC: Author.

American Nurses Association (2001). *Scope and standards of gerontological nursing practice* (2nd ed.). Washington, DC: Author.

American Nurses Association (2000). *Scope and standards of psychiatric-mental health nursing practice.* Washington, DC: Author.

American Nurses Association (1996). *Social policy statement.* Washington, DC: Author.

American Nurses Association (1998a). *Standards of clinical nursing practice.* Washington, DC: Author.

American Psychiatric Nurses Association (2003). Geropsychiatric grant awarded to APNA. Retrieved July 17, 2003, from http://www.apna.org/pdfs/Geropsych.pdf

American Psychiatric Nurses Association (n.d.). Frequently asked questions about psychiatric nursing. Retrieved May 30, 2003, from http://www.apna.org/faq/aboutnursing.html

Antonovsky, A. (1980). *Health, stress, and coping.* San Francisco: Jossey-Bass.

Antonovsky, A. (1987). *Unraveling the mysteries of health.* San Francisco: Jossey-Bass.

Bandura, A. (1977). *Social learning theory.* Englewood Cliffs, N J: Prentice-Hall.

Bandura, A. (1997). *Self-efficacy: The exercise of control.* New York: W. H. Freeman.

Berkman, L. F. & Syme, S. L. (1979). Social networks, host resistance, and mortality: A nine-year follow-up study of Alameda County residents. *American Journal of Epidemiology, 109,* 186–204.

Boissevain, J. (1979). Network analysis: A reappraisal. *Current Anthropology, 20*(2), 392–394.

Brandt, A. M. & Gardner, M. (2000). Antagonism and accommodation: Interpreting the relationship between public health and medicine in the United States during the 20th century. *American Journal of Public Health, 90*(5), 707–715.

Burgess, A. W. (1997). *Psychiatric nursing: Promoting mental health.* Stamford, CT: Appleton & Lange.

Buss, A. R. (1979). Dialectics, history, and development: The historical roots of the individual-society dialectic. *Life-span Development and Behavior, 2,* 313–333.

Caplan, G. (1964). *Principles of preventive psychiatry.* New York: Basic Books.

Department of Health and Human Services (2001). *Healthy people 2010.* Washington, DC: U.S. DHHS.

Edmands, M. S., Hoff, L. A., Kaylor, L., Mower, L., & Sorrell, S. (1999). Bridging gaps between mind, body and spirit: Healing the whole person. *Journal of Psychosocial Nursing, 37*(10), 1–7.

Eliopoulos, C. (1997). *Gerontological nursing* (4th ed.). Philadelphia: J.B. Lippincott.

Erikson, E. (1963). *Childhood and society* (2nd ed.). New York: Norton.

Estes, C. L. (1995). Mental health services for the elderly. Key policy elements. In M. Gatz (Ed.). *Emerging issues in mental health and aging* (pp. 303–327). Washington, DC: American Psychological Association.

Fadiman, A. (1997). *The spirit catches you and you fall down.* New York: Noonday Press.

Fee, E. & Brown, T. M. (2000). The past and future of public health practice. *American Journal of Public Health, 90*(5), 690–691.

Frankl, V. E. (1963). (I. Lasch, Trans.) *Man's search for meaning: An introduction to logotherapy.* New York: Washington Square Press.

Futrell, M. & Melillo, K. D. (2002). *Evidence-based protocol: Wandering*. Iowa City, IA: The University of Iowa Gerontological Nursing Intervention Research Center, Research Dissemination Core.

Gerdner, L. A., Buckwalter, K. C. & Reed, D. (2002). Impact of a psychoeducational intervention on caregiver response to behavioral problems. *Nursing Research, 51*(6), 363–374.

Gerdner, L. A., Hall, G. R., & Buckwalter, K. C. (1996). Caregiver training for people with Alzheimer's based on a stress threshold model. *Image: Journal of Nursing Scholarship, 28*(3), 241–246.

Greenspan, M. (1983). *A new approach to women and therapy*. New York: McGraw-Hill.

Hall, G. R. & Buckwalter, K. C. (1987). Progressively lowered stress threshold: A conceptual model for care of adults with Alzheimer's disease. *Archives of Psychiatric Nursing, 1*, 399–406.

Hall, G. R. & Laloudakis, D. (1999). A behavioral approach to Alzheimer's disease. *Advance for Nurse Practitioners, 7*(7), 39–46, 81.

Hansell, N. (1976). *The person in distress*. New York: Human Sciences Press.

Hoff, L. A. (1990). *Battered women as survivors*. London & New York: Routledge.

Hoff, L. A. (1993). Review essay: Health policy and the plight of the mentally ill. *Psychiatry, 56* (4), 400–419.

Hoff, L. A. (2001). *People in crisis: Clinical and public health perspectives* (5th ed.). San Francisco: Jossey-Bass.

Hoff, L. A. (1994). *Violence issues: An interdisciplinary curriculum guide for health professionals*. Mental Health Division, Health Services Directorate, Health Canada.

Hoff, L. A. & Adamowski, K. (1998). *Creating excellence in crisis care: A guide to effective training and program designs*. San Francisco: Jossey-Bass.

International Society for Education and Research in Psychiatric-Mental Health Nursing (n.d.). Divisions. Retrieved July 21, 2003, from http://ispn-psych.org/html/serpn.html

Jeste, D. V., Alexopoulos, G. S., Bartels, S. J., Cummings, J. L., Gallo, J. J., Gottlieb, G. L., Halpain, M. C., Palmer, B. W., Patterson, T. L., Reynolds, C. F., & Lebowitz, B. D. (1999). Consensus statement on the upcoming crisis in geriatric mental health: Research agenda for the next two decades. *Archives of General Psychiatry, 56*(9), 848–853. Retrieved January 21, 2003, from http://gateway1.ovid.com/ovidweb.cgi

Joint Commission on Mental Illness & Health (1961). *Action for mental health*. Report of the Joint Commission on Mental Illness and Health. New York: Basic Books.

John A. Hartford Foundation Institute for Geriatric Nursing (n.d.). *Fast facts: Emphasis needed on geriatric nursing*. Retrieved June 22, 2004, from http://hartfordign.org

John A. Hartford Foundation Institute for Geriatric Nursing and the American Association of Colleges of Nursing (2002). *Older adults: Recommended baccalaureate competencies and curricular guidelines for geriatric nursing care*. Retrieved June 19, 2002, from http://www.hartfordign.org/publications/bacc.html

John A. Hartford Foundation Institute for Geriatric Nursing. *The phase II renewal plan, strategies and tactics years 2001–2006*. New York: Author.

Kaseje, D. C. O., & Sempebwa, E. K. N. (1989). An integrated rural health project in Saradidi, Kenya. *Social Science and Medicine, 28*(10), 1063–1071.

Kovner, C. T., Mezey, M., & Harrington, C. (2002). Who cares for older adults? Workforce implications of an aging society. *Health Affairs, 21*(5), 78–89.

Lindemann, E. (1944). Symptomatology and management of acute grief. *American Journal of Psychiatry, 101*, 101–148.

Loustaunau, M. O. & Sobo, E. J. (1997). *The cultural context of health, illness , and medicine*. Westport, CT: Bergin & Garvey.

Marks, I., & Scott, R. (Eds.). (1990). *Mental health care delivery: Innovations, impediments and implementation*. Cambridge, UK: Cambridge University Press.

Maslow, A. (1970). *Motivation and personality* (2nd ed.). New York: Harper & Row.

McKinlay, J. B. (1990). A case for refocusing upstream: The political economy of illness. In

P. Conrad & R. Kern (Eds.). *The sociology of health and illness: Critical perspectives* (3rd ed.) (pp. 502–516). New York: St. Martin's Press.

Mezey, M. & Fulmer, T. (2002). The future history of gerontological nursing. *Journal of Gerontology: Medical Sciences, 57A*(7), M438–M441.

Mitchell, S. C. (Ed.). (1969). *Social networks in urban situations.* Manchester, UK: Manchester University Press.

Mosher, L. R. & Burti, L. (1989). *Community mental health: Principles and practice.* New York: W.W. Norton.

National Conference of Gerontological Nurse Practitioners (2003). *2002–2003 NCGNP health affairs agenda.* Retrieved November 26, 2002, from http://www.ncgnp.org/displaycommon.cfm?an=3

Orem, D. E. (1980). *Nursing: Concepts of practice.* New York: McGraw-Hill.

Orem, D. E., Taylor, S. G., & Renpenning, K. M. (2001). *Nursing: Concepts of practice* (6th ed.). St. Louis, MO: Mosby.

Peplau, H. E. (1952). Interpersonal relations in nursing: A conceptual frame of reference for psychodynamic nursing. New York: Putnam.

Peplau, H. E. (1991). Interpersonal relations in nursing: A conceptual frame of reference for psychodynamic nursing. New York: Springer.

Peterson's guide to colleges and universities (2003). Retrieved June 27, 2003, from http://iiswin-prd03.petersons.com/ugchannel/articles/asp

Rachlis, M., & Kushner, C. (1994) *Strong medicine: How to save Canada's health care system.* Toronto, Ontario: Harper Collins.

Rieker, P. P., & Carmen, E. H. (Eds.). (1984). *The gender gap in psychotherapy: Social realities and psychological processes.* New York: Plenum.

Robinson, D. (1971). *The process of becoming ill.* London: Routledge & Kegan Paul.

Rodriguez-Garcia, R. & Akhter, M. N. (2000). Human rights: The foundation of public health practice. *American Journal of Public Health, 90*(5), 693–694.

Rosenfeld, P., Bottrell, M., Fulmer, T., & Mezey, M. (1999). Gerontological nursing content in baccalaureate nursing programs: Findings from a national survey. *Journal of Professional Nursing, 15*(2), 84–94.

Sarason, A. G. & Sarason, B. R. (Eds.). (1985). *Social support: Theory, research, and application.* The Hague, Netherlands: Martinus Nijhof.

Scheper-Hughes, N. & Lovell, A. M. (1986). Breaking the circuit of social control: Lessons in public psychiatry from Italy and Franco Basaglia. *Social Science and Medicine, 23*(2), 159–178.

Selye, H. (1956). *The stress of life.* New York: McGraw-Hill.

Sullivan, H. (1947). *Conceptions of modern psychiatry.* Washington, DC: Wm. Alanson White Psychiatric Foundation.

Taylor, S. G., Compton, A., Eben, J. D., Emerson, S., Gashti, N. N., Tomey, A. M. et al. (1998). Dorothea E. Orem: Self-care defincit theory of nursing. In A. M. Tomey and M. R. Alligood (Eds.), *Nusing theorists and their work* (pp. 175–197). St. Louis, MO: C.V. Mosby.

Ustun, T. B. (1999). The global burden of mental disorders. *American Journal of Public Health, 89*(9), 1315–1321.

Walsh, M. R. (1987). *The psychology of women: Ongoing debates.* New Haven, CT: Yale University Press.

World Health Organization (2002). *Global burden of mental illness.* Geneva, Switzerland: Author.

CHAPTER 3

Comprehensive Mental Health Assessment: An Integrated Approach

Lee Ann Hoff, PhD, MSN, MA
Lisa Brown, MS, APRN, BC

Assessment, the first step in the nursing process, lays the foundation for diagnosis, planning crisis intervention and treatment, implementing the plan, and evaluating results through follow-up strategies. Lack of progress in meeting treatment goals, unanticipated complications, and provider frustration or burnout can often be traced to inadequate or incomplete assessment. Such barriers to effective service delivery are compounded in the psychiatric/mental health practice arena by a key factor in one's experience of emotional distress or mental illness: subjectivity. As discussed in Chapter 2, the meaning that people attach to life events and their emotional, physical, and social sequelae often constitutes a major influence on one's healthy or unhealthy response to life's hardships, challenges of role transition, and recovery from traumatic experiences.

In the physical realm, providers can rely on a variety of technological and other objective assessment and diagnostic tools. But in emotional and cognitive spheres, while structured assessment tools exist, they will never be as accurate as those available for diagnosing physical phenomena precisely because of the subjectivity of people's emotional, cognitive, and spiritual response to life events. To illustrate: the indifferent attitude of a provider ordering laboratory tests for diagnosing a physical problem will not affect the objective laboratory results, although it may exacerbate a client's distress, whereas an indifferent attitude of a provider aiming to ascertain a depressed person's risk of suicide may result in denial of suicidal plans and failure to obtain other data for assessing suicide risk. This means that, in addition to structured assessment guides, the nurse–patient relationship and the provider's communication skills constitute the most essential "tools" in the psychiatric/mental health assessment process (Peplau, 1993).

This chapter begins with an overview and critique of assessment methods and published instruments available to the geropsychiatric nurse: Nursing diagnosis, Mini-Mental State Examination (MMSE), Diagnostic and Statistical Manual of Mental Disorders (DSM), and the Comprehensive Mental Health Assessment tool (CMHA). The use of these tools is then illustrated with a case example, with the major focus on the CMHA. This tool (Hoff, 2001) is highlighted for its close correspondence to the emphasis on functional assessment of older persons whose welfare and treatment outcomes can be compromised by concentrating on pathology and psychiatric diagnostic labels at this stage of the life cycle. We also discuss the CMHA's complementarity with psychiatrist McHugh's (2001) "essentials" approach to psychiatric diagnosis.

A service contract form illustrates a client and provider intervention framework that complements the Comprehensive Mental Health Assessment tool. It lists the CMHA assessment items as a structured guide for a data-based crisis intervention and mental health service plan that emphasizes a collaborative nurse–patient relationship as a key factor in treatment outcomes. Continuing the client-empowerment focus of the CMHA, it spells out specific strategies that the client and provider will employ to address the items identified.

■■■■■ OVERVIEW OF
ASSESSMENT METHODS

The multifaceted process of aging complicates mental health assessment of older people. As with any age group, it is essential to rule out an organic cause for any mental status change before assigning a psychiatric diagnosis. Subsequent to ruling out all organic causes of changed mental status, a thorough psychiatric assessment is warranted.

Nursing Diagnosis

Nursing diagnosis addresses areas of life affected by an alteration in health status. Nursing diagnoses of mental health are grouped under the following categories of Gordon's functional health patterns: Cognitive–Perceptual Pattern, Self-Perception–Self-Concept Pattern, Role–Relationship Pattern, Sexuality–Reproductive Pattern, Coping–Stress Tolerance Pattern, Value–Belief Pattern, and Sleep–Rest Pattern. An example could be "Alteration in mental status related to postoperative procedure as evidenced by short-term memory loss, disorientation to time and place." The nursing diagnosis illustrates what

the problem is and how it is manifesting itself. Registered nurses are educated to provide comprehensive, holistic assessments. Since they practice in a multidisciplinary system, nurses should be familiar with medical diagnosis and treatment.

Diagnostic and Statistical Manual of Mental Disorders (DSM)

The Diagnostic and Statistical Manual of Mental Disorders (DSM) is currently published in its fourth edition with revisions (DSM-IV-TR). Physicians, advanced practice psychiatric nurses, social workers, and psychologists use the DSM-IV-TR as a guide for diagnosing mental disorders. It is important for geropsychiatric nurses to be familiar with this tool, its benefits, and limitations in practice.

The first Diagnostic and Statistical Manual, published in 1952, was a compilation of diagnostic categories and a description of each. Reflecting the influence of Adolf Meyer's psychobiological approach, the word *reaction* was used to depict his belief that each disorder was a reaction to psychological, social, or biological factors, or a combination of these factors. The DSM-II was very similar to the first edition except that it eliminated the term *reaction.*

The DSM-III, published in 1980, included explicit diagnostic criteria, a multiaxial system and a "descriptive approach that attempted to be neutral with respect to theories of etiology" (American Psychiatric Association, 2000, p. 26). One of the primary goals of creating the DSM-III was to provide a medical nomenclature for clinical providers and researchers. The DSM-IV was published in 1994, the fourth edition with text revision in 2000.

The DSM-IV has been widely accepted in clinical and research settings. Significant controversy surrounds the development of the DSM-III and the revised text (Caplan, 1995; Cooksey & Brown, 1998; Luhrmann, 2000). However, this appears to have abated with the fourth edition with text revision

(APA, DSM-IV-TR, 2000). The five axes of the multiaxis systems of the DSM-IV-TR are as follows:

Axis I Clinical disorders, such as major depression, schizophrenia. Other conditions, such as alcohol dependence, that may be a focus of clinical attention

Axis II Personality disorders and mental retardation

Axis III General medical conditions; for example, HIV infection may cause dementia (Axis I), or alcohol dependence (Axis I) may cause cirrhosis (Axis III)

Axis IV Psychosocial and environmental problems—includes events and stressors that may precipitate, result from, and/or affect mental status and treatment outcomes

Axis V Global assessment of functioning. This axis indicates the client's overall functional level, including psychologic, social, and occupational well-being on a scale of 1 to 100 (low numbers designating low-level functioning, and higher numbers revealing a higher functioning level) (APA, 2000, p. 27; O'Brien, Kennedy, & Ballard, 1999, pp. 64-65).

Axis V of the DSM corresponds most closely to the CMHA in use for charting a client's progress from admission to discharge.

The broad acceptance of the DSM-IV, often referred to as the "bible" of psychiatry, is evident in the lack of literature discussing its use, benefits, and limitations. This is most obvious in the area of nursing and the social sciences, including social work and clinical psychology. Dialogue is also limited in the medical arena; however, this is where most of the literature can be found.

The DSM-IV-TR is not a diagnostic tool. It provides an outline of criteria for each diagnosis. Cooksey and Brown (1998) note nurses'

criticism of the DSM in that it provides inadequate information regarding the client's individual experience. This is in direct contrast to a nursing diagnosis outlining an alteration in mental health. It is important for registered nurses to be familiar with the criteria for individual diagnosis and simultaneously complete a thorough biopsychosocial assessment of each individual. The DSM diagnosis does not provide information regarding how particular individuals are functioning in their daily life.

Mental health assessment tools are varied and generally are specific to certain elements of mental health. For example, there are mania scales, depression scales, suicide risk assessment scales, and so forth. Many of these were originally designed as research tools and therefore are not always suitable for clinical assessment, particularly in high-risk situations where time is of the essence.

Mini-Mental State Exam

The Mini-Mental State Exam (MMSE) is a screening instrument that provides a brief assessment of an individual's cognitive function (Folstein, Folstein, & McHugh, 1975). This tool is useful in that it is simple, brief, and can be administered by a variety of disciplines with minimal training.

The MMSE's use may be limited by the patient's individual presentation. To administer the exam correctly, the patient must possess the ability to interact verbally as well as read, and write. Its use, therefore, in assessing clients who may be blind, or have limited education, for example, is tentative.

As with any assessment tool, if the MMSE is administered in a mechanical way that contradicts the importance of interpersonal rapport and empathy as prerequisites for a thorough holistic assessment of a distressed human being, its findings will be limited. It is prudent to never lose sight of the cultural, social, educational, and medical/physical factors that may affect one's "mental status" (Peplau, 1993) (See appendix in this chapter for sample questions from the MMSE tool.)

Comprehensive Mental Health Assessment Tool

The Comprehensive Mental Health Assessment Tool (CMHA) was developed and tested in the 1970s in the Erie County Mental Health System, Buffalo, NY (see Hoff, 2001, pp. 87-98). A major impetus for this tool came from the New York State government's need for a record system to track the incidence of mental disorders, as well as the effectiveness of community-based services for a range of people in distress or with serious mental illness. The tool's origin coincided with a nationwide development of the community mental health system following Congressional legislation in 1963 and 1965. The entire CMHA record system consists of these forms:*

1. Initial Contact Sheet (includes crisis rating)
2. Client Assessment Worksheet
3. Significant Other Assessment Worksheet
4. Comprehensive Mental Health Assessment (summary of interview and worksheet data)
5. Termination Summary
6. Interagency Referral Form
7. Consultation Form
8. Follow-up Assessment
9. Child Screening Checklist
10. Service Contract

The CMHA forms provide a structured guide to the interview, assessment, and service planning process with clients. Their intended use is within a health service system that recognizes the intrinsic relationship between physical, emotional, and sociocultural factors affecting the mental health status of individuals. The underlying philosophy of this record system emphasizes three key assumptions:

1. The person in distress or crisis is a member of a social network.
2. The stability of a person's social attachments and gratification of basic human needs strongly influences his or her physical, emotional, and mental health and one's related ability to function within the community.
3. The provision of crisis prevention, early intervention, and social support services will conserve costly health care dollars by restoring and maintaining people in non-institutional settings and preventing readmission to psychiatric facilities whenever possible.

The current CMHA version builds on Hoff's (1990) research with abused women in which the tool was used to assess mental health sequelae of violence and victimization. Its updated edition was developed and pilot-tested by Lee Ann Hoff and psychiatric nursing graduate students at the University of Massachusetts Lowell (Hoff, 2001).

The CMHA assessment and planning tool emphasizes client-centered, goal-oriented treatment. It utilizes a five-point Likert-like scale (1=excellent/very high functioning, 3=fair; 5=very poor/very low functioning) to ascertain client stress levels in 21 areas of biopsychosocial functioning through active collaboration with the client and significant others. It also allows for systematic evaluation of treatment outcomes and follow-up planning.

The forms are designed to assist in the achievement of several objectives:

---

*The complete set of CMHA forms is available by contacting the authors (Hoff & Brown). Researchers are invited to collaborate in further testing of this assessment tool.

1. To provide health/mental health providers, clients, and collaborating agencies a standardized framework for gathering data, while including subjective, narrative-style information from the client and significant others that is relevant to mental health across the life cycle.

2. To organize this information in a way that sharply defines the client's level of functioning (emotional, cognitive, and behavioral) and life-threatening risk, and outlines complementary treatment goals and methods to evaluate progress toward desired outcomes in specified functional areas.

3. To assist in fostering continuity between service during acute crisis states and the longer-term mental health treatment needed by some clients. (This objective is especially relevant vis-à-vis the issue of "socially constructed suicidality" that is sometimes used as the only "ticket" to psychiatric in-patient admission when health system economic factors supercede client need in clinical decision making.)

4. To provide supervisory staff with the information necessary to monitor service and assure quality and continuity of client care.

5. To provide administrative staff with information for monitoring and evaluating achievement of crisis intervention, counseling or psychotherapy, and related services for individual clients, and cumulative data revealing service outcomes in relation to agency objectives.

In an era of providing cost-effective health care without compromising the quality of care, this assessment and planning tool is especially relevant in its focus on client-centered, goal-oriented treatment and systematic evaluation of service outcomes. Its design depicting a person's functional level also avoids the negative effects of psychiatric labeling. Data concerning a client's "Basic Life Attachments" and "Signals of Distress" (Hansell, 1976) offer a structured, holistic, humanistic framework for addressing a range of human experience and functioning affected by various life events and traumas and the emotional/mental illness or disabilities that may follow.

The 21 assessment items in the CMHA, with ratings from high to low functioning, can serve as a checklist to assure that a thorough evaluation has been done. The scaled items evaluate a person's physical, mental, emotional, behavioral, spiritual, and social concerns allowing for prioritizing issues for action. The tool can facilitate meeting the demands of cost-effective service delivery, emphasis on community-based treatment, client empowerment, and evaluation of observable treatment outcomes as manifested by the functional level of the client and his/her quality of life.

The CMHA allows for varying techniques in collecting data and exemplifies the importance of obtaining collateral information from other health care providers as well as significant others. Depending on the clinical situation, the Client Self-Assessment Worksheet can be given to and completed by the client before formal interview or used as an interview guide. Either way it serves to reinforce the idea of the client's active involvement in the assessment process. The complete assessment protocol includes data collection from a significant other(s) on the same 21 items.

The structured five-point Likert-like scale allows for formal comparative assessment at (1) initial, (2) interim, and (3) termination phases of counseling or treatment. Besides prioritizing problems, immediate risks, and goals, it presents visually the potential progress in a client's strengths, functional level, and/or stress reduction. The scales and descriptive comments also assist both client and mental health provider to keep focused and to chart progress toward meeting treatment goals. Finally, the tool is a guide for additional interventions or referrals that might follow from the crisis intervention and/or counseling process. [See Figure 3-1 for the complete CMHA protocol and rating scales. Contact the authors for operational definitions of the scales, and information about on-going evaluation of this tool.]

CMHA and McHugh's "Essentials": Description and Commonalities

Elements of the CMHA are complementary to the work of Dr. Paul McHugh of Johns Hopkins University. In his critique of psychiatric assessment tools, McHugh states: "At Johns Hopkins Department of Psychiatry we have long held that psychiatry needs a new conceptual structure that ties the mental disorders we treat to mental life as psychological science understands it today. Such a structure would insist on defining mental disorders by their essential natures rather than by their appearances alone" (McHugh, 2001, p. 2).

McHugh divides the 20th century of psychiatry into three segments, the first being Meyerian, based on the teachings of Adolf Meyer, who emphasized psychobiology. Psychobiology differs from biologic psychiatry by studying life from the psychological perspective. Next the psychoanalytic period emerged. The discovery of psychotropic medication in the 1950s put an end to this period, giving way to emphasis on the empirical. The empirical period focus is on the importance of reliability in diagnosis, revisiting comprehensive assessments as emphasized by Meyer; this led to the development of the current DSM. McHugh acknowledges advancements in the area of research while pointing out that the emphasis on reliability has neglected the validity of psychiatry.

McHugh takes issue with certain diagnoses such as multiple personality disorder and chronic posttraumatic stress disorder. He requests psychiatry to give up "appearance driven" diagnosis, as did internal medicine many years ago. McHugh (1999) refers to the "weaknesses inherent in a system of classification based on appearances—and contaminated by self-interest advocacy." He calls for a new method that can "comprehend several inter-

active sources of disorder and sustain a complex program of treatment and rehabilitation" (McHugh, 1999, p. 38).

McHugh (2001) illustrates an alternative approach to categorizing and treatment planning for mental disorder. In a structure consisting of interactive perspectives of psychiatry, he attempts to reunite psychosocial components with biology. These interactive sources of disorder include four perspectives for assessment and diagnosis in psychiatric practice: (1) the Disease Perspective, encompassing pathophysiology and pathogenesis; (2) the Dimensional Perspective, including personality, life circumstances, and neurotic symptoms; (3) the Behavioral Perspective, including physiologic drive, conditioned learning, and choice; (4) the Life Story Perspective, encompassing setting, sequence, and outcome (McHugh, 2001).

McHugh (2001) and colleagues at Johns Hopkins hold that these four distinct but interrelated levels of expression constitute the hierarchical organization of human psychological life from the most basic neurological to the most highly developed psychological functioning. Assessment skill demands ascertaining the particular way a person's psychological functioning can go awry as defined by the four perspectives.

The dynamic interactive sources of disorder McHugh proposes for assessing psychological functioning are highly complementary to assessment factors depicted in the CMHA. In particular, McHugh's four perspectives underscore two key concepts framing the CMHA tool: Basic Life Attachments, and Signals of Distress—concepts from ego psychology, sociocultural theory, crisis theory, and preventive psychiatry (Caplan, 1964; Hansell, 1976; Hoff, 2001).

The complementarity of McHugh's perspective and the CMHA will become more apparent in the following Case Example with application of both the Mini-Mental State Examination, Nursing Diagnosis, and DSM-IV-TR.

Case Study

Frank Kelly, first introduced in Chapter 2, is a 72-year-old widowed Caucasian male.

He had presented to the emergency room of a community hospital complaining of chest pain. The cardiac workup was negative and evaluation revealed that Frank had been depressed and having thoughts of suicide. A psychiatric evaluation was ordered. The crisis team was called and a clinician proceeded with assessment. The clinician asked to speak with Frank and then his daughter. Unfortunately his daughter needed to leave to care for her children and would return as soon as possible; therefore, the CMHA was only conducted with Frank.

Comprehensive Mental Health Assessment
Initial Contact sheet

Today's date: <u>September 2, 2004</u>   ID#: <u>9999</u>

Name: Kelly, Frank
Age: <u>72</u>   Relationship status: ___ Married   ___ Single   _X_ Widowed
Address: <u>7 Any Street, Anytown, USA</u>
Telephone: <u>555-1111</u>

Have you talked with anyone about this? No ___ Yes _X_

If yes, who? <u>Kate who is with him in ER</u>   Date of last contact: _____

Significant other (name & phone): <u>Kate Smith 555-2222 (daughter)</u>

Are you taking any medication now? No ___ Yes _X_
If yes, What? <u>ASA 81 mg daily, Hydrochlorothiazide 12.5 mg daily</u>

CRISIS RATING: 1   2   3   **4**   5

                    Not urgent   Very urgent

Probability of engaging for counseling treatment contract (1= high; 5= low)

                    1   **2**   3   4   5

Summary of presenting situation or problem and help-seeking goal:

Frank Kelly, a 72-year-old Caucasian, widowed male was brought to the emergency department by his daughter secondary to complaints of chest pain. The cardiac work up was negative. During his evaluation, a depressed mood and sad affect were observed and suicidal ideations were reported. Frank was cooperative with the mental health assessment but seemed surprised when the issue of counseling/ mental health care was raised.

Date of next contact/appointment: _____

Signature (intake/triage person): _____ Date: _____

continues

Case Study (*continued*)

Assessment Worksheet
(to be used as initial interview guide with client)
NOTE: Comments by client are italicized; comments by provider are [in brackets].

1. *Physical Health:* How do you judge your physical health in general?

1	**2**	3	4	5
Excellent	Good	Fair	Poor	Very poor

Comments: *Sometimes I have a lot of pain with the arthritis but most days it is tolerable.*

2. *Self-Acceptance/Self-Esteem:* How do you feel about yourself as a person?

1	2	3	**4**	5
Excellent	Good	Fair	Poor	Very poor

Comments: *I am proud of my marriage and we raised three good kids. I had a decent career as a pipe fitter. I am just not sure what to do with myself now.*

3. *Vocational/Occupational (includes student, homemaker, volunteer):* How would you judge your work/school situation?

1	**2**	3	4	5
Very good	Good	Fair	Poor	Very poor

Comments: *Retired, I guess I could use something to do.*

4. *Immediate Family:* How would you describe your relationship with your family?

1	**2**	3	4	5
Very good	Good	Fair	Poor	Very poor

Comments: *The kids come by to see me at least once a week. They have their own lives to lead now.* [Considerable low self-esteem and depression, he may feel unworthy of more attention]

5. *Intimacy/Significant Other Relationship(s):* Is there anyone you feel really close to and can rely on if you're very upset or in a life-threatening situation?

1	2	**3**	4	5
Always	Usually	Sometimes	Rarely	Never

Comments: *I could call my kids if I needed them in an emergency. I don't want to call them up crying, though. I have no interest in meeting women.*

6. *Residential/Housing:* How do you judge your housing situation?

1	2	3	4	5
Excellent	Good	Fair	Poor	Very poor

Comments: *We sold our house five years ago and bought a condo unit in a complex for seniors.*

7. *Financial:* How would you describe your financial situation?

1	**2**	3	4	5
Very good	Good	Fair	Poor	Very poor

Comments: *I don't have any problems paying my bills and I have enough money so it won't cost the kids to bury me.*

8. *Decision-Making Ability:* How satisfied are you with your ability to make life decisions?

1	2	3	4	5
Always very satisfied		Somewhat dissatisfied		Always very dissatisfied

Comments: *I wish I had my wife to talk to like I used to but I can make decisions just fine.*
[Correlate with MMSE]

9. *Problem-Solving Ability:* How would you judge your ability to solve everyday problems?

1	2	3	4	5
Very good	Good	Fair	Poor	Very poor

Comments: *Same thing—wish the wife was here but I can do it myself.*
[Although he prides himself on problem-solving, suicidal ideation suggests desperation and unhealthy problem-solving]

10. *Life Goals/Spiritual Values:* How satisfied are you with how your life goals (and things you value most) are working for you?

1	2	3	4	**5**
Always very satisfied		Somewhat dissatisfied		Always very dissatisfied

Comments: *My only goal now is to die and be with my wife. The problem is, if I kill myself I will go to hell and I will never be with her. I don't go to church as much as I used to with my wife. I still try to go. I do find it helpful; I feel better when I go.*

11. *Leisure Time/Community Involvement:* How satisfied are you with the availability of leisure time and ability to relax and take part in activities beyond everyday duties?

1	2	3	**4**	5
Always very satisfied		Somewhat dissatisfied		Always very dissatisfied

Comments: *I am bored; I watch TV, eat, and sleep. Crying—I don't know what to do without her (wife).*
[Needs help in finding social support and involvement beyond immediate family]

12. Feelings: How comfortable are you with your feelings? (for example, do you often feel anxious or fearful?)

1	2	3	4	**5**
Always comfortable	Sometimes uncomfortable			Always uncomfortable

Comments: *I cry all the time.*
[High correlation with low self-esteem and suicidality]

13. Violence/Abuse Experienced: To what extent have you been injured or troubled by physical, sexual, and/or emotional abuse?

1	2	3	4	5
Never		Several times recently		Routinely (every day or so)

Comment/describe:

Note: If rating of Item 13 is 2 or above, answer items 19, 20, & 21 below

continues

Case Study   *(continued)*

14. *Injury to Self:* Do you have any thoughts of suicide or a plan to hurt yourself in any way?

    　　　　1　　　　2　　　　3　　　　**4**　　　　5
    　　　No risk whatsoever　　Moderate risk　　Very serious risk

    Comments/describe: [Openly admits to suicidal ideations, has access to guns and drinks ETOH regularly; however, he does not have an explicit, immediate plan to hurt himself.]

15. *Danger to other(s):* Do you have any thoughts about violence or a plan to physically harm someone?

    　　　　1　　　　2　　　　3　　　　4　　　　5
    　　　No risk whatsoever　　Moderate risk　　Very serious risk

    Comments/describe: *I would never hurt anyone else.*

16. *Substance Use (alcohol and/or other drugs):* Does the use of alcohol and/or other drugs concern you or interfere with your life in any way (work, family)?

    　　　　1　　　　2　　　　3　　　　**4**　　　　5
    　　　Never　　Rarely　　Sometimes　Frequently　Constantly

    Comments/describe: *My wife hated me drinking so I quit about 20 years ago. I started drinking again six months after she died. I don't have a problem. I only drink at home. I don't drive after I have been drinking.* [Reports consuming 6–8 beers 3–4x/week. Denies other drug use. Blood alcohol 0 today and drug screen negative.]

17. *Legal:* What is your tendency to get into trouble with the law?

    　　　　1　　　　2　　　　3　　　　4　　　　5
    　　　None　　Slight　　Moderate　Great　　Very great

    Comments/describe: *I haven't been in any trouble since I was 17 and even then it was drinking in public.*

18. *Agency Use:* How satisfied are you with getting the help you need from doctors or other health providers?

    　　　　1　　　　2　　　　3　　　　4　　　　5
    　　Always very satisfied　　Somewhat dissatisfied　　Always very dissatisfied

    Comments: *I have no complaints.*
    Note: If Item 13, Violence/Abuse Experienced, is rated 2 or higher, answer Items 19, 20 & 21.

19. *Relationship with Abuser:* How would you describe your relationship with the person who has abused you?

    　　　　1　　　　2　　　　3　　　　4　　　　5
    　　No contact or conflict now　　Occasional conflict　　Great conflict & turmoil

    Comments:

20. *Safety—Self:* How safe do you feel now?

    　　　　1　　　　2　　　　3　　　　4　　　　5
    　　Very safe　　Somewhat safe　　Very unsafe

    Comments:

21. *(If there are children) Safety—Children:* How safe do you think your children are?

1	2	3	4	5
Very safe		Somewhat safe		Very unsafe

Comments:

Additional items: Do you have any other issues, concerns, or problems that you wish to discuss with a counselor?

> *No, I told you everything.*

Urgency/Importance: Among the items noted, which do you consider the most urgent and/or in need of immediate attention?

> *I want to feel better.*

CMHA Assessment Worksheet Highlights

Among the 18 functional items applicable to Mr. Kelly, the following should receive the most immediate attention and action, based on ratings between 3 and 5 (moderate to high stress). The number in parentheses ( ) indicates the rating for these priority items.

12:   Feelings (5)
10:   Life Goal/Spiritual Values (5)
14:   Injury to Self (4)
16:   Substance Use (4)
11:   Leisure Time/Community Involvement (4)
2:    Self-Acceptance/Self-Esteem (4)
5:    Intimacy/Significant Other (3)

Of particular note among these priority ratings is their interrelationship; for example, Mr. Kelly does not know what to do with himself, he just wants to die and be with his wife, his risk for suicide, feeling reluctant to reach out to family, and coping with excessive use of alcohol.

Planned actions (by provider and client) around these "basic life attachments" and "signals of distress" are illustrated in Table 3-1, the Service Contract.

Mini-Mental State Examination

Score 24, poor concentration noted, difficulty with recall. *Note:* See Appendix B for a sample of MMSE questions and information for obtaining the complete form.

Nursing Diagnoses

1. Risk for violence toward self as evidenced by suicidal ideations, access to guns, and frequent use of alcohol.
2. Dysfunctional grieving related to loss of wife and career as evidenced by inability to establish new relationships, activities, and goals.
3. Knowledge deficit related to signs and symptoms of depression as evidenced by his difficulty in accepting the recommendation for counseling/mental health care.

continues

Case Study   (*continued*)

4. Situational low self-esteem related to loss of marriage and career and evidenced by self-report, "I don't know what to do with myself now."
5. Family coping, potential for growth as evidenced by concern by children, regular visits, and opportunity to open up dialogue regarding increased needs of the family patriarch.
6. Social isolation as evidenced by lack of peers, time spent home alone drinking alcohol.

Diagnostic and Statistical Manual Diagnosis—DSM-IV-TR

Axis I	Major depressive disorder, single episode, alcohol dependence
Axis II	Not applicable
Axis III	Hypertension, gout, arthritis
Axis IV	Death of wife, retirement, lack of peer support
Axis V	Global Assessment of Functioning (GAF)=50

Data-Based Service Planning

Table 3-1 illustrates a service contract developed with Frank Kelly from assessment data. Problems and issues identified for counseling and treatment correspond to the numbered items in the CMHA assessment tool. Numbers in parentheses indicate the stress rating for particular items. Note that of the 21 CMHA items, the seven functional areas with ratings of 3, 4, or 5 (indicating high stress and/or low functioning) included here illustrate priority areas for crisis intervention and treatment.

TABLE 3-1   Service Contract—Frank Kelly

Date:
Code:

1. Physical health	8. Decision-making ability	15. Danger to other(s)
2. Self-acceptance/self-esteem	9. Problem-solving ability	16. Substance use/abuse
3. Vocational/occupational	10. Life goals/spiritual values	17. Legal
4. Immediate family	11. Leisure time/ community involvement	18. Agency use
5. Intimate relationship(s)	12. Feelings	19. Relationship with abuser
6. Residential/housing	13. Violence/abuse experienced	20. Safety-self
7. Financial security	14. Injury to self	21. Safety-children

Stress rating Code: 1= low stress/very high functioning   5= high stress/very low functioning

Item/Stress Rating	Problem/Issue Specification	Strategies/techniques (planned actions of client & health provider)
12. Feelings (5)	"I cry all the time."	1. Provide supportive environment, allowing patient to express feelings freely
		2. Provide education on depression
		3. Explore role of unresolved grief of multiple losses (wife, career, health)

10. Life goals/ (5) Spiritual values	"My only goal is to die and be with my wife." He believes he will "go to hell" and therefore not be with wife if he takes his own life.	1. Explore openness to including pastoral counseling 2. Discuss opportunities to become active in his church
14. Injury to self (4)	Suicidal ideation, possesses guns, consumes ETOH on regular basis	1. Recommend immediate removal of firearms from home 2. Assess risk for suicide every visit 3. Confer with family and discuss suicide risk
16. Substance use (4)	ETOH 6–8 beers, 3–4x/wk	1. Assess if patient believes ETOH to be a problem 2. Provide education regarding ETOH and depression 3. Reevaluate frequently
11. Leisure time/ (4) Community involvement	"I am bored, I watch TV, eat, and sleep."	1. Integrate above strategies to increase activity, decrease isolation therefore increasing self-esteem/acceptance, increase possibility of peer relationships and explore options to set goals and achieve them.
2. Self-acceptance/ Self-esteem (4)	Was proud of marriage and career and both are now gone; "not sure what to do with myself now"	1. Explore areas of interest 2. Set small attainable goals to foster feeling of worth and accomplishment
5. Intimacy/ (3) Significant other	Has ongoing, reliable relationship with children but does not want to burden them. No peer support.	1. Discuss attending a grief support group 2. Explore social options available in his community 3. Explore having joint session with family as additional suicide prevention measure

Signatures: Client _____   Crisis worker _____

This service contract example suggests a cautionary note regarding suicide prevention. The "no-suicide contract" is a technique employed by some health providers in which the client promises not to harm him- or herself between sessions. While widely practiced (especially by providers without specialty training in crisis intervention), such contracts offer no special protection against suicide, nor legal protection for the therapist or other provider. Any value the contract may have is only as good as the quality of the therapeutic relationship in which we convey caring and concern for the client. A no-suicide contract should never be used as a convenient substitute for time spent in empathic listening to and planning nonlethal alternatives with a suicidal person (Clark & Kerkhof, 1993; Hoff, 2001, pp. 212-219). The service contract with Frank Kelly highlights such alternatives, as well as attention to Mr. Kelly's losses, his unhealthy coping with alcohol, and other issues fueling his despair.

REFERENCES

American Psychiatric Association (2000). *Diagnostic and statistical manual of mental disorders* (4th ed., Rev.). Washington, DC: Author.

Caplan, G. (1964). *Principles of preventive psychiatry.* New York: Basic Books.

Caplan, P. (1995). *They say you're crazy.* Reading, MA: Perseus Books.

Clark, D. C. & Kerkhof, A. J. F. M. (1993). No-suicide decisions and suicide contracts in therapy. *Crisis, 14*(3), 98–99.

Cooksey, E. C. & Brown, P. (1998). Spinning on its axes: DSM and the social construction of psychiatric diagnosis. *International Journal of Health Services, 28*(3), 525–554.

Folstein, M. F., Folstein, S. E., & McHugh, P. R. (1975). Mini-mental state. A practical method for grading the cognitive state of patients for the clinician. *Journal of Psychiatric Research, 12*(3), 189–198.

Hansell, N. (1976). *The person in distress.* New York: Human Sciences Press.

Hoff, L. A. (1990). *Battered women as survivors.* London: Routledge.

Hoff, L. A. (2001). *People in crisis: Clinical and public health perspectives* (5th ed.). San Francisco: Jossey-Bass.

Luhrmann, T. M. (2000). *Of two minds: An anthropologist looks at American psychiatry.* New York: Vintage Books.

McHugh, P. R. (1999). How psychiatry lost its way. *Commentary, 108*(5), 32–39.

McHugh, P. R. (2001). Beyond DSM-IV: From appearances to essences. *Psychiatric Research Report, 17*(2), 1–5.

O'Brien, P. G., Kennedy, W. Z., & Ballard, K. A. (1999). *Psychiatric nursing.* New York: McGraw-Hill.

Peplau, H. (1993). *Interpersonal relations in nursing.* New York: Springer.

FIGURE 3-1

Comprehensive Mental Health Assessment Data: Initial, Interim, and Termination Status

Rating Code: 1 = Excellent/very high functioning/low stress
3 = Fair
5 = Very poor/very low functioning/high stress

BASIC LIFE FUNCTIONS

1. *Physical Health*   Medical information (chronic/acute illnesses, surgeries, OB/Gyn Hx, accidents, sexual dysfunction, allergies)

Current primary care provider: Yes _____ No _____
If yes, name: _____ Agency: _____
Telephone: _____ Date of last visit: _____

Medications:

Name	Dosage	Duration	Prescriber
1.			
2.			
3.			
4.			
5.			
6.			

ASSESSMENT RATINGS

Initial Comments:	1	2	3	4	5
Interim Comments:	1	2	3	4	5
Termination Comments:	1	2	3	4	5

2. *Self-Acceptance/Self-Esteem*:

Initial Comments:	1	2	3	4	5
Interim Comments:	1	2	3	4	5

continues

FIGURE 3-1	(*continued*)

Termination   1   2   3   4   5
Comments:

3. *Vocational/Occupational*   Employed _____ Student _____ Homemaker _____ Volunteer _____
   Other _____

Initial   1   2   3   4   5
Comments:

Interim   1   2   3   4   5
Comments:

Termination   1   2   3   4   5
Comments:

4. *Immediate Family*   Parental status: Children: Yes _____ No _____ How many? _____ Ages _____
   (Refer to Child Screening Checklist)

Initial   1   2   3   4   5
Comments:

Interim   1   2   3   4   5
Comments:

Termination   1   2   3   4   5
Comments:

5. *Intimacy/Significant Others*   Marital status: Never married _____ Married _____ Widowed _____
   Divorced _____ Separated _____ Living together _____ How long? _____

Initial   1   2   3   4   5
Comments:

Interim   1   2   3   4   5
Comments:

Termination   1   2   3   4   5
Comments:

6. *Residential/Housing*   Living situation: Lives alone _____ Lives with family _____ Other _____
   (specify) _____

Significant Other Information
Within household:
Name _____ Age _____ Nature of relationship _____
Supportive: Yes _____ No _____

Outside household:
Name _____ Age _____ Relationship _____
Address _____ Telephone _____

Initial Comments:	1	2	3	4	5
Interim Comments:	1	2	3	4	5
Termination Comments:	1	2	3	4	5

7. *Financial Security*   Source of income _____

Initial Comments:	1	2	3	4	5
Interim Comments:	1	2	3	4	5
Termination Comments:	1	2	3	4	5

8. *Decision-Making Ability*

Initial Comments:	1	2	3	4	5
Interim Comments:	1	2	3	4	5
Termination Comments:	1	2	3	4	5

9. *Problem-Solving Ability*

Initial Comments:	1	2	3	4	5
Interim Comments:	1	2	3	4	5
Termination Comments:	1	2	3	4	5

continues

FIGURE 3-1   *(continued)*

10. *Life Goals/Spiritual Values*

Initial   1   2   3   4   5
Comments:

Interim   1   2   3   4   5
Comments:

Termination   1   2   3   4   5
Comments:

11. *Leisure Time/Community Involvement*   Primary leisure & self-care
    activities _____

Initial   1   2   3   4   5
Comments:

Interim   1   2   3   4   5
Comments:

Termination   1   2   3   4   5
Comments:

12. *Feeling Management*   (coping with anxiety)

Initial   1   2   3   4   5
Comments:

Interim   1   2   3   4   5
Comments:

Termination   1   2   3   4   5
Comments:

SIGNALS OF DISTRESS

13. *Violence Experienced*   History of physical and/or sexual assault
    Date of last assault _____ Description _____
    Abuser/assailant (stranger, family) _____ Outcome _____

    ____ within last month   ____ medical treatment only
    ____ within last 6 months   ____ hospital intensive care
    ____ within last year   ____ hospital psychiatric
    ____ over 1 year ago   ____ outpatient follow-up
    ____ began in childhood   ____ survivor support group
    ____ multiple occasions   ____ no treatment or support

Initial   1   2   3   4   5
Comments:

| Interim | 1 | 2 | 3 | 4 | 5 |
Comments:

| Termination | 1 | 2 | 3 | 4 | 5 |
Comments:

14. *Injury to Self*   History of suicide attempts, ideation, threats, and current risk of suicide
     Date of last injury _____ Method _____ Outcome _____
     Ideation/threat, no specific plan _____

     ____ within last month   ____ medical treatment only
     ____ within last 6 months   ____ hospital intensive care
     ____ within last year   ____ hospital psychiatric
     ____ over 1 year ago   ____ outpatient follow-up
                       ____ no treatment

| Initial | 1 | 2 | 3 | 4 | 5 |
Comments:

| Interim | 1 | 2 | 3 | 4 | 5 |
Comments:

| Termination | 1 | 2 | 3 | 4 | 5 |
Comments:

15. *Danger to Others*   History of injury to others, threats, and antisocial behavior
     Date of last assault _____ Method/description _____
     Outcome (victim injury, arrest, etc.) _____
     Ideation/threat, no specific plan _____
     Context of assault/aggression (e.g., alcohol abuse) _____

     ____ within last month   ____ psychotropic drug treatment only
     ____ within last 6 months   ____ hospital psychiatric
     ____ over 1 year ago   ____ outpatient follow-up
     ____ began in adolescence   ____ batterers treatment group
     ____ began with intimate partner   ____ no treatment

| Initial | 1 | 2 | 3 | 4 | 5 |
Comments:

| Interim | 1 | 2 | 3 | 4 | 5 |
Comments:

| Termination | 1 | 2 | 3 | 4 | 5 |
Comments:

16. *Substance Use*   (alcohol or other drugs)

continues

FIGURE 3-1 *(continued)*					

Type	Present Use				Past Use	Duration
1.						
2.						
3.						
4.						
5.						

Initial   1   2   3   4   5
Comments:

Interim   1   2   3   4   5
Comments:

Termination   1   2   3   4   5
Comments:

17. *Legal*

    1. Pending court action: Yes ____ No ____ When _____
    2. On probation: Yes ____ No ____ Probation officer _____
    3. On parole: Yes ____ No ____ Parole officer _____
    4. Conditional discharge: Yes ____ No ____ Requirement _____
    5. Other (describe): _____

Initial   1   2   3   4   5
Comments:

Interim   1   2   3   4   5
Comments:

Termination   1   2   3   4   5
Comments:

18. *Agency Use*

    Previous Mental Health Service Contacts

    Outpatient: Agency _____ Phone # _____
             Contact person _____
             Address _____

    Inpatient: Agency _____ Phone # _____
             Contact person _____
             Address _____ Date last Hosp. _____
             Reason for admission _____
             How often? _____ How long? _____ Avg. length of stay _____

Initial   1   2   3   4   5
Comments:

Interim   1   2   3   4   5
Comments:

Termination   1   2   3   4   5
Comments:

Optional Information
Religious concerns: No _____ Yes _____ What? _____
Ethnic/cultural concerns: No _____ Yes _____ What? _____

Note: **Following items to be addressed if rating on Item 13 is 2 or higher**

19. *Relationship with Abuser*

    Living with abuser _____
    Living in a shelter _____
    Living with relative or friend _____
    In process of divorce _____
    Restraining order in effect _____
    In process of seeking counseling _____
    No contact with abuser now _____
    Other (describe) _____

Initial   1   2   3   4   5
Comments:

Interim   1   2   3   4   5
Comments:

Termination   1   2   3   4   5
Comments:

20. *Safety—Self*

Safety plan (describe) _____

Initial   1   2   3   4   5
Comments:

Interim   1   2   3   4   5
Comments:

Termination   1   2   3   4   5
Comments:

21. *Safety—Children*

    Children abused: No _____ Yes _____ Date _____ Outcome _____
    Children witnessed parental violence: No _____ Yes _____ Date _____
    Children in protective custody: No _____ Yes _____ How long? _____
    Safety plan for children (describe): _____

Initial   1   2   3   4   5
Comments:

continues

FIGURE 3-1 *(continued)*					
Interim Comments:	1	2	3	4	5
Termination Comments:	1	2	3	4	5

A. Do you have any other issues, concerns, or problems that we have not addressed?
    Explain:

B. Major problems—client goals

C. Narrative summary

Databased Problem Prioritizing, Goal Setting, and Service Planning: Items with ratings of 5, 4, & 3 are priority areas for intervention/service (see Service Contract Form)

Appendix

MMSE Sample Items

Orientation Time
"What is the date?"

Registration
"Listen carefully. I am going to say three words. You say them back after I stop.
Ready? Here they are . . .
HOUSE (pause), CAR (pause), LAKE (pause). Now repeat those words back to me."
[Repeat up to 5 times, but score only the first trial.]

Naming
"What is this?" [Point to a pencil or pen.]

Reading
"Please read this and do what it says. [Show examinee the words on the stimulus form.]
CLOSE YOUR EYES

CHAPTER 4

Ethnic Elders

Jane Cloutterbuck, PhD, RN
Lin Zhan, PhD, RN, FAAN

Dramatic changes in the nation's demographic and immigration patterns are rapidly transforming the United States into a multicultural, multiracial, and multilingual society. As the US population ages and becomes more ethnically and culturally diverse, mental health professionals will increasingly encounter ethnic elders in their practice. Population aging and multicultural change have major implications for the mental health field (Abramson, Trejo, & Lai, 2002). The growing presence of ethnic elders in the population, coupled with the high level of disparities that they experience in mental health care, places moral and ethical pressure on mental health planners, administrators, and frontline providers to critically evaluate psychiatric assessment and management for these groups. The need to integrate concepts of culture and ethnicity into mental health services and provide culturally competent care to this chronically underserved and often clinically misunderstood population is both immediate and imperative.

DEMOGRAPHICS

The older adult population is rapidly increasing in diversity. The number of ethnic elders age 65 and older has doubled with each census since 1960, and this pattern is expected to continue well into the 21st century. The federal government has officially designated four major racial or ethnic minority groups in the United States: African Americans (blacks), Hispanic Americans (Latinos), Asian American and Pacific Islanders, and Native American and Alaska Natives. These four broad groups comprise many distinct subgroups that are characterized by a wide array of cultural differences. The designation *Asian/Pacific Islanders*, for example, embraces at least 32 separate groups and includes among others Chinese, Korean, Japanese, Filipino, and Samoan. The category *Native American* includes the highly heterogeneous population of American Indians, Aleuts, and Inuits from approximately 278 federally recognized reservations, 500 tribes, bands of native villages, and 100 nonrecognized tribes. The *Hispanic* category, while unified by linguistic and some cultural traditions, shows significant differences between Mexican American, Cuban, Puerto Rican, South American, and Central American populations. Persons of Hispanic origin may also be of any race. The African-American group, largely native to the United States, may variously have as their country of origin a Caribbean island, Africa, or South America (Scharlach, Thompson-Fuller, & Kramer, 1992).

Although white Americans presently comprise the largest segment of the older adult population, their proportion is projected to decline over the next 50 years as the proportion of ethnic elders increases. At present, about 29.2 million of the nation's elders are white, 2.8 million are African-American, 1.74 million are of Hispanic origin, 815,000 are Asian/Pacific Islander, and 125,000 are American Indian/Eskimo/Aleut (Table 4-1). Between the years 2000 and 2030, the white population age 65 and older is projected to increase by 81% as compared with a 219% increase for older ethnic minorities, with Hispanics increasing by 328%, Asian American/ Pacific Islanders by 285%, African-Americans by 147%, and American Indian/Alaskan Natives by 131%. Of the 3.1 million foreign-born persons age 65 and older, over half (56%) are from non-European countries (U.S. Bureau of the Census, 2002). By the year 2030, ethnic elders are projected to represent 25% of the older adult population, up from 16.4% in 2000. By the year 2050, approximately one-third of the older adult population will be black, Hispanic, or other minority ethnicities (Administration on Aging, 2001; Angel & Hogan, 1991; U. S. Bureau of the Census, 1996, 2002).

Ethnic elders can be generally characterized as belonging to groups whose language and/or physical and cultural characteristics make them visible and identifiable. They each have special histories in the United States and/or from their countries of origin. Collectively, they have experienced differential and unequal treatment in America and regard themselves as objects of collective discrimination and oppression because of their racial and/or ethnocultural characteristics (Kiyak & Hooyman, 1994). Their histories are reflected in their current economic, social and political status. A great variety exists within and between the four major groups in terms of age, education, socioeconomic status, phenotype, region or country of origin, immigration status, family structure/function, living arrangements, level of acculturation/assimilation, literacy/linguistic fluency, and personal expe-

TABLE 4-1 Number and Percent of Persons 65+ by Race and Hispanic Origin—2000		
Total 65+	**Numbers**	**Percent**
Non-Hispanic African-American	2,787,427	8.0%
Native American/ Alaskan Native	124,797	0.4%
Native Hawaiian/ Pacific Islander	19,085	0.1%
Asian	796,008	2.3%
Hispanic (any race)	1,733,591	5.6%
TOTAL MINORITY	5,746,893	6.4%
White (Alone—Non-Hispanic)	29,244,860	83.6%
TOTAL 65+	34,991,753	100%

Adapted from: Administration on Aging (2001). Facts and figures: Statistics on minority aging in the United States, number and percent of persons 65+ by race and Hispanic origin, 2000; projected distribution of the population age 65 and older, by race and Hispanic origin, 2000 and 2050. Retrieved August 23, 2003, from http://www.aoa.dhhs.gov/prof/Statistics/minority_aging/facts_minority_aging.asp

rience with the health care system and its providers. As a result, ethnic elders cannot be thought of as being monolithic. Care must be taken not to overgeneralize the four groups or to perpetuate stereotypes about them. At the same time, one must be knowledgeable about the potential issues and patterns in their lives that give both strength and support and/or place them at risk and make them vulnerable to mental and physical problems.

A substantial body of evidence exists regarding mental health and the provision of mental health services to ethnocultural minorities in the United States. Recently synthesized (Department of Health and Human Services [DHHS], 2001), this literature reveals the dire disparities in mental health treatment for ethnocultural minority populations in access, utilization, quality, and intensity of mental health services, and representation in mental health research as compared to their white counterparts (DHHS, 2001, Smedley, Stith, & Nelson 2002). Ethnocultural minorities experience at least as many mental health problems as do European Americans (Atkinson, Morton, & Sue, 1998), but a large proportion do not seek professional help for mental health problems. When they do, they often fail to receive quality care (DHHS). Misdiagnosis, premature termination of treatment, suboptimal treatment, and other negative outcomes are common for those who do utilize formal mental health services (Atkinson, Morten, & Sue, 1998; Cloutterbuck & Mahoney, 2003; DHHS, 2001; Smedley, Stith, & Nelson, 2002; Virnig, Huang, Lurie, Musgrave, McBean, & Dowd, 2004; Zhan, 2003b). Disparities among ethnocultural minorities in mental health care are considered to be one of the most persistent and pressing public health problems in the United States today.

Rates of mental disorders among ethnic elders who live in the community are comparable to those of community-dwelling older whites after controlling for differences in education, income and marital status (DHHS, 2001, Omotade, 2003). Some researchers suggest, however, that being both old and a member of an ethnocultural minority group may result in extra vulnerability for mental health problems (Deeg, Karduan, & Fozard, 1996). This may be attributable, in part, to the considerably greater level of social and material adversity that ethnic elders have experienced across a lifetime, compared to their white counterparts. They are likely to have less education, less money, less adequate housing, poorer health, and fewer years of life. They may have suffered long-term discrimination and may, in addition, be discriminated against for being old. The effects of these factors and more contribute to increased risk of mental disorders. Ethnocultural minorities also bear a heavier burden of disability from behavioral disorders than their white counterparts because they receive less and poorer quality mental health care (DHHS, 2001).

Mental health professionals are only recently beginning to understand the complex relationship between cultural issues and mental health care. This chapter provides an introduction to and overview of issues important to this understanding including social and ethnocultural/sociostructural (systemic) factors that influence mental health help-seeking behavior, access to and utilization of formal mental health services, and the quality of mental health care received by ethnic elders. In addition, it highlights the practice of culturally competent care and makes recommendations for future research. Before moving ahead, it is important to define the concepts of *race, culture, ethnicity,* and *minority group* as they are used in this chapter.

DEFINITIONS OF RACE, CULTURE, ETHNICITY, AND MINORITY GROUP

The differences betweeen the terms *race, culture, minority group,* and *ethnicity,* which are often used interchangeably in the literature and have different interpretations depending on the context in which they are used, are often confusing. *Race,* once used as a biological classification system determined by phenotypic characteristics of genetic origin such as skin color, hair texture, and body shape, has fallen into disuse as a meaningful descriptor to clearly distinguish subgroups of humankind (Sue, 2003). *Race* is now more a sociological and political construct than a scientific one. Despite the limitations inherent in the concept, federal agencies continue to collect data on racial groups for administrative and political purposes.

Culture describes nonbiologically determined, socially learned attitudes and patterns of behavior that are transmitted from generation to generation. *Culture* is "an integrated pattern of human behavior that includes thoughts, communications, languages, practices, beliefs, values, customs, courtesies, rituals, manners of interacting, roles, relationships, and expected behaviors of a racial, ethnic, religious, or social group" (Goode, Sockalingam, Bronheim, Brown, & Jones, 2000, p. 1).

Ethnicity identifies broad population groups and refers to "social groupings which distinguish themselves from other groups based on ideas of shared descent and aspirations as well as behavioral norms and forms of personal identity associated with such groups" (Mezzich et al., 1993, p. 7). Lu, Lim, and Mezzich (1995) expand upon this definition and suggest that ethnicity includes an individual's sense of belonging to a group, sharing a common origin or history, and holding similar cultural and social beliefs with others in the group. Ethnicity is also thought to be closely linked to an individual's self-image and personal identity and may imply national or geographic origin, as well as religious beliefs. Some authors (Cose, 1997; Feagin & Feagin, 1999; Hacker, 1995) warn that use of the more generic term *ethnicity* to

describe groups formerly referred to as ethnic–racial minorities may cloud or ignore the day-to-day realities that American bias, racism, and discrimination do influence the delivery of health care. Further, caution is needed to avoid making assumptions about a client's ethnicity based on language and appearance alone. Such assumptions, if incorrect, could lead to misunderstanding and misdiagnosis (Gaw, 2001). Finally, Gaw warns that the concept of ethnicity should not be exoticized and viewed as a subspecialty thought to apply to ethnic minority groups only. The concept has universal application across all ethnic groups, including European Americans.

Minority group is a subgroup within a population. From the perspective of social science, minority groups receive differential and unequal treatment and suffer subordination and discrimination within society, usually based on their race, ethnicity, or national origin. The federal government describes minority groups as protected or disadvantaged ethnic or racial populations (Yeo, 2000).

MENTAL ILLNESS: SOCIAL AND ETHNOCULTURAL CONTEXTS

In order to provide effective mental health services to ethnic elders, mental health professionals must pay attention to the social, historical, and ethnocultural context that shapes their worldview and within which mental disorders occur. This context includes individuals' and clinicians' explanatory models of mental illness, the influence exerted by families, stigma associated with mental illness, and level of trust in the health care system and its providers. How an individual explains the cause of mental illness, manifests or presents its symptoms, manages the disorder within the family or community context, and utilizes formal mental health services, is partially determined by social and ethnocultural factors. The social and ethnocultural context clearly influences help-seeking behaviors and pathways taken toward the utilization of formal mental health services and subsequent satisfaction with care (Loustunau & Sobo, 1997).

Explanatory Models of Mental Illness

An individual's subjective interpretation of the nature of his or her problem, its cause, its severity, prognosis, and treatment preference, as well as his or her response to a specific illness experience (Kleinman, Eisenberg, & Good, 1978) is influenced by social environment, culture, and ethnicity (McSweeney, Allan, & Mayo, 1997). In traditional Western culture, the origin of mental illness is attributed to two main sources: psychological–psychiatric stress/trauma, and organic causes, such as chemical imbalances in the brain that lead to the manifestation of a disease. Western medicine conceptualizes mental illness within a biomedical framework of scientific reductionism that is characterized by a "mechanistic model of the human body, separation of the mind and body, [and a] discounting of spirit or soul" (Yeo, 2000, p. 22). Therapies within this explanatory model of mental health are based on monocultural, Western European and North American concepts, values, and beliefs; a view of the client as autonomous, egalitarian, rational, self-assertive, and self-aware; and an intrapsychic etiology model that requires an open-verbal style of communication (Veach, 2000).

Ethnocultural minority groups, conversely, may conceptualize the causes of mental problems and related behaviors differently (Kirmayer, Young, & Robbins, 1994). Although mental illness is thought of by some as being caused by a disease (natural illness), it is often attributed to wider social, religious, and/or metaphysical factors. Spirit possession, witchcraft, divine retribution, breaking of religious taboos, the loss of a vital body

essence, capture of the soul by a spirit, and disharmony in the biological, spiritual, family, or community realm are included in the many etiological explanations (Gaines, 1991; Landrine & Klonoff, 1994). Mental problems in non-Western groups have, in addition, been attributed to a lack of personal willpower, character weakness, God's will, or as punishment for an evil committed by the individual in a former life, by a family member, or by ancestors (Damon-Rodriguez, Wallace, & Kingston, 1994; Flaskerud, 2000; Green, Jackson, & Neighbors, 1993; Herrick & Brown, 1998; Leininger, 1991; McGoldrick, Giordano, & Pearce, 1996; Rogler & Cortez, 1993). Explanations for mental disturbances attributed to etiologies outside of the Western biomedical model have, until recently, received little attention in modern therapy, and more needs to be known about how they are used by individuals to explain, organize, and manage episodes of impaired well-being.

While rigorous methodological research in this area is lacking (DHHS, 2001), illustrations of ethnocultural minorities' purported explanatory models of mental distress do appear in the literature. Tseng (2001) cites, for example, a Hispanic woman who presented for treatment with the problem of "losing her soul," and an American Indian woman who could not escape her "spirit song." David Milne (2002, p. 18) cites an African-American truck driver who reported that he frequently "saw the devil sitting beside him warning that life was about to take a turn for the worse." An uninformed clinician assessing these examples at face value might suspect psychosis or a delusional disorder. Misinterpretation of such behaviors can result from not considering the cultural context within which they occur and their unique meaning. The truck driver in the latter vignette explained later that he had used a colloquialism common to many southern communities in the United States (Tseng), and that his statement should not be taken literally, but rather be viewed within its cultural context (Milne).

Conceptualization of mental illness within ethnocultural groups is not uniform and varies widely depending on other important factors such as age, education, socioeconomic status, regional location or country of birth, length of time in the United States, and level of acculturation. Although most ethnocultural minorities in the United States have been exposed to Western medicine and have some information about it (Applewhite, 1995; Patcher, 1994), traditional folk beliefs are still prevalent to varying degrees, especially among members of the older population. When working with individuals from ethnocultural minority backgrounds, it is helpful to elicit their explanation of what they believe is causing their mental distress (Klienman, Eisenberg, & Good, 1978). Having a clear understanding of the individual's view of what is causing their mental distress is important in helping the clinician differentiate his or her own assessment of etiology from that of the client's. This clarity provides the basis for negotiating treatment and setting mutual goals that encompass the perspective of both the client and the clinician.

Patcher's Awareness–Assessment–Negotiation model (1994) may be useful when dealing with individuals whose presentation of symptoms does not fit a standard biomedical model. Its application calls for the clinician to: (1) be familiar with the health beliefs and practices commonly held by individuals in the population served, (2) determine whether the individual subscribes to these common beliefs and practices, and (3) negotiate how to safely incorporate indigenous practices into a treatment plan that both the clinician and the individual see as being useful.

Idioms of Distress/Culture-Bound Syndromes

There is clear evidence of variations in the symptomatic expression of mental disorders by culture and locality (Guarnaccia & Rogler, 1999). Each culture has established a set of interpretive behaviors that its group members can accept and use with each other to describe what is wrong. These symptomatic or interpretive behaviors are known as "idioms of distress" (Nichter, 1981). Idioms of distress can be thought of as ways of accounting for misfortune or expressing distress. *Ataque de nerviosis*, an example of an "idiom of distress," is prominent among the Hispanic population from the Caribbean and other Hispanic groups. A general feature experienced by most sufferers is feeling out of control. Symptoms associated with *ataque de nerviosis* commonly include attacks of crying, uncontrollable screaming, trembling, and becoming verbally or physically aggressive. Following the *ataque*, individuals may experience amnesia but quickly return to their usual level of functioning. The *ataque* is thought to be a direct result of a stressful life event related to the family or significant others (Guarnaccia, Rivera, Franco, Neighbors, & Allende-Ramos, 1996).

According to the Surgeon General's report (DHHS, 1999), African-Americans, Asian Americans and Hispanics are more likely than non-Hispanic whites to express mental distress through physical symptoms (somatization). The presentation of somatic symptoms may differ according to the ethnocultural group in which they exist and are considered to be culturally acceptable expressions of mental distress. Somatization, an expression of mental suffering, is the most common "idiom of distress" worldwide. Care should be taken to differentiate it from psychosomatic disease, which has a verifiable physiologic disturbance (Isacc, Janca, & Orley, 1996; Tseng & Streltzer, 1997). *Somatization* describes symptoms caused by stress but experienced as bodily sensations that cannot be defined biomedically. The most common somatic symptoms of depression and anxiety are musculoskeletal pain, fatigue, stomach pain, chest pain, and dizziness. Some somatic symptoms may seem bizarre when encountered outside of a client's cultural context and may lead clinicians to mistakenly diagnose them as delusional or psychotic disorders. The mental distress that causes somatization may or may not be consciously conceptualized by an individual or may not be discussed because of the social stigma often associated with mental problems. A culturally uninformed primary care provider caring for an ethnocultural minority individual presenting with somatic symptoms may miss the opportunity to refer them for further investigation. The root problem of the distress goes unexamined and untreated.

The "culture-bound syndrome" is another important concept for mental health care providers who serve individuals from ethnocultural minority groups (Al Issa, 1995; Stewart, 1998). Culture-bound syndromes are defined as recurrent, locality-specific patterns of aberrant behavior and troubling experience that do not occur worldwide (American Psychiatric Association [APA], 2000) (Table 4-2). Similar to idioms of distress, they are culturally influenced expressions of mental distress and reflect the underlying values, morals, and traditions embedded in the social and cultural context within which they exist (Mezzich & Lewis-Fernandez, 1997; Kirmayer & Young, 1999). These syndromes may not, however, correspond directly with the disorders listed in the DSM-IV-TR (APA, 2000) and can be misdiagnosed as mental illness. *Koro* and *ghost sickness* are two examples of unique behavior observed in certain cultural environments. *Koro* (genital retraction syndrome) occurs in China and Southeast Asia. It is a sudden intense anxiety that the penis will recede into the body and possibly cause death. This phenomenon is explained as a sign of fatal exhaustion of the yang element within the framework of the yin-yang balance, and is attributed to guilt and anxiety over real or imagined sexual excess, especially autoerotic (Bartholomew, 1998; Hall, 1998). *Ghost sickness* occurs among American Indian groups in the

United States and is a preoccupation with death and the dead and is thought to be associated with witchcraft. Symptoms include loss of appetite, nightmares, weakness, fear and anxiety, confusion, a sense of being suffocated, hopelessness, and fainting (Hall).

Until fairly recently, Western mental health professionals have been generally unaware of or insensitive to ethnocultural differences in symptom expressions of emotional distress (Neighbors, 1997) and have tended to assume universal (etic) applications of their concepts and goals to the exclusion of culture-specific (emic) views (Veach, 2000). The *Outline for Cultural Formulation* (OCF), of the DSM-IV, Text Revision (APA, 2000) attempts to bring better awareness of the importance of the cultural dimension of the individual's clinical presentation. The OCF supplements the multiaxial diagnostic assessment and helps the clinician systematically evaluate and report the impact of the individual's context in the illness experience during the clinical encounter. It consists of five components: assessing cultural identity, cultural explanations of the illness, cultural factors related to the psychosocial environment and levels of functioning, and the overall impact of culture on diagnosis and care.

Family Influence

Although family characteristics among ethnocultural minority families have not yet been empirically linked to service use, they are thought to exert a great influence on an individual's help-seeking behavior and pathway toward formal mental health treatment (Ho, Rasheed, & Rasheed, 2003; Okun, 1996). Until fairly recently, the concept of family in the United States has been synonymous with traditional Western culture's nuclear structure based on immediate family membership and an individualistic worldview. The individualistic worldview emphasizes the self as autonomous and the primacy of individual rights and personal goals. Ethnocultural minority

TABLE 4-2 Components of Cultural Formulation	
Cultural formulation section	**Subheading**
Cultural identity of the individual	—Individual's ethnic or cultural reference group(s) —Degree of involvement with both the culture of origin and the host culture (for immigrants and ethnic minorities) —Language abilities, use, and preference
Cultural explanations of the individual's illness	—Predominant idioms of distress through which symptoms, or the need for social supports, are communicated —Meaning and perceived severity of the individual's symptoms in relation to norms of the cultural reference group(s) —Local illness categories used by the individual's family and community to identify the condition —Perceived causes and explanatory models that the individual and the reference group(s) use to explain illness —Current preferences for and past experiences with professional and popular sources of care
Cultural factors related to psychosocial environment and levels of functioning	—Culturally relevant interpretations of social stressors, available social supports, and levels of functioning and disability —Stresses in the local social environment —Role of religion and kin networks in providing emotional, instrumental, and informational support
Cultural elements of the relationship between the individual and the clinician	—Individual differences in culture and social status between the individual and the clinician —Problems that these differences may cause in diagnosis and treatment (for example: difficulties in relating or eliciting symptoms and understanding their cultural significance, in determining whether a behavior is normal or pathological, etc.)
Overall cultural assessment for diagnosis and care	—Discussion of how cultural considerations specifically influence comprehensive diagnosis and care

Summarized with permission from: American Psychiatric Association (2000). *Diagnostic and statistical manual of mental disorders* Text revision (DSM-IV-TR) (4th ed., pp. 897–898). Washington, DC: American Psychiatric Association.

groups tend to hold a more collectivist world-view that favors an extended family structure that goes beyond the bounds of the nuclear family. The collectivist worldview is characterized by subordination of personal goals and a high regard for in-group (family, community, nation) norms. Familial obligation supersedes the primacy of the individual, and ascribed statuses and strong bonds of mutual obligation exist (Kagitcibasi, 1997). While all four of the major ethnocultural minority groups tend toward collectivism in their worldview, family decision making is more formalized and hierarchical in Asian American and Hispanic families than in the African-American and Native American groups, where roles tend to be more egalitarian and flexible (Geiger & Davidhizer, 2004; Goldenberg & Goldenberg, 2002; Hurtado,1995; Purnell & Paulanka, 1998; Sue & Sue, 2003).

The problems of individual family members in ethnocultural minority groups are thought to be best supported and managed within the family (Garcia-Preto, 1996) and community. Ethnocultural minority families tend to experience more pronounced feelings of shame and embarrassment about having a mentally ill member of the family than do the nonminority members of the general population. This sense of stigma is especially prominent in Asian American and Hispanic American families (Lin, Inui, Kleinman, & Womack, 1992; DHHS, 2001).

Stigma Associated with Mental Illness

The association of stigma with mental illness in the United States is common. Feelings of shame and embarrassment are, however, much more intense among ethnocultural minority groups (Atkinson, Morten, & Sue, 1998; Diala, Muntaner, Walrath, Nickerson, LaVeist, & Leaf, 2001). *Stigma* is defined as "a mark or token of infamy, disgrace, or reproach" (The American Heritage Dictionary of English Language, 1992). The stigma associated with mental illness results from negative attitudes and beliefs held by the general public that cause fear, rejection, avoidance, and discrimination (Corrigan & Penn, 1999; Farina, 1998). Understanding the intense degree of stigma associated with mental illness among ethnocultural minority groups may help explain their help-seeking behavior and low level of utilization of formal mental health care services. The negative effects of stigma range from denial of mental health problems and expression of psychological distress through the body rather than the mind (Zhan, 2003a), to lack of disclosure of psychological distress to significant others or health care professionals, to serious delay in seeking formal help, to irreparable damage of family relationships (Baker & Adelman, 1994; Cheng, Leong, & Geist, 1993). Stigma associated with mental illness can extend beyond the individual to the entire family and ruin its public image and respect in the community (Lin,

Inui, Kleinman, & Womack 1992). Ethnocultural families with a mentally ill member may be marginalized within their community because it is assumed that the entire family has "bad blood" (Sue & Morishima, 1982). This places family members at risk of not having chances for employment and/or having good marriages ruined. Stigma serves as a powerful barrier among ethnocultural minority individuals' utilization of formal mental health services.

Level of Trust

The past and current experience of many ethnic elders with the health care system has been heavily marked by disregard, disrespect, lack of access, and abuse (Shavers, Lynch, & Burmeister, 2000). These factors shape attitudes and behaviors regarding the utilization of formal health care (Gamble, 1997). Fear and mistrust of the health care system and its providers by ethnic elders is yet another important factor that influences their help-seeking behavior and the utilization of formal mental health services. The Institute of Medicine publication *Unequal Treatment: Confronting Racial and Ethnic Disparities in Health Care* (Smedley, Stith, & Nelson, 2003) documents lower levels of trust in health care when patients are nonwhite and poor. Bloche (2001), Byrd and Clayton (2000, 2001), Cloutterbuck and Mahoney (2003), Gamble (1993), Sue (2003), and Swanson and Ward (1995) document past and present differentiation in the allocation of health care made on the basis of factors such as race, ethnicity, and class. Most of today's ethnocultural elders, who were born in the United States, have spent much of their lives under a separate but unequal system of segregated health care, and have been directly scarred by a history of discrimination and racism, especially during the pre-Civil Rights era (Byrd & Clayton, 2001). Elders, who have experienced lifelong humiliation and subordination in health care and other societal venues, may hesitate to seek needed help within what they perceive to be a hostile environment. The legacies of atrocities such as the Tuskegee Syphilis Study have produced a lingering distrust of the health care system and its providers. Ethnocultural minority elders, who have immigrated to the United States from countries with oppressive and authoritarian governments, may also lack trust because health care is provided through bureaucratic systems by persons who know little of their country of origin, migration history, and who may be—or may be perceived to be—biased against their language or culture.

Help-Seeking Behavior

According to Srebnik, Cauce, and Baydar (1997), an individual's help-seeking behavior in mental health arises out of a dynamic interaction between individual and family choice, cultural values and beliefs regarding mental health, and contextual and systemic factors such as the availability of services. What triggers an individual to seek help for mental distress, when, and from whom, is highly variable across ethnocultural minority groups (Cauce, Paradise, Domenech-Rodriguez, Cochran, Shea, & Srebnik, 2002; Lin & Cheung, 1999; Pescosolido, Brooks-Gardner, & Lubell, 1998). Help-seeking occurs in three stages. An individual must first recognize that he or she has a problem; second, decide to seek help; and third, select a provider (Srebink, Cauce, & Baydar, 1997). According to Gaines (1991) and Yeo (2000), the typical help-seeking pathway toward obtaining formal mental health care services for ethnocultural minority groups is as follows: (1) no care is sought, (2) the problem is managed through personal coping and/or interfamilial support and intervention, (3) consultation is sought from trusted extended family and friends, (4) outside help is sought from an indigenous healer or from the faith-based community, and (5) presentation of a

somatic complaint is made to a primary care provider. According to this model, help is finally sought from formal mental services only after multiple alternative attempts to address suffering have been tried but were unsuccessful. This help-seeking behavior helps, too, to explain why ethnocultural minorities in the United States are less likely than whites to seek formal mental health treatment, and contributes to their underrepresentation in most mental health services (DHHS, 2001; Kessler et al., 1996).

Other social and ethnocultural factors affecting utilization of mental health services by ethnocultural minority elders include: (1) literacy level and speaking a language other than English as a primary language, (2) fatalism, (3) lack of knowledge about services, (4) concern about confidentiality and adverse effects of medication, (5) fear of being hospitalized involuntarily, (6) lack of awareness of mental health services, and (7) negative experience in the mental health service system.

Sociostructural Contexts of Mental Health Care

The social and ethnocultural context of mental health care is *internal* to the individual. The sociostructural or systemic context of mental health care refers to those aspects of mental health care that are *external* and include the financing, organization, and availability of mental health services, provider behavior, client–provider interaction, and clinical decision making. In common with all Americans, ethnocultural minority groups encounter structural barriers such as cost, system fragmentation, and lack of available services (DHHS, 2001). They also face, however, additional barriers related to institutional and provider characteristics that may negatively affect the quality of care received (Damon-Rodriguez, Wallace, & Kingston, 1994; DHHS, 2001).

Zhan's Access Barrier Model (2003b) proposes three major types of barriers that ethnic elders face as they seek and utilize health care services: demographic, ethnocultural, and structural–systemic (see Figure 4-1).

Access to Care

When an individual seeks or needs service, he or she should be able to obtain it in a direct and timely way (La Roche & Turner, 2002). Many ethnocultural minorities needing mental health care are unlikely to receive care when they need it, and if they do, the care may be substandard or sought too late (Virnig, Huang, Lurie, Musgrave, McBean, & Dowd, 2004). The 1987 National Medical Expenditure Study reports that African-Americans were only 61% and Hispanic Americans only 49% as likely as non-Hispanic whites to have received mental health care (Vega & Rumbaut, 1991). The landmark report *Mental Health: A Report of the Surgeon General* (DHHS, 1999) found that Asian Amer-

icans were only one fourth as likely as non-Hispanic white Americans and half as likely as African-American and Hispanic Americans to have sought mental health services, even when socioeconomic differences were controlled (La Roche & Turner, 2002). In 2001, David Sacher, Surgeon General to the United States, issued a supplement to *The Surgeon General's 1999 Report on Mental Health* (DHHS 1999), *Mental Health: Culture, Race, and Ethnicity* (DHHS, 2001). This and other reports (Pescosolido, 1992; Rogler, 1999) document the nature and extent of disparities in mental health care for ethnocultural minorities that exist in access to and quality of mental health care.

Quality of Care

The effect of the clinician's attitude on the quality of care provided to ethnocultural minorities has not been well documented (Pi, Gutierrez, & Gray, 1993), but it is thought to play an important role in clinical decision

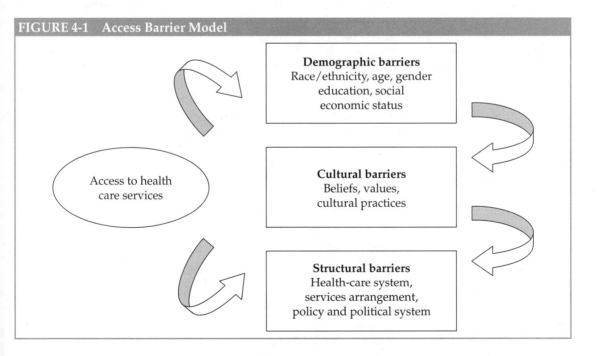

FIGURE 4-1   Access Barrier Model

Access to health care services

Demographic barriers
Race/ethnicity, age, gender education, social economic status

Cultural barriers
Beliefs, values, cultural practices

Structural barriers
Health-care system, services arrangement, policy and political system

making. The Institute of Medicine's (2003) report on unequal treatment in health care documents a large body of published research which reveals that racial and ethnic minorities experience a lower quality of health services, are less likely to receive even routine care, and have worse outcomes than their white counterparts (DHHS, 2001; Kales, Blow, Bingham, Roberts, Copeland, & Mellow, 2002). The quality of care for ethnocultural minorities is determined by many factors, including clinician bias and clinical uncertainty. Clinician bias with ethnic elders during the clinical encounter may be based on the clinician's attitude toward ethnic elders, be it for reason of ageism or cultural distance. Such bias may be unintentional and unconscious, and emerge from an inability to communicate due to linguistic barriers, unexamined racial stereotypes, class differences, and/or from notions of racial superiority. A classic example of clinical bias in general health care is reported by a seminal study conducted by van Ryn and Burke (2000). This study investigated physicians' attitudes toward African-Americans, who were being treated for cardiovascular disease. They found that physicians tended to rate African-Americans as less intelligent, less well educated, more likely to abuse drugs and alcohol, less likely to comply with medical advice, less likely to have social supports, and less likely to participate in cardiac rehabilitation—even after the patient's income, education, and personality characteristics were taken into account.

A number of studies in mental health care show that when an ethnocultural minority client is identical to a mainstream client in every way except for racial or ethnic minority group identification, a significantly more severe diagnosis may be assigned (Gaw, 1993). Abreu (1999) reports, for example, that African-Americans were evaluated more negatively than a hypothesized patient with the same symptoms whose race was not identified. Finally, Fabrega, Mulsant, and

Rifal (1994) found that the diagnosis of psychosis was significantly higher in African-American older adults than in European Americans. Such differential diagnosis patterns are thought to be more related to clinician bias than to the actual severity of an individual's condition. (Atkinson, Morten, & Sue, 1998). Ethnocultural minority group mental health clients experience more incorrect diagnoses, involuntary hospitalization, and less preferred forms of treatment than European American populations (DHHS, 2001; Flaskerud & Hu, 1992). Clinician bias may also result in the lack of a proactive approach (Priest, 1991). Ethnocultural minority individuals may be more likely to have fewer sessions with a clinician, and receive more medications than whites with comparable symptoms.

Quality care outcomes can be further affected by the clinician's etiquette and style of interaction during the clinical encounter. Clinicians who encounter clients from cultural groups other than their own must learn about these groups' normative cultural values, as the relationship established between the clinician and individual will often determine the success of the clinical encounter. Cultural values are behaviors, beliefs, and ideas that a group shares and expects to see observed in their dealings with others. Cultural etiquette and general style of interaction, respect, and rapport (or lack thereof) between the individual and the clinician all have an important effect on the clinical encounter, the care that is delivered therein, and the quality of the outcome. Considerations such as the use of surnames, the appropriate degree of personal interaction, attitudes toward authority figures, education, class differences, language facility, and terminology usage are extremely important when establishing a therapeutic alliance with ethnic elders. Clinicians who are unfamiliar with certain cultural values run the risk of offending ethnic elders during the clinical encounter, resulting in poor outcomes (Abramson, Trejo, & Lai, 2002).

A final area of bias in mental health care is the use of screening instruments, evaluation tools, psychological tests, and rating scales that have not been validated for use among ethnic minority populations (Lopez & Guarnaccia, 2000; Rogler, 1999). Most instruments in use today to help diagnose mental illness or disorders were developed on white European Americans and are heavily based on Eurocentric views. Any instrument being considered for use with ethnocultural minority older adults should be tested and found reliable for the population group (Baker & Bell, 1999). The use of inappropriate screening instruments is an ongoing problem, as only a few have been validated for use. A culturally sensitive assessment is extremely important for an accurate diagnosis among ethnocultural minority clients, especially for non-English-speaking persons who are primary candidates for misdiagnosis.

■ CULTURAL COMPETENCE

Cultural competence is defined as "a set of cultural behaviors and attitudes integrated into the practice methods of a system, agency, or its professionals, that enable them to work effectively in cross-cultural situations" (Administration on Aging, 2001, p. 9). Cultural competence is achieved by the willingness and ability of a system to value the importance of culture in the delivery of services to all segments of the population. It is the use of a systems perspective that values differences and is responsive to diversity at all levels of an organization.

One important step for achieving cultural competence involves careful consideration of the cultural bases and biases of contemporary psychiatric practice and clinicians' knowledge of their own ethnocultural identities and the implicit biases this brings (Kirmayer, 2001). Cultural competence is developmental,

community-focused, and family oriented. In particular, it is the promotion of quality services to underserved or ethnocultural groups through the valuing of differences to support the delivery of culturally relevant and competent care. It is also the development and continued promotion of skills and practices important in clinical practice, cross-cultural interactions, and systems to support the delivery of culturally relevant and competent care. Training in cultural competence is available through workplace in-service programs, courses offered at institutions of higher education, and through self-study. A number of excellent resources on cultural competence and mental health care are available on the Internet and in journal articles and textbooks.

Cultural competence activities include the development of knowledge, attitudes and skills through training, use of self-assessment for providers and systems, and implementation of objectives to ensure that governance, administrative policies and practices, and clinical skills and practices are responsive to the culture and diversity within the population served. It is a process of continuous quality improvement.

■ SUMMARY

As the population of older adults becomes a richer cultural and ethnic mix, mental health professionals are gaining in appreciation of the implications, challenges, and benefits of such diversity for care. The social–ethnocultural and sociostructural contexts of ethnic elders significantly determine their help-seeking behavior, access to and utilization of mental health services, and quality of care. The development of cultural competence is a critical element in the provision of safe, appropriate care and quality outcomes for this historically underserved and clinically misunderstood population.

Major gaps in the nursing literature regarding the mental health care of ethnic elders by geropsychiatric nurses continue to exist. An investigation of clinician bias and approaches that will best help geropsychiatric nurses to become more aware of their own assumptions and behaviors regarding older adults of different ethnocultural backgrounds may be a good place to begin. Geropsychiatric nursing models that address social and ethnocultural factors in mental health care of older adults in the areas of prevention, outreach, engagement, assessment, and intervention should be designed and tested to facilitate quality outcomes.

REFERENCES

Abramson, T. A., Trejo, L., & Lai, D. W. L. (2002). Culture and mental health: Providing appropriate services for a diverse older population. *Generations, 26*(1), 21–27.

Abreu, J. M. (1999). Conscious and non-conscious African American stereotypes: Impact on first impressions and diagnostic ratings by therapists. *Journal of Consulting and Clinical Psychology, 67*(3), 387–393.

Administration on Aging (2001). *Achieving cultural competence: A guidebook for providers.* Retrieved December 19, 2004, from http://www.aoa.gov/prof/addiv/cultural/cc-guidebook.pdf

Administration on Aging (2001). *Facts and figures: Statistics on minority aging in the U.S., Number and percent of persons 65+ by race and Hispanic origin—2000; Projected distribution of the population age 65 and older, by race and Hispanic origin, 2000 and 2050.* Retrieved August 23, 2003, from http://www.aoa.dhhs.gov/prof/Statistics/minority_aging/facts_minority_aging.asp

Al Issa, I. (1995). *Handbook of culture and mental illness: An international perspective.* Madison, CT: International Universities Press.

American Heritage Dictionary of the English Language (1992). (3rd ed.) Boston: Houghton and Mifflin.

American Psychiatric Association (2000). *Diagnostic and statistical manual of mental disorders.* (Rev. ed.) Washington, DC: Author.

Angel, J. L. & Hogan, D. P. (1991). The demography of minority aging populations. In L. K. Harootyan (Ed.), *Minority elders*, (pp. 1–13). Washington, DC: Gerontological Society of America.

Applewhite, S. L. (1995). Curanderismo: Demystifying the health belief and practices of elderly Mexican-Americans. *Health and Social Work Journal, 20*(4), 247–253.

Applewhite, S. L. (1998). Culturally competent practice with elderly Latinos. *Journal of Gerontological Social Work, 30*(1–2), 1–15.

Atkinson, D. R., Morten, G., & Sue, D. W. (1998). *Counseling American minorities* (5th ed.), Boston: McGraw Hill.

Baker, F. M. (1990). Ethnic minority elderly: Differential diagnosis, medication, treatment, and outcomes. In M. S. Harper, (Ed.), *Minority aging: Essential curricula content for selected health and allied health professionals*, (DHHS Pub. No. HRS P-V-90-4, pp. 449–577). Washington, DC: United States. Department of Health and Human Services.

Baker, F. M & Bell, C. C. (1999). Issues in the psychiatric treatment of African Americans. *Psychiatric Services, 50*, 362–368.

Barker, L. A. & Adelman, H. S. (1994). Mental health and help-seeking among ethnic minority adolescents. *Journal of Adolescence, 17*, 251–263.

Bartholomew, R. E. (1998). The medicalization of exotic deviance: A sociological perspective on epidemic koro. *Transcultural Psychiatry, 35*(1), 5–38.

Bloche, M. G. (2001). Race and discretion in American medicine. *Yale Journal of Health Policy, Law, and Ethics, 1*, 95–131.

Byrd, W. M. & Clayton, L. A. (2000). *An American health dilemma: A medical history of African Americans and the problems of race. Beginnings to 1900.* New York: Routledge.

Byrd, W. M & Clayton, L. A. (2001). *An American health dilemma: Race, medicine, and health care in the United States. 1900–2000.* New York: Routledge.

Cauce, A. M., Paradise, M., Domeneche-Rodriquez, M., Cochran, B. N., Shea, J. M. Srebnik, D. et al. (2002). Cultural and contextual influences in mental health help seeking: A focus on ethnic minority youth. *Journal of Counseling and Clinical Psychology, 70*(1), 44–55.

Cheng, D., Leong, F. T. & Geist, R. (1993). Cultural differences in psychological distress between Asian and Caucasian American college students. *Journal of Multicultural Counseling and Development, 21,* 182–190.

Chun, C., Enomoto, K. & Sue, S. (1996). Health care issues among Asian Americans: Implications for somatization. In M. Kata & T. Mann (Eds.), *Handbook of Diversity Issues in Health Psychology* (pp. 347–366), New York: Plenum.

Cloutterbuck, J. & Mahoney, D. F. (2003). African American dementia caregivers: The duality of respect. *Dementia, 2*(2), 221–243.

Corrigan, P. W. & Penn, D. L. (1999). Lessons from social psychology on discrediting psychiatric stigma. *American Psychologist, 54,* 765–776.

Cose, E. (1997). *Color blind: Seeing beyond race in a race-obsessed world.* New York: Harper Collins.

Damon-Rodriguez, J., Wallace, S., & Kingston, R. (1994). Service utilization and minority elderly: Appropriateness, accessibility and acceptability. *Gerontology and Geriatrics Education, 15,* 45–63.

Deeg, J., Karduan, P., & Fozard, J. W. (1996). Health behavior and aging. In J. E. Birren & K. W. Schaie (Eds.), *Handbook of the psychology of aging* (4th ed.), pp. 129–149. San Diego, CA: Academic Press.

Department of Health and Human Services. (1999). *Mental health: A report of the Surgeon General.* Rockville, MD: Author.

Department of Health and Human Services (2001). *Mental health: Culture, race and ethnicity – supplement to mental health, a report of the surgeon general.* Rockville, MD: U. S. Department of Health and Human Services, Substance Abuse and Mental Health Services, National Institutes of Health, National Institute of Mental Health.

Diala, C. C., Muntaner, C., Walrath, C, Nickerson, K., La Viest, T., & Leaf, P. (2001) Racial/ethnic differences in attitudes toward seeking professional mental health services. *American Journal of Public Health, 91*(5), 805–807.

Fabrega, H., Mulsant, B. M., Rifal, A. H., Sweet, R. A., Pasternak, R., Ulrich, R. et al. (1994). Ethnicity and psychopathology in an aging hospital-based population. *Journal of Nervous and Mental Disease, 182,* 136–144.

Farina, A. (1998). Stigma. In K. T. Tarrier and N. Tarrier (Eds.), *Functioning in schizophrenia.* Boston: Allyn & Bacon.

Feagin, J. R. & Feagin, C. B. (1999). *Racial and ethnic relations* (6th ed.). Upper Saddle River, NJ: Prentice-Hall.

Flaskerud, J. H. (2000). Ethnicity, culture and neuropsychiatry. *Issues in Mental Health Nursing, 21,* 5–29.

Flaskerud, J. H. & Hu, L. (1992a). Racial/ethnic identity and amount and type of psychiatric treatment. *American Journal of Psychiatry, 149,* 379–384.

Flaskerud, J. H. & Hu, L. (1992b). Relationship of ethnicity to psychiatric diagnosis. *Journal of Nervous and Mental Disease, 180*(5), 296–303.

Gaines, A. (1991). *Ethnopsychiatry.* Honolulu, HI: University of Hawaii Press.

Gamble, V. (1993). Legacy of distrust: African Americans and medical research. *American. Journal of Preventive Medicine, 9,* 35–37.

Gamble, V. (1997). Under the shadow of Tuskegee: African Americans and health care. *American Journal of Public Health, 87*(11), 1773–1777.

Garcia-Preto, N. (1996). Latino families: An overview. In M. McGoldrick, J. Giordano, & J. K. Pearce. (Eds.), *Ethnicity and family therapy* (pp. 141-154). New York: Guilford Press.

Gaw, A. C. (2001). *A concise guide to cross-cultural psychiatry.* Washington, DC: American Psychiatric.

Gaw, A. C. (Ed.). (1993). *Culture, ethnicity and mental illness.* Washington, DC: American Psychiatric Press.

Geiger, J. N. & Davidhizar, R. E. (2004). *Transcultural nursing: Assessment and intervention* (4th ed.). Philadelphia: Mosby.

Golderberg, I. & Goldenberg, H. (2002). *Counseling today's families* (4th ed.). Pacific Grove, CA: Brooks/Cole.

Goode, T., Sockalingam, S., Bronheim, S., Brown, M., & Jones, W. (2000). *Planner's guide: Infusing principles, content and themes related to cultural and linguistic competence into meetings and conferences* [Electronic version]. Washington, DC: Georgetown University, National Center for Cultural Competence, Center for Excellence in Developmental Disabilities. Retrieved August 22, 2003, from http://www.dml.georgetown.edu/depts/pediatrics/gucdc

Green, R. L., Jackson, J. S., & Neighbors, H. W. (1993). Mental health and help-seeking behaviors. In J. S. Jackson, L. M. Chatters & R. J. Taylor (Eds.), *Aging in Black America* (pp. 185–200). Newbury Park, CA: Sage.

Guarnaccia, P. J., Rivera, M., Franco, F., Neighbors, C., & Allende-Ramos, C. (1996). The experiences of attaques de nervios: Towards anthropology of emotion in Puerto Rico. *Culture, Medicine, and Psychiatry, 20,* 343–367.

Guarnaccia, P. J. & Rogler, L. H. (1999). Research on culture-bound syndromes: New directions. *American Journal of Psychiatry, 156*(9), 1322–1327.

Hacker, A. (1995). *Two nations: Black and White, separate, hostile, unequal.* New York: Balantine Books.

Hall, T. M. (1998). *Glossary of culture-bound syndromes.* Retrieved December 24, 2003, from http://weber.uscd.edu/~thall/cbs_glos.html

Herrick, C. A. & Brown, H. N. (1998). Underutilization of mental health services by Asian-Americans residing in the United States. *Issues in Mental Health Nursing, 19,* 225–240.

Ho, M. K., Rasheed, J. M., & Rasheed, M. N. (2003). *Family therapy with ethnic minorities* (2nd ed). Thousand Oaks, CA: Sage.

Hurtado, A. (1995). Variations, combinations, evolutions: Latino families in the U.S. In R. E. Zambrana (Ed.), *Understanding Latino families: Scholarship, policy, and practice* (pp. 40–61). Thousand Oaks, CA: Sage.

Issac, M., Janca, M., & Orley, J. (1996). Somatization—a culture-bound or universal syndrome: *Journal of Mental Health, 5*(3), 219–222.

Kagitcibasi, C. (1997). Individualism and collectivism. In J. Berry, M. H. Segall & C. Kagitcibasi (Eds.), *Handbook of cross-cultural psychology, Volume 3, Social and behavioral applications* (pp. 1–49). Boston, MA: Allyn & Bacon.

Kales, H. C., Blow, F. C., Bingham, R., Roberts, J. S., Copeland, L. A., & Mellow, A. M. (2002). Race, psychiatric diagnosis and mental health care in older patients. *American Journal of Geriatric Psychiatry, 8*(4), 301–309.

Kessler, R. C., Berglund, P. A., Zhao, S., Leaf, P. J., Kouzis, A. C., Bruce, M. L. et al. (Eds.). (1996). The 12-month prevalence and correlates of serious mental illness. In R.W. Manderscheid and M.A. Sonnenschein (Eds.), *Mental health, United States, 1996* (DHHS Publication No. SMA 96-3089, pp. 59–70). Washington, DC: U.S. Government Printing Office.

Kirmayer, L. J. (2001). Cultural variations in the clinical presentation of depression and anxiety: Implications for diagnosis and treatment. *Journal of Clinical Psychiatry, 62*(13), 22–28.

Kirmayer, L. J. & Young, A. (1999). Culture and context in the evolutionary concept of mental disorders. *Abnormal Psychology. 108,* 446–452.

Kirmayer, L. J., Young, A., & Robbins, J. M. (1994). Symptom attribution in cultural perspective. *Canadian Journal of Psychiatry, 39*(10), 584–595.

Kiyak, H. A. & Hooyman, N. R. (1994) Minority and socioeconomic status: Impact on quality of life in aging. In R. P. Ables, H. C. Gift, & M. G. Ory (Eds.), *Aging and quality of life.* New York: Springer.

Kleinman, A., Eisenberg, L., & Good, B. (1978). Culture, illness and care: Clinical lessons from anthropologic and cross-cultural research. *Annals of Internal Medicine, 88,* 251–258.

Landrine, H. & Klonoff, E. A. (1994). Cultural diversity in the causal attributions for illness: The role of the supernatural. *Journal of Behavioral Medicine, 17,* 181–193.

La Roche, M. J. & Turner, C. (2002). At the crossroads: Managed mental health care, the ethics code and ethnic minorities. *Cultural Diversity and Ethnic Minority Psychology, 8*(3), 187–198.

Leininger, M. M. (Ed.). (1991). *Culture care diversity and universality: A theory of nursing.* New York: National League for Nursing Press.

Lin, K. M. & Cheung F. (1999). Mental health issues for Asian Americans. *Psychiatric Services, 50,* 774–780.

Lin, K., Inui, T. S., Kleinman, A. M., & Womack, W. M. (1982). Sociocultural determinants of the help-seeking behavior of patients with mental illness. *Journal of Nervous and Mental Disease, 170,* 78–85.

Lopez, S. R. & Guarnaccia, P. J. (2000). Cultural psychopathology: Uncovering the social world of mental illness. *Annual Review of Psychology, 51,* 571–598.

Loustaunau, M. O. & Sobo, E. J. (1997). *The cultural context of health and illness and medicine.* Westport, CT: Bergin & Garvey.

Lu, F. G., Lim, R., & Mezzich, J. E. (1995). Issues in the assessment and diagnosis of culturally diverse individuals. In J. M. Oldman & M. B. Riba (Eds.), *Review of psychiatry, 14* (pp. 477–510). Washington, DC: American Psychiatric Press.

McGoldrick, M., Giordano, J., & Pearce, J. K. (Eds.). (1996). *Ethnicity and family therapy.* New York: Guilford Press.

McSweeny, J., Allan, J., & Mayo, K. (1997). Exploring the use of explanatory models in nursing research and practice. *Image: Journal of Professional Scholarship, 29*(3), 243–248.

Mezzich, J.W., Kleinman, A., Fabrega, H., Parron, D. L., Good, B. J., Lin, K. et al. (1993). *Revised cultural proposals for DSM-IV technical report.* Pittsburgh, PA: National Institute of Mental Health.

Mezzich, J. E. & Lewis-Fernandez, R. (1997). Cultural considerations in psychopathology. In A. Tasman, J. Kay & J. A. Leiberman (Eds.). *Psychiatry.* W. B. Saunders.

Milne, D. (2002). Culture cannot be divorced from psychiatric care [Electronic version]. *Psychiatric News, 37*(21), 18. Retrieved August 30, 2003, from http://pn.psychiatryonline.org/cgi/content/full/37/21/18

Neighbors, H. W. (1997). The (mis) diagnosis of mental disorders in African Americans. *African American Research Perspectives, 3*(1), 1–11.

Nichter, M. (1981). Idioms of distress: Alternatives in the expression of psychosocial distress, a case study form south India. *Culture, Medicine and Psychiatry, 5,* 379–408.

Okun, B. F. (1996). *Understanding diverse families: What practitioners need to know.* New York: Guilford Press.

Omatade, A. O. (2003). SNMA's presidential initiative: Mental health and minority communities. *Journal of the National Medical Association, 95*(4), 296–297.

Patcher, L. M. (1994). Culture and clinical care: Folk illness, beliefs and behaviors, and their implications for health care delivery. *Journal of the American Medical Association, 271*(9), 690–694.

Pescosolido, B. A. (1992). Beyond rational choice: The social dynamics of how people seek help. *American Journal of Sociology, 97,* 1096–1138.

Pescosolido, B. A., Brooks-Gardner, C., & Lubell, K. M. (1998). How people get into mental health services: Stories, choices, coercion and "muddling through" from "first timers." *Social Science and Medicine, 46,* 275–286.

Pi, E. H., Gutierrez, M. A., & Gray, G. E. (1993). Tardive dyskenesia: Cross-cultural perspectives. In K. M. Lin, R. E. Poland & F. Nakasaki (Eds.), *Psychopharmacology and psychobiology of ethnicity* (pp. 153–167). Washington, DC: American Psychiatric Press.

Priest, R. (1991). Racism and prejudice as negative impacts on African American clients in therapy. *Journal of Counseling and Development, 70,* 213–215.

Purnell, L. D. & Paulanka, B. J. (1998). *Transcultural health care: A culturally competent approach.* Philadelphia: F. A. Davis.

Rogler, L. H. (1999). Methodological sources of cultural insensitivity in mental health research. *American Psychologist, 54,* 424–433.

Rogler, L. H. & Cortez, D. E. (1993). Health seeking pathways: A unifying concept in mental health care. *American Journal of Psychiatry, 150,* 554–561.

Scharlack, A., Thompson-Fuller, E., & Kramer, B. J. (1992). *Curriculum modules on aging and ethnicity.* Berkeley, CA: University of California, School of Social Welfare, Center for the Advanced Study of Aging Services.

Shavers, V. L., Lynch, C. F. & Burmeister, L. F. (2000). Knowledge of the Tuskegee study and its impact on willingness to participate in medical research studies. *Journal of the National Medical Association, 92,* 563–572.

Smedley, B., Stith, A. & Nelson, A. (Eds.). (2002). *Unequal treatment: Confronting racial and ethnic disparities in health care.* Washington, DC: National Academy Press.

Srebnik, D., Cauce, A. M., & Baydar, N. (1997). Help-seeking pathways for children and adolescents. *Journal of Emotional and Behavioral Disorders, 4,* 210–220.

Stewart, M. (1998). Mental disorders and culture-bound syndromes. *AJN Nursing World.* Retrieved January 23, 2004, from http://www.nursingworld.org/tan/98janfeb/mental.htm

Sue, D. W. (2003). *Overcoming our racism: The journey to liberation.* San Francisco, CA: Jossey-Bass.

Sue, D. W. & Sue, D. (2003). *Counseling the culturally diverse: Theory and practice.* (4th ed.). New York: John Wiley.

Sue, S. (1994). Mental health. In N. W. S. Zane, D. T. Takeuchi & K. N. J. Young (Eds.). *Confronting critical health issues of Asian and Pacific Islander Americans* (pp. 266–288). London: Sage Publications.

Sue, S. & Morishima, J. (1982). *The mental health of Asian Americans.* San Francisco,: Jossey-Bass.

Tseng, W. S. (2001). *Handbook of cultural psychiatry.* San Diego, CA: Academic Press.

Tseng, W. S. & Streltzer, J. (Eds.). (1997*). Culture and psychopathology: A guide to clinical assessment.* New York: Bruner/Mazel.

United States Bureau of the Census. (1996). *Population projections of the U.S. by age, sex, race, and Hispanic origin, 1995–2050,* Table B-1. Washington, DC: U.S. Government Printing Office.

United States Bureau of the Census (2002). *The older foreign-born population of the United States.* Washington, DC: U.S. Government Printing Office.

van Ryn, M. & Burke, J. (2000). The effect of patient race and socio-economic status on physicians' perceptions of patients. *Social Science and Medicine, 50,* 813–828.

Veach, R. (Ed.). (2000). *Cross-cultural perspectives in medical ethics.* Sudbury, MA: Jones & Bartlett.

Vega, W. A., Kolody, B., Aguilar-Gaziola, S., & Catalano, R. (1999). Gaps in service utilization by Mexican Americans with mental health problems. *American Journal of Psychiatry, 156*(6), 928–934.

Vega, W. A. & Rumbaut, R. G. (1991). Ethnic minorities and mental health. *Annual* Review of Sociology, 17, 351–383.

Virnig, B., Huang, Z., Lurie, N., Musgrave, D., McBean, A. M., & Dowd, B. (2004). Does Medicare managed care provide equal treatment for mental illness across races? *Archives of General Psychology, 61,* 210–205.

Whaley, A. L. (2001). Cultural mistrust of white mental health clinicians among African Americans with severe mental illness. *American Journal of Orthopsychiatry, 71*(2), 252, 256.

Yeo, G. (Ed.). (2000). *Core curriculum in ethnogeriatrics* (2nd ed.). Palo Alto, CA: Stanford Geriatric Center.

Zhan, L. (2003a). Culture, health, and health practices. In L. Zhan (Ed.), *Asian Americans: Vulnerable populations, model interventions, and clarifying agendas* (pp. 3–18). Sudbury, MA: Jones & Bartlett.

Zhan, L. (2003b). Improving health for older Asian Pacific Islander Americans. In L. Zhan (Ed.), *Asian Americans: Vulnerable populations, model interventions, and clarifying agendas* (pp. 283–316). Sudbury, MA: Jones & Bartlett.

CHAPTER 5

Mental Health Promotion

Charles Blair, PhD, RN, CS, LNFA

MENTAL HEALTH AND WELLNESS

The number and proportion of the population age 65 years and older will grow rapidly after 2010 (Department of Health and Human Services [DHHS], 2000). As the nation ages, the mental health needs of older adults must be addressed because their needs will continue to grow. Mental health is a state of successful performance of mental functioning, resulting in productive activities, fulfilling relationships with other people, and the ability to cope with and adjust to the recurrent stresses of every-day living in an acceptable way. It is a state of balance that individuals establish within themselves and between themselves and their social and physical environments. Mental health is indispensable to personal well-being, family and interpersonal relationships, and one's contributions to community and society (DHHS).

To gain a deeper understanding of the meaning of mental health for older adults, Hedelin (2001) interviewed 16 women between the ages of 71 and 92. Participants in this study indicated that mental health is the experience of confirmation, trust, and confidence in the future, as well as a zest for life, development, and involvement in one's relationship to oneself and others.

Mental wellness is the capacity to perform well in any endeavor, to love and have friends, and to enjoy life with relative freedom from internal stress without causing stress to others. Promoting mental health is both any action to enhance the mental well-being of individuals, families, organizations, and communities, and a set of principles that recognize the mental health impact of how services, in the widest sense, are planned, designed, delivered, and evaluated. Mental health promotion works at three levels: (1) strengthening individuals or increasing emotional resilience through interventions designed to promote self-esteem, life skills, and coping skills, e.g., communicating, negotiating, and relationship skills; (2) strengthening communities by promoting social inclusion and participation, improving neighborhood environments, developing health and social services that support mental health, workplace health, community safety, and self-help networks; and (3) reducing structural barriers to mental health through initiatives to reduce discrimination and inequalities, and to promote access to education, meaningful employment, housing, services, and support for those who are vulnerable.

At each level, mental health promotion is relevant to the whole population, individuals at risk, vulnerable groups, and people with mental health problems. At each level, interventions may focus on strengthening factors known to protect mental health (e.g., social support, physical health) or to reduce factors known to increase risk (e.g., racial discrimination and loneliness). Mental health promotion has a role in preventing certain mental health problems in older adults, notably depression, anxiety, and substance abuse. Also, mental health promotion may foster recovery from mental illness and improve the quality of life of older adults with mental health problems (Hogstel, 1995).

STRESSORS IMPACTING MENTAL HEALTH

Older adults' lives are not free of stress. Stressors are events that either have a direct effect on the body or an indirect effect through various mediators. The individual's reaction to stressors is an attempt at adaptation, and if the stressors are not extreme or chronic, the attempt is usually successful. In that sense, stress reactions are good, in that they are a part of the homeostatic mechanism of the body to transient disruptions of equilibrium. If, however, the stressor becomes chronic, the individual's ability to successfully adapt is often compromised with resulting undesirable consequences such as mental ill health. Stressors that may challenge the lives of older adults include physical health problems, financial issues, difficulty accessing social services, transportation barriers, isolation, and finding affordable long-term care services.

However, it makes little sense to speak of, or to consider, older adults as a homogeneous group. Cook and Kramek (1986) suggested that older adults could be viewed as two distinct groups: those who are both financially poor and subject to chronic illness, and those who are both physically and financially well off. Moreover, issues of gender, race, and ethnicity create further distinctions. Ruiz (1995) noted, for example, that old men and old women are treated differently in the United States, as are older adults of various races and ethnic backgrounds. What is of interest here is that each of these variables may be considered a stressor, and to some degree may affect the mental health of older adults. From a mental health perspective, becoming aware of the basis of these stressors may be the first step toward mental health promotion and illness prevention.

Gender

Longevity and living arrangements have a significant impact on all older adults' quality of life and mental health, but more so on older women's. Because many more women than men survive into old age, the role of gender deserves special consideration in any discussion of mental health promotion in older adults. Women who reach age 65 can expect to live nearly 20 more years, whereas men at age 65 can only expect about 15 years (Moody, 2002). The typical fate is for men to die early and for women to survive with chronic disease. Because women tend to marry men who are older than they are, women are more likely to be widowed and live alone in old age than men. Because the family caregiving role of women often has the consequence of removing them from the paid labor force, they accumulate lower pension benefits than men. Retirement income for older women is on average only about 55% of what it is for older men, and nearly three out of four older Americans who fall below the poverty line are women (Moody). Divorce is also becoming an increasingly prevalent influence on older women's living arrangements (Moody). Divorced women usually experience a sudden reduction in their financial circumstances and they, unlike men, are less likely to remarry. For older women, socioeconomic stressors, patterns of inequality involving social class, race, ethnicity, and gender reinforce one another. If women earn less than men, and if minority group members are subject to prejudice over their lifetime, it is not surprising that an older, divorced, or widowed woman, who is from a lower socioeconomic class and a member of a minority racial or ethnic group, would experience problems in the area of health status, income, and housing that could negatively affect her mental health.

Race and Ethnicity

The poor socioeconomic position of many individuals in minority ethnic populations in the United States is a major cause of poor mental health, and highlights the need for policies and programs to reduce inequalities in mental health services between the majority and minority populations (Chow, Jaffee, &, Snowden, 2003). In studies conducted in South London, based on contact with psychiatric services over a 10-year period, Boydell et al. (2001) and Sharpley, Hutchinson, Murray, and McKenzie (2001) found that the incidence of schizophrenia in nonwhite minority groups increased significantly as the proportion of such minorities in the local population fell. The authors concluded that the increase may have been due to reduced protection against stress and life events due to isolation and fewer social networks. They suggested that people from minority racial and ethnic groups may be more likely to be singled out or to be more vulnerable when they are few in number or dispersed. These findings point to the importance of social factors as an explanation for the increased rate of schizophrenia among British-born minority racial and ethnic individuals.

Psychosocial factors may have particular significance for minority racial and ethnic populations because of the impact of racism and discrimination on individual and collective self-esteem. Racism affects mental well-being in two main ways: (1) It contributes to mental distress and can lead to feelings of isolation, fear, intimidation, low self-esteem, and anger. Depression may be caused by feelings of rejection, loss, helplessness, hopelessness, and an inability to have control over external forces (Bhugra & Bahl, 1999), and (2) it can act as a barrier to the access and provision of appropriate services. Minority racial and ethnic individuals may feel excluded from services because of direct discrimination by staff or through indirect discrimination such as being unable to access services because of language barriers.

Challenges of Late Life

During their later years, adults are confronted with what are possibly the greatest number of challenges in their lives, often with their lowest level of emotional resources and financial means due to fixed and limited incomes. It is a time when they may feel psychologically and physically fragile, in the midst of what constitutes, for many individuals, a very difficult period: aging and impending mortality. Issues of loss, disability, and identity are just a few of the many biopsychosocial concerns that older adults need to address for a continued sense of well-being. In facing these issues, older adults often find their biological and social families fractured or missing due to death, illness, or relocation.

Changes or loss in health, family, society, and finances can foster psychological disequilibrium and promote stress in older adults. According to Neugarten and Datan (1975), the stressful impact of an event is less intense when change is expected as opposed to when it is not expected. For example, the sudden onset of illness can be traumatic and can result in older adults feeling that their health is out of their control, creating a very stressful experience. Seligman (1992) pointed out that generally, adults with limited emotional and financial resources, who perceive their lives as having progressive and unexpected problems, often experience their situation as unstable and unpredictable and are more inclined to become depressed.

Successful aging implies that individuals are satisfied or content with their lives; that is, they have found ways of maximizing the positives in their lives while minimizing the impact of inevitable age-related losses. Maintaining connections with others is an important aspect of adult life. Mitchell (1990) found that older adults often affirm themselves through interrelationships. Maintaining such connections can become increasingly difficult during older adulthood as significant others die or are relocated. Physical deficits that occur with aging may also limit access to others. Visual impairment may limit older adults' ability to travel independently outside their immediate surroundings, thereby reducing their ability to drive or use public transportation and thus reducing their opportunity to leave their homes.

Chronic Illness

Events such as chronic illness, physical decline, and functional disability exert enormous strain on the mental health of older adults. Also, depressive symptoms are associated with many drugs used to manage chronic illness (Lueckenotte, 2000). Some chronic conditions such as cataracts and hearing impairment can be limiting but not life threatening. Other conditions such as hypertension and heart disease can lead to fatal disorders. Alzheimer's disease is probably one of the leading causes of disability and death afflicting people over age 65. Arthritis is the most familiar and the most prevalent chronic disease of later life, and it is the most important cause of physical disability in the United States (Moody, 2002). The joint and bone

degeneration that occurs as a result of arthritis and osteoporosis is a major problem for many sufferers, causing a loss of strength, weakened bones which are more likely to break, and reduced ability to perform independent activities of daily living, a major source of self-esteem for older adults (Blair, 1999). Parkinson's disease, characterized by a loss of control over body movements, affects mainly older people. Dementia is quite prevalent, and depression is common among people with Parkinson's disease. Cancer is overwhelmingly a disease of old age, and depressive symptoms occur as a side effect of the medications used to control the disease. Cardiovascular disease, which includes stroke and heart disease (Moody), is one of the leading causes of death among people over age 65. A stroke may cause immediate death or permanent disability including language or speech disturbance. For the disabled, the loss of quality of life can lead to frustration, anger, and depression. Alzheimer's disease involves progressive loss of the ability to think and remember. In its early stage, the symptoms of Alzheimer's disease may be severe enough to interfere with usual activities of daily living, work, or social relationships, the consequence of which may be emotional distress and depression.

Financial Problems

Morgan and Kunkel (2001) noted that there have been striking improvements in the economic well-being of the average older American in the past three decades. However, many still remain near or below the poverty level. Being African-American, Hispanic, or a female living alone are related to serious economic disadvantage. The rate of poverty for older African-Americans and Hispanic Americans is about three times that of European Americans. Women of all racial and ethnic backgrounds have poverty rates almost twice the rate of their male counterparts. This difference in economic well-being is reflected in differences in psychological well-being, with those who are economically distressed showing greater signs of depression (Morgan & Kunkel).

Admission to Nursing Home

Despite a decline in health and functional ability, older adults prefer to remain in their own homes and receive care there (Moody, 2002). But, because of the high cost of health care services, most older adults are forced to depend on federally funded services purchased through the Medicare and Medicaid financing programs. For many, nursing home placement is seen as a negative experience and viewed as institutionalization. Reliance on Medicare and Medicaid for payment of nursing home services is also stressful for some older adults.

There is an increased and immediate sense of loss for older adults upon admission to nursing homes. Relocation to such an institution can be fraught with emotional and psychological turmoil. As a result, depression is widespread among residents (Lueckenotte, 2000). Often this is due to fear of losing one's identity, friends, possessions, lifestyle, history, and personal space. Allen (2003) noted that, because residents live in an institutional setting, personal losses are inevitable. For many residents, the loss of control over their daily lives and the lack of decision-making opportunities constitute stressful living conditions. As far back as 1988, Phan and Reifler reported a high percentage of decreased interest, decreased energy, difficulty concentrating, feelings of helplessness and hopelessness, and psychomotor retardation in nursing home residents. Moody (2002) suggested that depression in nursing home residents may be a reaction to the fact that it is impossible for them to "start over" at this later stage of life.

▬ COMPREHENSIVE MENTAL HEALTH ASSESSMENT IN CLINICAL PRACTICE

Nursing assessment calls for information about the nature and scale of clients' problems. The method in which assessment information is collected often depends on the problem involved. Because of the need to understand the "whole person," mental health nurses are required to assess all aspects of the person—biophysical, psychosocial, and spiritual. In this sense, mental health assessments may be formal or informal, but should always be rigorous and comprehensive (Campbell, 1995; Ritter & Watkins, 1997). Comprehensive assessment of older adults should identify not just weaknesses and problems, but also strengths and potentials. Comprehensive assessment of capabilities and incapacities, as well as social functioning and support systems, establishes a rational basis for the development of treatment plans tailored to the client's physical, psychological, and social needs. Accordingly, the essential components of comprehensive assessment should comprise physical functioning, mental and emotional functioning, family and social support, and living environmental characteristics.

Physical Functioning

A health history and assessment is essential to the psychiatric nursing assessment. Some physical problems can present with psychiatric complications. Similarly, some psychiatric disorders can present with physical problems. Loss of physical health has direct effects on the quality of life of older people. Bodily systems featured in the physical assessment include the cardiovascular, respiratory, endocrine, genitourinary, gastrointestinal, and musculoskeletal systems. Functional status is considered an important and significant component of an older adult's quality of life. Functional assessment determines the older person's capabilities in performing basic activities of daily living (ADLs) and the more complex instrumental activities of daily living (IADLs). Functional assessment also determines the person's nutritional status, ability to mobilize, sleep patterns, hearing and vision, and medication behavior. A widely used instrument for assessing ADLs is the Barthel Index (Mahoney & Barthel, 1965). A widely used instrument for assessing IADLs is the Instrumental Activities of Daily Living Scale (Lawton & Brody, 1969).

Pain history and assessment should be included in the assessment of physical functioning. Pain interferes with the proper physical functioning of older adults, especially their ability to mobilize, and this has a profound effect on perception of well-being. Pain correlates with less socialization with colleagues (Ritter & Watkins, 1997). The daily pain diary (McCaffery & Pasero, 1999) and the Self-Care Pain Management log (Ferrell & Ferrell, 1995) are useful tools for measuring pain in older adults.

Mental and Emotional Functioning

The mental status examination, one of the most important diagnostic screening measures available to nurses, is designed to assess the client's mental functioning level and estimate the effectiveness of the clients' mental capacity. The purpose of the mental status assessment in the older adult is to determine the client's level of cognitive functioning, the degree of cognitive impairment, and the effect of that impairment on functional ability. Cognitive functioning is the aspect of mental functioning most affected by aging (Moody, 2002).

Cognition refers to the mental organization or reorganization of information. Assessment of cognitive functioning is concerned with evaluating the older person's conscious processes: thoughts, memory, judgment, comprehension, reasoning, and problem-solving strategies used in daily living. Responses to cognitive demands may be tested in several ways. Abstract thinking, decision making, problem solving, and reasoning ability may be observed through activities such as budgeting, shopping, and other IADLs. Abstract reasoning involves the ability to think beyond a concrete way. Abstract reasoning may be tested by the interpretation of proverbs or the identification of similarities between items. Level of comprehension may be determined by the client's engagement and attentiveness to the interview and by the relevance and accuracy of the client's responses to questions and tasks. Memory may be tested in a simplistic way by asking the client to memorize and retrieve from memory a piece of information such as a name or an address. Judgment is the end result of the client's ability to assess a situation, analyze it, come to an appropriate conclusion, and make sound decisions. Judgment can be assessed by listening as the client relates actual life events that required gathering and interpreting data, formulating a decision, and carrying out a plan. Judgment can be assessed by asking the client to make a decision about a hypothetical problem. Assessment of judgment also relies on observation and reports of informants who know the client well.

Older adults' cognitive functioning may be diminished by anxiety and worry, which may negatively influence recall and concentration (Morgan & Kunkel, 2001). Because of stereotypes of cognitive decline with aging that are held by society and the older adults themselves, mood and self-esteem of older adults are important factors to consider when measuring cognitive functioning. Ritter and Watkins (1997) noted that older clients tend to judge their memory as defective despite objective reports to the contrary. Consequently, self-report may not be a reliable way of estimating change in the cognitive functioning of older adults. Also, since diminished cognitive function in older adults is associated with lower educational achievement and lower socioeconomic status (Luis, Loewenstein, Acevedo, Barker, & Duara, 2003), any assessment of an elderly person's cognitive ability should include independent information about family patterns, as well as about the person's educational achievement, so that individual measures are interpreted within their true social context.

Although the mental status examination done by the nurse may provide good subjective evidence of the client's mental functioning, it provides only a baseline that identifies the need for the administration of one of the standardized mental status tests. Tests that nurses can use clinically include the Mini-Mental State Examination (Folstein, Folstein, & McHugh, 1975) and the Short Portable Mental Status Questionnaire (Pfeiffer, 1975).

Emotional Functioning

The feeling element is perhaps the most commonly recognized aspect of the emotional dimension. Emotion refers to affective states and feelings. Each individual has the capacity to experience the entire realm of feelings, which is meant to be experienced, not ignored. Feelings such as joy, anger, sadness, and fear occur most naturally in young children who are not yet restricted, through social learning, in expressing their feelings. Adults, however, often attach judgments to their feelings and consequently ignore uncomfortable ones.

As with the young, older adults are not passive receptacles of emotional experiences. A related social event can elicit and define the nature of a particular emotional experience, such as fear in response to a loss of power. The emotional status of the client is assessed in terms of affect, appropriateness of the affect

to the situation, quality and stability of the mood, physical signs of emotion, and emotional response patterns. The appropriateness of affect to the situation is based on the congruency between the affect the client is displaying and the client's culturally expected affective response in a particular situation. Both affect and appropriateness of affect are culturally determined in part; also, emotional status is commonly altered in acute and chronic illness. Consequently, these circumstances must be considered in any interpretation by the nurse. Tools that may be used by nurses to measure affect include the Beck Depression Inventory, Short Form (Beck & Beck, 1972) and the Geriatric Depression Scale (Yesavage & Brink, 1983).

Family and Social Support

According to Morgan and Kunkel (2001), family members in all generations are involved in giving and receiving various types of assistance, including assistance during illness, child care, financial support, emotional support, and household management. Older adults who lack supportive ties on whom they can rely for assistance are at greatest risk for institutionalization when they can no longer care for themselves. Dwyer (1995) estimated that 80% of informal care to frail and disabled elders is provided by family caregivers. However, there are differences in the quality and quantity of support given to older adults by family members from different race, class, and ethnic groups.

The quality of life an older person experiences is closely linked to social functioning. Social support needs of older adults tend to increase with advancing years and functional limitations as a result of declining health. Although most older adults are assisted by family, many depend on friends and nonfamily social networks to maintain their independence and decrease loneliness and social isolation. Because many elderly individuals confront most of life's difficulties by seeking out information, advice, and support from trusted others, the contributions of this social support can positively influence their performance of everyday functional activities. But social interactions may also have negative consequences for the older adult. Interactions that are unwanted or unpleasant may be detrimental to social relationships.

Because social factors can be so influential in the mental health status of older adults, it is important that nurses take an adequate social history. The nurse must be careful to consider both familial and nonfamilial sources of social support when assessing older adults' social systems. Neff (1996) suggested nurses assess the client's living environment characteristics to determine how it is perceived by the client, and whether it is conducive to maximum functional abilities. The client's financial resources should also be assessed for change in income and ability to meet need for food, clothing, shelter, recreational activities, or trips. The client's daily, weekly, and regular contacts should be noted. The client's verbalized insights into needs for services are also important. Client and family integration into the community should also be noted. Methods of transportation and the way the client spends a typical day should be assessed. Screening tools that nurses can use to assess clients' family and social support include the Family APGAR (Smilkstein, Ashworth, & Montano, 1982) and the OARS Social Resource Scale (Duke University Center for the Study of Aging and Human Development, 1988).

ASSERTIVENESS AND PROBLEM-SOLVING SKILLS TRAINING AS PART OF SOCIAL SKILLS TRAINING

Assertiveness is the ability to express one's needs and desires directly to the appropriate person in an appropriate manner. It involves standing up for personal rights and expressing thoughts, feelings, and beliefs, and making requests in direct, honest, and appropriate ways that respect the rights of others. It involves assuming responsibility for one's self and one's emotions and not projecting these onto others. In older adults, lowered interpersonal assertiveness has been found to be correlated with depression (Donohue, Acierno, Hersen, & Van Hasselt, 1995).

Since older adults with little or no effective interpersonal behaviors may be at risk of becoming depressed, it is incumbent upon the nurse to help them to gain the skills or to make a referral for skills training to develop effective interpersonal behaviors and increased interpersonal assertiveness. Skills training may be provided by clinicians including nurses, psychologists, and social workers who have been trained in behavioral principles and procedures. Skills training may involve anything from teaching clients how to shake hands to practicing conversational skills. Evidence of effective interpersonal functioning includes being goal-directed, showing signs of perception and integration of social signals, self-presentation, ability to take the role of others, use of appropriate social behavior, and the ability to provide feedback to others.

Teaching older adults to behave in a highly assertive yet appropriate manner through social skills training may reduce their chances of developing depression. Specific techniques of assertiveness training include repeated modeling of appropriate skills, role playing, high levels of descriptive verbal reinforcement, and in vivo rehearsal-based homework assignments which require that the individual rehearse assertiveness in assigned real-life situations, rather than in his or her imagination. The outcome of assertiveness training may be an increase in the perceived, if not the actual, level of control in interpersonal relationships.

LATE LIFE CHALLENGES THAT CAN CONTRIBUTE TO MENTAL HEALTH PROBLEMS

Caregiving Role and Stressors

Increasingly, older adults are taking on informal caregiving roles for individuals who become dependent or need assistance because of physical or mental effects of chronic illness. One notable chronic illness is that due to HIV infection. Research conducted in the past decade suggests that of the many adults living with HIV infection, half depend on older relatives for financial, physical, medical, or emotional support (Allers, 1990; Ory & Zablotsky, 1989). An estimated 50,000 to 100,000 adult Americans with AIDS receive help from older caregivers. In addition, there is a growing population of orphans whose caregiving parents have died, that are cared for by grandparents through standby adoption or guardianship (Goodkin et al., 2003). About 80% of the youths who are orphaned by HIV infection are people of color, and most older caregivers are members of minority ethnic groups. An estimated 70% of these caregivers are women, with 35% older than 65 years. As informal caregivers, older minority women face the multiple disadvantages of racial or ethnic inequities, compromised health status, poverty, aging, and sexism (Goodkin et al.). Despite the obvious benefits to care recipients, and regardless of their race, the stress experienced by most elderly caregivers often decreases their physical and psychological health (Given, Kozachik, Collins, DeVoss, & Given, 2001).

Dysphoria

Dysphoria is a disorder of affect characterized by distress and depression. Generally, the individual is in this state for understandable reasons. In older adults, the reasons may include the many losses and subsequent changes with which they are struggling to cope. The loss of physical health and independence, employment and income, family and friends, house and comfortable environment are difficult to accept, especially if they all occur within a relatively short period. These losses may overwhelm some older adults, causing them to worry and preventing them from feeling in control of their lives. This type of disorder usually calls for major psychosocial intervention (Sadock & Sadock, 2000).

Loneliness and Isolation

Loneliness is a strong indicator that an individual is feeling isolated from others. A number of conditions support the notion that loneliness is more widespread among older adults. Social isolation and loneliness negatively affect older adults' physical and psychological well-being. Behaviors and symptoms associated with loneliness are similar to those of mild depressive mood and include isolation, constipation, weight loss, insomnia, fatigue, and loss of appetite (Allen, 2003).

Death of family and friends, retirement, relocation, and other life changes can reduce opportunities for social contacts and place older adults at risk for social isolation. Physical limitations such as sensory deficits that limit communication or mobility may prevent visiting friends and family. In studying the impact of loneliness on older adults, Pinquart and Sorensen (2001) noted that: (1) the old-old and oldest-old tend to experience the highest levels of loneliness due to physical and sensory decrements and loss of their spouse and friends, and (2) older women, due to their higher risk of widowhood, tend to experience more loneliness than older men. Opportunities for social interaction also decrease with widowhood.

Lack of a social network may lead to nursing home admission. Pinquart and Sorensen

(2001) found that older adults in nursing homes are lonelier than those in community dwellings. Allen (2003) noted that loneliness has a profound effect on the mental health of nursing home residents.

Role Loss, Change, and Coping

The mental, emotional, and physical health of people of all ages is related to their ability to cope with and adapt to the changes in their lives. Most changes in early life are often voluntary and involve assumption of greater responsibility. For the older adult the opposite is true (Bunten, 2001). Change in this group often represents a loss, and some interpret it as a role loss. Losses such as leaving a valued position in the workforce, losing parental authority as children leave home, losing physical ability because of chronic illness, and experiencing bereavement with the death of family and friends, can create problems for those who are unable to successfully grieve their losses and establish new resources of morale and satisfaction (Moody, 2002).

Burden of Illness and Disability

Compared with the general population, older people on average have twice as many days in which activities are restricted because of chronic conditions such as arthritis and heart conditions. Living with a chronic illness affects a person's lifestyle and interactions with others. Many chronically ill older adults become homebound, and this decreases contact with the community and leads to social isolation. As with other age groups, older adults with chronic illnesses typically have repeated hospitalization to treat exacerbations of their illnesses. Inability to control an illness or disability produces feelings of powerlessness, especially when there is realization of a loss of function and the loss of one's former self. Feelings of powerlessness can lead to a loss of hope and depression.

Common Maturational and Situational Crises of Older Adults

A crisis is an internal imbalance that results from a perceived threat to one's well-being. Crises are usually precipitated by situations of loss, transition, or change. When such situations arise, a series of behaviors are activated that lead either to mastery of the situation or to crisis. Blazer (1990) noted that some degree of cognitive and physical loss is expected as we mature into old age. These losses may provoke anxiety and depression in older adults whose coping resources are taxed beyond their customary capacity. As we slip into old age, occasional forgetfulness, especially of the recent past, and an increase in the time needed for processing information may occur. Likewise, older adults may take longer to respond to questions and requests, and to process multiple stimuli. Decrease in physical strength and changes in physical appearance such as graying of the hair, wrinkled skin, and sagging bodies may be difficult for some older adults to accept. Hearing difficulty is both the most common and the most disabling sensory problem of aging: a decrease in both pitch discrimination and hearing acuity may occur. Decreased visual acuity, accommodation, and adaptation to darkness, and increased sensitivity to glare are likely to occur. Presbyopia is one of the most common visual problems; however, age-related macular degeneration, cataracts, and glaucoma are more serious. Decline in cognitive and physical ability may lead to other problems, such as lessened ability to independently perform ADLs and IADL tasks, including driving and shopping, and may increase the chance of social isolation.

A situational crisis may be thought of as a sudden unexpected threat to or loss of basic resources or life goals. In the older adult, these crises may be more common than the maturational ones. Much of the depression and anxiety in older adults is caused by situational factors in the environment, such as the deaths of family and friends, loss of or relocation from home, and loss or decline in economic stability. Losses such as the death of a spouse, or a divorce, are commonly accompanied by a transition to being single. Loss of a job or retirement may mean the loss of not only financial resources, but also companionship and a major source of pride and self esteem.

THERAPEUTIC INTERVENTIONS TO ADDRESS MENTAL HEALTH PROMOTION AND WELLNESS

Counseling and Support

Counseling is the act of providing advice and guidance to clients. The task of counseling is to give the client an opportunity to explore, discover, and clarify ways of living more resourcefully and toward greater well-being. Minardi and Hays (2003a) noted that an important aspect of counseling is the formation of a unique therapeutic relationship with the client in which an agreement is made as to the type of psychological work that will take place. Counseling involves using skills such as active and attentive listening, paraphrasing, questioning, and responding in such a way as to demonstrate to the client that the counselor is genuine, empathetic, and trying to understand the client's concerns, while not supporting unhealthy behaviors the client may exhibit. Because counseling is not therapy (Minardi & Hays), and therefore does not require specialized training, geriatric nurses are amply qualified to use counseling skills within their work settings to assist older adults in the process of reminiscence, and to deal with their numerous losses. Through counseling, older adults can be helped to face the reality of the losses, deal with the effects, break down barriers to readjusting to those losses, and make healthy choices in selecting replacements or substitutes for them.

Crisis Intervention

Crisis intervention is an active entering into the life situation of the client who is experiencing the crisis, to decrease the impact of the crisis event, and to assist the individual to mobilize his or her resources and regain equilibrium (Jacobs, 1989). Though related to it, crisis intervention is not psychotherapy. It is the provision of short-term help by crisis workers, including nurses. The goal of crisis intervention is to resolve the most pressing problems within the shortest possible time through focused, directed intervention aimed at helping the older adult develop new adaptive coping methods. No attempt is made at in-depth analysis.

Older adults in crisis situations need to be provided immediate attention by therapists. Nothing will raise these clients' hope more than an immediate offer of help. An essential characteristic of a crisis is the highly motivated nature of clients. No one has to persuade them to accept help. Often, they plead for it and uncritically accept it when it is offered. Such trust among older adults allows maximum caregiver–client interaction.

The purpose of crisis intervention is to restore in the person the level of functioning that existed before the current crisis. Burgess (1998) suggests five therapeutic goals. The first deals with safety and security. If there is danger of suicide, the family or significant others need to be informed and urged to exercise vigilance. In situations where the chance of self-harm is significant, the patient should be referred for emergency admission into the nearest hospital with an inpatient psychiatric service. Victims of crises often experience such intense turmoil that they fear they are going insane. For this reason, the second goal is to allow victims the opportunity to ventilate and to have their reactions validated. A third goal is to assist the individual to examine the circumstances related to the crisis and help him or her to prepare for dealing with similar situations in the future. Individuals should be encouraged to talk or write about the crisis experience and to identify a person to whom he or she could turn in the event of impending disaster. A fourth goal is to practice role-playing responses to a variety of calamitous scenarios. This is considered a practical way to plan for future events. The fifth goal is to provide educational opportunities for the individual through writing and reading assignments, self-assessment exercises, crisis intervention and supportive counseling, and peer support groups.

Pharmacological Therapies

Pharmacotherapy is the use of substances to alleviate symptoms, maintain improvements, and prevent relapse in psychiatric clients. Psychotropic agents can be used to control violence, dangerous or destructive behavior, improve the client's subjective feelings, shorten inpatient treatment time, and hasten the recovery of some clients. Because many nursing home residents have diagnosed psychiatric problems, psychotropic medications are more likely to be prescribed for this group of older adults. Psychotropic agents used with the older adult population include neuroleptics or major tranquilizers, antidepressants, and sedative–hypnotics.

Appropriate indications for neuroleptic prescriptions include treatment of psychoses, such as schizophrenia, paranoia, major depression and mania, and psychotic symptoms, such as hallucinations and delusions, which may occur in other conditions. Because of the potentially severe side effects of these medications, they should be prescribed only where a clear need exists.

Antidepressants are used to treat depressive symptoms in clients. Three major groups of these medications are used: tricyclic antidepressants (TCAs), selective serotonin reuptake inhibitors (SSRIs), and monoamine oxidase inhibitors (MAOIs). The choice of antidepressant is dependent on its side-effect profile.

Those with minimum potential for orthostatic hypotension, sedation, and anticholinergic effects are preferred. Antidepressants may be prescribed for dysthymia in older adults. For those with minor depression, it is suggested that antidepressants be given only when there is evidence of severe impairment as demonstrated by clients' need to make significantly increased effort to accomplish near-normal functioning in social, occupational, or other important areas of life.

Sedatives or antianxiety medications are used primarily to reduce anxiety in older adults. The major group of antianxiety agents is the benzodiazepines, which are used also to treat acute alcohol withdrawal and impending delirium tremens. Some benzodiazepines are used primarily to induce sleep and not to treat anxiety. Because older adults may be more sensitive to toxic effects of these medications due to accumulation of their active metabolites, they are generally prescribed the lowest possible dosages and for time-limited periods. SSRIs may also be used in the treatment of anxiety in older adults.

Individual, Group, and Family-Focused Interventions and Treatment Modalities

Nurses are well placed to use psychosocial interventions therapeutically with older adults in institutional and community settings to promote mental health and wellness. Many psychosocial interventions—the psychotherapeutic interventions—are designed to help clients alter dysfunctional relationship patterns and to develop more effective problem-solving skills. Development of insight or awareness of factors that motivate feelings, thoughts, and behavior is generally seen as a necessary precondition for change. Because older adults' capacity for insight may vary, some psychosocial interventions may serve to stimulate change without the active participation of clients in the process. Minardi and Hays (2003a, 2003b) point to several individual and group psychosocially based therapies available for use with older adults. These include psychotherapy, psychodynamic therapy, cognitive–behavioral therapy, reminiscence therapy, validation therapy, and the activity-based therapies: music, art, dance, drama, and exercise. Some of these psychosocial interventions are clearly within the nurse's role, while psychotherapies would require advanced training to conduct. Minardi and Hays noted that, in using these interventions, nurses must establish a therapeutic relationship with the older clients so that the clients feel psychologically safe enough to participate freely. An important aspect of using these therapies is the need for nurses to recognize the relationship boundaries between themselves, the clients, and the clients' significant others as they move in and out of the different interventions.

Psychotherapy, psychodynamic therapy, and cognitive behavioral therapy may be provided in either group or individual formats. The facilitators are trained therapists and the sessions are structured with precise start and end times. However, the principles upon which these therapies are based can be accommodated easily by nurses, since they already possess some of the necessary skills and knowledge.

The activity-based therapies, such as music, art, dance, and exercise therapies, may be delivered formally or informally, as when they are incorporated into interventions to promote relaxation or increase self-esteem and a sense of achievement. These therapies may be used in individual or group formats. When used formally, it may be necessary to leave interpretations of client's behaviors to qualified therapists, who are more competent to appropriately examine and interpret issues in depth.

Reminiscence therapy may be used by nurses to assist older adults to reexamine the life they have lived. It may be useful in helping clients to remember their accomplish-

ments, their failures, and their contribution to society. It may be an important process for boosting client's self-esteem. Validation therapy is used with demented older adults to relieve the client's distress and restore self-worth (Feil, 1992, 1999). Validation is a communication process. When using this therapy, the nurse focuses on the client's verbal and nonverbal communication and, rather than making interpretations based on the factual information presented in that communication, the nurse attempts to interpret only the emotions expressed in the communication. If the client's communication on a particular topic is repetitious, the nurse explores the client's feelings about the topic by prompting and shaping the client's communication on the topic. Minardi and Hays (2003b) noted that by not allowing factual errors to interrupt meaningful dialogue, nurses may use validation therapy to help demented older adults review their past and express feelings that may have been buried for a long time.

Complementary and Alternative Therapies

Older adults are taking herbal and other types of dietary supplements in record numbers (National Council for Reliable Healthy Information [NCRHI] Newsletter, 2000). While traditional therapies are the backbone of mental health care, botanical and nonbotanical complementary and alternative therapies, along with nontraditional psychosocial therapies, provide a break from the more regimented programs. These therapies encourage many of the same goals as traditional therapies and are thought to provide sensory and mental stimulation along with therapeutic benefits. According to McCabe (2002), an estimated one in three adults in the United States, including older adults, use botanical and nonbotanical complementary and alternative therapies to help promote mental wellbeing.

Botanical and Nonbotanical Therapies

Botanical agents include St. John's wort, a common weed that grows in the United States, that is frequently used for the treatment of depression. Despite its questionable efficacy, many take it on a regular basis. Ginkgo biloba comes from the leaves of a decorative tree. It is indicated for memory problems, and for this reason its common psychiatric use is with demented clients. Kava, a psychoactive derivative of the pepper plant, is used most often to treat anxiety and on some occasions insomnia. Ginseng has no focused use, but rather is indicated broadly for improved quality of life and generalized well-being. Valerian, grown abundantly in most parts of the world, may be used as a sedative and hypnotic (Hodges & Kam, 2002; McCabe, 2002). Passion flower, a compound derived from the dried flowers of the passion flower plant, is used as a mild sedative and antianxiety agent (McCabe, 2002; Starbuck, 1999). Nonbotanical mineral–vitamin agents include the dietary supplement SAMe (S-adenosylmethionine), an amino acid compound used widely as an antidepressant, and Omega-3 fatty oils, which are thought to promote mood stability and decreased aggression (McCabe).

Nontraditional Psychosocial Therapies

Pet and Plant Therapy This approach, dubbed the "Eden Alternative" (Thomas, 1994), is an effort to address the three major plagues of nursing home life: loneliness, helplessness, and boredom. Birds, dogs, cats, rabbits, and plants are introduced to the nursing home environment. Here, the residents have the opportunity to gain physical, emotional, spiritual, sensory, and intellectual benefits while experiencing natural, living things. Plants and animals not only provide the older residents a link with nature, but also create an opportunity for a more meaningful, homelike atmosphere.

Dance and Movement Therapy Dance/movement can allow older adults to improve mobility, circulation, and self-esteem. It also strengthens the body, making it easier to effectively deal with mental and physical stressors. Dance/movement may help participants to experience an inner awareness of self while having open interaction with the environment. This interaction provides a therapeutic self-help process that can release tension and anxiety, reduce confusion, stimulate memory, decrease depression, and rechannel anger and frustration.

Music and Art Therapy Music therapy is one of the most popular alternative therapies that allows older adults with various levels of cognition to experience many happy memories. Art therapy gives them the chance to express themselves and their emotions whether they can or cannot verbalize those emotions.

Consultation and Referral

Consultation in the mental health field involves the collaborative activity of professionals in the management of mental health problems. Generally, the problems presented for consultation are complex and potentially expensive. Caplan's (1970) model of mental health consultation identifies four types of consultation: program-centered administrative consultation, consultee-centered administrative consultation, client-centered case consultation, and consultee-centered case consultation. The latter two are the most relevant to our purpose here.

The essence of consultation is personal and professional respect. The consultant's expertise in a specific area is sought by the consultee who needs help or advice to manage a client's mental health problem. The consultant and consultee may or may not be mental health professionals.

Referral in the mental health field is the process by which clients are introduced to other professionals for mental health-related services. Referral of clients may be from one mental health professional to another, from a nonmental health professional to a mental health specialist, or from a mental health professional to a nonmental health professional. Many psychiatric mental health nurses have a specialty focus to their work, and there is a wide range of medical settings—including critical care and burns units—and long-term care settings for older adults—including nursing homes and assisted living facilities—where consultant mental health nurses can employ their expertise directly or indirectly to promote mental health care of older adults.

Education

Nurses are in a prime position to utilize education as a method of promoting mental health of older adults. Individual, family, and community-focused education intervention programs can be used to forge a partnership between mental health professionals, individuals, families, and communities, and thereby facilitate improved long-term mental health outcomes. Major objectives of these programs should be increasing knowledge of mental health promotion and illness prevention of the community at large, and supporting the self-care and daily management of mentally ill older adults by families.

Some educational interventions may be offered as formal stand-alone educational programs on mental health-related issues. Focus areas may include: (1) coping needs that result from the decrements that occur naturally in the process of aging, (2) support systems, (3) socioeconomic changes due to retirement and decreased earning ability, (3) ageism, and (4) community resources for the prevention or treatment of mental disorders. Some educational interventions may be imbedded in treatment programs for mentally ill clients, or physically ill clients at risk of mental illness. Emphasis should be placed on clients' and significant others' strengths rather than their weaknesses. Presentation formats may involve oral presentations, question-and-answer periods, discussion, and distribution of written materials. With the widening and almost universal availability of electronic media, presentation formats should include audiovideo formats, such as television, and the Internet.

▪ FAMILY AND COMMUNITY RESOURCES TO ENHANCE MENTAL WELLNESS

The presence of a family has a positive influence upon coping with aging. Family relationships are not only salient, but the support available within them is a key variable predicting well-being in older persons (Qualls, 2000). Often family members provide instrumental as well as intangible support to their elderly members, including assistance with activities of daily living, transportation, finances, and so forth. The average family caregiver provides 18 hours of unpaid care weekly to older adults within the family (National Family Caregivers Association, 1997). The average amount of out-of-pocket money spent monthly on care recipients by family caregivers was $171; those who provide 40 or more hours of care weekly spend an average of $357 (National Alliance for Caregiving & American Association of Retired Persons, 1997). Social support systems, such as the family, can buffer the negative effects of stress on the mental health status of older adults, thus reducing their vulnerability to mental illness and institutionalization.

The community approach to mental health promotion in older adults requires an appropriate mix of resources and service (Buckwalter, Weiler, & Stolley, 1995).

Community resources and services may be professional or nonprofessional in nature. Nonprofessional services may be offered by voluntary or state-funded agencies and include home-delivered meals, transportation services, and home upkeep services. Private-pay services include geriatric day care and assisted living centers. Professional resources include personnel such as physicians and nurses, psychologists, social workers, and academic educators who provide appropriate health, psychological, social, and academic services. Structural resources for supporting mental health promotion include hospitals, psychiatric day care centers, nursing homes, community colleges and universities, senior centers, and places of worship. Ideally, professional and nonprofessional services should complement each other and strive to satisfy the service needs of older adults.

▇ CLINICAL RESEARCH PERTAINING TO MENTAL HEALTH PROMOTION IN OLDER ADULTS

Clinical Issues

Silvera and Allebec (2001) conducted face-to-face interviews with 28 male Somali immigrants, aged 60 years and older, to explore views on mental health and well-being and identify sources of stress and support so as to gain a greater understanding of factors leading to life satisfaction and depression in this population. Social isolation, low level of con-

trol over one's life, helplessness, ageism, perceived racial or religious discrimination, and racial harassment were identified in people who were depressed. Family support was the main buffer against depression.

Reijneveld, Westhoff, and Hopman-Rock (2003), in a randomized clinical trial, assessed the effect of eight, two-hour long sessions consisting of health education and physical exercises on the health of 126 elderly Turkish immigrants living in the Netherlands. Results showed an improvement in the mental health of the subjects in the intervention group.

In a six-month-long program, Matuska, Giles-Heinz, Flinn, Neighbour, and Bass-Haugen (2003) taught 65 older adults from three senior apartment complexes the importance to the quality of their lives of participation in meaningful social and community work. As a result, subjects had significantly higher scores on vitality, social functioning, and mental health over baseline. Participants reported increased frequency of social and community participation. Participants who benefited the most were older, attended more classes, and were nondrivers.

Watt and Cappeliez (2000) tested the effectiveness of integrative and instrumental reminiscence therapies, implemented in a short-term group format, and active socialization on decreasing depression in 26 older adults. Evaluation of the clinical significance of the results showed that both reminiscence therapies led to significant improvements in the symptoms of depression at the end of the intervention.

REFERENCES

Allen, J. E. (2003). *Nursing home administration* (4th ed.) New York: Springer Publishing.

Allers, C. T. (1990). AIDS and the older adult. *Gerontologist, 30*, 405–407.

Beck, A.T. & Beck, R. W. (1972). Screening depressed patients in family practice: A rapid technique. *Postgraduate Medicine, 52*(6), 81–85).

Bhugra, D. & Bahl, V. (1999). *Ethnicity: An agenda for mental health.* London: Gaskell.

Blair, C. E. (1999). Effect of self-care ADLs on self-esteem of intact nursing home residents. *Issues in Mental Health Nursing, 20*, 559–570.

Blazer, D. (1990). *Emotional problems in later life: Intervention strategies for professional caregivers.* New York: Springer.

Boydell, J., Van Os, J., McKenzie, K., Allardyce, J., Goel, R., McCreadie, R. G. et al. (2001). Incidence of schizophrenia in ethnic minorities in London: Ecological study into interactions with environment. *British Medical Journal, 322,* 1336.

Buckwalter, K. C., Weiler, K., & Stolley, J. (1995). Community programs. In M. O. Hogstel (Ed.), *Geropsychiatric nursing* (2nd ed., pp. 341-365). St. Louis, MO: Mosby.

Bunten, D. (2001). Normal changes with aging. In Maas et al. (Eds.), *Nursing care of older adults: Diagnoses, outcomes & interventions.* St. Louis, MO: Mosby.

Burgess, A. W. (1998). *Advanced practice psychiatric nursing.* Stamford, CT: Appleton & Lange.

Campbell, J. M. (1995) Assessment. In M. O. Hogstel (Ed.), *Geropsychiatric nursing* (2nd ed., pp. 73–95). St. Louis, MO: Mosby.

Caplan, G. (1970). *The theory and practice of mental health consultation.* New York: Basic Books.

Chow, J. C., Jaffee, K., & Snowden, L. (2003). Racial/ethnic disparities in the use of mental health services in poverty areas. *American Journal of Public Health, 93,* 792–797.

Cook, F. L. & Kramek, L. M. (1986). Measuring economic hardship among older Americans. *The Gerontologist, 26,* 38–47.

Department of Health and Human Services (2000). *Healthy People 2010* (2nd ed, two vols.). Washington, DC: U.S. Government Printing Office.

Donohue, B., Acierno, R., Hersen, M., & Van Hasselt, V. B. (1995). Social skills training for depressed, visually impaired older adults. *Behavior Modification, 19,* 379–424.

Duke University Center for the Study of Aging and Human Development (1988). *OARS multidimensional functional assessment questionnaire.* Durham, NC: Duke University.

Dwyer, J. W. (1995). The effects of aging on the family. In R. Blieszner & V. H. Bedford (Eds.), *Handbook on aging and the family* (pp. 401–421). New York: Greenwood Press.

Feil, N. (1992). Validation therapy with late-onset dementia populations. In G. M. Jones & B. M. Miesen (Eds.), *Care-giving in dementia: Research and applications* (pp. 199–218). New York: Routledge.

Feil, N. (1999). Current concepts and techniques in validation therapy. In M. Duffy (Ed.), *Handbook of counseling and psychotherapy with older adults* (pp. 590–613). New York: John Wiley and Sons.

Ferrell, B. R. & Ferrell, B. A. (1995). Pain in the elderly. In D. B. McGuire, C. H. Yarbro, & B. R. Ferrell, *Cancer pain management* (2nd ed., pp. 273–287). Boston: Jones and Bartlett.

Folstein, M. F., Folstein, S. E., & McHugh, P. R. (1975). Mini-Mental State: A practical method for grading the cognitive state of patients for the clinician. *Journal of Psychiatric Research, 12,* 189–198.

Given, B. A., Kozachik, S. L., Collins, C. E., DeVoss, D. N., & Given, C. W. (2001). Caregiver role strain. In M. L. Mass, K. C. Buckwalter, M. A. Hardy, T. Tripp-Reimer, M. G. Titler, J. P. Specht (Eds.), *Nursing care of older adults: Diagnoses, outcomes, & interventions* (pp. 679–695). St. Louis, MO: Mosby.

Goodkin, K., Heckman, T., Siegel, K., Linsk, N., Khamis, I., Lee, D., et al. (2003). "Putting a face" on HIV infection/AIDS in older adults: A psychosocial context. *JAIDS, 33*(Suppl 2), S171–S184.

Hedelin, B. (2001). The meaning of mental health from elderly women's perspectives: A basis for health promotion. *Perspectives in Psychiatric Care, 37,* 7–14.

Hodges, P. F. & Kam, P. C. (2002). The peri-operative implications of herbal medicines. *Anaesthesia, 57,* 889–899.

Hogstel, M. O. (1995). *Geropsychiatric nursing* (2nd ed.). St. Louis, MO: Mosby.

Jacobs, L. S. (1989). Crisis screening and diversion services. *Hawaii Medical Journal, 48,* 73.

Lawton, H. P. & Brody, E. M. (1969). Assessment of older people: Self maintaining and instrumental activities of daily living. *Gerontologist, 9,* 179–186.

Lueckenotte, A. G. (2000). *Gerontologic nursing* (2nd ed.). St. Louis, MO: Mosby.

Luis, C. A., Loewenstein, D. A., Acevedo, A., Barker, W. W., & Duara, R. (2003). Mild cognitive impairment: Directions for future research. *Neurology, 61,* 438–444.

McCabe, S. (2002). Complementary herbal and alternative drugs in clinical practice. *Perspectives in Psychiatric Care, 38,* 98–107.

McCaffery, M. & Pasero, C. (1999). *Pain: Clinical manual* (2nd ed.). St. Louis, MO: Mosby.

Mahoney, F. I. & Barthel, B. W. (1965). Functional evaluation: The Barthel Index. *Maryland State Medical Journal, 14,* 61–65.

Matuska, K., Giles-Heinz, A., Flinn, N., Neighbour, M., & Bass-Haugen, J. (2003). Outcomes of a pilot occupational therapy wellness program for older adults. *American Journal of Occupational Therapy, 57,* 220–224.

Minardi, H. & Hays, N. (2003a). Nursing older adults with mental health problems: Therapeutic interventions—Part 1. *Nursing Older People, 15*(6), 22–28.

Minardi, H. & Hays, N. (2003b). Nursing older adults with mental health problems: Therapeutic interventions—Part 2. *Nursing Older People, 15*(7), 20–24.

Mitchell, G. J. (1990). The lived experience of taking life day-by-day in later life: Research guided by Parse's emergent method. *Nursing Science Quarterly, 3,* 29–36,

Moody, H. R. (2002). *Aging: Concepts and controversies.* Thousand Oaks, CA: Sage.

Morgan, L. & Kunkel, S. (2001). *Aging: The social context (2nd ed.).* Boston: Pine Forge Press.

National Alliance for Caregiving & American Association of Retired Persons. (1997). *Family caregiving in the U.S.: Findings from a national survey.* Bethesda, MD: Author.

National Family Caregivers Association (1997). *A national report on the status of caregiving in America.* Kensington, MD: National Family Caregivers Association.

National Council for Reliable Health Information [NCRHI] Newsletter (2000). The herbal hype of dietary supplements among the elderly. *NCRHI Newsletter, 23*(4), 1–2.

Neff, D. F. (1996). Gerontological counseling. In S. Lego (Ed.), *Psychiatric nursing: A comprehensive reference* (pp. 165–174). Philadelphia: Lippincott.

Neugarten, B. L. & Datan, N. (1975). Sociological perspectives on the life-cycle. In P. B. Baltes & K. W. Schaie (Eds.), *Lifespan developmental psychology: Personality and socialization* (pp. 53–69). New York: Academic Press.

Ory, M. G. & Zablotsky, D. (1989). Notes for the future: Research, prevention, care, public policy.

In M. W. Riley, M. G. Ory, & D. Zablotsky (Eds.). *AIDS in an aging society: What we need to know* (pp 202–216.). New York: Springer.

Pfeiffer, E. (1975). A short portable questionnaire for the assessment of organic brain deficit in elderly patients. *Journal of the American Geriatrics Society, 23,* 433–441.

Phan, T. T. & Reifler, B. V. (1988). Psychiatric disorders among nursing home residents. *Clinical Geriatric Medicine, 4,* 601–611.

Pinquart, M. & Sorensen, S. (2001). Influence on loneliness in older adults: A meta-analysis. *Basic and Applied Social Psychology, 23,* 245–266.

Qualls, S. H. (2000). Therapy with aging families: Rationale, opportunities and challenges. *Aging & Mental Health, 4,* 191–199.

Reijneveld, S. A., Westhoff, M. H., & Hopman-Rock, M. (2003). Promotion of health and physical activity improves the mental health of elderly immigrants: Results of a group randomized controlled trial among Turkish immigrants in the Netherlands aged 45 and over. *Journal of Epidemiology and Community Health, 57,* 405–411.

Ritter, S. & Watkins, M. (1997) Assessment of older people. In I. J. Norman & S. J. Redfern (Eds.), *Mental health care for older people* (pp. 99–130). New York: Churchill Livingstone.

Ruiz, D. S. (1995). Demographic and epidemiological profile of the ethnic elderly. In D. K. Padgett (Ed.), *Handbook of ethnicity, aging, and mental health* (pp. 3–21). Wesport, CT: Greenwood Press.

Sadock, B. J. & Sadock, V. A. (2000). *Kaplan and Sadock's comprehensive textbook of psychiatry* (7th ed.). Baltimore: Williams & Wilkins.

Seligman, M. E. P. (1992). *Helplessness: On depression, development and death.* San Francisco: Freeman.

Sharpley, M. S., Hutchinson, G., Murray, R. M., & McKenzie, K. (2001). Understanding the excess of psychosis among the African-Caribbean population in England: Review of current hypotheses. *British Journal of Psychiatry, 178*(Suppl. 40), 60–68.

Silvera, E. & Allebec, P. (2001). Migration, ageing, and mental health: An ethnographic study on perceptions of life satisfaction, anxiety and depression in older Somali men in East London. *International Journal of Social Welfare, 10,* 309–320.

Smilkstein G., Ashworth, C., & Montano, M. A. (1982) Validity and reliability of the Family APGAR as a test of family functioning. *Journal of Family Practice, 15*, 303–311.

Starbuck, J. J. (1999). Calming herbs. *Better Nutrition, 61*(2), 50–52.

Thomas, W. (1994). *The Eden alternative: Nature, hope, and nursing home.* Cherburne, NY: Eden Alternative.

Watt, L. M. & Cappeliez, P. (2000). Integrative and instrumental reminiscence therapies for depression in older adults: Intervention strategies and treatment effectiveness. *Aging & Mental Health, 4* (2), 166–177.

Yesavage, J. A. & Brink, T. L. (1983). Development and validation of a geriatric depression screening scale: A preliminary report. *Journal of Psychiatric Research, 17*, 37–49.

CHAPTER 6

Psychopharmacology

Barbara Edlund, RN, PhD, ANP-BC
James Sterrett, BS, Pharm D, CDE
Geoffry McEnany, PhD, APRN, BC

INTRODUCTION

While prevalence data vary widely, approximately 25% of adults over age 65 have significant mental health symptoms (Jeste, Okamoto, Napolitano, Kane, & Martinez, 2000; Sadock & Sadock, 2003). In 2000, an estimated nine million older adults suffered from some form of mental illness. This number is expected to increase to 20 million by the middle of the century given our aging demographics (U.S. Bureau of the Census, 2000). It is anticipated that this number will equal the number of younger adults (ages 30–44) with mental health problems over the next 30 years (Jeste et al., 2000). In addition, the composition of the population over 65 will shift to a more ethnically, racially, and culturally diverse group of older adults due to a significant growth in minority populations.

Currently, older adults suffer more chronic illnesses, are hospitalized more frequently, and take more medications than any other age group (Schretzman & Strumpf, 2002). Approximately 40% of all prescriptions written in the United States each year are for those 65 and older (Walker & Foreman, 1999). Psychotropics are the second-most-commonly prescribed class of drugs in geriatric patients and the most frequently associated with adverse drug reactions (Ives, 2001). Symptoms that become the focus of treatment include insomnia, agitation, aggression, and other disruptive behaviors. Commonly treated syndromes or disorders include anxiety, depression, mood cycling, psychosis, and cognitive disorders with associated dysregulations in sleep across all of these disorders (Keltner & Folks, 2001; Kornstein & McEnany, 2000). In addition to prescribed medications, it is estimated that approximately 90% of older adults take over-the-counter medications at least occasionally (Finucane, 1994). As a result, nearly three million adults 65 and older may be at risk for herb/vitamin/medication interactions (Dossey, 1997). Given the commonplace use of herbal preparations among the general population and elders in particular, clinicians often need a reliable source of reference in understanding the implications of these compounds. A resource such as the *Physician's Desk Reference for Herbal Medications* (Gruenwald, Brendler, & Jaenicke, 2000) is a helpful compendium of information that can serve as a guide to clinicians who have questions related to the use of these medications separately or in combination with other drugs.

Undiagnosed and untreated mental illness can lead to unnecessary and costly procedures and hospitalizations, increased disability, premature death, increased morbidity, increased risk of institutionalization, and a significant decrease in quality of life for older adults. Changing demographics, combined with the disproportionate rate at which older adults use medical resources and the pressures to contain costs, will require that health care providers become increasingly knowledgeable in the care of a diverse older population (Edlund, 2004) and vigilant in diagnosing and treating mental illness in this population. It is essential that clinicians working with older adults aggressively address the mental health issues of this population in order to meet the goals for *Healthy People 2010*, which seek to increase quality years of life and eliminate health disparities (USDHHS, 2000).

CHALLENGES IN PRESCRIBING FOR OLDER ADULTS

Mental health problems in older adults often differ in clinical manifestations, pathogenesis, and pathophysiology from mental health problems of younger adults (Sadock & Sadock, 2003). Thus, the diagnosis and treatment of older adults can present more difficulties than treating younger adults. Factors contributing to such difficulties include normal age-related changes, the coexistence of chronic medical problems and disabilities, the use of multiple medications, and the presence of cognitive impairment (Edlund & Spain, 2003). In addition, the signs and symptoms of health problems in the older adult may not be as obvious as in the younger adult, given the complexities presented by medical comorbidities and natural changes incurred in the course of aging. There may also be differences in the quantity and quality of symptoms with older persons. Older adults may present with

vague versus specific complaints. For example, lightheadedness may be the only symptom reported by an older adult experiencing anxiety, or multiple general somatic complaints may be the predominant presentation of an older adult experiencing depression. Older adults may also hesitate to mention changes in their bodies associated with health problems, because they perceive these changes as normal aging (Edlund & Haight, 1992). Clearly, changes need to be explored in order to determine whether there is underlying disease or whether the changes are age-related and normal. Additionally, older adults often perceive their health based on their ability to function rather than on the number of health problems. This population is unique in that they may be diagnosed with two or more chronic diseases, take a number of medications, and still function at a high level of health (Kane, Ouslander, & Abrass, 2004; Michocki, 2001). These cohort-related trends may reflect both cultural and generational patterns of response.

Prescribing a psychotropic drug for an older adult should be based on a thorough assessment, target symptoms, stages and progression of illness, provider's knowledge of drug choices, and the pharmacokinetic and pharmacodynamic changes that accompany aging. In addition, a review of current medications that may interact or contribute to adverse drug reactions should be conducted. A dose appropriate for the older adult should be prescribed in a dosing schedule that enhances compliance. Individualizing treatment plans that include psychoeducation, and evaluating responses to drug interventions, are essential due to the great deal of variability among the older adult population (American Nurses Association, 1994). The following table references several Web-based resources that may be helpful sources of information for clinicians working with elders who have diagnosed psychiatric conditions.

Web-Based Resources: Geriatric Psychiatry & Gerontology

The Gerontological Society of America (www.geron.org). This is an excellent resource that disseminates research-based information on many topics related to gerontology. Full text journals are accessible from the Web page.

National Institute on Aging (www.nih.gov/nia). This site contains an impressive compilation of information-related public education, as well as biomedical, behavioral, and social research related to aging. A variety of publications for professionals are available through this site.

Drug Interactions (www.drug-interactions.com). This is a particularly helpful Web site that offers the clinician some pragmatic information related to potential drug interactions. Downloadable resources are available free of charge.

American Psychiatric Association (www.psych.org). This Web site is an excellent resource for the clinician who is seeking information related to practice guidelines and evidence-based approaches to the treatment of psychiatric illnesses.

FACTORS INFLUENCING PHARMACOTHERAPY IN OLDER ADULTS

Pharmacotherapy in older adults may be complicated by multiple factors, among them the pharmacokinetic (drug absorption, distribution, metabolism, excretion) and pharmacodynamic changes associated with aging (Table 6-1). These changes involve altered receptor response.

Pharmacokinetics are a source of concern from a variety of perspectives for clinicians who work with elders. The following section aims to assist clinicians in the understanding of such pharmacokinetic-based concerns, and will address these issues according to the categories of absorption, distribution, metabolism, and excretion.

Absorption

While there is an age-related decrease in small bowel surface and an increase in gastric pH, changes in drug absorption appear to be the pharmacologic parameter least affected by increasing age (Kane et al., 2004). In contrast, the distribution of a drug is influenced by age-related changes in body composition of water (total and intracellular) and lean body mass

relative to body fat. Specifically, the percentage of total body water decreases by 10 to 15% between the ages of 20 and 80 years. This relative decrease in total body water leads to a higher blood and tissue concentration of some water-soluble drugs. In addition, the ratio of lean mass to body fat decreases with age. Thus, a drug distributed only in lean tissue, such as lithium, should be given in a lower dose due to the decrease in lean body mass with aging (Lueckenotte, 1996).

Distribution

While the percentage of lean body mass to body fat decreases with age, the percentage of body fat increases from 18 to 36% in men and from 33 to 45% in women. An increase in total body fat increases the volume of distribution for lipophilic drugs such as the long-acting benzodiazepines, diazepam (Valium), and chlordiazepoxide HCl (Librium). Thus, many lipid-soluble psychotropic drugs are distributed more widely, prolonging the action of the drug and increasing the likelihood of serious adverse consequences (Keltner & Folks, 2001; Stahl, 2001).

In addition to changes in total body water and body fat, the distribution of drugs into the peripheral circulation and tissues is

TABLE 6-1 Age-Related Pharmacokinetic Changes	
Absorption	**Metabolism**
Delayed gastric emptying	Decreased liver size
Increased gastric pH	Decreased hepatic blood flow
Decreased intestinal motility	Decreased level of drug metabolizing enzymes
Decreased mucosal surface area	
Distribution	**Excretion**
Decreased lean body (muscle) mass	Decreased blood flow
Increased body fat	Decreased glomeruli
Decreased total body water	Decreased glomerular filtration
Decreased albumin	Decreased tubular secretion
Decreased alpha 1–acid glycoprotein	Decreased creatinine production
	Decreased creatinine clearance

Note. Adapted from: *Essentials of Clinical Geriatrics,* R. Kane, J. Ouslander, & I. Abrass, 2004, New York: McGraw-Hill; and from *Psychotropic Drugs* (3rd ed.), by N. Keltner & D. Folks, 2001, St. Louis, MO: Mosby.

influenced by serum albumin (protein binding) and alpha 1–acid glycoprotein levels. With age, there may be a decrease in serum albumin levels. This results in increased fractions of free drug (not bound to protein) circulating in the body. "It is the free, unbound drug that exerts pharmacodynamic actions whether they are desirable or adverse" (Keltner & Folks, 2001, p. 52). In contrast to decreasing levels of serum albumin, alpha 1–acid glycoprotein levels increase with age, resulting in the increased binding of drugs that normally bind to this protein. An increase in alpha 1–acid glycoprotein levels may affect the distribution of a number of psychotropic drugs such as the tricyclic antidepressants, resulting in a prolonged half-life of these drugs. However, the clinical consequences of an increase in alpha 1–acid glycoprotein have not been well studied in older adults (Keltner & Folks, 2001; Stahl, 2001).

Metabolism

Drug metabolism in the older adult is complex, difficult to predict, and affected by age-related hepatic changes. These include a decrease in liver size, blood flow, and hepatic microsomal enzyme (CYP P-450) activity. In addition, a variety of other factors can influence hepatic drug metabolism, such as caffeine, tobacco, foods that act as CYP P-450 inducers or inhibitors such as grapefruit juice, cruciferous vegetables, or charbroiled meats, alcohol, current disease state, nutritional status, gender, genetic determinants, and lifelong exposure to various chemicals (Johnson, 2000; Bezchlibnyk-Butler & Jeffries, 2004). There is evidence that the first phase of drug metabolism declines with age, while the second phase appears to be less affected. However, as Kane et al. (2004) noted, "It is not safe to assume that an older adult with normal liver function tests can metabolize drugs as efficiently as a younger individual" (p. 362).

Excretion

Excretion of drugs by the kidneys is better understood than hepatic drug metabolism in the older adult. Age-related changes in renal function include decreases in renal blood flow, glomerular filtration rate, production of creatinine, and creatinine clearance. Because of an age-related decline in muscle mass resulting in the decreased production of creatinine, a serum creatinine level is not a reliable marker of renal function in the older adult. The serum creatinine, however, is used to calculate the creatinine clearance, a more accurate reflection of renal function in this patient population. "Thus a drug such as lithium that depends on renal excretion for its elimination is likely to accumulate to potentially toxic levels unless the dosage is adjusted downward" (Keltner & Folks, 2001, p. 53). Other factors such as intrinsic renal disease, state of hydration, and cardiac output also can affect the renal clearance of a drug. Thus, it is important to calculate a baseline estimate of creatinine clearance before initiating drug therapy in older adults.

In addition to the pharmacokinetic changes that occur with aging, pharmacodynamic changes occur as well. These changes deal with an individual's responsiveness to the concentration of a given drug (altered receptor response). It is known that sensitivity to both the therapeutic and toxic effects of many medications, especially centrally acting medications, increases with age. This sensitivity is heightened in the very frail and the very old individual. Kane et al. (2004) noted that this sensitivity was true for certain drugs, such as sedating medications, but not true for other drugs, such as blood pressure medications mediated by beta-adrenergic receptors, which appear to decline with age. While considerably less is known about the pharmacodynamic changes that occur with aging, increased sensitivity to the concentration of a particular drug must be considered, particularly when the medication has serious adverse side effects.

It is also important to understand the types of drug interactions in order to prevent the potential detrimental effect from two or more drugs that can interact with each other (Hansten, 1998). One type of interaction

occurs when one drug interferes with another drug's ability to interact with the receptor responsible for effect. Another is when one drug enhances another's therapeutic or adverse effect by stimulation of the receptor by both drugs. Two agents that have properties of lowering blood pressure, when combined, may lead to greater chances of hypotension. The other general type of drug interaction occurs when one medication affects the plasma concentration of another medication by affecting absorption, distribution, metabolism, or elimination. This is termed a *pharmacokinetic interaction.*

The cytochrome (CYP) P-450 isoenzymes are located mostly in the liver and the small intestine. They are responsible for the first phase of biotransformation, the rate-limiting step in drug clearance. A CYP P-450 drug interaction occurs when a drug either speeds up (induction) or slows down (inhibition) enzymatic activity. The most clinically relevant isoenzymes include CYP1A2, CYP2C9, CYP2C19, CYP2D6, and CYP3A4 (Cadieux, 1999). Competitive inhibition of the cytochrome (CYP) P-450 hepatic isoenzymes is an example of this type of interaction and is common in psychotropic drug use. Visit www.drug-interactions.com for a review of the rudiments of the P-450 system, as well as pragmatic information related to assessment for potential drug interactions.

The choice, dose, and dosing frequency of a medication for an older adult must be carefully planned in light of the pharmacokinetic and pharmacodynamic changes that occur with aging. This is true for all medications prescribed for this population but even more critical for the prescription of psychotropic medications, the second most common category of drugs prescribed for older adults after cardiac medications. Psychoactive drugs are prescribed for 65% of nursing home residents, with some residents using three or more psychoactive drugs concurrently (Beers & Berkow, 2004).

Voyer and colleagues (2004) point out that the prevalence of psychotropic drug use among community-dwelling older persons (usually defined as those 65 years and older) varies from about 20% to 48%, and that many of these elders use the psychotropic medications for more than six months. This time period may often exceed the time period for which the drug is needed, e.g., with benzodiazepines. Along with the protracted use of these drugs may be the associated liabilities that are common to drug accumulation in elders, due to changes in pharmacokinetics, as was previously discussed. Such trends are noteworthy from the perspective that the use of these drugs may fall outside of evidence-based recommendations, and as such create liabilities for both the patient and the clinician who prescribes the drugs.

Bartels and colleagues (2003) noted that until recently there has been little information available to guide the practitioner in choosing appropriate clinical interventions for older adults. Most clinical trials have excluded older adults, particularly those with medical comorbidities and disabilities (Banerjee & Dickinson, 1997). Recent advances in mental health treatment have led to the development of an evidence base specific to older adults (Bartels et al., 2003). Thus, prescribing a psychoactive medication for an older adult with multiple comorbidities, who is taking an average of four to five medications, requires a thorough knowledge of the psychotropic drug, as well as the latest consensus data specific for prescribing for this population, particularly in light of the pharmacokinetic and pharmacodynamic issues addressed previously.

To successfully accomplish a goal of maximizing outcomes while minimizing adverse events requires a multifactorial approach to prescribing psychotropic agents in older adults. The practitioner must consider medical comorbidity and polypharmacy, age-related physiologic changes, cognitive ability, caregiver status, as well as psychosocial factors. Medical comorbidity and polypharmacy (9 or more medications or 12 or more doses per day) are common in the geriatric population. Polypharmacy has been shown to be a risk factor for developing adverse drug events in the older adult (Cadieux, 1989; Catterson, Preskorn, & Martin, 1997). Proper education of patients and caregivers and monitoring medication regimens are important for early identification of adverse events and adherence problems. Equally important is the communication between different prescribers to avoid drug interactions and maximize outcomes.

Among elders, as is the case with large numbers of the adult population in the United States, both over-the-counter (OTC) medications and herbal supplements are commonly used in attempts to relieve symptoms (McEnany 2000a, 2000b, 2001). Unfortunately, what many consumers do not realize is that "herbal" or "naturopathic" remedies are not benign substances, and are often cleared through hepatic metabolism, specifically by P-450 mechanisms. As such, the potential for drug interactions with prescribed medications is significant, and merits the attention of the prescriber. The clinician needs to closely assess usage patterns of both OTC and herbal remedies in an attempt to reduce the chances of a drug interaction and associated adverse event for the patient.

The assessment of medication cost and insurance coverage is an important factor to be considered in order to assure adherence feasibility. Sometimes the prescriber is forced to make medication choices based on external factors such as insurance formularies or restrictions and on the patient's ability to pay for medications. It is essential for clinicians to recognize that good prescribing practice is a multifaceted process as depicted in Figure 6-1.

Clinicians may find the Web site http://www.atdn.org/access/pa.html helpful when dealing with patients who are uninsured or who have limited resources available for med-

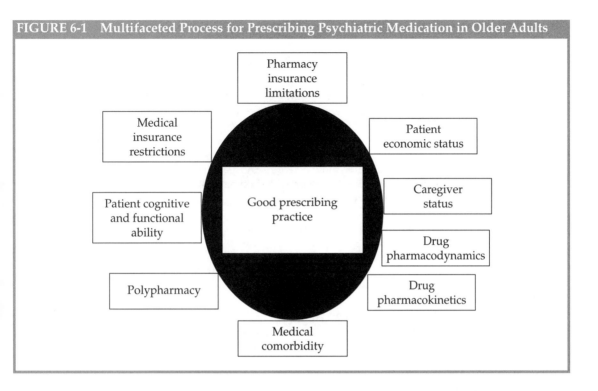

FIGURE 6-1 Multifaceted Process for Prescribing Psychiatric Medication in Older Adults

ications. This online resource contains all of the details for how to access patient assistance programs for medications free of cost to the medically disadvantaged or indigent. The site has direct links to many of the pharmaceutical companies offering patient assistance programs, along with detailed descriptions of the procedures related to ordering medications.

Although psychiatric conditions are often underdiagnosed in the older adult, health care providers should carefully examine the necessity of pharmacotherapy before prescribing new medications. In addition, the necessity and compatibility of all long-term medications should be periodically reexamined. If deemed necessary, prescriptions, dosages, and intervals should be based on the patient's age, renal and hepatic function, and concomitant diseases and medications. In an effort to increase the quality of care and limit the inappropriate use of psychotropic medications in residents of long-term-care facilities, the Omnibus Budget

Reconciliation Act (OBRA) was passed in 1987. The interpretive guidelines enforcing OBRA were implemented in 1990 and updated in 1999. While proper documentation of necessity and attempted withdrawal trials of medications became the requirements, the outcome of OBRA has been increased attention to appropriate prescribing of psychotropic medication in such a fashion as to minimize adverse events and detrimental effects on physical and cognitive function.

PSYCHOTROPIC DRUGS

Psychotropic drugs can be broadly categorized as antidepressants, anxiolytics, sedative–hypnotics, antipsychotics and mood stabilizers. These categories of drugs, their characteristics, and the drugs included in each class are listed in Table 6-2. Each category of psychotropic drugs will be discussed in detail

TABLE 6-2	Categories of Psychotropic Drugs	
Category	Characteristics	Drug Classes
Antidepressants	Equally effective but differ based on side-effect profile and potential for drug interactions	Tricyclic antidepressants (TCAs) Monoaminine oxidase inhibitors (MAOIs) Selective serotonin reuptake inhibitors (SSRIs) Non-SSRI second generation antidepressants SNRI (serotonin norepinephrine reuptake inhibitors)
Anxiolytics	Short-acting agents without active metabolites preferred in older adults to minimize lasting adverse events	Short-acting benzodiazepines Long-acting benzodiazepines
Sedative–hypnotics	Should be avoided due to side-effect profiles	Barbiturates Miscellaneous hypnotic/sedatives
Antipsychotics	Atypical agents in low doses preferred due to less anticholinergic and extrapyramidal system (EPS) side effects	Typical antipsychotics Atypical antipsychotics
Mood stabilizers	Both on-label (FDA) and off-label uses of medications aimed to stabilize mood	Lithium carbonate Divalproate Lamotrigine Others

Note. Adapted from: "Appropriate Use of Psychotropic Drugs in Nursing Homes," by T. Gurvich, & J. Cunningham, 2000, *American Family Physician, 61*, pp. 1437–1446.

with recommendations for their use in older adults.

Antidepressants

The goal of antidepressant therapy includes improving and maintaining mood, physical and social daily functioning, and quality of life while minimizing side effects. Doses should be started low and titrated slowly to the desired effect. Antidepressants typically take 2–4 weeks before benefits can be discerned in the younger population, but 6–12 weeks in the older-adult population. Titration, therefore, should be adjusted based on tolerability of side effects and effectiveness.

Antidepressants can be subdivided into four categories: tricyclic antidepressants (TCAs), monoamine oxidase inhibitors

(MAOIs), selective serotonin reuptake inhibitors (SSRIs), and non-SSRI second generation antidepressants (Table 6-3).

Although the older TCAs are effective for treating depression, most should be avoided in the older adult due to their substantial side-effect profile, which includes excessive sedation, anticholinergic effects (dry mouth, constipation, urinary retention, blurred vision, and confusion), and cardiovascular effects (orthostasis, tachycardia, and EKG changes). Because of their cardiovascular effects, TCAs are lethal in overdose, which is always a serious concern in depressed patients. If the decision is to use a TCA, then the best choices are desipramine and nortriptyline, because these agents have the least anticholinergic side-effect profile. Interestingly, the TCAs have fallen out of fashion as first-line agents for the treatment

TABLE 6-3 Categories of Antidepressants and Mode of Action	
Drug Class	**Mode of Action**
Tricyclic antidepressants (TCAs)	Increase the synaptic concentration of serotonin and/or norepinephrine in the CNS by inhibition of their uptake by the presynaptic neuronal membrane
Monoamine oxidase inhibitors (MAOIs)	Inhibits the monamine oxidase A and B enzymes responsible for the intraneuronal metabolism of norepinephrine and serotonin
Selective serotonin reuptake inhibitors (SSRIs)	Inhibits CNS neuronal reuptake of serotonin
Non-SSRI second generation antidepressants	Variety of modes of action, including effects on serotonin, norepinephrine, and/or dopamine

Note. Adapted from: *Geriatric Dosage Handbook*, (8th ed.), by T. Semla, 2003, Hudson, OH: Lexi-comp.

of depression. However, their use is on the rise in off-label applications in the treatment of migraines, chronic pain, sleep disturbances, and various neuropathic pain syndromes. The concerns related to use in depression apply to off-label uses as well.

Although MAOIs, such as phenelzine (Nardil) and tranylcypromine (Parnate), have been found to be useful for some patients with atypical depression and in those resistant to the other antidepressants, they do have significant drug and food interactions and potentially can cause serious side effects. They can lead to a life-threatening rise in blood pressure, especially if combined with certain foods containing tyramine, such as wines, cheeses, smoked fish, beef or chicken liver, sausage, yeast, or certain bean pods. MAOIs also can potentiate many categories of drugs, such as CNS stimulants and sympathomimetics, and lead to hypertensive crisis. They can add to the effect of sulfonyureas and can lower blood sugar to dangerous levels. Combining with other antidepressants has the potential to cause either seizures or serotonin syndrome, which may result in nausea, anxiety, tremor, and/or difficulty sleeping. MAOIs, therefore, are generally avoided in elderly patients due to their significant side-effect profile and food–drug and drug–drug interactions.

There are two types of monoamine oxidase inhibitors (types A and B), and the conventional MAOIs in use in the United States target type B. An expansion on the use of a newer type of monoamine oxidase inhibitors, referred to as reversible inhibitors of monoamine oxidase, type A, sometimes abbreviated as RIMAs, has provided an MAOI option with significantly fewer liabilities. Because RIMAs are reversible, they clear the body more quickly and have significantly fewer interactions with other drugs and foods. An example of a RIMA is moclobemide. Unfortunately, RIMAs are not available in the United States.

The SSRIs, noted in Table 6-4, create a more attractive alternative, although not without flaws. On a positive note, they have good efficacy data and, because of an extended half-life, an advantage to adherence is once-daily dosing. However, they can cause a serious adverse event such as serotonin syndrome, SIADH (hyponatremia), and withdrawal syndrome if cessation is not titrated downward. Tolerability can be adversely affected by gastrointestinal effects, sexual dysfunction, and sleep disturbances. While side effects tend to be an effect of the class of medication, drug–drug interactions are more individualized. Sleep disturbance, weight gain, and sexual dysfunction are very common to these agents.

TABLE 6-4   Common SSRIs, Dosing, and Hepatic Enzyme Affected

Medication	Starting Dose in Older Adults/Day	Maintenance Dose in Older Adults/Day	Oral Solution Available	Hepatic Enzyme Affected
Citalopram (Celexa)	10 mg	20–40 mg	Yes	Minimal
Escitalopram (Lexapro)	5 mg	5–20 mg	No	Minimal
Fluoxetine (Prozac)	10 mg	20–40 mg	Yes	CYP2C9, CYP2C19
Fluvoxamine (Luvox, Solvay)	50 mg	50–200 mg	No	CYP1A4, CYP2C9, CYP2C19
Paroxetine (Paxil, Paxil CR)	10 mg	20–30 mg	Yes	CYP2D6
Sertraline (Zoloft)	25 mg	50–150 mg	Yes	Minor CYP2D6, CYP3A4, CYP2C19

Note. Adapted from: "Antidepressant Drug Interactions in the Elderly: Understanding the P-450 System is Half the Battle in Reducing Risks," by R. J. Cadieux, 1999, *Postgraduate Medicine*, 106(6), pp. 231–49; and from *Geriatric Dosage Handbook*, (8th ed.), by T. Semla, 2003, Hudson, OH: Lexi-comp.

TABLE 6-5   Non-SSRIs, Dosing, and Hepatic Enzyme Affected

Medication	Starting Dose in the Older Adults	Maintenance Dose in Older Adults/Day	Hepatic Enzyme Affected
Venlafaxine (Effexor, Effexor XR)	25 mg BID; XR 37.5 mg QD	75–150 mg	CYP2D6, CYP2E1
Bupropion (Wellbutrin, Wellbutrin SR, Wellbutrin XL)	37.5 mg BID; SR100 mg QAM; XL 150 mg QAM	100–150 mg	CYP2B6, CYP2D6
Mirtazapine (Remeron, Remeron SolTab)	7.5 mg QHS	15–30 mg	CYP1A2, CYP2D6, CYP3A4
Trazodone (Desyrel)	25 mg QHS	25–50 mg	CYP3A4
Nefazodone (Serzone—brand no longer available in the U.S.)	50 mg BID	200–400 mg	CYP3A4, CYP2D6
Duloxetine (Cymbalta)	20 mg	20–60 mg	CYP2D6, CYP1A2

Note. Adapted from: *Geriatric Dosage Handbook*, (8th ed.), by T. Semla, 2003, Hudson, OH: Lexi-comp.

The non-SSRI second generation agents listed in Table 6-5 include venlafaxine, bupropion, mirtazapine, trazodone, and nefazodone. In 2004, Bristol-Meyers Squibb, the manufacturers of Serzone (nefazodone) made the decision to remove this drug from the market due to issues of hepatotoxicity (Choi, 2003). A newer antidepressant, Cymbalta (duloxetine HCl), is also an SNRI, but has a longer half-life than venlafaxine. Each agent has unique characteristics relevant to prescribing in the older adult. Venlafaxine (Effexor) inhibits the reuptake of serotonin and, with higher doses, norepinephrine. Effexor is available in both immediate- and extended-release preparations, and documentation states that the extended-release form of the medication has an improved side-effect profile, which may enhance adherence (Nemeroff, 2003). It is the only agent similar in action to the older TCAs but without their anticholineric side effects. It has approved uses in both depression and generalized anxiety disorder. Like other antidepressants that interfere with serotonin reuptake, venlafaxine may interact pharmacodynamically with other serotonergic agents (e.g., tryptophan, dextromethorphan) and should be avoided due to potential serotonin syndrome. Side effects with venlafaxine are similar to the SSRIs, with the addition of dose-related elevated blood pressure. Proper monitoring of blood pressure should be performed initially and at follow-up visits due to the prevalence of hypertension and cardiovascular diseases in the older adult. Elevated serum levels and toxicity can occur if combined with either CYP2D6 (paroxetine, amiodarone, cimetidine, quinidine), or CYP3A4 (clarithromycin, erythromycin, diltiazem, grapefruit juice, ketoconazole) inhibitors (Semla, 2003). While dosage adjustment for age alone is unnecessary, dosing should be started low and increased gradually (Wyeth-Ayerst, 2003). A 25% decreased dosage adjustment is required with renal impairment and 50% with moderate hepatic impairment (Semla, 2003).

Bupropion is a weak serotonin and norepinephrine reuptake inhibitor and it has some dopamine reuptake inhibition (Glaxo Smith-Kline, 2003). It offers the advantages of no sedative side effects, no cardiotoxicity, and no sexual side effects. Buproprion, however, can increase agitation, headache, tremor, insomnia, and anorexia. The primary safety issue with buproprion is its ability to cause seizures. Coadministration of bupropion with drugs that lower the seizure threshold, such as typical antipsychotics, TCAs, fluoroquinolones, theophylline, as well as any drug

that can increase buproprion levels or toxicity (2D6 substrates, levodopa, MAOIs), should be avoided because of the seizure risk. Dosage adjustment must be made due to hepatic or renal disease. Bupropion is available in immediate-release (IR), sustained-release (SR), and once-a-day (XL) formulations and there is some evidence in the literature that the extended-release formulation may have a more tolerable side-effect profile, possibly contributing to greater adherence (Nemeroff, 2003).

Mirtazapine (Remeron) antagonizes alpha 2-adrenergic receptors, blocks two serotonin receptor subtypes, and has a strong affinity for histaminic receptors. It causes somnolence, particularly at lower doses, which relates to its effect on antihistamine receptors and should therefore be dosed at bedtime. Mirtazapine has limited clinical data in geriatric populations but does have low risks of drug interactions and no cardiotoxicity. It also has been associated with weight gain and can therefore be useful in depressed anorexic older patients. In rare instances, it can cause agranulocytosis. It is, therefore, important to monitor WBC and neutrophil counts if the patient presents with associated signs or symptoms such as infection or fever. Mirtazapine clearance is decreased up to 40% in older adults, particularly with males, when compared to younger males, so dosing should be started low (Organon, 2002). Nicholas and colleagues (2003) have documented the possibility of elevated total cholesterol with the use of this agent.

Trazodone and nefazodone hydrochloride (Serzone) are serotonin reuptake inhibitors and serotonin 5-HT2 receptor antagonists. Trazodone causes significant sedation without significant anticholinergic activity and should therefore be reserved for use at bedtime for patients with insomnia. Nefazodone has less sedative effect, but has significant drug interactions, and has also been known to cause hepatic failure. Nefazodone inhibits the

CYP3A4 isoenzyme and also increases blood levels of digoxin, a drug with a narrow therapeutic index (Bristol-Myers Squibb, 2001).

Discontinuing antidepressants too quickly can lead to a withdrawal syndrome. Antidepressant withdrawal syndromes have been reported with the TCAs, the SSRIs, and the newer agents (Dilsaver, Greden, & Snider, 1987; Haddad, 1997). The syndrome can consist of a cluster of symptoms that may include headaches, nausea, dizziness, unstable moods, gastrointestinal upset, recurrence of depression, bizarre dreams, stroke-like symptoms, abnormal sensations of burning, prickling, tingling, or auditory hallucinations. TCA-related withdrawal also can include cardiac arrhythmias (Dilsaver et al., 1987). Reeves and Beddingfield (2003) have documented discontinuation syndrome with selective serotonin and norepinephrine reuptake inhibitors as well. Other investigators have discussed atypical symptoms of antidepressant discontinuation, including discontinuation-associated mania (Andrade, 2004). What is clear from this body of literature is the fact that clinicians need to be well apprised of these potential manifestations of discontinuation syndrome in order to assure comfort and safety during antidepressant withdrawal.

While it is important to recognize the individual differences between the classes and individual antidepressants, it should be understood there are no clear directives for choosing an antidepressant based on the summary of current clinical trials in the older-adult population (Alexopoulos, Katz, Reynolds, Carpenter, & Docherty, 2001). All antidepressant classes demonstrate superiority over placebos in the older-adult population. While the newer agents were expected to have greater efficacy, they have failed to show superiority when compared to TCAs (Williams et al., 2000). Despite there being empirical reasons for poorer tolerability of TCAs, there are no differences between the newer agents and older agents based on

patient dropout rates. The provider's responsibility in prescribing, therefore, is to choose the best particular antidepressant based primarily on the potential for adverse effects, drug–drug interactions, and cost for each individual patient.

One topic that merits some attention from clinicians is the issue of tachyphylaxis related to the use of antidepressants. This phenomenon is best described as a precipitous or insidious loss of therapeutic effect from the use of the antidepressant. It is not well understood and there have been no studies published to document predictors of this loss of effect. Clinicians are well advised to review the practice guidelines available from the American Psychiatric Association (APA), including the guideline on the treatment of depression (www.psych.org) (APA, 2000). These guidelines offer evidence-based guidance related to the community standard for the treatment of select psychiatric disorders, including depression.

Antipsychotics

Experts recommend antipsychotics in several geriatric psychiatric disorders, including agitated dementia, late-life schizophrenia, delusional disorder, and psychotic mood disorders (Alexopoulos, Streim, Carpenter, & Docherty, 2004). Providers must assess if these symptoms are the result of treatable etiologies. These may include the use of pharmacologic agents such as beta-blockers, anticholinergics, or steroids, dosage additions, or changes of other medications, or conditions such as fluid or electrolyte loss or infections. Correction by addressing the underlying cause, such as removing offending agents or treating a disease state, should be the primary goal of therapy. If symptoms continue, an antipsychotic may be temporarily considered. Frequent attempts to withdraw the agent at appropriate intervals based on the disease state are important (Alexopoulos et al., 2004).

Gradual reduction is key with attempts to discontinue antipsychotics. Abrupt discontinuation can lead to cholinergic rebound, withdrawal dyskinesias, and relapse or rebound syndrome.

Both typical and atypical antipsychotics have been clinically evaluated with older adults. The two classes of antipsychotics differ in both side-effect profiles and documented efficacy and can be considered for use in the older population. However, atypical agents generally are considered first line due to a more favorable side-effect profile (Alexopoulos et al., 2004; Bartels et al., 2003). The atypical agents include clozapine (Clozaril), risperidone (Risperdal), olanzapine (Zyprexa), quetiapine (Seroquel), ziprasidone (Geodon), and aripiprazole (Abilify). These drugs, with dosing schedule and adverse effects, are featured in Table 6-6. The drug interactions of the atypical antipsychotics and geriatric considerations are noted in Table 6-7.

The typical agents include haloperidol, fluphenazine, trifluoperazine, chlorpromazine, and thioridazine.

The "conventional" or "typical" antipsychotics offer a relatively poor benefit-to-risk ratio because of significant side-effect, drug–drug and drug–disease interaction profiles in the older-adult population (Kastrup, 2004; Malhotra, Litman, & Pickar, 1993; Pollock & Mulsant, 1995). They have considerable anticholinergic and sedative properties, both of which raise serious concerns in older adults. They can lead to falls, fractures, weight loss, pressure ulcers, incontinence, urinary tract infections, and decreased cognition. In addition, they are associated with movement disorders, such as tardive dyskinesia (TD) and extrapyramidal symptoms (EPS). Tardive dyskinesia is a troubling side effect characterized by involuntary and abnormal movements. EPS can cause patients to experience restlessness, an inability to sit still, or muscle

TABLE 6-6 Atypical Antipsychotics, Dosing, and Adverse* Effects			
Medications	**Starting Dose**	**Maintenance Dose**	**Adverse Effects**
Clozapine (Clozaril)	25 mg/day	Up to 300–450 day over slow titration	Agranulocytosis, anticholinergic side effects, cognitive and motor impairment, orthostasis, tachycardia
Risperidone (Risperdal)	0.25–0.5 mg once or twice daily	0.75–1.5 mg /day	EPS, anticholinergic effects, orthostasis, sedation (all increased at higher dosages), slight increased risk of stroke
Olanzapine (Zyprexa)	5 mg/day	10–20 mg/day	Hyperprolactinemia, dose-related somnolence, headache, diabetes, dyslipidemia, slight increased risk of stroke
Quetiapine (Seroquel)	25 mg twice daily	150–750 mg/day	Somnolence, dyslipidemia, diabetes, slight increased risk of stroke, seizures, thyroid dysfunction, orthostasis
Ziprasidone (Geodon)	20 mg twice daily	20–80 mg twice daily	QT prolongation, cognitive and motor impairment, rash, orthostasis
Aripiprazole (Abilify)	5 mg daily	10–30 mg/day	Headache, orthostasis, anxiety, and insomnia

* Neuroleptic Malignant Syndrome (NMS) has been reported with all atypicals.

Note. Adapted from: *Geriatric Dosage Handbook*, (8th ed.), by T. Semla, 2003, Hudson, OH: Lexi-comp.

TABLE 6-7	Atypical Antipsychotics: Drug Interactions and Geriatric Considerations	
Medications	**Drug Interactions**	**Geriatric Considerations***
Clozapine (Clozaril)	Benzodiazepines, antihypertensives, anticholinergics, CYP1A2	Not recommended for nonpsychotic patients
Risperidone (Risperdal)	CYP2D6 and CYP3A4, increased hypotension with antihypertensives, decreased levels with inducers, St. John's wort	Oral solution can be mixed with water, orange juice, or low-fat milk but not with cola, grapefruit juice, or tea
Olanzapine (Zyprexa)	CYP1A2, CYP2D6, increased hypotension with antihypertensives, decreased levels with inducers, St. John's wort	Half-life 1.5 times that of younger adults
Quetiapine (Seroquel)	CYP3A4, clearance increased with phenytoin	No oral solution available
Ziprasidone (Geodon)	Increased hypotension with antihypertensives, other agents that affect QTc prolongation	No dosage adjustment recommended. Start low and titrate slowly based on response, avoid in patients with cardiac disease
Aripiprazole (Abilify)	CYP2D6, CYP3A4, highly protein bound	Once-daily dosing, does not cause weight gain or EKG changes

*Metoclopamide (Reglan), because of its affinity for dopamine, increases EPS, while the effects of levadopa may be antagonized by antipsychotics.

Note. Adapted from: "Use of Pharmacologic Agents in the Elderly," by A. Desai, 2003, *Clinics in Geriatric Medicine, 19*(4), pp. 697–719; and from *Geriatric Dosage Handbook,* (8th ed.), by T. Semla, 2003, Hudson, OH: Lexi-comp.

rigidity. Conventional agents also cause increased prolactin secretion, which can lead to problems such as sexual and reproductive dysfunction, breast pathology, bone demineralization, depression, memory deficits, and damage to the cardiovascular endothelium (Arana, 2000).

While the newer atypical antipsychotics have become an attractive alternative, they are not devoid of side effects. Each drug in the class has slightly different characteristics, all of which are important to consider in the older adult population. Possible adverse effects of this class include headache, orthostatic hypotension, falls, cardiovascular effects, weight gain, dyslipidemia, diabetes, and to a lesser extent, TD and EPS. As a class, however, the atypical agents have a lower affinity for the dopamine D_2 receptor, which accounts for the relatively low incidence of EPS, TD, and prolactinemia. The faster the drug disso-

ciates from the D_2 receptor, the lower the rates of these treatment-induced D_2-related side effects. Clozapine and quetiapine have fast dissociation from the D_2 receptor. Olanzapine and risperidone have slower dissociation and the typical antipsychotics have even slower dissociation. Therefore, the typical agents have the highest dopamine D_2-related side effects, followed by olanzapine and risperidone. The dopamine-related side-effect profiles of some atypicals are dose-dependent because of loss of specificity. For example, increasing doses of olanzapine, risperidone, and ziprasidone raise relative D_2 occupancy and can begin to resemble side-effect profiles of typical agents at higher dosages. In older adults, this can be more problematic and occur at lower dosages than in younger age groups (Jeste, 2004).

Atypical antipsychotics have been studied much more extensively in younger populations than in older age groups and have been found to differ from typical agents in that they have greater ability to treat negative symptoms. Since the newer atypical agents have a different side-effect profile that is potentially less detrimental to the older adult in lower doses, they are being examined more closely for use in this population to determine their efficacy. A base of studies is beginning to establish the benefit of these agents, especially in low dosages, but the decision to prescribe requires drug knowledge in the absence of large-scale randomized control trials (Chan, Pariser, & Neufeld, 1999; Defilippi & Crismon, 2000). The use of several of the atypical agents, including risperidone, olanzapine, and quetiapine, have been studied in patients with psychosis and Alzheimer's disease in the Clinical Antipsychotic Trials of Intervention Effectiveness Study (CATIE) (http://www.catie.unc.edu). A brief review of the individual atypical antipsychotic agents follows.

In 2004, Marder and colleagues published a consensus paper on physical health monitoring with persons treated with second generation antipsychotics. This paper discusses the potential problems with lipid dysregulation, insulin resistance, and potential for type 2 diabetes in conjunction with these agents. In many ways, these problems are the equivalent of what tardive dyskinesia was to the conventional antipsychotic agents, and need to be addressed by any clinician who is working with patients receiving these agents as part of their treatment plan. There are specific guidelines for monitoring weight, lipids, and glucose, and these guidelines have become a dimension of the community standard of practice to which all clinicians are accountable. Additionally, the FDA requires that second generation antipsychotic medications carry a warning related to risk of hyperglycemia and diabetes (Rosack, 2003). Such changes carry significant implications for the monitoring of elders who are treated with these agents.

Clozapine has been studied for the treatment of psychotic symptoms, including those associated with dementia, and demonstrates overall benefit in over half of the older-adult patients treated, especially at low doses. It has minimal effect in the striatal area, which explains its relative low potential for extrapyramidal side effects. Clozapine, however, does have other serious potential side effects in older adults, such as seizures, hypotension, and potent anticholinergic effects. Even more limiting is the potential of clozapine-induced agranulocytosis, which can have an incidence as high as 1.3% per year (Novartis, 2002), and which increases with age (Alvir, Lieberman, Safferman, Schwimmer, & Schaaf, 1993). The risk of fatal agranulocytosis requiring frequent blood monitoring makes it more restrictive to use than other atypicals. Clozapine may be considered in older adults refractory to all other choices and possibly in patients with Parkinson's disease, because it does not increase the motor symptoms, like many of the other agents (Barak, Wittenberg, Naor, Kutzuk, & Weizman, 1999; Pitner, Mintzer, Pennypacker, & Jackson, 1995; Salzman, Vaccaro, Lieff, & Weiner, 1995).

Risperidone affects both serotonin and dopamine and has been shown to improve both negative and positive symptoms of psychoses while reducing the incidence of EPS (Jeste et al., 2000). Risperidone should be dosed as low as possible to maintain efficacy and prevent dose-related D_2 motor side effects. Risperidone has been evaluated in several open-label studies and case studies, as well as one large randomized controlled trial in older adults with positive benefit (Katz et al., 1999; Madhusoodanan, Brenner, Araujo, & Gupta, 1995; Raheja, Bharwani, & Penetrante, 1995; Zarate et al., 1997).

Olanzapine is thought to work through an antagonism of both dopamine and serotonin receptors. It does affect muscarinic, histamine, and alpha-1 receptors to a degree, which explains potential anticholinergic side effects, sedation, and hypotension. Studies of olanzapine use in the older adult have been conducted primarily in dementia patients, demonstrating beneficial effects on behavior (Solomons & Geiger, 2000; Street et al., 2000). Olanzapine can increase the potential for development of diabetes and associated problems. Olanzapine can also contribute to the development of dyslipidemia. Therefore, proper monitoring for these two conditions is necessary.

Quetiapine is thought to work through a combination of dopamine and serotonin antagonism. It has no appreciable affinity for muscarinic or benzodiazepine receptors but does cause some blockade at histamine and alpha-1 receptors. Therefore, quetiapine can cause somnolence and orthostatic hypotension. Quetiapine does have a good EPS tolerability profile across the entire dose range (AstraZeneca Pharmaceuticals LP, 2004). The most common adverse events exhibited across placebo-controlled trials included headache, somnolence, and dizziness (Tariot, Salzman, Yeung, Pultz, & Rak, 2000). Quetiapine has been shown to be effective in the treatment of psychosis in older adults and in patients with Parkinson's disease. Effective doses are often lower when used in the older adults (Friedman & Factor, 2000; McManus, Arvanitis, & Kowalcyk, 1999; Targum & Abbott, 2000; Tariot et al., 2000).

Very few data are available on the use of newer atypical antipsychotic medications in the older-adult population, such as ziprasidone and aripiprazole. In general, there is no indication of any different tolerability of ziprasidone or for reduced clearance of ziprasidone in older adults compared to younger adults. However, dosages should still be started low and titrated slowly to therapeutic response with careful monitoring of potential side effects, such as orthostasis (Pfizer, 2002). Aripiprazole, another new antipsychotic, has common side effects of somnolence and orthostatic hypotension (Bristol-Myers Squibb,

2003; Burris et al., 2002) Aripiprazole is the first antipsychotic agent on the market whose mechanism of action includes dopamine partial agonism and serotonin antagonism. This unique mechanism of action places it in a class by itself and may be the first "atypical" atypical antipsychotic agent. The alleged benefits of aripiprazole include an absence of hyperprolactimenia, reduced risk for weight gain and type 2 diabetes, and absence of dyslipidemia (Davies, Scheffler, & Roth, 2004).

It is important to note that the misuse of antipsychotics in older adults, particularly in long-term-care settings, prompted the passage of the Omnibus Budget Reconciliation Act (OBRA) in 1987 with modifications in 1990. This act mandated nursing home reform. Among its many stipulations, it stated that residents had the right to be free from chemical and physical restraints imposed for the purpose of convenience or discipline and not required to treat a medical condition. Further, there must be documented need for the use of this category of drugs to treat a specific condition. This act focused on improving quality of life and eliminating the unnecessary use of antipsychotic, anxiolytic, and sedative–hypnotic drugs as a means of chemically restraining older adults in long-term-care settings.

Anxiolytics

Proper treatment of anxiety in older adults requires proper diagnosis by addressing organic causes, comorbid psychiatric conditions, or a medication that causes anxiety-related side effects. There is very little evidence-based data to guide anxiolytic therapy (Bartels et al., 2003). However, antianxiety medications should be prescribed based on the suitability of the drug for an individual patient, taking into account potential side effects and compatibility with the existing medication profile (Burke, Folks, & McNeilly, 1998). Antidepressants may be recommended as first line therapy for anxiety disorders, but a short course of a benzodiazepine sometimes is considered (Alexopoulos et al., 2004). If a benzodiazepine is prescribed, it is important to appreciate the potential risks associated with its use.

Benzodiazepines have a side-effect profile particularly dangerous in older adults. Benzodiazepines are likely to cause sedation and a decrease in hand-eye coordination. The outcome of benzodiazepine use at modest doses impairs driving performance in the older driver to a level similar to the legal definition of alcohol intoxication (Beers & Berkow, 2004). Ataxia, slurred speech, impaired coordination, confusion, poor concentration, memory loss, sleep disturbances, and depressive symptoms also may occur. Patients should be monitored closely for adverse effects.

OBRA guidelines for benzodiazepine use with residents of long-term-care facilities are fairly specific related to use with proper diagnoses, which drugs to avoid, duration of treatment, attempts at withdrawal of medication, and maximum daily dose (Omnibus Budget Reconciliation Act, 1987). Generally, geriatric patients will experience fewer adverse effects from shorter-acting drugs without active metabolites such as alprazolam, lorazepam, and oxazepam. Longer-acting drugs, such as diazepam and chlordiazepoxide, should be avoided. Short-acting benzodiazepines are listed in Table 6-8 with the recommended dosing schedule. It is generally recommended to use low regularly scheduled doses, but as-needed dosing (prn) may be beneficial in certain patients. Clinicians need to consider when and how to discontinue the antianxiety medications once they are started. A brief period of 4 to 6 weeks may be all that is required for treatment, but benzodiazepines may require an additional 3 to 4 weeks to be gradually tapered. Older adults should be aware of the need for short-term treatment with these agents, to better prepare them for proper titration off the drug at the appropriate time. Tapering a benzodiazepine too quickly can lead to rebound anxiety or even a withdrawal syndrome with possible seizures.

An alternative to benzodiazepines is buspirone (Buspar). Buspirone is less sedating than the benzodiazepines and is not

TABLE 6-8 Preferred Benzodiazepines and Dosing Schedule*				
Medication	Initial Dose	Recommended Maximum Daily Dose*	Dosing in Hepatic and Renal Disease	Dosage Forms
Short-Acting Benzodiazepines				
Alprazolam (Xanax)	0.125–0.25 mg BID	0.75 mg	Decrease 50% in hepatic impairment, avoid in cirrhosis, caution in renal disease	Tablet, liquid
Lorazepam (Ativan)	0.25–0.5 mg BID	2 mg	Caution if renal or hepatic disease	Tablet, liquid, IM injection
Oxazepam (Serax)	10 mg BID	30 mg	Avoid in hepatic disease, caution yet safer option in renal impairment	Tablet, capsule

*Per HCFA guidelines for residents of long-term-care facilities.

Note. Adapted from: *Geriatric Dosage Handbook*, (8th ed.), by T. Semla, 2003, Hudson, OH: Lexi-comp.

addicting. Efficacy and safety of this drug is reported to be equal in older adults compared to younger adults (Semla, 2003). The initial dose is 5 mg twice daily and titrated by 5 mg daily up to an average dose of 20 to 30 mg divided into two or three doses per day. Buspirone will take longer to show subjective benefit than benzodiazepines; it usually begins to show benefit after 2 weeks and maximum benefit after 4 weeks of continuous therapy. Because of this delay in effect, patients who have used benzodiazepines in the past may be resistant to using buspirone. Concomitant use of benzodiazepines with buspirone will reduce the effectiveness of the buspirone.

▆▆▆▆ SUMMARY

Psychotropic medications are the second-most-commonly prescribed class of drugs in the geriatric population and the class most frequently associated with adverse drug reactions (Ives, 2001). It is essential for clinicians to recognize that good prescribing practice is a multifaceted process. This process not only involves the clinician's knowledge of pharmacotherapeutics, but takes into account patient and caregiver status, as well as financial concerns and insurance restrictions. The treatment of mental illness in older adults, as noted in this chapter, presents challenges unique to this patient population. By carefully considering and weighing the many factors that influence the treatment of mental illness in older adults, clinicians will evidence the very best prescribing practice as they address the mental health needs of older adults.

REFERENCES

Alexopoulos, G. S, Katz I. R., Reynolds, C. F., Carpenter D., & Docherty, J. P. (2001). Pharmacotherapy of depressive disorders in older patients. The Expert Consensus Guideline Series [Special report]. *Postgraduate Medicine, 2001,* 1–82.

Alexopoulos, G. S., Streim, J., Carpenter, D., & Docherty, J. P. (2004). Introduction: Methods, commentary, and summary. *The Journal of Clinical Psychiatry, 65* (Suppl. 2), 5–19.

American Nurses Association (1994). Psychiatric mental health nursing psychopharmacology project. Washington, DC: American Nurses.

American Psychiatric Association (2000). *Practice guideline for the treatment of patients with major depressive disorder* (2nd ed.). Retrieved January 10, 2005, from www.psych.org.

Alvir, J. M., Lieberman, J. A., Safferman, A. Z., Schwimmer, J. L., & Schaaf, J. A. (1993). Clozapine-induced agranulocytosis. Incidence and risk factors in the United States. *New England Journal of Medicine, 329*(3), 204–205.

Andrade, C. (2004). Antidepressant-withdrawal mania: A critical review and synthesis of the literature. *Journal of Clinical Psychiatry, 65*(7), 987–93.

Arana, G. W. (2000). An overview of side effects caused by typical antipsychotics. *The Journal of Clinical Psychiatry, 61*(Suppl. 8), 5–11.

AstraZeneca Pharmaceuticals LP. (2004). Seroquel [Product insert]. Wilmington, DE: Author.

Banerjee, S., & Dickinson, E. (1997). Evidence-based health care in old age psychiatry. *The International Journal of Psychiatry in Medicine, 27*(3), 283–292.

Barak, Y., Wittenberg, N., Naor, S., Kutzuk, D., & Weizman, A. (1999). Clozapine in elderly psychiatric patients: Tolerability, safety, and efficacy. *Comprehensive Psychiatry, 40,* 320–325.

Bartels, S., Dums, A., Oxman, T., Schneider, L., Areán, P., Alexopoulos, G., et al. (2003). Evidence-based practices in geriatric mental health care: An overview of systematic reviews and meta-analyses. *The Psychiatric Clinics of North America, 26,* 971–990.

Beers, M., & Berkow, R. (Eds.). (2004). *Merck manual of geriatrics.* Whitehouse Station, NJ: Merck Research Labs.

Bezchlibnyk-Butler, K. Z., & Jeffries, J. J. (2004). *Clinical handbook of psychotropic drugs* (14th ed.). Seattle: Hogrefe & Huber.

Bristol-Myers Squibb. (2001). Serzone [Package insert]. Princeton, NJ: Author.

Bristol-Myers Squibb. (2003). Abilify [Package insert]. Princeton, NJ: Author.

Burke, W. J., Folks, D. G., & McNeilly, D. P. (1998). Effective use of anxiolytics in older adults. *Clinics in Geriatric Medicine, 14,* 47–65.

Burris, K., Molski, T., Xu, C., Ryan, E., Tottori, K., & Kikuchi, T. (2002). Aripiprazole, a novel antipsychotic, is a high-affinity partial agonist at human dopamine D2 receptors. *The Journal of Pharmacology and Experimental Therapeutics, 302*(1), 381–389.

Cadieux, R. J. (1989). Drug interactions in the elderly: How multiple drug use increases risk exponentially. *Postgraduate Medicine, 86*(8), 179–86.

Cadieux, R. J. (1999). Antidepressant drug interactions in the elderly: Understanding the P-450 system is half the battle in reducing risks. *Postgraduate Medicine, 106*(6), 231–49.

Catterson, M. L., Preskorn, S. H., & Martin, R. L. (1997). Pharmacodynamic and pharmacokinetic considerations in geriatric psychopharmacology. *The Psychiatric Clinics of North America, 20*(1), 205–218.

Chan, Y. C., Pariser, S. F., & Neufeld, G. (1999). Atypical antipsychotics in older adults. *Pharmacotherapy, 19*(7), 811–822.

Choi S. (2003). Nefazodone (Serzone) withdrawn because of hepatotoxicity. *Canadian Medical Association Journal, 169*(11), 1035.

Davies, M. A., Sheffler, D. J., Roth, B. L. (2004). Aripiprazole: A novel atypical antipsychotic drug with a uniquely robust pharmacology. *CNS Drug Review, 10*(4), 317–36.

Defilippi, J. L., & Crismon, M. L. (2000). Antipsychotic agents in patients with dementia. *Pharmacotherapy, 20*(1), 23–33.

Desai, A. (2003). Use of pharmacologic agents in the elderly. *Clinics in Geriatric Medicine, 19*(4), 697–719.

Dilsaver, S. C., Greden, J. F. & Snider, R. M. (1987). Antidepressant withdrawal syndromes: Phenomenology and pathophysiology. *International Clinical Psychopharmacology, 2,* 1–19.

Dossey, B. (1997). Complementary and alternative therapies for our aging society. *Journal of Gerontological Nursing, 23*(9), 45–51.

Edlund, B. (2004). Medication use and misuse. *Journal of Gerontological Nursing, 30*(7), 4.

Edlund, B., & Haight, B. (1992). Assessment of the older adult. In J. Bellack & B. Edlund (Eds.), *Nursing assessment and diagnosis.* (pp. 776–808). Boston: Jones and Bartlett.

Edlund, B., & Spain, M. (2003). Geriatric assessment. *Advance for Nurses, 5*(4), 13–17.

Finucane, T. E. (1994). Geriatric medicine: Special considerations. In L. R. Barker, J. R. Burton, & P. D. Lieve (Eds.), *Principles of ambulatory medicine* (4th ed., pp. 72–88). Baltimore: Williams & Wilkins.

Friedman, J. H. & Factor, S. A. (2000). Atypical antipsychotics in the treatment of drug-induced psychosis in Parkinson's disease. *Movement Disorders, 15*(2), 201–211.

Glaxo SmithKline. (2003). Wellbutrin XL [Package insert]. Research Triangle Park, NC: Author.

Gruenwald J., Brendler T., & Jaenicke, C. (Eds.). (2000). *PDR for herbal medicines.* Montvale, NJ: Medical Economics.

Gurvich, T., & Cunningham, J. (2000). Appropriate use of psychotropic drugs in nursing homes. *American Family Physician, 61,* 1437–1446.

Haddad, P. (1997). Newer antidepressants and the discontinuation syndrome. *Journal of Clinical Psychiatry, 57*(7), 17–21.

Hansten, P. D. (1998). Understanding drug–drug interactions. *Science and Medicine, 5,* 16–25.

Ives, T. J. (2001). Pharmacotherapeutics. In R. Ham, P. Sloane, & G. Warshaw (Eds.), *Primary care geriatrics: A case-based approach,* (4th ed.) (pp. 137–148). St. Louis: MO: Mosby.

Jeste, D. V. (2004). Tardive dyskinesia rates with atypical antipsychotics in older adults. *Journal of Clinical Psychiatry, 65*(Suppl. 9), 21–24.

Jeste, D. V., Okamoto, A., Napolitano, J., Kane, J. M., & Martinez, R. A. (2000). Low incidence of persistent tardive dyskinesia in elderly patients with dementia treated with risperidone. *American Journal of Psychiatry, 157,* 1150–1155.

Johnson, J. (2000). Pharmacologic management. In A. Lueckenotte (Ed.), *Gerontological nursing* (2nd ed., pp. 425–447). St. Louis, MO: Mosby.

Kane, R., Ouslander, J., & Abrass, I. (2004). *Essentials of clinical geriatrics.* New York: McGraw-Hill.

Kastrup, E. (2004). *Drug facts and comparisons.* St. Louis, MO: Kluwer Health.

Katz, I. R., Jeste, D. V., Mintzer, J. E., Clyde, C., Napolitano, J., & Brecher, M. (1999). Comparison of risperidone and placebo for psychosis and behavioral disturbances associated with dementia: A randomized, double-blind trial. Risperidone Study Group. *The Journal of Clinical Psychiatry, 60,* 107–115.

Keltner, N., & Folks, D. (2001). *Psychotropic drugs* (3rd ed.). St. Louis, MO: Mosby.

Kornstein, S. G., & McEnany, G. W. (2000). Enhancing pharmacologic effects in the treatment of depression in women. *Journal of Clinical Psychiatry, 61*(Suppl. 11), 18–27.

Madhusoodanan, S., Brenner, R., Araujo, L., & Gupta, S. (1995). Efficacy of risperidone treatment for psychoses associated with schizophrenia, schizoaffective disorder, bipolar disorder, or senile dementia in 11 geriatric patients: A case series. *The Journal of Clinical Psychiatry, 56,* 514–518.

Malhotra, A., Litman, R., & Pickar, D. (1993). Adverse effects of antipsychotic drugs. *Drug Safety, 9,* 429–436.

Marder, S. R., Essock, S. M., Miller, A. L., et al. (2004). Physical health monitoring of patients with schizophrenia. *American Journal of Psychiatry, 161*(8), 1334–1349.

McEnany, G. W. (1999). Herbal psychotropics (Part 1): Focus on St. John's wort and SAMe. *Journal of the American Psychiatric Nurses Association, 5*(6), 192–196.

McEnany, G. W. (2000a). Herbal psychotropics (Part 2): Focus on inositol and omega-3 fatty acids. *Journal of the American Psychiatric Nurses Association, 6*(1), 93–96.

McEnany, G. W. (2000b). Herbal psychotropics (Part 3): Focus on kava, valerian and melatonin. *Journal of the American Psychiatric Nurses Association, 6*(2), 126–130.

McEnany, G. W. (2001). Herbal psychotropics (Part 4): Focus on ginko biloba, L-carnitine, lactobacillus/acidophilus and ginger root. *Journal of the American Psychiatric Nurses Association, 7*(1), 22–25.

McManus, D. Q., Arvanitis, L. A., & Kowalcyk, B. B. (for the Seroquel Trial 48 Study Group). (1999). Quetiapine, a novel antipsychotic: Experience in elderly patients with psychotic disorders. *The Journal of Clinical Psychiatry, 60,* 107–115.

Michocki, R. (2001). Polypharmacy and principles of drug therapy. In A. Adelman & M. Daly (Eds.), *20 common problems in geriatrics* (pp. 69–81). New York: McGraw-Hill.

Nemeroff, C. B. (2003). Improving antidepressant adherence. *Journal of Clinical Psychiatry, 64* (Suppl. 18), 25–30.

Nicholas, L. M., Ford, A. L., Esposito, S. M., Ekstrom, R. D., Golden, R. N. (2003). The effects of mirtazapine on plasma lipid profiles in healthy subjects. *Journal of Clinical Psychiatry, 64*(8), 883–889.

Novartis. (2002) Clozaril [Package insert]. East Hanover, NJ: Author.

Omnibus Budget Reconciliation Act. (1987) Subtitle C, nursing home reform: PL100-203. Washington, DC: National Coalition for Nursing Home Reform.

Organon. (2002). Remeron SolTab [Package insert]. West Orange, NJ: Author.

Pfizer. (2002). Geodon [Package insert]. New York: Author.

Pitner, J. K., Mintzer, J. E., Pennypacker, L. C., & Jackson, C. (1995). Efficacy and adverse effects of clozapine in four elderly patients. *The Journal of Clinical Psychiatry, 56,* 180–185.

Pollock, B., & Mulsant, B. (1995). Antipsychotics in older patients. A safety perspective. *Drugs & Aging, 6,* 312–23.

Raheja, R., Bharwani, I., & Penetrante, A. (1995). Efficacy of risperidone for behavioral disorders in the elderly: A clinical observation. *Journal of Geriatric Psychiatry and Neurology, 8,* 159–161.

Reeves, R. R., Beddingfield, J. J. (2003). Shock-like sensations during venlafaxine withdrawal. *Pharmacotherapy, 23*(5), 678–81.

Rosack, J. (2003). FDA to require diabetes warning on antipsychotics. *Psychiatric News, 38*(20), 1.

Sadock, B., & Sadock, A. (2003). *Synopsis of psychiatry.* Philadelphia: Lippincott, Williams, & Wilkins.

Salzman, C., Vaccaro, B., Lieff, J., & Weiner, A. (1995). Clozapine in older patients with psychosis and behavioral disruption. *American Journal of Geriatric Psychiatry, 3*, 26–33.

Schretzman, D., & Strumpf, N. (2002). Principles guiding care of older adults. In V. Cotter & N. Strumpf, *Advanced practice nursing with older adults* (pp. 5–25). New York: McGraw-Hill.

Semla, T. (2003). *Geriatric dosage handbook* (8th ed.). Hudson, OH: Lexi-comp.

Solomons, K., & Geiger, O. (2000). Olanzapine use in the elderly: A retrospective analysis. *The Canadian Journal of Psychiatry, 45*, 151–155.

Stahl, S. M. (2001). Essential psychopharmacology: Neuroscientific basis and practical applications (2nd ed.). Cambridge, UK: Cambridge University Press.

Street, J., Clark, W., Gannon, K., Cummings, J., Bymaster, F., Tamura, R., et al. (2000). Olanzapine treatment of psychotic and behavioral symptoms in patients with Alzheimer's disease in nursing care facilities: A double-blind, randomized, placebo-controlled trial. The HGEU Study Group. *Archives of General Psychiatry, 57*, 968–976.

Targum, S. D., & Abbott, J. L. (2000). Efficacy of quetiapine in Parkinson's patients with psychosis. *Journal of Clinical Psychopharmacology, 20*, 54–60.

Tariot, P. N., Salzman, C., Yeung, P. P., Pultz, J., & Rak, I. W. (2000). Long-term use of quetiapine in elderly patients with psychotic disorders, *Clinical Therapeutics, 22*(9), 1068–1084.

US Bureau of the Census. (2000). [Demographic data]. Available at: www.census.gov/popest/estimates.php.

US Department of Health and Human Services. (2000). *Healthy People 2010: Understanding and improving health.* Retrieved March 16, 2004, from http://www.health.gov/healthypeople/

Voyer, P., Cohen, D., Lauzon, S. & Collins, J. (2004). Factors associated with psychotropic drug use among community dwelling older persons: A review of empirical studies. *BMC Nursing, 3*(1), 3.

Walker, M. K., & Foreman, M. D. (1999). Medication safety: A protocol for nursing action. *Geriatric Nursing, 20*(1), 34–39.

Williams, J. W., Jr., Mulrow, C. D., Chiquette, E., Noel, P. H., Aguilar, C., & Cornell J. (2000). A systematic review of newer pharmacotherapies for depression in adults: Evidence report summary. *Annals of Internal Medicine, 132,* 743–56.

Wyeth-Ayerst. (2003). Effexor [Package insert]. Philadelphia: Author.

Zarate, C. A., Jr., Baldessarini, R. J., Siegel, A. J., Nakamura, A., McDonald, J., Muir-Hutchinson, L., et al. (1997). Risperidone in the elderly: A pharmacoepidemiologic study. *The Journal of Clinical Psychiatry, 58,* 311–17.

SECTION II

Psychopathology of Late Life

CHAPTER 7

Nursing Assessment and Treatment of Depressive Disorders of Late Life

Eve Heemann Byrd, MSN, MPH, APRN-BC

> Depression is a disorder of mood, so mysteriously painful and elusive in the way it becomes known to the self—to the mediating intellect—as to verge close to being beyond description. It thus remains nearly incomprehensible to those who have not experienced it in its extreme mood, although the gloom, "the blues" which people go through occasionally and associate with the general hassle of everyday existence are of such prevalence that they do give many individuals a hint of the illness in its catastrophic form.
>
> —William Styron, *Darkness Visible: A Memoir of Madness* (1990)

Depression is one of the most common, often the most debilitating yet the most treatable, illnesses seen in older adults. According to the World Health Organization (1990), unipolar major depression will be the second leading cause of disability worldwide, second to ischemic heart disease, and is expected to be the leading cause of disability for women and developing countries by the year 2020. Older adult women are twice as likely to suffer from depression as older adult men. The 2000 Cache County, Utah, study of more that 4500 nondemented older adults revealed a 4.4% rate of major depression in women and a 2.7% rate in men (Steffens et al., 2000).

Depression is not only disabling; there is increasing evidence that depression is a fatal illness in older adults. Depression is the leading risk factor for suicide. The suicide rate for persons 65 years and older is greater than any other age group. Older adults account for 18% of all suicides, while they only make up 13% of the population in the United States (National Institute of Mental Health, 1999). The highest frequency is found among white males 65 years and older at 62 per 100,000 (Blazer, 2003).

Depression in older adults costs the nation an estimated $43 billion per year, not includ-ing the pain, suffering, and poor quality of life that results from depression (American Association of Geriatric Psychiatry, 2001). Older adults with symptoms of depression have 50% higher health care costs (Unutzer, 1997). We live in an aging society and as the average age of the population increases, there will be an increased cost to the American public as a result of unnecessary disability and mortality should late-life depression go undiagnosed and inadequately treated.

Nurses are in a position to play a significant role in decreasing older adult disability and mortality. However, nurses must first assess their own prejudices toward persons with mental illness. Ageism and the stigma associated with depression are among the underlying reasons for the numerous barriers that older adults encounter in attempting to receive treatment for depression. Older adults themselves think depression is a normal part of aging. According to a 1996 survey conducted by the National Mental Health Association, 58% of people 65 years of age and older believe it is normal for persons to get depressed as they get older. American culture and health care delivery perpetuates this belief. Medicare currently reimburses only 50% of the Medicare allowable amount for psychological health services. Less than 50% of adults exhibiting depressive symptoms receive treatment from their primary care provider for their depressive illness (Sadovsky, 1998). This is further magnified by the fact that there is a shortage of health care providers for older adults, particularly geriatric mental health professionals.

The Surgeon General's Report (Department of Health and Human Services [DHHS], 1999) states that the only way the mental health needs of America will be met is for "non-mental health professionals" to be educated and participate in the mental health care of persons suffering from mental illness. Nurses must educate themselves regarding depression and its treatments and must recognize that frequently they are the health care provider who spends the most time with an older client; therefore, nurses are often in a key position to assess for symptoms of depression. Nurses need to advocate for health care services and environments aimed at prevention and early recognition of depression. Finally, nurses must also advocate for adequate treatment. The nurse's goal in treating an older adult with depression is full remission from the illness.

Depression is insidious. It invades all aspects of the older adult's life—physical, mental, social, and spiritual. Symptoms of depression, such as loss of interest in activities, social withdrawal, irritability, anxiety, chronic aches and pains that do not respond to treatment, and increased dependency, are often incorrectly explained as a normal part of aging. Older adult women have described depression as "the reexperiencing of a severe personal insult" that results in feelings of worthlessness, increased vulnerability or insecurity, a loss of self-respect, and feelings of inferiority or incompetence (Hedelin & Strandmark, 2001, p.407). The symptoms of depression are also too often attributed to neurologic or other physical illnesses by both physicians and patients themselves. Neurovegetative symptoms such as sleep distur-

bances, loss of appetite, poor concentration, and low energy are frequently explained as symptoms of a comorbid illness. There is a growing body of evidence that depression not only contributes to poor medical outcomes because of unhealthy behavior but it is also an etiologic factor in illnesses such as cardiovascular disease, stroke, cancer, and epilepsy (Evans et al., 2003). Depression, the "unwanted cotraveler," a phrase coined at the March 2001 National Institute of Mental Health Forum, also affects the progression of chronic illnesses such as cardiovascular, cerebrovascular, neurological disorders, diabetes, cancer, and HIV/AIDS (Evans et al.). Therefore, a strong case can be made for the development and implementation of depression prevention, early detection, and adequate treatment strategies.

ETIOLOGY

Typically, depression is multifactorial in origin and evaluated from a biopsychosocial model. Depression in late life can either be the recurrence of an illness experienced earlier or it can show up for the first time later in life—after the age of 55. Depression in older adults is most frequently associated with physiological changes or abnormalities of the brain (Lebowitz et al., 1997). These changes are thought to be of vascular origin or the result of early changes caused by dementing illnesses such as Alzheimer's disease or vascular dementia. These physiological changes affect synaptic activity causing fewer serotonin receptor sites or impaired receptor response (Blazer, 2003). Hormonal changes have also been associated with depression. Low levels of estrogen and dehydroepiandrosterone in women (DHEA) and low levels of total testosterone in older men have been shown to be associated with depressive symptoms; however, the efficacy of treating either has not been established (Blazer; Lebowitz et al., 1997; Tweedy, Morrison, & DeMichele, 2002).

In addition to the biological etiology of depression in older adults, there are clearly psychological contributing factors. The older adult's life events and the interpretation and response to the events, contribute to the risk for developing depression. The predominant life events that put an older adult at risk for depression, as well as contribute to the older adult's experience and receptiveness to treatment for depression, are medical illness, bereavement or death of a loved one, disability, trauma, and impaired social support (Bruce & Pearson, 1999). These risk factors do not necessarily individually cause depression, rather it may be the chain of events that results in depression (Bruce & Pearson). Risk factors, coupled with behavioral, psychodynamic, and negative thoughts surrounding life events, appear to contribute to late-life depression (Blazer). For instance, older adults' interpretation of their situation may be that no matter what they do, bad things continue to happen and/or they continue to experience losses, so they assume a helpless position. Older adults also may not adapt to physical changes that occur with aging and may have unrealistic expectations and feel as if they continue to fail (Blazer, 2003). The current culture that places value on one's accomplishments or one's physical ability to "do," versus an individual's contribution to the greater good, may compound the older adult's feelings of inadequacy. Impaired social support is also associated with depression in older adults (Blazer).

ASSESSMENT AND SCREENING OF LATE-LIFE DEPRESSION

Most older adults fall into one or more at-risk groups for depression. Many, however, do not recognize their symptoms as depression and do not request an evaluation. Older adults may be resistant to seeking treatment because of the stigma of mental illness. As a result, all older adults should be screened for depres-

sion whether they present in a primary care office, hospital, long-term care home, or community senior center. The Geriatric Depression Screening (GDS) tool (Yesavage & Brink, 1983) is a useful self-rated screening instrument (Table 7-1). The GDS is a valid tool and is used frequently for detecting depression in older adults who have co-occuring medical illness as well as in older adults with mild to moderate cognitive impairment. A score of 10–11 or greater out of 30 yes-or-no questions is considered to be significant for depression and warrants a more thorough evaluation. There is also a 15-item or short form version of the GDS. One drawback of the GDS is that it does not include a question on suicidal thought or intent. Another screening instrument recommended for use in persons with dementia is an interviewer-rated scale called the Cornell Scale for Depression in Dementia (Table 7-2) (Alexopoulos, Abrams, Young & Shamoian, 1988; Alexopoulos, Katz, Reynolds, Carpenter & Docherty, 2001). It is a 19-item questionnaire that takes approximately 20–30 minutes to administer. A score of 12 or greater indicates depression.

DIAGNOSIS OF MOOD DISORDERS

The Diagnostic and Statistical Manual of Mental Disorders (DSM-IV) (American Psychiatric Association [APA], 2000) outlines the criteria for major depression, dysthymia, and minor depression. A diagnosis of major depression requires that for a two-week period, the individual either exhibits: (1) a sad, depressed mood, or (2) a loss of interest or pleasure in usual activities, and five or more of the following symptoms: significant weight loss or an increase or decrease in appetite, insomnia or hypersomnia nearly every day, psychomotor agitation or retardation observable by others nearly every day, fatigue or loss of energy nearly every day, feelings of worthlessness or excessive guilt, diminished ability

TABLE 7-1	Geriatric Depression Screening Tool		
	Yes	**No**	
1	X	☐	Are you basically satisfied with your life?
2	☐	X	Have you dropped many of your activities and interests?
3	☐	X	Do you feel that your life is empty?
4	☐	X	Do you often get bored?
5	X	☐	Are you hopeful about the future?
6	☐	X	Are you bothered by thoughts that you can't get out of your head?
7	X	☐	Are you in good spirits most of the time?
8	☐	X	Are you afraid that something bad is going to happen to you?
9	X	☐	Do you feel happy most of the time?
10	☐	X	Do you feel helpless?
11	☐	X	Do you often get restless and fidgety?
12	☐	X	Do you prefer to stay at home, rather than going out and doing new things?
13	☐	X	Do you frequently worry about the future?
14	☐	X	Do you feel you have more problems with your memory than most?
15	X	☐	Do you think it is wonderful to be alive now?
16	☐	X	Do you often feel downhearted and blue?
17	☐	X	Do you feel pretty worthless the way you are now?
18	☐	X	Do you often worry a lot about the past?
19	X	☐	Do you find life very exciting?
20	☐	X	Is it hard for you to get started on new projects?
21	X	☐	Do you feel full of energy?
22	☐	X	Do you feel that your situation is hopeless?
23	☐	X	Do you think that most people are better off than you are?
24	☐	X	Do you frequently get upset over little things?
25	☐	X	Do you frequently feel like crying?
26	☐	X	Do you have trouble concentrating?
27	X	☐	Do you enjoy getting up in the morning?
28	☐	X	Do you prefer to avoid social gatherings?
29	X	☐	Is it easy for you to make decisions?
30	X	☐	Is your mind as clear as it used to be?

Scoring System

Note: The boxes indicate response indicating depressive symptom and each is equivalent to 1. Score of 10–11 indicates an evaluation for depression is indicated. (Yesavage & Brink, 1983)

Note: From "Development and Validation of a Geriatric Depression Scale: A Preliminary Report," by J. A. Yesavage and T. L. Brink, 1983, *Journal of Psychiatric Research, 17*, pp. 37–49. Reprinted with permission.

to think or concentrate or make decisions nearly every day, and/or recurrent thoughts of death (not just fear of dying or developmentally appropriate thoughts of death as a part of growing old), recurrent suicidal ideation without a specific plan, or a suicide attempt, or a specific plan for committing suicide (APA, 2000).

The diagnostic criteria for dysthymia is exhibiting a depressed mood for more days than not for two years and two or more of the following: poor appetite or overeating, insomnia or hypersomnia, low energy or fatigue, low self-esteem, poor concentration or difficulty making decisions, and/or feelings of hopelessness (APA, 2000).

TABLE 7-2   Cornell Scale for Depression in Dementia

A. Mood-Related Signs

1. Anxiety: anxious expression, ruminations, worrying	a 0 1 2
2. Sadness: sad expression, sad voice, tearfulness	a 0 1 2
3. Lack of reactivity to pleasant events	a 0 1 2
4. Irritability: easily annoyed, short-tempered	a 0 1 2

B. Behavioral Disturbance

5. Agitation: restlessness, hand-wringing, hair-pulling	a 0 1 2
6. Retardation: slow movement, slow speech, slow reactions	a 0 1 2
7. Multiple physical complaints (score 0 if GI symptoms only)	a 0 1 2
8. Loss of interest: less involved in usual activities (score only if change occurred acutely, i.e., in less than 1 month)	a 0 1 2

C. Physical Signs

9. Appetite loss: eating less than usual	a 0 1 2
10. Weight loss (score 2 if greater than 5 lb. in 1 month)	a 0 1 2
11. Lack of energy: fatigues easily, unable to sustain activities (score only if change occurred acutely, i.e., in less than 1 month)	a 0 1 2

D. Cyclic Functions

12. Diurnal variation of mood: symptoms worse in the morning	a 0 1 2
13. Difficulty falling asleep: later than usual for this individual	a 0 1 2
14. Multiple awakenings during sleep	a 0 1 2
15. Early morning awakening: earlier than usual for this individual	a 0 1 2

E. Ideational Disturbance

16. Suicide: feels life is not worth living, has suicidal wishes, or makes suicide attempt	a 0 1 2
17. Poor self-esteem: self-blame, self-depreciation, feelings of failure	a 0 1 2
18. Pessimism: anticipation of the worst	a 0 1 2
19. Mood congruent delusions: delusions of poverty, illness, or loss	a 0 1 2

Scoring System
a = unable to evaluate
0 = absent
1 = mild or intermittent
2 = severe
Ratings should be based on symptoms and signs occurring during the week prior to interview. No score should be given if symptoms result from physical disability or illness. Scores of 12 or greater indicate probable depression.

Note: From "Cornell Scale for Depression in Dementia," by G. S. Alexopoulos, J. R. Young, and C. A. Shamoian, 1988, *Biological Psychiatry, 23*, pp. 271–284. Reprinted with permission from the Society for Biological Psychiatry.

In recent years, more attention has been paid to the importance of diagnosing and treating subsyndromal or minor depression. It is diagnosed with the occurrence of one or more periods of depressive symptoms that are identical to major depressive periods in duration, but which involve fewer symptoms and less impairment. A minor depressive episode includes either a period of sad or "blue" mood or a loss of interest in activities and at least two additional depressive symptoms (APA, 2000).

There is growing evidence that supports aggressive treatment of minor depressive episodes. Twenty-five percent of persons with minor depression will go on to experience a major depression episode (Lyness, King, Cox, Yoediono, & Caine, 1999; Oxman, Barrett, & Gerber, 1990). Parmelee, Katz, and Lawton (1992) demonstrated that over time nursing home residents who exhibited minor depressive symptoms went on to develop major depression at a greater rate than those who did not exhibit depressive symptoms.

The DSM-IV criteria for major depression, dysthymia, and minor depression do not capture symptoms distinctive of geriatric depression. Older adults tend to have more somatic and cognitive complaints (Alexopoulos et al., 2002). They may not report a sad feeling but instead complain of a lack of feeling or emotion, apathy, or fatigue. Anxiety, nervousness, or increased worry are also common complaints of older adults experiencing depression. This presentation may be described as "depression without sadness" (Gallo & Rabins, 1999). For example, the primary complaint of an older adult may be anxiety or difficulty with concentration or memory. When evaluated further, additional symptoms are present that add up to a diagnosis of depression.

The DSM-IV criteria for depression require that for a diagnosis of major depression, dysthymia, or minor depression, symptoms are not the result of a medical condition (e.g.,

hypothyroidism, vitamin deficiency) or a substance (e.g., medication, alcohol). Assessing depression in older adults is complicated by the fact that more frequently than not, the older adult is also experiencing the symptoms of chronic illnesses and/or symptoms of dementia.

Brown, Lapane, and Luisi (2002) found that nursing home residents with several diagnoses, including cancer, were all less likely to receive pharmacological treatment for depression. The tendency is to attribute symptoms of depression to other physical conditions because of the stigma associated with a depression diagnosis. Residents of nursing homes who were female, Black, or cognitively impaired were less likely to receive treatment (Brown et al., 2002). Because depression in older adults is underrecognized and undertreated, it is recommended that all older adults be screened using a structured instrument, such as the GDS or Cornell Scale for Depression. If a screening tool is not used, then an "inclusive" approach, in which all depressive symptoms are indicative of depression, should be adopted. If depression is suspected, a referral should then be made for a more thorough medical/psychiatric evaluation, diagnosis, and treatment plan. The medical evaluation for depression includes a thorough evaluation of the causes for the depressive symptoms guided by a review of systems, a physical examination, including a neurologic examination, and laboratory work. The laboratory examination should include, but not be limited to (depending on findings in the review of symptoms): serum electrolytes, complete blood count with platelets, thyroid panel with thyroid-stimulating hormone, B12, and folate. The evaluation for depression includes an evaluation of medical conditions that contribute to depressive symptoms (Table 7-3) and medications that can cause depressive symptoms (Table 7-4). The *Nursing Standard of Practice Protocol: Depression in Older Adult Patients* is a refer-

TABLE 7-3 Physical Illnesses Associated with Depression in Older Adults

Metabolic Disturbances

Dehydration
  Azotemia, uremia
  Acid-base disturbances
  Hypoxia
  Hyponatremia and hypernatremia
  Hypoglycemia and hyperglycemia
  Hypocalcemia and hypercalcemia
Endocrine Disorders
  Hypothyroidism and hyperthyroidism
  Hyperparathyroidism
  Diabetes mellitus
  Cushing's disease
  Addison's disease
Infections
  Viral: pneumonia, encephalitis
  Bacterial: pneumonia, urinary tract, meningitis, endocarditis
  Other: tuberculosis, brucellosis, fungal, neurosyphilis
Cardiovascular Disorders
  Congestive heart failure
  Myocardial infarction, angina
Pulmonary Disorders
  Chronic obstructive lung disease
  Malignancy
Gastrointestinal Disorders
  Malignancy (especially pancreatic)
  Irritable bowel
  Other organic causes of chronic abdominal pain, ulcer, diverticulosis, hepatitis
Genitourinary Disorders
  Urinary incontinence
Musculoskeletal Disorders
  Degenerative arthritis
  Osteoporosis with vertebral compression or hip fractures
  Polymyalgia rheumatica
  Paget's disease
Neurologic Disorders
  Cerebrovascular disease
  Transient ischemic attacks
  Stroke
  Dementia (all types)
  Intracranial mass: Primary or metastatic tumors
  Parkinson's disease
Other Illnesses
  Anemia (of any cause)
  Vitamin deficiencies
  Hematologic or other systemic malignancy

Note: From "Nursing Standard of Practice Protocol: Depression in Older Adult Patients," by L. H. Kurlowicz, 1997, *Geriatric Nursing* 18(5), p. 197. Reprinted with permission from Elsevier.

TABLE 7-4   Drugs that Cause Symptoms of Depression in Older Adults

Antihypertensives
    Reserpine
    Methyldopa
    Propranolol
    Clonidine
    Hydralazine
    Guanethidine
    Diuretics (by causing dehydration or electrolyte imbalance)
Analgesics
    Narcotics
    Morphine
    Codeine
    Meperidine
    Pentazocine
    Propoxyphene
Nonnarcotic
    Indomethacin
Antiparkinsonian agents
    L-dopa
Antimicrobials
    Sulfonamides
    Isoniazid
Cardiovascular agents
    Digitalis
    Lidocaine (toxicity)
Hypoglycemic agents (by causing hypoglycemia)
Steroids
    Corticosteroids
    Estrogens
Others
    Cimetidine
    Cancer chemotherapeutic agents

Note: From Kurlowicz, 1997, p. 198. (See Note, Table 7-3)

ence tool that provides a systematic approach to assessing older adults for depression (Kurlowicz et al., 1997).

SUICIDE

Older adults who are widowed, live alone, have poor sleep quality, lack someone in whom they can confide, are grieving, are experiencing family discord, perceive themselves to be physically ill, suffer from chronic depression, and who have a history of prior suicide attempts are at high risk for suicide (Blazer, 2003; Conwell, Duberstein, & Caine, 2002). The consensus of expert clinicians is that the severity of the depressive illness, the presence of psychosis, alcoholism, a recent loss or bereavement, abuse of sedatives or hypnotics, and the development of disability are the greatest risk factors for suicide in older adults (Alexopoulos et al., 2001). "Older adult suicides give fewer warnings to others of their suicide plans, use more violent and potentially deadly methods to commit suicide, and apply those methods with greater planning and resolve" (Conwell et al., p. 194). It is imperative that nurses assess for suicidal ideation or intent, keeping in mind that noncompliance with medical recommendations may be suicidal behavior (Conwell et al.). A patient who speaks of wanting to die, who states they would be better off dead, or who exhibits behavior that indicates they are preparing for their imminent death, including not following medical treatment, must be further assessed by asking poignant questions that determine the older adult's intentions. The nurse must be open to hearing and seeing this behavior among older adults, as there is great reluctance among nurses to ask patients if they are suicidal. As health care providers, nurses must assess their own beliefs and prejudices surrounding suicide as these can interfere with the ability to provide a complete assessment of a patient suffering from a potentially life-threatening illness.

Having a suicide protocol in place that clearly defines how the nurse will intervene should the nurse receive an affirmative response to the questions, "Do you have thoughts of ending your life? Or do you have a plan and intend to carry it out?" will increase the nurse's comfort in completing a full assessment of the depressed patient. The protocol must include the involvement of others responsible for the care of the patient, such as the physician, nursing supervisor, family members, and others with whom the patient has a trusting relationship, such as a clergy person. If the patient has the intent to commit suicide and a plan to carry it out, then he or she must undergo constant supervision until hospitalization and the potential for carrying out the intent has been eliminated. If there is suicidal thought or ideation, then the nurse must, in conjunction with other health care providers, including a psychiatrist, develop a plan for keeping the patient safe. Involving

someone in whom the patient feels comfortable confiding is important. The plan should include removing all lethal weapons or other means of suicide, consistent companionship, or day treatment, if hospitalization is not possible, and close monitoring of the depression by a mental health specialist or the health care provider.

■ TREATMENT OPTIONS

The treatment options for depression are pharmacological, psychotherapeutic and psychosocial interventions, and electroconvulsive therapy. Novel treatment options such as transcranial magnetic stimulation are currently being investigated. The most effective treatment is a combination of pharmacological therapy and psychotherapy (DHHS, 1999). The goal of treatment is for the patient to return to his or her baseline prior to the depression episode or to where the residual physiological symptoms are clearly related to a chronic illness.

Depression is a recurring illness and the use of a combination of treatments such as medications, psychotherapy, and the adoption of positive psychosocial behaviors will help prevent relapse and assist the client and his or her family to detect relapse early.

Recovery or obtaining a remission is not immediate. It may take longer for older adults to respond to treatment (Nelson, 2001). Generally, medications take four to six weeks to be effective and often months to reach optimal treatment. Some trial and error is involved in the treatment of depression requiring several different medication trials or combinations of medications. Frequently patients are the last to recognize their improvement despite family members being able to see positive changes; therefore, reassurance, as well as identification and discussion of areas of improvement with the older adult may be beneficial and facilitate continuation of treatment. Older adults may blame a relapse or the recurrence of symptoms on other physical illnesses or life situations, continuing to deny their psychiatric illness. On the other hand, because of the pain and disability experienced when depressed, some patients will become hypersensitive to their mood by becoming concerned that they are becoming depressed again whenever they have a "down" day or two as the result of normal life experiences. Patients need to be taught and reminded of the signs and symptoms of depression and their own presentation. They also may need to be reminded of the self-care strategies they have learned and when to seek professional care.

▓▓▓ PHARMACOLOGIC TREATMENT OPTIONS

Recommendations for pharmacotherapy in older adults are based on expert consensus because the majority of clinical trials are conducted in younger patients (Alexopoulos, Katz, Reynolds, Carpenter & Docherty, 2001). Clinicians treating older adults must apply what is known from clinical trials to a population of patients who generally have a number of coexisting medical conditions, metabolize medications more slowly, and are taking other medications that contribute to their depressive symptoms (Alexopoulos et al., 2001). Antidepressant medications most frequently used in older adults include the selective serotonin reuptake inhibitors (SSRIs), serotonin and norepinephrine reuptake inhibitors or modulators (SNRIs), and unicyclic aminoketone (e.g., bupropion). Medications used less frequently in older adults include piperazine (e.g., trazodone, nefazodone), tricyclic antidepressants (TCAs) and monoamine oxidase inhibitors (MAOIs). Although individuals will respond differently to medications, all of the medications are 60%–80% effective (McDonald, 2000).

The Expert Consensus Guideline Series (Alexopoulos et al., 2001) supports the use of SSRIs or Venlafaxine XR in combination with psychotherapy as the first line of treatment for unipolar nonpsychotic major depression (Table 7-5). This is largely due to the presumed low side-effect profile of the SSRIs. The currently available data, particularly that which pertains to older adults, does not support the use of hypericum perforatum (St. John's wort) or other herbals and botanicals over standard clinical care for the treatment of depression (Alexopoulos et al., 2001; Desai & Grossberg, 2003; Davidson et al., 2002). Table 7-6 provides an overview of the antidepressants most commonly recommended for older adults.

The familiar geriatric axiom "start low, go slow" holds true when prescribing antidepressants. However, a common mistake is to undertreat or not raise the dosage to its higher limits in order to eliminate all depressive symptoms or obtain full remission. Anxiety is a common residual symptom of depression, and it is recommended that the dose of antidepressant medication, other than TCAs, be raised to its highest therapeutic level in an attempt to treat the anxiety (Alexopoulos et al., 2001). The patient should be maintained on the dose of that medication that adequately treated the depressive illness for at least one year if it is their first episode of depression (Alexopoulos et al.). Experts vary in their recommendations as to how long a patient should be maintained on the antidepressant if it is their second or third depressive episode. Alexopoulos et al. note that in addition to the number of depressive episodes, other factors such as severity of the illness and how well the illness responded to treatment will play a role in the decision to continue treatment for three years or longer.

For patients with symptoms of minor depression or dysthymia, which have persisted for two to three months, the first line of treatment is medication with psychotherapy or medication or psychotherapy alone (Alexopoulos et al., 2001). Watchful waiting

TABLE 7-5   Medication and Treatment Selection Strategies for Unipolar Nonpsychotic Major Depression (Mild and Severe) and Unipolar Psychotic Major Depression

Mild Depression

Preferred	Alternate
Antidepressant medication and psychotherapy	Antidepressant medication alone or psychotherapy alone
SSRI Venlafaxine XR	Bupropion Mirtazapine

Severe Depression

Preferred	Alternate
Antidepressant medication and psychotherapy Antidepressant medication alone	ECT
SSRI Venlafaxine XR	TCAs Mirtazapine Bupropion

Psychotic Depression

Preferred	Alternate
Antidepressant (SSRI or Venlafaxine XR) plus antipsychotic (risperidone, olanzapine, quetiapine) or electroconvulsive therapy	Medication plus psychotherapy Antidepressant: TCA Antipsychotics: Ziprasidone or Aripiprazole*

* Ziprasidone had just been released at the time of the Expert Consensus Guidelines Survey and Aripiprazole had not yet been released.

Note: From The Expert Consensus Guideline Series: Pharmacotherapy of Depressive Disorder in Older Adults. A Postgraduate Medicine Special Report, pp. 24–25, by G. S. Alexopoulos, I. R. Katz, C. F. Reynolds, D. Carpenter, and J. P. Docherty, 2001. Minneapolis, MN: McGraw-Hill. Adapted with permission.

and psychoeducation or psychotherapy is recommended for patients who exhibit dysthymic disorder or minor depressive symptoms for a few weeks or more.

The most common side effects of the SSRIs are mild nausea, stomach upset, and a slight jittery feeling similar to what caffeine may cause. These common but mild side effects will usually go away in seven to ten days and are minimized by slow titration of dosage. Serotonergic drugs can cause a "serotonin syndrome," which can be mild to severe nausea, tremor, difficulty sleeping, and anxiety. This occurs most frequently when a medication is started, possibly at too high of

a dose or when added to another serotonergic medication, such as L-tryptophan, hypericum (St. John's wort), MAOIs, or lithium (McDonald, 2000). This should be addressed by decreasing or eliminating a serotonergic medication. More notable side effects indicating a need to discontinue the medication include rash, agitation, headaches, insomnia, and loss of appetite. The SSRIs are not associated with cardiac effects and they do not potentiate medications that are central nervous system depressants. SSRIs should not be abruptly discontinued. When stopped abruptly, the patient can experience flu-like symptoms.

TABLE 7-6   Dosing and Duration of Medication

Antidepressant	Average starting dose (mg/day)	Average target dose after 6 weeks of treatment (mg/day)	Usual highest final acute dose (mg/day)
SSRIs			
Citalopram	10–20	20–30	30–40
Fluoxetine	10	20	20–40
Lexapro*	5–10	10	20
Paroxetine	10–20	20–30	30–40
Paroxetine CR	12.5	25–37.5	50
Sertraline	25–50	50–100	100–200
SNRI			
Venlafaxine XR	25–75	75–200	150–300
Others			
Bupropion SR	100	150–300 (in divided doses)	300–400 (in divided doses)
Bupropion XL	150	300	450
Mirtazapine	7.5–15	15–30	30–45
TCA			
Nortriptyline**	10–30	40–100	75–125
Desipramine**	10–40	50–100	100–150

*Was not on the market at the time of the Expert Consensus Survey. Dosages given are based on pharmaceutical recommendations.

**Recommended target blood levels:
    Nortriptyline: 50–150 ng/ml
    Desipramine: 115–200 ng/ml
Note: Adapted from Alexopoulos et al., 2001. (See Note, Table 7-5)

Venlafaxine (Effexor), a serotonin–norepinephrine inhibitor (SNRI), does not have any effect on seizure threshold or cardiac side effects. It has a low incidence of sexual dysfunction and drug-induced anxiety that is sometimes seen when starting the SSRIs, and it has a more rapid onset of effectiveness (McDonald, 2000). Similar to the SSRIs, side effects such as nausea, difficulty sleeping, or mild headaches can be minimized by starting the medication at a low dose and titrating up slowly. In some patients, SSRIs and venlafaxine are stimulating and therefore should be given in the morning. If a patient finds the medications to be a little sedating, then they should be dosed in the evening. Venlafaxine should be used with caution in persons with uncontrolled hypertension because it is associated with dose-related hypertension. The patient's blood pressure should be monitored each time the dose is increased.

Bupropion and Mirtazapine are considered high second-line alternatives (Alexopoulos et al., 2001). Bupropion (Wellbutrin), a unicyclic aminoketone, has a side-effect profile similar to the SSRIs. Unlike the SSRIs, it does not cause sexual dysfunction. The medication can be somewhat activating or stimulating, therefore it should not be dosed in the evening because it could interfere with sleep. Bupropion is associated with an increased risk of seizure. The risk of seizure has been significantly decreased with the newer sustained release (SR) and extended release (XL) formulas.

Mirtazapine (Remeron), a piperazinoazepine or serotonin and norepinephrine reuptake modulator, also does not have significant sexual or cardiac side effects. Mirtazapine can cause weight gain. It also is sedating at lower doses. Dosing is counterintuitive with Remeron in that it is more sedating at lower starting doses than at target doses. Remeron is often selected as a treatment because of its side effects of weight gain and sedation, which can be helpful in an older adult with a poor appetite, weight loss, and difficulty sleeping.

Although more difficult to use in older adults because of their side effect profile, tricyclics (TCAs) may be considered an option when treating depression that is unresponsive to the newer antidepressants (SSRIs, SNRIs, and others) that have a more favorable side-effect profile and are better tolerated in older adults (Alexopoulos et al., 2001). The Expert Consensus agrees with research showing the SSRIs are as effective as the TCAs with a better side-effect profile (Alexopoulos et al., 2001). Tricyclic antidepressants are associated with anticholinergic side effects, including dry mouth, tachycardia, increased or decreased sweating, impaired visual accommodation or blurred vision, constipation and urine retention, orthostatic hypotension, and sedation (McDonald, 2000). Older adults are at risk of an anticholinergic-induced delirium in which the patient becomes confused, agitated, or more withdrawn. This could be confused with a worsening of their depression. Most importantly, TCAs can cause heart block and arrhythmias. A TCA overdose is likely to be fatal.

Monoamine oxidase inhibitors (MAOIs) are effective antidepressants but are not used often in older adults because of the risk of severe drug interactions. Like with TCAs, close monitoring for drug interaction is rec-

ommended when prescribing MAOIs (Alexopoulos et al., 2001). Hypertensive crisis can occur when MAOIs are taken with foods that contain tyramine, sympathomimetic medications, narcotics, TCAs, nefazodone (Serzone), and SSRIs.

Finally, piperazines, nefazodone (Serzone), and trazodone (Desyrel), are not frequently used with older adults because they cause orthostatic hypotension and sedation at doses that are needed to have an antidepressant effect. Trazodone, however, may be used as a treatment for insomnia (Alexopoulos et al., 2001) and can be helpful in decreasing agitation in older adults (McDonald, 2000). When these medications are used, the patient needs to be carefully assessed for hypotension and instructed regarding the risk of falls. Neither medications are associated with cardiotoxicity or sexual dysfunction.

PSYCHOTHERAPY

The Expert Consensus Guidelines (Alexopoulos et al., 2001) consider cognitive–behavioral therapy, supportive psychotherapy, problem-solving psychotherapy, and interpersonal therapy to be first-line psychotherapy options. The two forms of psychotherapy that have been studied the most and have been shown to be the most effective in treating depression are cognitive–behavioral therapy (CBT) and interpersonal therapy (Arean & Cook, 2002; Blazer, 2003). There is some evidence that brief dynamic therapy and reminiscence therapy are somewhat effective in treating late-life depression (Arean & Cook). CBT has also been shown to help prevent relapse and improve psychosocial functioning in younger patients (Fava, Grandi, Zielenzny, Canestrari, & Morphy, 1994; Paykel et al., 1999; Scott et al., 2000). Psychotherapy is effective for individuals or in groups. Group therapy is one way of providing a peer group for older adults who have lost their social network or support.

The skilled psychotherapist can treat almost all of the symptoms of depression and the resulting behaviors associated with depression (i.e. hopelessness, anhedonia, anxiety, interpersonal problems, treatment compliance, poor energy, negative thoughts). However, a moderate to severe depressive episode, which may include sleep disturbance, change in appetite, suicidal thoughts and/or psychosis, will almost always require pharmacotherapy as well. Licensed therapists such as clinical nurse specialists, psychiatric nurse practitioners, psychologists, licensed clinical social workers, licensed professional counselors, licensed marriage and family counselors, pastoral counselors, and psychiatrists, are all psychotherapists. However, not all specialize in the therapies proven to be effective in treating depression and not all are skilled at working with older adults.

All advanced practice nurses treating older adults with depression can use CBT techniques (when a therapist is not available or in collaboration with a therapist) with the goal of altering negative behaviors and thought patterns. The basic premise of behavioral therapy is to influence or change behavior that contributes negatively to an individual's depression. Someone who suffers from depression for any length of time will adopt behaviors that exacerbate or perpetuate the symptoms of depression. A hallmark symptom of depression is loss of interest in activities that were pleasurable (anhedonia). Clearly, the depressed person who no longer enjoys things will over time lose social contacts and become less physically active. Being separated from others socially and becoming less physically active, contributes to depressive symptoms. Persons who have been cut off from family and friends and who are inactive because of their depression frequently need to be provided guidance and support to change behaviors. Chronically depressed persons or older adults who are transitioning from work to retirement, or from living independently to

assisted living, may need assistance in identifying activities they enjoy and that provide them with a sense of satisfaction. Likewise, the changing of roles that are the result of retirement, loss of a spouse or friend, or a change in lifestyle can benefit from cognitive therapy where they are assisted with changing their thoughts or perceptions of their changing roles and contributions.

One behavioral therapy strategy is *activity scheduling* (France & Robson, 1997). Activity scheduling requires the patient keep a diary of the activities they were involved in over the week (e.g., watching TV, bathing, grocery shopping). Once the nurse has a clear picture of the patient's level of activity, the patient should be asked to evaluate the activities for themselves, as to whether they are considered an achievement or a pleasurable experience. This information, in addition to the patient's psychosocial history, is used to help the patient identify which activities affect their mood positively and to set goals for increasing those activities. During this process, the older adult might identify numerous barriers to assuming an active lifestyle (e.g., immobility, pain, lack of transportation). Here lies the challenge to the nurse. These barriers should be discussed and the nurse can provide valuable guidance to the older adult in identifying ways to overcome the barriers or alternative activities that will be enjoyable to that individual.

While implementing the "activity scheduling" technique, the nurse is certain to identify the depressed patient's negative or fatalistic attitudes. These negative thoughts are a hallmark of depression. Frequently depression contributes negatively to the patient's self esteem and the negativity becomes a conditioned or an automatic response. Cognitive therapy helps the depressed person recognize his or her negative thoughts and challenges those thoughts with a positive response (France & Robson, 1997). What one thinks about or how one interprets life's events affects mood. France and Robson suggest that even though a thought may be fleeting, the mood it creates may linger. The same is true with a negative interpretation of events.

One cognitive therapy strategy is a *negative automatic thoughts record* (France & Robson, 1997). The patient is instructed to keep record of negative thoughts, including the negative meaning they have assigned to events and images and their mood during that day. The nurse can help the patient evaluate how their thoughts correlate with their moods. The patient is challenged to think about their automatic thoughts regarding an event, if their response (thought) is rational and if not, what is a rational response. A plan to carry out the more positive rational response is developed.

ELECTROCONVULSIVE THERAPY

Electroconvulsive therapy (ECT) is a highly effective treatment for major depression. Published research and expert clinicians support the safety and efficacy of ECT in older adults (Salzman, Wong, & Wright, 2002; Alexopoulos et al., 2001). ECT is most appropriate in psychotic depression and when depression has failed to respond to an antidepressant and antipsychotic medication or in a severe depression that has failed to respond to adequate trials of two antidepressants (Alexopoulos et al., 2001). It is also appropriate for severe depression with acute suicidal risk that may include refusing medication and food (Alexopoulos et al., 2001). Unfortunately, ECT is postponed or not considered a viable treatment option by many patients, families, and clinicians because of its historical negative depiction. Likewise, there are persons who have had negative experiences with ECT and are opposed to the use of ECT. However, similar to many medical procedures, ECT has been developed over past years such that side effects are minimized. The most common side effect of ECT is disturbance of memory

around the time of the course of treatment and possibly loss of memory of isolated events. Cognition is closely monitored during the course of treatment.

Prior to being treated with ECT, the patient undergoes a full medical evaluation including labs, electrocardiogram, and a CT scan of the brain. A recent stroke is a contraindication for ECT. With close monitoring, persons with severe cardiovascular disease can be successfully treated with ECT (Zielinski, Roose, Devanand, Woodring, & Sackeim, 1993).

ECT is administered while the patient is asleep and their muscles are totally relaxed using medication. An electrical stimulus that causes a seizure is administered through the electrodes that are placed on the depressed person's head. The patient does not feel any pain. The patient awakes approximately five to ten minutes following the seizure. The patient is closely monitored for confusion, agitation, headache, and changes in cognition or memory. Any changes are addressed medically as indicated.

NURSING INTERVENTIONS

Nurses can be instrumental in arranging for comprehensive and thus more effective treatment of depression. In addition to pharmacotherapy and psychotherapy, psychosocial interventions need to be considered and included in the treatment plan as appropriate. Psychosocial interventions such as psychoeducation, family counseling, visiting nursing services, bereavement groups, and senior citizen center activities are all strongly recommended as first-line intervention options (Alexopoulos et al., 2001). Kurlowicz (1997) provides a comprehensive list of nursing interventions for the management of depression (Table 7-7).

Depressed older adults need an advocate and someone to provide ongoing supportive counseling that reinforces what they have been taught about the illness. They also need

TABLE 7-7   Nursing Care Parameters

For all levels of depression, develop an individualized plan integrating the following nursing interventions:

1. Institute safety precautions for suicide risk as per institutional policy (in outpatient settings, ensure continuous surveillance of the patient while obtaining an emergency psychiatric evaluation and disposition).
2. Remove or control etiologic agents.
   a. Avoid/remove/change depressogenic medications.
   b. Correct/treat metabolic/systemic disturbances.
3. Monitor and promote nutrition, elimination, sleep/rest patterns, physical comfort (especially pain control).
4. Enhance physical function (i.e., structure regular exercise/activity, refer to physical, occupational, recreational therapies); develop a daily activity schedule.
5. Enhance social support (i.e., identify/mobilize a support person(s) [e.g., family, confidante, friends, hospital resources, support groups, patient visitors]); ascertain need for spiritual support and contact appropriate clergy.
6. Maximize autonomy/personal control/self-efficacy, (e.g., include patient in active participation in making daily schedules, short-term goals).
7. Identify and reinforce strengths and capabilities.
8. Structure and encourage daily participation in relaxation therapies, pleasant activities.
9. Monitor and document response to medication and other therapies; readminister depression screening tool.
10. Provide practical assistance; assist with problem solving.
11. Provide emotional support (i.e., empathic, supportive listening, encourage expression of feelings, instill hope), support adaptive coping, encourage pleasant reminiscences but do not "force" happiness.
12. Provide information about the physical illness and treatment(s) and about depression (i.e., that depression is common, treatable, and not the person's fault).
13. Educate about the importance of adherence to prescribed treatment regimen for depression (especially medication) to prevent recurrence; educate about specific antidepressant side effects and any dietary restrictions.
14. Ensure mental health community link-up; consider psychiatric nursing home care intervention.

Note: Adapted from Kurlowicz et al., 1997, p.195. (See Note, Table 7-3)

assistance in combating the stigma of the illness, problem solving and setting goals, and ongoing reassurance. Just knowing that there is someone to talk to who understands their illness and is available to answer questions and provide reassurance is extremely therapeutic for both the patient and their caregiver.

MODELS OF CARE DELIVERY

Numerous efforts, including the recommendation that all primary care providers screen for depression and the advent of antidepressant medications with fewer side effects, have increased the number of older adults receiving treatment for depression. However, the "expertise gap" (primary clinicians are unable to be experts in all areas) has been cited as the primary reason for older adults not receiving adequate treatment for depression (Bartels et al., 2002). Studies have shown that older adults whose primary care practitioners collaborate with a specialist as opposed to simply consulting a specialist, such as a psychiatrist, psychologist, psychiatric clinical nurse specialist, or other mental health provider, are more adequately treated (Katon et al., 1995; Unutzer, 2002). Similarly collaborative models of care such as Prevention of Suicide in the Primary Care Older Adults Collaborative Trial (PROSPECT) and Improving Mood: Promoting Access to Collaborative Treatment for Late-Life Depression (IMPACT) have been effective by utilizing specially trained nurses within primary care (Bruce & Pearson, 1999; Unutzer et al., 2002). Important components of nursing interventions are patient education regarding the illness and treatment options as well as education regarding support services and ongoing supportive counseling. Similar models of care that utilize specially trained nurses to assess for depression, provide care management, liaison with primary care and mental health specialists, and train residential community staff to recognize depression, have been shown to be effective in decreasing depressive symptoms among older adults in older adult residential communities (Blanchard, 1995; Llewellyn-Jones et al., 1999; Rabins et al., 2000).

An important component of nursing care of older adults with depression that should not be overlooked is the care of the primary caregiver of the depressed person. Caregivers, particularly those caring for a person with a mental illness, are themselves at risk for depression (Horton-Deutsch, Farran, Choi, & Fogg, 2002). Caregivers must be included in the treatment plan and be assessed for symptoms of depression. The PLUS intervention, which provides education, assistance in identification and strengthening of resources and supportive counseling for caregivers, was shown to benefit the depressed patient by improving their personal activities of daily living while decreasing the amount of time the caregiver spent in direct caregiving activities (Horton-Deutsch et al., 2002). By decreasing the caregiver burden, the nurse has taken steps to prevent disability in both the caregiver and the depressed older adult.

REFERENCES

Alexopoulos, G. S., Abrams, R. C., Young, J. R., & Shamoian, C. A. (1988). Cornell scale for depression in dementia. *Biological Psychiatry, 23,* 271–284.

Alexopoulos, G. S., Borson, S., Cothbert, B. N., Devanand, D. P., Mulsant, B. H., Olin, J. T., et al. (2002). Assessment of late life depression. *Biological Psychiatry, 52*(3), 164–174.

Alexopoulos, G. S., Katz, I. R., Reynolds, C. F., Carpenter, D., & Docherty, J. P. (2001). The expert consensus guideline series: Pharmacotherapy of depressive disorders in older adults. *A Postgraduate Medicine Special Report.* Minneapolis, MN: McGraw-Hill.

American Association of Geriatric Psychiatry. (2001). Depression fact sheet. Retrieved November 24, 2004 from http://www.aagponline.org/p_c/depression.asp.

American Psychiatric Association. (2000). *Diagnostic and Statistical Manual of Mental Disorders.* (4th ed.). Washington, DC: Author.

Arean, P. A., & Cook, B. L. (2002). Psychotherapy and combine psychotherapy/ pharmacotherapy for late life depression. *Biological Psychiatry, 52*(3), 293–303.

Bartels, S. J., Dums, A. R., Oxman, T. E., Schneider, L. S., Arean, P. A., Alexopoulos, G. S., et al. (2002). Evidence-based practices in geriatric mental health care psychiatric services, *Psychiatric Services, 53*(11), 1419–1431.

Blanchard, M. R. (1995). The effect of primary care nurse intervention upon older people screened as depressed. *International Journal of Geriatric Psychiatry, 10,* 289–298.

Blazer, D. G. (2003). Depression in late life: Review and commentary. *Journal of Gerontology, 58*(3), 249–265.

Brown, M. N., Lapane, K. L., & Luisi, A. F. (2002). The management of depression in older nursing home residents. *Journal of the American Geriatrics Society, 50,* 69–76.

Bruce, M. L., & Pearson, J. L. (1999). Designing an intervention to prevent suicide: PROSPECT (Prevention of Suicide in Primary Care Older Adults: Collaborative Trial). *Dialogues in Clinical Neuroscience, 1*(2), 100–112.

Conwell, Y., Duberstein, P. R., & Caine, E. D. (2002). Risk factors for suicide in later life. *Biological Psychiatry, 52*(3), 193–204.

Davidson, J. R., Gadde, K. M., Fairbank, J. A., Krishnan, R. R., Califf, R. M., Binanay, C., et al. (2002). Effect of hypericum perforatum (St. John's Wort) in major depressive disorder: A randomized controlled trial. *Journal of the American Medical Association, 287*(14), 1807–1814.

Department of Health and Human Services. *Mental Health. A Report of the Surgeon General.* (1999). Rockville, MD: U.S. Department of Health and Human Services, Substance Abuse and Mental Health Services Administration, Center for Mental Health Services, National Institute of Mental Health.

Desai, A. K., & Grossberg, G. T. (2003). Herbals and botanicals in geriatric psychiatry. *American Journal of Geriatric Psychiatry, 11*(15), 498–506.

Evans, D. L., Charney, D. S., Lewis, L., Golden, R. N., Gorman, J. M., Krishnan, R. R., et al. (2003). Depression Bipolar Support Alliance consensus statement on the diagnosis and treatment of mood disorders in the medically ill. Unpublished manuscript.

Fava, G. A., Grandi, S., Zielenzny, M., Canestrari, R., & Morphy, M. A. (1994) Cognitive behavioral treatment of residual symptoms in primary major depressive disorder. *American Journal of Psychiatry, 151*(9), 1295–1299.

France, R., & Robson, M. (1997). The management of depression. *Cognitive Behavioral Therapy in Primary Care: A Practical Guide.* London: Jessica Kingsly.

Gallo, J. J., & Rabins, P. V. (1999). Depression without sadness: Alternative presentations of depression in late life. *American Family Physician, 60*, 820–826.

Hedelin, B., & Strandmark, M. (2001) The meaning of depression from the life-world perspective of older adult women. *Issues in Mental Health Nursing, 22*, 401–420.

Horton-Deutsch, S. L., Farran, C. J., Choi, E. E., & Fogg, L. (2002). The PLUS intervention: A pilot test with caregivers of depressed older adults. *Archives of Psychiatric Nursing, 16*(2), 61–71.

Katon, W., Korff, M. V., Lin, E., Walker, E., Simon, G. E., Bush, T., et al. (1995). Collaborative management to achieve treatment guidelines: Impact on depression in primary care. *The Journal of the American Medical Association, 273*(13), 1026–1031.

Kurlowicz, L. H., & NICHE faculty. (1997). Nursing standard of practice protocol: Depression in older adult patients. *Geriatric Nursing, 18*(5), 192–199.

Lebowitz, B. D., Pearson, J. L., Schneider, L. S., Reynolds, C. F., Alexopoulos, G. S., Bruce, M. L., et al (1997). Diagnosis and treatment of depression in late life: Consensus statement update. *Journal of the American Medical Association, 278* (14), 1186–1190.

Llewellyn-Jones, R. H., Baikie, A., Smiters, H., Cohen, J., Snowdon, J., Tennant, C. C. (1999). Multifaceted shared care intervention for late-life depression in residential care: Randomized controlled trial. *British Medical Journal, 319*, 676–682.

Lyness, J. M., King, D. A., Cox, C., Yoediono, Z., & Caine, E. D. (1999). The importance of subsyndromal depression in older primary care patients: Prevalence and associated functional disability. *Journal of the American Geriatrics Society, 47*, 757–758.

McDonald, W. M. (2000). Geriatric Psychiatry. In K. R. R. Krishnan, (Ed), *Educational Review Manual In Psychiatry* (pp. 1–44). New York: Castle Connolly Graduate Medical.

National Institute of Mental Health. (1999). Older adults: Depression and suicide facts. Retrieved November 24, 2004 from http://www.nimh.nih.gov/publicat/elderlydepsuicide.cfm.

National Mental Health Association. (1996). American attitudes about clinical depression and its treatment survey. Washington, DC: Author.

Nelson, J. C. (2001). Diagnosing and treating depression in the elderly. *Journal of Clinical Psychiatry, 62* (suppl 24), 18–22.

Oxman, T. E., Barrett, J., & Gerber, P. (1990). Symptomatology of late-life minor depression among primary care patients. *Psychosomatics, 31*, 174–180.

Parmelee, P. A., Katz, I. R., & Lawton, M. P. (1992). Incidence of depression in long-term care settings. *Journal of Gerontology: Medical Sciences, 47,* 189–196.

Paykel, E. S., Scott, J., Tesdale, J. D., Johnson, A. L., Garland, A., & Moore, R., et al. (1999). Prevention in relapse in residual depression by cognitive therapy. *Archives of General Psychiatry, 56*(9), 829–835.

Rabins, P. V., Black, B. S., Roca, R., German, P., McGuire, M., Robbins, B., et al. (2000). Effectiveness of a nurse-based outreach program for identifying and treating psychiatric illness in the older adults. *Journal of the American Medical Association, 283*(21), 2802–2809.

Sadovsky, R. (1998) Prevalence and recognition of depression in older adult patients. *American Academy of Family Physicians, 57*(5), 1096–1097.

Salzman, C., Wong, E., & Wright, B. C. (2002). Drug and ECT treatment of depression in older adults, 1996–2001: A literature review. *Biological Psychiatry, 52*(3), 265–284.

Scott, J., Tesdale, J. D., Paykel, E. S., Johnson, A. L., Abbott, R., Hayhurst, H., et al. (2000). Effects of cognitive therapy on psychological symptoms and social functioning in residual depression. *British Journal of Psychiatry, 177,* 440–446.

Steffens, D. C., Skoog, I., Norton, M. C., Hart, A. D., Tschanz, J. T., Plassman, B. C., et al. (2000). Prevalence of depression and its treatment in an elderly population: The Cache County study. *Archives of General Psychiatry, 57,* 601–607.

Styron, W. (1990). *Darkness Visible: A Memoir of Madness.* New York: Random House.

Tweedy, K., Morrison, M. F., DeMichele, S. G. (2002). Depression in older women. *Psychiatric Annals, 327,* 417–429.

Unutzer, J. (1997). Depression symptoms and the cost of health services in HMO patients aged 65 years and older: A 4-year prospective study. *Journal of the American Medical Association, 277*(20), 1618–1623.

Unutzer, J. (2002). Diagnosis and treatment of older adults with depression in primary care. *Biological Psychiatry, 52*(3), 285–292.

Unutzer, J., Katon, W., Callahan, C. M., Williams, J. W., Hunkeler, E., Harpole, L., et al. (2002). Collaborative care management of late-life depression in the primary care setting. *Journal of the American Medical Association, 288*(22), 2836–2845.

World Health Organization. (1990). *The global burden of disease.* Retrieved April 7, 2004, from http://www.who.int/msa/mnh/ems/dalys/intro.htm.

Yesavage, J. A., & Brink, T. L. (1983). Development and validation of a geriatric depression scale: A preliminary report. *Journal of Psychiatric Research, 17,* 37–49.

Zielinski, R. J., Roose, S. P., Devanand, D. P., Woodring S., & Sackeim, H. A. (1993). Cardiovascular complications of ECT in depressed patients with cardiac disease. *American Journal of Psychiatry, 150*(6), 904-908.

CHAPTER 8

Nursing Assessment and Treatment of Anxiety in Late Life

Marianne Smith, MS, ARNP, CS

INTRODUCTION

The experience of anxiety symptoms is often a complex phenomenon in older adults. Anxiety is a diffuse, unpleasant, and vague feeling of apprehensive expectation and worry that is accompanied by a range of behavioral symptoms such as restlessness, fatigue, difficulty concentrating, irritability, muscle tension, and sleep disturbance (American Psychiatric Association [APA], 2000). Anxiety is the primary symptom in a diverse array of anxiety disorders, regularly occurs as a comorbid condition or symptom in both late-life depression and dementia, is the direct consequence of a wide variety of physical health conditions that are common among aging individuals, and is aroused in response to a wide variety of social, environmental, personal, and health-related stressors that tend to cluster in later life (Blazer, 1997; Lenze, Mulsant, Shear, Houck, & Reynolds, 2002; Small, 1997; Stanley & Beck, 2000).

Understanding and managing anxiety symptoms and disorders in late life is challenging for a number of reasons. Of perhaps most importance, anxiety symptoms exist on a continuum from "normal" reactions to life experiences to "pathological" levels that im-

pair function and create substantial suffering. All people experience anxiety symptoms, to a greater or lesser extent, throughout their lives. Use of diagnostic hierarchies and arbitrary "caseness" criteria that reflect problems of young adults are questionable at a time when little is known about "normal" anxiety in older adults, and in turn, how much anxiety constitutes a "case" (Krasucki, Howard, & Mann, 1999).

Distinguishing appropriate anxiety and worry from excessive anxiety and worry is often difficult for older adults themselves, as well as for mental health and primary care providers who provide treatment for diverse health complaints (Blazer, 1997). In addition, the literature is inconsistent regarding the characteristics of anxiety disorders in older adults, its prevalence in late life (particularly new-onset anxiety disorders), and the extent to which comorbid psychiatric and medical illness account for the observed frequency of anxiety symptoms. Unlike depression and dementia, considerably less research has been conducted specifically with older adults who experience anxiety symptoms and disorders (Dunner, 2000; Flint, 1994). Although older adults are increasingly included in mixed age studies of anxiety, their numbers are too few to draw any reasonable conclusion. As a result, assumptions about diagnosis and treatment are based primarily on studies of younger persons (Blazer).

In spite of the dearth of empirical research to guide clinical practice, anxiety symptoms are commonly observed among older adults, often have profound and negative effects, and regularly result in both increased use of health services and diminished quality of life for both the person who experiences the distress and his or her caregivers (Dugue & Neugroschl, 2002). Nurses and other allied heath providers are challenged to recognize and understand the wide array of problems and health conditions that serve as antecedents to anxiety-related symptoms; to conduct comprehensive, interdisciplinary assessments that use a biopsychosocial framework and examine complex interactions between physical, mental, personal, social, and environmental factors; and to devise effective and lasting interventions that maximize function and comfort.

This chapter emphasizes the often unique problems and issues that may arise in the identification and treatment of late-life anxiety symptoms and disorders, and assumes that the reader has a basic understanding of both anxiety disorders and treatment strategies used with younger age groups. Anxiety symptoms, which are defined here as distressing physical and emotional experiences that often occur as a cluster, but do not meet criteria for diagnosis as a disorder, are an important focus of nursing care and are considered throughout the chapter. Commonly occurring comorbid conditions, including depression, cognitive impairment, physical health conditions, and life stressors, are described. Assessment methods, including factors to consider in the diagnostic workup, presentation of anxiety symptoms in late life, interviewing techniques, and scales that may assist in quantifying symptoms, are addressed. Finally, treatment strategies, including nonpharmacological and pharmacological interventions

that target late-life anxiety disorders, are reviewed.

◼ ANXIETY DISORDERS IN LATE LIFE

A number of important issues are essential to consider if nurses and allied health care providers hope to accurately identify, assess, and treat anxiety symptoms and disorders in older adults. Frequently quoted statistics note that prevalence rates of anxiety disorder are lower in older adults compared to younger ones (Regier et al., 1988; Robins & Regier, 1991). Knowledge of these statistics, combined with prevailing views that new-onset anxiety disorders are uncommon in late life (Flint, 1994; Regier et al.), may inadvertently reduce clinicians' attention to important symptom clusters that are representative of diagnosable disorders, and more importantly, distressing experiences that warrant intervention. Phobias, particularly agoraphobia associated with a specific event, such as falling, generalized anxiety disorders (GAD), and posttraumatic stress disorders associated with trauma earlier in life are all increasingly recognized as emerging for the first time in late life (Blazer, 1997; Flint, 1994; Sadavoy & LeClair, 1997; Stanley & Beck, 2000).

Moreover, anxiety disorders are the most common psychiatric disorders among people of all ages and affect a substantial number of older adults (Stanley & Beck, 2000). Variation in the rates of anxiety vary considerably from study to study, from a low of 0.7% to rates as high as 18.6% (Small, 1997), suggesting that methods used to detect anxiety disorder are highly influential in determining its presence. Thus, appropriate assessment methods and understanding of factors that may confound presentation of late-life anxiety, are essential for accurate detection.

A wide variety of factors are recognized as potentially complicating identification of anxiety disorders in late life. An important perspective to keep in mind is that diagnostic criteria for anxiety disorders, like other psychiatric illness, are largely based on knowledge about younger adults and may not reflect unique problems of late life (Stanley & Beck, 2000). Questions remain about whether anxiety is qualitatively different in older adults compared to younger ones (Christensen et al., 1999), particularly in light of commonly observed subthreshold syndromes that create substantial distress but do not meet current diagnostic criteria (Angst, Merkangas, & Preisig, 1997; Carmin, Wiegartz, & Scher, 2000).

Characteristics of older adults may also influence accurate identification of anxiety, including potential somatization of symptoms (i.e., focus on physical complaints), attribution of symptoms to physical health problems, and unwillingness to acknowledge and report anxiety (Carmin et al., 2000; Krasucki, Howard, & Mann, 1998). For example, older patients with GAD are more likely to present with physical complaints, such as aching, soreness, sweating, trembling, or nausea, rather than psychological complaints of anxiety or worry (Gorman, 2001). Table 8-1 presents commonly expressed anxiety-related

TABLE 8-1   Anxiety Symptoms in Older Adults

Cognitive	Vigilance/Scanning	Motor Tension	Autonomic Arousal/ Somatic
Anxiety	Hyperattentiveness	Shakiness	Anorexia
Worry	Feeling "on edge"	Jitteriness	Body aches and pains
Apprehensive expectation	Impatience	Jumpiness	Diaphoresis, sweating
Rumination	Irritability	Trembling	Diarrhea
Anticipation that something	Distractibility	Tension	Dizziness
bad is about to happen:	Difficulty concentrating	Muscle aches	Dry mouth
• Fear of fainting	Insomnia	Fatigability	Dyspnea
• Fear of losing control	Difficulty falling asleep	Inability to relax	Headache
• Fear of dying	Interrupted sleep	Eyelid twitch	Faintness
• Fear that family members	Fatigue on awakening	Furrowed brow	Fatigability
are ill or injured		Strained face	Flushing
		Fidgeting	Frequent urination
		Restlessness	Insomnia
		Easy startle	Heart pounding
		Sighing	Hot or cold spells
			Light-headedness
			Nausea, upset stomach
			Palpitations
			Pallor
			Paresthesias
			Pulse increased at rest
			Tremor
			Vomiting

From *Diagnostic and Statistical Manual of Mental Disorders* (3rd ed.), APA, 1980, Washington, DC; Also from "Generalized Anxiety Disorder in the Elderly," by F. Dada, S. Sethi, and G. T. Grossberg, 2001, *Psychiatric Clinics of North America*, 24(1), pp. 155–164; also from "Overview and Clinical Presentation of Generalized Anxiety Disorder," by K. Rickels and M. Rynn, 2001, *Psychiatric Clinics of North America*, 24(1), pp. 1–177; also from "Recognizing and Treating Anxiety in the Elderly," by G. W. Small, 1997, *Journal of Clinical Psychiatry*, 58(Suppl. 3), pp. 41–50.

symptoms in the older adult. The fact that late-life anxiety disorders are largely under-recognized and undertreated in primary care settings suggests that both patients and providers have difficulty recognizing anxiety symptoms and disorders in the older adult (Harman, Rollman, Hanusa, Lenze, & Shear, 2002; Small, 1997).

COMORBID CONDITIONS

Depression (Beekman et al., 2000; Flint & Rifat, 2002; Lenze et al., 2000), cognitive impairment, physical health problems, alcohol abuse (Devanand, 2002; Dunner, 2000), and longstanding personality disorder (Coolidge, Janitell, & Griego, 1994) are also widely recognized as complicating the identification and treatment of anxiety disorders in older adults. Each creates similar yet somewhat different anxiety symptoms that must be distinguished as a separate anxiety disorder, or understood as being the result of the comorbid mental or physical health problem. Treatment approaches are largely guided by underlying causal factors, making this differentiation an important first step in care planning.

Depression and Anxiety

Some clinicians and researchers suggest that anxiety symptoms are the result of late-life depression (Gorman, 2001), producing what is often labeled as "anxious depression." Others observe that anxiety disorders commonly co-exist with depression in late life, constituting a condition of comorbid anxiety and depression (Beekman et al., 2000; Lenze et al., 2001). Still others note that the overlap between diagnostic criteria for GAD and major depression, both of which include fatigue, concentration impairment, sleep disturbance, and restlessness, creates substantial diagnostic confusion (Rickels & Rynn, 2001). Irrespective of the position taken, prominent anxiety symptoms affect as many as 50% of patients with depres-

sion and rates of comorbid anxiety disorder and depression range from 2.5% to 38% (Alexopoulos, 1990; Lenze et al., 2001; Lenze et al., 2000; Mulsant, Reynolds, Shear, Sweet, & Miller, 1996).

Most importantly, comorbid anxiety and depression in older adults produces greater severity of illness and poorer treatment responses than is observed in either condition alone (Lenze et al., 2001). Older adults with comorbid anxiety and depression have more severe somatic symptoms, poorer social function, and greater suicidal ideation (Lenze et al., 2000). In addition, medically ill older patients who experience anxiety and depression have greater disability and poorer outcomes compared to those who do not experience psychiatric symptoms (Lenze et al., 2001). Emerging treatment research suggests that the most important factor in improving anxiety symptoms is reduction of depression severity (Flint & Rifat, 2002), an important consideration for providers when formulating care plans and interventions.

Cognitive Impairment and Anxiety

Anxiety symptoms associated with cognitive impairment, early dementia, and/or behavioral symptoms in middle to later dementia are another area of concern in the nursing care of older adults. Although anxiety and anxiety-related symptoms are often the focus of clinical care (Mahoney, Volicer, & Hurley, 2000), limited research focuses on anxiety and anxiety-related symptoms in Alzheimer's disease (AD) and related disorders (Ferretti, McCurry, Logsdon, Gibbons, & Teri, 2001).

Anxiety-related symptoms affect as many as 40% to 80% of individuals with AD (Teri et al., 1999). Table 8-2 provides an overview of common indicators and examples of anxiety in dementia. Anxiety may arise as an emotional response to confusing or uncomfortable aspects of the environment, be the result of medical conditions or their treatments, stem from overlapping psychiatric conditions like depression or psychosis, or be directly caused by pathological changes associated with dementia (Hall & Buckwalter, 1987; Mahoney et al., 2000). Recognition of diverse behaviors that may represent apprehension and worry among individuals who are unable to clearly formulate their fears is essential to devising interventions to reduce or eliminate possible sources of discomfort, and to providing needed reassurance and comfort measures.

Physical Health Conditions and Anxiety

Another challenging area for nurses and other allied health personnel is the differentiation of anxiety stemming from an anxiety disorder and anxiety related to general medical conditions that tend to cluster in later life. Physical and mental illness are connected and interact in several important ways (Buckwalter, Smith, & Mitchell, 1993; Kogan, Edelstein, & McKee, 2000; Sable & Jeste, 2001). First, physical illness can *directly cause* the symptoms of anxiety, as reflected in the diagnosis "Anxiety due to . . . [a specific general medical condition]" (APA, 2000, p. 479). As illustrated in Table 8-3, a wide variety of physical health problems are known to cause anxiety symptoms. Physical illness and its treatment may trigger a *reaction* of apprehension and worry. This is especially true of illnesses that cause fear of pain or

---

TABLE 8-2 Indicators and Examples of Anxiety in Dementia

Verbal Indicators
- *Asking repeated questions*: "Is it all right?" "Where is my [daughter]?" "When are we going?"
- *Repeated statements indicating distress*: "Oh dear, oh dear, oh dear . . ." "Help me, help me, help me."
- *Quivering tone of voice*: Vocal inflections sound uncertain, fearful, apprehensive.

Facial Indicators
- *Facial tension, frowning*: appears worried, as if something bad is about to happen
- *Angry or suspicious expressions*: signals self-protective response to threat of harm
- *Watchfulness, glancing about*: self-protective monitoring of environment

Emotion Indicators
- *Wariness*: expectation that you, others, are about to do harm; cannot be trusted
- *Fearfulness*: cannot name source of threat but is afraid
- *Crying, tearfulness*: expression of distress and apprehension, more than sadness; says "I don't know what is wrong" when asked
- *Irritability*: easily upset with little provocation; on edge; may blame caregiver, e.g., "It's YOU! You did it!"
- *Angry outbursts, resistiveness*: self-protective reaction to unclear threat of harm; pulls back, tries to "escape" from caregiver or situation

Motor Indicators
- *Reduced eye contact*: looks away, averts eyes as if to avoid contact with harm
- *Restlessness, fidgeting, inability to sit still*: gets up and down from chair, checks doors or windows, wiggles or squirms; can't get comfortable due to sense of threat
- *Repetitive movements*: tapping, rubbing hands together
- *Pacing*: purposeless wandering seeking reassurance or safety; checking behaviors
- *Shadowing*: closely following caregivers to assure personal safety
- *Escalation*: unrelieved anxiety increases and results in verbally and physically agitated behaviors

TABLE 8-3 General Medical Conditions That Cause Anxiety Symptoms		
Metabolic	**Endocrine**	**Neurological**
Acidosis	Cushing's Syndrome	Cerebral anoxia
Dehydration	Hyper- and hypothyroidism	Cerebral neoplasm
Electrolyte imbalance	Hyperadrenocorticism	Delirium
(e.g., hypercalcemia)	Hypo- or hyperparathyroidism	Dementia
Hyperthermia	Hypoglycemia, hyperinsulinism	Epilepsy
Porphyria	Pheochromocytoma	Parkinson's disease
	Vitamin B-12 deficiency	Post-concussion disorders
		Vestibular dysfunction
		Encephalitis
Cardiovascular	**Respiratory**	**Other conditions**
Angina pectoris	Chronic obstructive pulmonary	Influenza
Arrhythmia	disease	Hepatitis
Cerebral atherosclerosis	Pneumonia	Constipation
Congestive heart failure	Hyperventilation	Pain
Mitral valve prolapse	Hypoxia	
Pulmonary embolism		

Note: From *Diagnostic and Statistical Manual of Mental Disorders* (4th ed.), 2000, Washington, DC: APA; also from "Anxiety Disorders. Helping Patients Regain Stability and Calm," by M. Dugue and J. Neugroschl, 2002, *Geriatrics, 57*(8), pp. 27–31; also from "Recognizing and Treating Anxiety in the Elderly," by G. W. Small, 1997, *Journal of Clinical Psychiatry, 58*(Suppl. 3), pp. 41–50.

cause chronic pain, disability, or loss of function, that affect self-esteem, increase dependence, or cause fear of death in relation to severe illness (Buckwalter et al.). Of importance, anxiety disorders may also be antecedent to physical health problems, such as gastrointestinal disorders (Stoudemire, 1996). Older adults tend to present with somatic rather than psychological complaints, which can further confuse whether problems are due to anxiety or physical problems. Medications that are commonly used to treat physical and mental health conditions may cause anxiety-like symptoms, as illustrated in Table 8-4. Anxiety disorders are widely recognized as existing comorbidly with health conditions (Stoudemire).

The importance of interactions between physical health conditions and anxiety is underscored by the potential downward spiral of disability that may occur as anxiety symptoms interfere with daily function in a kind of "self-fulfilling prophecy." For example, the person who has fallen is anxious about falling again, so restricts his or her activity. Activity restriction in turn causes disuse atrophy, which increases the risk of falling again, places him/her more at risk for problems associated with immobility, and creates an even greater sense of apprehension about abilities. One problem complicates another and so the spiral turns downward.

Late-Life Change and Anxiety

Psychosocial issues and changes that occur in later life, including frailty, social isolation, financial changes, caregiving responsibilities,

TABLE 8-4	Medications and Substances Associated with Anxiety Symptoms		
Intoxication	**Withdrawal**	**Medications**	**Heavy Metal & Toxins**
Alcohol	Alcohol	Analgesics / Anesthetics	Carbon dioxide
Amphetamines	Anxiolytics	Anticholinergics	Carbon monoxide
Cannabis	Barbituates	Anticonvulsants	Gasoline, paint, other volatile
Cocaine	Cocaine	Antidepressants	substances
Hallucinogens	Hypnotics	Antihistamines	Nerve gases
Inhalants	Narcotics	Antihypertensives	Organophosphate insecticides
Phencyclidine	Nicotine	Antiparkinsonian medications	
	Sedatives	Antipsychotics, atypical antipsychotics	
		Bronchodilators (e.g., albuterol, terbutaline)	
		Caffeine	
		Corticosteroids	
		Digoxin	
		Insulin	
		Lithium carbonate	
		Meclizine HCL	
		Nonsteroidal anti-inflammatory agents	
		Over-the-counter cough/cold preparations (e.g., pseudoephedrine, caffeine)	
		Over-the-counter hypnotics	
		Tobacco	
		Theophylline	
		Thyroid preparations (e.g., thyroxine)	

Note: From APA, 2000; Dugue & Neugroschl, 2002; Small, 1997. (See Note, Table 8-3)

safety issues and other age-related changes, may also arouse anxious feelings and behaviors and thus contribute to diagnostic difficulties. As noted earlier, determining what is "excessive" worry is sometimes difficult when the older person faces a number of real-life problems and stressors.

Because anxiety disorders are widely recognized as having an onset in adolescence and early adulthood, thoughtful examination of longstanding patterns of behavior is essential. For a variety of historical and social reasons, many older adults who experienced mental illness during their lifetime were not identified, diagnosed, or treated. As a result, life review that includes assessment of long-

standing patterns of coping, social history, and both treated and untreated physical health problems, are often essential to establishing a diagnosis of anxiety disorder.

ASSESSMENT OF ANXIETY IN LATER LIFE

The confounding factors that may mimic, precipitate, and coexist with anxiety disorders in late life emphasizes the importance of comprehensive physical, social, and environmental assessment. Like assessment of other health problems in older people, use of a biopsychosocial framework and attention to both current and historical factors is essential to the accurate identification and treatment of anxiety.

History and Physical

Careful and comprehensive history, physical exam, and routine laboratory studies are recommended as part of the diagnostic workup for anxiety disorder in later life (Gorman, 2001; Sable & Jeste, 2001). If assessment is conducted in a mental health setting, collaboration and consultation with the patient's primary care provider, including review of relevant medical records, is warranted (Kogan et al., 2000). Similarly, collateral history from a family member or caregiver who knows the person well can provide important information about current symptoms and past history (Sable & Jeste). Other components that are

important to consider in geropsychiatric assessment of anxiety are briefly described in Table 8-5.

As with assessment of other psychiatric and mental health conditions in late life, avoiding use of medical jargon, and adopting terms and descriptions used by the patient himself or herself to describe the problem (including exploration of somatic symptoms), may be particularly useful. History of anxiety symptoms that existed earlier in life and are now exacerbated due to social or personal changes (e.g., symptoms were "managed" through family or work habits) is important to consider. Likewise, the presence of traumatic life events (e.g., combat, holocaust, prisoner of war) that may serve as antecedents to late-life onset of posttraumatic stress disorder (Stanley & Beck, 2000), or history of anxiety disorder in

---

TABLE 8-5   Components of the Diagnostic Workup

Medical History
- Current and past medical disorders
- Drug and alcohol use; caffeine intake
- Prescribed and over-the-counter medications; use of herbal or home remedies
- Recent changes in health conditions and their treatment (e.g., change in medications)

Psychiatric History and Assessment
- Past psychiatric history, including "nervous breakdowns" or other untreated mental illness
- Rule out or establish coexistence of mood disorders, psychotic disorders, delirium, and dementia
- Consider changes that may represent subsyndromal conditions or early impairment

Laboratory
- Complete blood count, electrolytes, serum glucose, hepatic and renal function tests, thyroid function tests, vitamin B-12 and folate levels, urinalysis, urine toxicology

Other tests
- Electrocardiogram, chest X-ray
- Brain imaging and neuropsychological testing if cognitive impairment is suspected

Collateral history
- Substantiation of symptom onset, range, duration, intensity by family or close friends
- Long-standing personality, coping, life history
- Recent events that may contribute

a first-degree relative (Gorman, 2001), may also contribute to understanding the current clinical picture.

Phrasing of questions is an important consideration when interviewing older adults who may not consider their distress as the result of anxiety. For example, "Have you been concerned about or fretted over a number of things?" or "Do you have a hard time putting things out of your mind?" may be more fruitful than traditional questions about worry, rumination, or obsessive thoughts (Lang & Stein, 2001). Likewise, assistance may be needed to place distressing experiences in a temporal framework to understand the duration of problems. In this instance, offering the person a significant date or event to cue memories is often helpful (e.g., "Were you having this experience before [Christmas]?" vs. "When did this first happen?"). Adjusting questions that target possible antecedents to symptoms (e.g., "What were you doing when you noticed the chest pain?") or associated features (e.g., "When you can't sleep, what is usually going through your head?") may also produce meaningful clinical data (Lang & Stein).

Anxiety Symptoms

The wide range of anxiety symptoms that may occur as the result of an anxiety disorder, anxious depression, cognitive impairment, physical illness or psychosocial stress emphasizes the importance of a comprehensive approach until the nature of the person's distress is better understood.

The context of worries is often used to differentiate pathological anxiety (which is excessive) from "normal" worries. As in other age groups, apprehension, anxiety, or worry may be associated with a variety of stressors (e.g., financial changes, health conditions, family changes or problems). Unlike chronic worry that is excessive and disabling, this type of normal anxiety is often situational and

temporary, and may even contribute to effective coping by anticipating future needs (Dugue & Neugroschl, 2002; Gorman, 2001). Clinicians regularly have difficulty deciding what is "justified" given the nature and extent of problems an older adult has experienced. For example, the rationale offered for an older person's fear of leaving home may be related to crime rates and fear of mugging. Whether that fear is reasonable or excessive largely depends on rates of crime in the older person's community, a question that may only be answered with collateral information from family or caregivers.

Assessment Scales

Although a number of well-established instruments exist for the measurement of anxiety, few are validated using older adults, and even fewer are developed with the specific problems and needs of older people in mind. Anxiety assessment scales are categorized as self-report, clinician-rated, or involving direct observation. Just as variability in prevalence rates may be related to the diagnostic classification system used, the range and type of symptoms detected often depends on the measurement method undertaken. For example, some scales purposely remove symptoms that may represent physiological arousal or somatic complaints that might be caused by a comorbid health condition, while others specifically include those symptoms (Sinoff, Ore, Zlotogorsky, & Tamir, 1999). Similarly, clinician-rated diagnostic methods based on current diagnostic criteria may produce different results than self-report measures that include a wider, or different, array of anxiety symptoms. In short, keeping the purpose of the assessment measure clearly in mind, and weighing the value of the rating against other data (e.g., patient complaints, physical exam, collateral interview data), reduces the risk of faulty conclusions about the presence of anxiety disorder in older adults (Kogan et al., 2000).

No matter which tool, scale, or method is used, clinicians must be alert to the fact that serious questions remain about the nature of anxiety in late life. Additional research is needed to better understand and quantify late-life anxiety. In the meantime, cautious use of existing methods and thoughtful attention to the type of anxiety symptoms being measured (e.g., anxious depression, in cognitive impairment, in medically ill patients, "true" anxiety disorders) is essential.

TREATMENT OF ANXIETY IN LATE LIFE

The treatment methods used with late-life anxiety disorders may include cognitive–behavioral, psychodynamic, supportive, and/or pharmacological interventions. The application of these modalities is based on research with younger age groups that is extrapolated, with or without adaptation, to older people (Krasucki et al., 1999). Late-life anxiety treatment research, like epidemiological and measurement research, is in a relatively early stage.

As in the treatment of younger age groups, the selection of interventions depends largely on the specific anxiety diagnosis, individualized symptom presentation, and concomitant medical conditions and medications being taken by the patient. No matter what type of intervention is used, the relationship between the older person and the therapist or health provider is often critically important in treatment effectiveness.

The value of the therapeutic alliance is a particularly salient issue in treatment of late-life anxiety disorders. The nature of anxiety, which includes apprehensive expectations, worry, fearfulness, and the feeling that one is either dying or going crazy, creates a special need for reassurance and psychological comfort measures (e.g., encouragement, support, reality testing). Additional time is often needed to discuss problems and experiences, explore possible alternative explanations for

symptoms, and provide support for "staying the course" in treatment when relief is slow to develop.

Nonpharmacological Interventions

In general, nonpharmacologic interventions are preferred in the treatment of most anxiety disorders, and are often used in combination with medication. This preference is especially appropriate for older adults who experience age-related changes that affect pharmacokinetics and are likely to be taking an array of medications for physical health conditions that increase risk of drug interactions (Small, 1997). Although little research supports the specific effectiveness of nonpharmacological treatments in older adults, most agree that there is little evidence that strategies used with middle-aged individuals would not also work well with older adults. Unlike medication interventions, nonpharmacological therapies have few, if any, side effects, and may easily be adapted to the unique needs of older people.

A substantial body of literature supports the effectiveness of nonpharmacological interventions for treatment of anxiety in younger age groups. National treatment guidelines for panic disorder (PD) strongly support the efficacy of cognitive–behavioral therapy (CBT), and effective treatment of generalized anxiety disorder (GAD) includes CBT, relaxation, and unstructured therapy techniques. In spite of the known effectiveness of various treatments, several large-scale studies indicate that adults with probable anxiety (and depressive) disorders often do not receive appropriate care (Young, Klap, Sherbourne, & Wells, 2001).

Cognitive–Behavioral Therapy Table 8-6 outlines nonpharmacological and pharmacological therapeutic interventions identified in a review of literature on treatment of late-life anxiety. CBT takes many forms, and generally includes structured therapy to identify, evaluate, control, and modify negative thoughts and cognitive distortions and attributions

TABLE 8-6 Interventions for Anxiety in Older Adults		
	Nonpharmacologic Interventions	**Pharmacologic Interventions**
General Principles	*Systematic treatment studies exploring treatments among older adults are limited* Meta-analysis of 15 studies indicates psychological interventions are more effective than no treatment for older adults (Nordhus & Pallesen, 2003), including • Cognitive–behavioral interventions • Supportive therapy • Progressive muscle relaxation • Pleasant events participation • Imaginal training • Personal construct therapy • Rational emotive therapy Lack of research is not a deterrent to use with older people, as few psychological interventions have side effects. Cognitive–behavioral and other interventions are often the first line of treatment in anxiety disorders, and are often recommended in combination with medication. Adjustments to accommodate older adults' physical and cognitive capacity (e.g., shorter sessions, use of age-relevant coping statements) are indicated.	*Medication side effects are a key consideration in geriatric prescribing* • Benzodiazepines are generally avoided due to associated risk of cognitive impairment, gait instability and falls, psychomotor impairment, daytime sedation, disinhibition, and dependency. • Low dose benzodiazepines are used sparingly, often for short-term relief using short-acting agents, and are monitored closely. • Selective serotonin reuptake inhibitor (SSRI) antidepressants are often the drug of choice, but may also produce side effects and must be monitored. • Tricyclic antidepressants are limited to secondary amines like nortriptyline [Pamelor] and desipramine [Norpramine]. • Monoamine oxidase (MAO) inhibitors may be useful. • Azaspirones like buspirone [Buspar] may be useful. • Medication management follows general geriatric rules of "start low, go slow" but also "target and achieve therapeutic benefits."
Phobias	*Behavioral Interventions* Exposure techniques • Systematic desensitization: confront fear, promote habituation Anxiety management • Progressive muscle relaxation • Controlled breathing *Cognitive-behavioral Interventions* Structured therapy to identify, evaluate, control, and modify negative thoughts and cognitive distortions and attributions • Cognitive restructuring • Positive self-talk • Imagery • Social skills training • Distraction • Thought stopping	Cognitive–Behavioral Therapy is treatment of choice, often in combination with medication [1,3,4] SSRIs [1,3] • Paroxetine [Paxil] * [2] MAO Inhibitors [1,4] • Phenelzine [Nardil] [3] Benzodiazepines [1,3,4] Beta-blockers [3,4] Buspirone [BuSpar] [3]

continues

TABLE 8-6 Interventions for Anxiety in Older Adults (*continued*)		
	Nonpharmacologic Interventions	**Pharmacologic Interventions**
Generalized Anxiety Disorder (GAD)	*Interactive Computer Programs* Use virtual reality techniques to provide modeling and exposure *Supportive Therapy* • Promote therapeutic alliance: interest, availability, predictability, accessibility, empathy, understanding of therapist *Eclectic therapeutic approaches* often in combination, targeting specific symptoms • Biofeedback • Relaxation training • Cognitive–behavioral approaches • Reminiscence therapy • Recreational therapy • Therapeutic touch • Progressive muscle relaxation • Controlled breathing • Thought stopping • Cognitive restructuring • Positive imagery *Psychodynamic therapy* Talk therapy oriented at identification of conflicts and resolution of problems such as • Coping with chronic illness • Death and dying • Understanding aging processes • Sexuality, love, marriage • Ethnicity	Treatment of depression, which is commonly comorbid with GAD, is a primary focus Nonpharmacological interventions are recommended in combination with medication SSRIs[1, 2] • Paroxetine [Paxil] * [2] • Citalopram [Celexa] [2] Unique property antidepressants [1] • Venlafaxine [Effexor] * [1, 2] • Trazodone [Desyrel] [1] Tricyclic antidepressants [1] Azaspirones • Buspirone [BuSpar] [1, 3, 4] Benzodiazepines
Panic Disorders (PD)	*Cognitive–Behavioral Approaches* • Psychoeducational strategies to facilitate increased understanding • Relaxation training • Controlled (diaphragmatic) breathing • Cognitive restructuring	SSRIs [1, 2, 3, 4] • Paroxetine [Paxil] * [2] • Sertraline [Zoloft] * [2] • Citalopram [Celexa] [2] Tricyclic antidepressants [1, 3, 4] MAO inhibitors [1, 3, 4] Benzodiazepines [1, 4]
Obsessive Compulsive Disorder (OCD)	*Behavioral Interventions* • Exposure • In vivo desensitization • Response prevention *Psychodynamic therapy* *Electroconvulsive therapy (ECT)* • OCD symptoms associated with depression	SSRIs [1, 2, 3, 4] • Sertraline [Zoloft]* [2] • Paroxetine [Paxil]* [2] • Citalopram [Celexa] [2] Tricyclic antidepressants [1]

Posttraumatic Stress Disorder (PTSD)	*Psychodynamic Therapy* • Individual therapy • Group therapy (war veterans) • Family therapy • Brief therapy *Cognitive–Behavioral Therapy* • Imagined and in vivo flooding • Thought stopping • Guided self dialogue • Combination approaches: psychoeducation, symptom management, relaxation, group therapy, family education *Supportive Therapeutic Alliance*	SSRIs [1, 2, 3] • Paroxetine [Paxil] * [2] • Sertraline [Zoloft] * [2] Tricyclic antidepressants [1, 2] MAO inhibitors [1, 2]

Note. Asterisks are placed by FDA-approved drugs for treatment of the specific anxiety disorder. Other drugs are listed that are prescribed for off-label purposes in clinical practice because of their potential efficacy. Footnotes placed by drugs indicate the source of information with related citations provided below. Inclusion here does not indicate endorsement of any drug for any purpose.

[1] From "Core Concepts in Geriatrics. Anxiety disorders.," by A. J. Flint, 2001. *Clinical Geriatrics*, 9(11), 21. Paper adapted from the American Geriatrics Society's *Geriatrics Review Syllabus: A Core Curriculum in Geriatric Medicine*, (4th ed.)

[2] From "Beyond Depression: Evaluation of Newer Indications and Off-label Uses for SSRIs," by K. C. Lee, M. D. Feldman, and P. R. Finley, 2002. *Formulary*, 37, 240–251.

[3] From "Treatment of Anxiety Disorders in the Elderly: Issues and Strategies," by J. I. Sheikh and E. L. Cassidy, 2000, *Journal of Anxiety Disorders*, 14(2), 173–190.

[4] From "Treatment of Anxiety Disorders in Late Life, by J. Sadavoy and J. K. LeClair, 1997, *Canadian Journal of Psychiatry—Revue Canadienne de Psychiatrie*, 42(Suppl. 1), 28SN–34SN.

Also from Blazer, 1997; Dugue & Neugroschl, 2002; Krasucki, Howard, & Mann, 1999; Nordhus & Pallesen, 2003; Stanley & Beck, 2000.

combined with behavioral strategies to confront fears and promote habituation. Cognitive–behavioral strategies are often the first line of intervention for treatment of many anxiety disorders (Stanley & Beck, 2000). As indicated in the table, a wide variety of both cognitive, behavioral, and combined cognitive–behavioral strategies can be applied to older individuals using both individual and group modalities.

Several studies shed additional light on the value of talking therapies with older adults. A recent randomized trial comparing CBT to supportive counseling reports that both interventions resulted in improvement in older adults with panic disorder with and without agoraphobia, social phobia, GAD, and anxiety disorder not otherwise specified (Barrowclough et al., 2001). While 71% of subjects receiving CBT showed good improvement, so did 39% of those receiving supportive counseling. This general finding was replicated in a second randomized study of older adults with GAD that compared CBT to a discussion group that focused on worry-provoking topics, and a third group that included individuals who were on a waiting list for therapy (Wetherell, Gatz, & Craske, 2003). Participants in both CBT and the discussion group improved substantially relative to those on the waiting list. Thus, supportive interventions that encourage sharing problems, discussion, and problem solving may be viable alternatives when treating anxiety in late life.

The effectiveness of CBT in late life may rely on adaptations that target the unique problems and issues of older people. Adjustments to therapy include increased structure during sessions, progressing at a somewhat slower rate to promote incorporation of ideas, use of memory aides and prompts (e.g., notebooks, tape recording), and more frequent reinforcement of learning (Wilkinson, 1997). Recent pilot investigations comparing standard CBT to CBT enhanced with learning and memory aids provide support for adapting standard CBT (Mohlman et al., 2003). Other researchers applying standardized CBT without adaptation to older adults with GAD report fair to good results (Durham, Chambers, MacDonald, Power, & Major, 2003; Stanley et al., 2003). A meta-analysis of psychological intervention studies conducted with older adults (10 of 15 involved CBT) reports that these interventions are more effective than placebo (Nordhus & Pallesen, 2003).

Psychodynamic Therapy   No systematic studies of the effectiveness of psychodynamic, insight-oriented psychotherapy for treatment of anxiety disorders in later life were found in the literature. Nevertheless, the benefits of such therapy cannot be ruled out, and may even be of specific value in treating older adults who experience uncomfortable, but not disabling, anxiety, and who are motivated to consider their problems in a psychodynamic framework (Blazer, 1997).

The potential benefits of insight-oriented therapy are perhaps best illustrated in case studies that detail the often complicated life courses that result in late-life mental illness and emotional distress. As told in the story of Maggie, a 65-year-old who presented with anxiety and depression, "creative integrationism" therapy that involves diverse methods oriented at insight about, and resolution

of, long-standing life traumas, can be extremely effective (Edmands & Marcellino-Boisvert, 2002). The following personal communication from Maggie emphasizes the power of both the therapeutic relationship and insight-oriented approaches.

> We seem to have to tell our stories over and over, like a hawk circling. My experience was that we were together in some place other than the now. It began to seem that what I suffered alone I now suffered with "M." [the therapist]. Therein lay my healing. (Edmands & Marcellino-Boisvert, p. 112)

Supportive Therapy   No research targeting supportive methods as an intervention with late-life anxiety disorders is reported in the literature. As noted earlier, however, use of these methods in two "comparison" situations of CBT research lends credence to their use. Nonspecific but supportive methods that encourage description of current problems, feelings, and experiences in a caring atmosphere may be viable alternative interventions.

Use of supportive therapy is consistent with both provision of care to individuals with chronic mental disorders and use of the therapeutic alliance as a curative factor. In some situations, nondirective talking therapy in which the therapist takes a more active role by providing encouragement, support, gentle direction, and/or guidance, education, and reassurance may be beneficial in the treatment of older people. In practice, most therapists working with older adults combine supportive methods with other therapeutic methods like CBT or psychodynamic therapy (Blazer, 1993).

Psychoeducational Strategies   Education about symptoms and symptom management is often a component of anxiety management, and is regularly provided as part of cognitive therapy in which the person is helped to understand their experiences by reframing or restructuring symptoms. Psychoeducational approaches may be particularly useful with older adults who are not familiar with psychological concepts, tend to present with somatic complaints and symptoms, and attribute their distress and discomfort to physical, not mental, health problems.

A promising group intervention uses psychoeducation and skills training with older women who experience anxiety and depression (Schimmel-Spreeuw, Linssen, & Heeren, 2000). Women between 56 and 85 years of age were provided a "course" that targeted enhanced overall knowledge, comfort, symptom management, and function. An overwhelming majority of participants reported improvements in coping with (85.7%) and understanding of (70.6%) their problems as a result of attending the course. In addition, statistically significant decreases in anxiety and depression were observed over time. Thus, educational methods that support understanding, adaptation, and coping among older adults may be effective interventions.

Alternative Therapies and Interventions   A host of supportive and alternative therapies are reviewed in the literature and may be valuable in treating older adults with anxiety symptoms or disorders. An exploratory study of the use of eye movement desensitization and reprocessing (EMDR) in combination with short-term dynamic psychotherapy suggests that these methods may be effective with older, as well as younger, adults (McCullough, 2002). Likewise, a preliminary study of a computer-assisted program that offers psychoeducation, socialization to cognitive and behavioral methods, and promotes self-help exercises suggests that this form of intervention may be an effective treatment tool for older adults with anxiety and depressive disorders (Wright, Wright, Beck, & Salmon, 2004; Wright et al., 2002).

Other therapies are regularly described in the context of treating anxiety-provoking medical conditions (e.g., cancer, myocardial infarct), or anxiety that is associated with medical settings (e.g., critical care) or procedures (e.g., pre-, peri-, postsurgery). In this context, nursing interventions to reduce anxiety states include music therapy, aromatherapy, massage (e.g., foot, back), therapeutic touch, light therapy, pet therapy, exercise therapy, self-hypnosis, distraction/redirection (e.g., reminiscence, life review, current events, television viewing), acupuncture, acupressure, and auricular acupressure, as well as cognitive–behavioral strategies such as guided imagery, relaxation exercises and therapy, and other stress-reduction methods.

In spite of the common-sense appeal of many of these interventions, there is little empirical research to support their use for treatment of anxiety disorders. However, several have demonstrated effectiveness with older individuals who experience anxiety (and agitation) as a consequence of dementia (Beck, Modlin, Heithoff, & Shue, 1992; Clair & Bernstein, 1994; Denney, 1997; Whall et al., 1997). Treatment of anxiety symptoms, whether or not they are representative of a true anxiety disorder, is often a nursing challenge. These supportive, therapeutic, "hands on" interventions may be particularly salient to nurses working in day-to-day caregiving settings, and as such, make an important contribution to the care and treatment of frail older people.

Pharmacological Interventions

Medication interventions continue to be the mainstay of treatment for anxiety disorders in both younger and older adults. Regrettably, many medications used with younger people have adverse consequences when used with older adults (e.g., benzodiazepines). A wide variety of normal aging changes influence drug actions in older people: cardiovascular changes contribute to pharmacokinetic alterations; respiratory system changes increase sensitivity to sedative effects; sensitivity to both peripheral and central anticholinergic effects is more likely with advancing age; glomerular filtration rate declines and effects renal clearance; and, perhaps most important, volume of drug distribution (e.g., the ratio of total drug in the body to the amount circulating in the plasma) is altered by decreased total body water, reduced lean body mass and increased body fat, which in turn increases the drug's half-life and extends the time needed for drugs to reach steady state. If liver disease is present, reduced hepatic blood flow and metabolism further compound problems, particularly with benzodiazepines that undergo hydroxylation (e.g., diazepam).

Additional problems are often created by the presence of multiple comorbid medical conditions and medications used to treat them. Potential drug-to-drug interactions that worsen side effects, alter plasma concentrations, and otherwise negatively influence medication performance and/or create toxicity, are all important factors to consider with older people. Furthermore, as the sheer number of medications increases, the complexity of the regimen often also increases (e.g., number of times per day medications are taken, number and type of medications taken at different times of day), creating additional risks for misunderstanding, confusion, and mismanagement of the medication regimen. Because medications have both benefits and associated hazards, geriatric-conscious providers strive to reduce the number of medications used by older people, simplify medication regimens, educate patients regarding the purpose and side-effect profiles of medications prescribed, and provide alternative nonpharmacological interventions whenever possible.

Rational treatment of anxiety disorders in late life demands use of a biopsychosocial framework that blends supportive, assistive, and nonpharmacological interventions with prudent use of medications that are carefully prescribed and monitored. Cognitive–behav-ioral and other psychotherapies should be combined with education and support for patients and family members. Interventions should address significant life stressors and optimize both mental health and physical function, including attention to sleep, exercise, and nutrition needs in order to facilitate best response to medication interventions (Sable & Jeste, 2001).

As in the treatment of other late-life mental disorders, medication interventions are often specifically selected for the type of disorder the person experiences, taking into consideration unique symptom presentations and other conditions and medications currently in use. General principles that apply to the selection and use of medications in older adults also apply to anxiolytic medications. Although use of nonpharmacological interventions as the first line of intervention is always desirable, use of medications is guided by the individual's level of distress and the presence of specific indications, such as anxious depression. Development of clear therapeutic goals and outcome criteria facilitate decision making as doses are titrated, medications are changed, and decisions to augment therapy are made. Clinicians must be confident that a maximum trial with a specific agent is completed without adequate response before making changes. Medications are selected within a classification using the medication's side-effect profile as a basis for decision making. For example, selective serotonin reuptake inhibiting (SSRI) antidepressants are first-line treatment for many anxiety disorders, but within that group of medications, the specific choice is guided by the individual medication's side effects in relation to the patient's symptom profile. For most anxiety disorders, medications with sedating qualities are preferred and those with stimulant properties are avoided. The adage "start low and go slow" applies, but should include additional recommendations to monitor symptom improvement carefully, watch for untoward side effects, offer

encouragement to patients and families because symptom reduction may take time, and
persist in treatment to achieve optimal therapeutic outcomes. The last point is underscored by research that reports older patients
receive "some" but not appropriate levels of
treatment (Young et al., 2001).

As with psychosocial interventions, little
research on medication effectiveness has been
conducted directly with older adults. Most
recommendations are extensions of research
conducted with younger age groups. While
there is some degree of consensus related to
medication use, tremendous variability in
opinion is observed. Medications commonly

recommended for the treatment of specific
anxiety disorders are referenced in Table 8-6
with specific dosing information in Table 8-7.

Benzodiazepines are commonly used with
younger adults who have anxiety disorders,
but must be applied carefully in treatment of
late-life disorders. A number of risks are associated with benzodiazepine use in older
adults. Most stem from normal aging changes
that alter pharmacokinetics and potentiate
negative side effects, such as cognitive impairment, gait instability and increased risk
of falls and hip fractures, psychomotor impairment, sedation, disinhibition, and dependency. Physical dependency may result in

TABLE 8-7   Antianxiety Medications: Drugs and Doses for Older Adults

Name	Starting Dose	Step-Up Dose	Target Dose	Maximum Dose	FDA Approval	Comments
First Line						
Citalopram (Celexa)	10 mg/d	10 mg/d	20 mg/d	40 mg/d	PD	Has minimal cyto-chrome p450 drug interactions
Paroxetine (Paxil)	10 mg/d	10 mg/d	20 mg/d	40 mg/d	GAD, PD, OCD, PTSD, social phobia	Slightly sedating; has cytochrome p450 interactions
Sertraline (Zoloft)	25 mg/d	25 mg/d	100 mg/d	200 mg/d	PD, OCD, PTSD	Has minimal p450 interactions
Venlafaxine XR (Effexor XR)	37.5 mg/d	37.5 mg/d	75–100 mg/d	225 mg/d	GAD	May increase blood pressure at higher doses
Second Line						
Alprazolam (Xanax)	0.125 mg/ bid	0.125 mg/ bid	0.25 mg/ PRN	1 mg/d		Short onset and duration of action; difficult to taper
Lorazepam (Ativan)	0.5 mg/ tid-qid	0.5 mg/d	1.0 mg/tid	4 mg/d		Short onset and duration of action; difficult to taper
Mirtazapine (Remeron)	15 mg/d	15 mg/d	30–45 mg/d	45 mg/d		Sedating properties may help to en-hance sleep

Note: From *DRUGDEX System* (Vol. 121), Greenwich Villge, CO: Also from "A Contemporary Protocol to Assist Primary Care Physicians in the Treatment of Panic and Generalized Anxiety Disorders," by B. L. Rollman, B. H. Belnap, C.
F. Reynolds, III, H. C. Schulberg, and M. K. Shear, 2003, *General Hospital Psychiatry, 25*, pp. 74–82, also from S. Schultz,
personal communication, September 10, 2004.

rebound symptoms when medications are discontinued. Abuse potential, which is a consideration in younger adults, is less often a threat with older adults. In short, there are many reasons to avoid or minimize use of benzodiazepines, particularly older drugs like diazepam (Valium) or chlordiazepoxide (Librium) that are more likely to accumulate and create toxicity.

Additionally, some suggest that tricyclic (TCA) and monoamine inhibiting (MAO) antidepressants should be avoided due to anticholinergic and cardiotoxic side effects (Sable & Jeste, 2001). Yet Flint, a seasoned researcher and clinician who specializes in late-life anxiety disorder, offers these drug categories as alternatives based on the results of controlled clinical trials with mixed age groups (Flint, 2001).

In summary, considerable variation in the management of anxiety in older adults exists, suggesting that the best medication and psychosocial interventions are devised by interdisciplinary teams composed of nurses, social workers, psychologists, psychiatrists, and other ancillary personnel who have expertise in geriatric psychiatry, and who work together to assess and treat older adults using a biopsychosocial framework.

Community and Family Resources

A final consideration in the identification and treatment of late-life anxiety symptoms and disorders relates to accessing sources of assistance. At present, the blended specialization of geriatric psychiatric care in nursing, psychology, social work, and psychiatry is limited to a small group of specialists and services. Although geropsychiatric specializations are growing, day-to-day care and treatment of late-life anxiety disorders is more often provided by generalist health providers in primary care settings, by psychiatric specialists who lack geriatric expertise, or geriatric specialists who lack psychiatric exper-

tise. As a result, access to more specialized information may be needed to promote quality of care.

Several national resources are worthy of mention. Perhaps most important is the Anxiety Disorder Association of America (ADAA), which offers a wide variety of resources that target education and advocacy, including informational materials (some of which are specific to late-life anxiety), an online bookstore, self-help tools, and assistance to find treatment in accessible locations. The ADAA sponsors an annual conference, offers full- and half-day professional workshops, and maintains an easy-to-use Website at http://www.adaa.org.

Although not specific to late-life anxiety disorders, several other national organizations offer assistance related to anxiety disorders. The National Institute of Mental Health (NIMH) provides a wide variety of educational products, including books, fact sheets, and summaries that can be accessed from its Website (http://www.nimh.nih.gov/health information/anxietymenu.cfm). Its free publication, *Anxiety Disorders*, provides a brief overview of various anxiety disorders and lists organizations to contact for further information. The American Psychiatric Association provides an informational page about anxiety (http://www.psych.org/public_info/anxiety.cfm), the American Psychological Association (http://www.apa.org) provides important links and information about anxiety disorder, and the American Association of Geriatric Psychiatry (http://www.agp online. org/links.asp) provides a comprehensive list of links to diverse aging and mental heath organizations, advocacy groups, governmental programs, and professional organizations.

Collectively, these resources provide a wide variety of educational materials that may be used directly or adapted for use with older adults and their families, health care professionals, and community service providers who may be unfamiliar with anxiety disorders. A common theme throughout the literature is underidentification of anxiety disorders that results in unnecessary suffering for older individuals and their families or caregivers. Use of educational resources such as these may be essential to promote appropriate referral and treatment.

◼ SUMMARY

The question of whether anxiety disorders are rare or common in late life will not soon be resolved. In the meantime, evidence supports the fact that distressing, and often disabling, anxiety symptoms are a problem for a substantial number of older people. Nurses are in a key position to identify anxiety-related symptoms and initiate assessment that will lead to appropriate management and treatment. Although some older adults will have long-standing experiences with anxiety disorders that have persisted throughout their lives, others will experience these symptoms for the first time in later life. Whether symptoms represent a diagnosable anxiety disorder is perhaps less important than the fact that the individual will suffer needlessly if assessment and treatment are not addressed. Comprehensive assessment using a biopsychosocial framework, and maximizing the benefits of the therapeutic alliance with the anxious, and often frightened, older person, offers the opportunity to understand the anxiety the older adult is experiencing, and to devise appropriate interventions.

REFERENCES

Alexopoulos, G. S. (1990). Anxiety-depression syndromes in old age. *International Journal of Geriatric Psychiatry, 5,* 351–353.

American Psychiatric Association (1980). *Diagnostic and Statistical Manual of Mental Disorders,* (3rd ed.). Washington, DC: Author.

American Psychiatric Association (2000). *Diagnostic and Statistical Manual of Mental Disorders,* (4th ed.) Washington, DC: Author.

Angst, J., Merkangas, K. R., & Preisig, M. (1997). Substhreshold syndromes of depression and anxiety in the community. *Journal of Clinical Psychiatry, 58(Suppl. 8),* 6–10.

Barrowclough, C., King, P., Colville, J., Russell, E., Burns, A., & Tarrier, N. (2001). A randomized trial of the effectiveness of cognitive-behavioral therapy and supportive counseling for anxiety symptoms in older adults. *Journal of Consulting & Clinical Psychology, 69*(5), 756–762.

Beck, C., Modlin, T., Heithoff, K., & Shue, V. (1992). Exercise as an intervention for behavior problems. *Geriatric Nursing, 13*(5), 273–275.

Beekman, A. T., de Beurs, E., van Balkom, A. J., Deeg, D. J., van Dyck, R., & van Tilburg, W. (2000). Anxiety and depression in later life: Co-occurrence and communality of risk factors. *American Journal of Psychiatry, 157*(1), 89—95.

Blazer, D. G. (1993). *Depression in late life*. St. Louis, MO: Mosby.

Blazer, D. G. (1997). Generalized anxiety disorder and panic disorder in the elderly: A review. *Harvard Review of Psychiatry, 5*(1), 18–27.

Buckwalter, K. C., Smith, M., & Mitchell, S. (1993). When you are more than down in the dumps: Depression in the elderly. In K. C. Buckwalter, M. Smith, & S. Mitchell (Eds.), *The Geriatric Mental Health Training Series*. Iowa City, IA: Hartford Center for Geriatric Nursing Excellence.

Carmin, C. N., Wiegartz, P. S., & Scher, C. (2000). Anxiety disorders in the elderly. *Current Psychiatry Reports, 2*(1), 13–19.

Christensen, H., Jorm, A. F., Mackinnon, A. J., Korten, A. E., Jacomb, P. A., Henderson, A. S., et al. (1999). Age differences in depression and anxiety symptoms: A structural equation modelling analysis of data from a general population sample. *Psychological Medicine, 29,* 325–339.

Clair, A. A., & Bernstein, B. (1994). The effect of no music, stimulative background music, and sedative background music on agitated behaviors in persons with severe dementia. *Activities, Adaptation & Aging, 19*(1), 61–70.

Coolidge, F. L., Janitell, P. M., & Griego, J. A. (1994). Personality disorders, depression, and anxiety in the elderly. *Clinical Gerontologist, 15*(2), 80–83.

Dada, F., Sethi, S., & Grossberg, G. T. (2001). Generalized anxiety disorder in the elderly. *Psychiatric Clinics of North America, 24*(1), 155–164.

Denney, A. (1997). Quiet music: An intervention for mealtime agitation? *Journal of Gerontological Nursing, 23*(7), 16–23.

Devanand, D. P. (2002). Comorbid psychiatric disorders in late life depression. *Biological Psychiatry, 52*(3), 236–242.

DRUGDEX System. *Thomson Micromedex,* (Vol. 121). Greenwich Village, Colorado: [Edition expires 09/04.] Retrieved from http://www.micromedex.com.

Dugue, M., & Neugroschl, J. (2002). Anxiety disorders. Helping patients regain stability and calm. *Geriatrics, 57*(8), 27–31.

Dunner, D. L. (2000). Management of anxiety disorders: The added challenge of comorbidity. *Depression & Anxiety, 13,* 57–71.

Durham, R. C., Chambers, J. A., MacDonald, R. R., Power, K. G., & Major, K. (2003). Does cognitive-behavioural therapy influence the long-term outcome of generalized anxiety disorder? An 8–14 year follow-up of two clinical trials. *Psychological Medicine, 33*(3), 499–509.

Edmands, M. S., & Marcellino-Boisvert, D. (2002). Reflections on a rose: A story of loss and longing. *Issues in Mental Health Nursing, 23*(2), 107–119.

Ferretti, L., McCurry, S. M., Logsdon, R., Gibbons, L., & Teri, L. (2001). Anxiety and Alzheimer's disease. *Journal of Geriatric Psychiatry & Neurology, 14*(1), 52–58.

Flint, A. J. (1994). Epidemiology and comorbidity of anxiety disorders in the elderly. *American Journal of Psychiatry, 151,* 640–649.

Flint, A. J. (2001). Core concepts in geriatrics. Anxiety disorders. Adapted from the *American Geriatrics Society's Geriatrics Review Syllabus: A Core Curriculum in Geriatric Medicine* (4th ed.). *Clinical Geriatrics, 9*(11), 21, 24–25, 28–30.

Flint, A. J., & Rifat, S. L. (2002). Factor structure of the hospital anxiety and depression scale in older patients with major depression. *International Journal of Geriatric Psychiatry, 17*(2), 117–123.

Gorman, J. M. (2001). Generalized anxiety disorder. *Clinical Cornerstone, 3*(3), 37–46.

Hall, G. R., & Buckwalter, K. C. (1987). Progressively lowered stress threshold: A conceptual model for care of adults with Alzheimer's disease. *Archives of Psychiatric Nursing, 1*(6), 399–406.

Harman, J. S., Rollman, B. L., Hanusa, B. H., Lenze, E. J., & Shear, M. K. (2002). Physician office visits of adults for anxiety disorders in the United States, 1985–1998. *Journal of General Internal Medicine, 17*(3), 165–172.

Kogan, J. N., Edelstein, B. A., & McKee, D. R. (2000). Assessment of anxiety in older adults: Current status. *Journal of Affective Disorders, 14*(2), 109–132.

Krasucki, C., Howard, R., & Mann, A. (1998). The relationship between anxiety disorders and age. *International Journal of Geriatric Psychiatry, 13*(2), 79–99.

Krasucki, C., Howard, R., & Mann, A. (1999). Anxiety in the elderly. Anxiety and its treatment in the elderly. *International Psychogeriatrics, 11*(1), 25–45.

Lang, A. J., & Stein, M. B. (2001). Anxiety disorders: How to recognize and treat the medical symptoms of emotional illness. *Geriatrics, 56*(5), 24–27, 31–34.

Lee, K. C., Feldman, M. D., & Finley, P. R. (2002). Beyond depression: Evaluation of newer indications and off-label uses for SSRIs. *Formulary, 37,* 240–251.

Lenze, E. J., Mulsant, B. H., Shear, M. K., Alexopoulos, G. S., Frank, E., & Reynolds, C. F. (2001). Comorbidity of depression and anxiety disorders in later life. *Depression & Anxiety, 14*(2), 86–93.

Lenze, E. J., Mulsant, B. H., Shear, M. K., Houck, P., & Reynolds, C. F. (2002). Anxiety symptoms in elderly patients with depression: What is the best approach to treatment? *Drugs & Aging, 19*(10), 753–760.

Lenze, E. J., Mulsant, B. H., Shear, M. K., Schulberg, H. C., Dew, M. A., Begley, A. E., et al. (2000). Comorbid anxiety disorders in depressed elderly patients. *American Journal of Psychiatry, 157*(5), 722–728.

Mahoney, E. K., Volicer, L., & Hurley, A. (2000). *Management of challenging behaviors in dementia.* Baltimore: Health Professions Press.

McCullough, L. (2002). Exploring change mechanisms in EMDR applied to "small-t trauma" in short-term dynamic psychotherapy: Research questions and speculations. *Journal of Clinical Psychology, 58*(12), 1531–1544.

Mohlman, J., Gorenstein, E. E., Kleber, M., de Jesus, M., Gorman, J. M., & Papp, L. A. (2003). Standard and enhanced cognitive-behavior therapy for late-life generalized anxiety disorder: Two pilot investigations. *American Journal of Geriatric Psychiatry, 11*(1), 24–32.

Mulsant, B. H., Reynolds, C. F., Shear, M. K., Sweet, R. A., & Miller, M. (1996). Comorbid anxiety disorders in late-life depression. *Anxiety, 2*(5), 242–247.

Nordhus, I. H., & Pallesen, S. (2003). Psychological treatment of late-life anxiety: An empirical review. *Journal of Consulting & Clinical Psychology, 71*(4), 643–651.

Regier, D. A., Boyd, J. H., Burke, J. D., Rae, D. S., Myers, J. K., Kramer, M., et al. (1988). One-month prevalence of mental disorders in the United States: Based on five epidemiologic catchment area sites. *Archives of General Psychiatry, 38*, 381–398.

Rickels, K., & Rynn, M. (2001). Overview and clinical presentation of generalized anxiety disorder. *Psychiatric Clinics of North America, 24*(1), 1–17.

Robins, L. N., & Regier, D. A. (1991). *Psychiatric Disorders in America: The Epidemiological Catchment Study.* New York: Free Press.

Rollman, B. L., Belnap, B. H., Reynolds, C. F., Schulberg, H. C., & Shear, M. K. (2003). A contemporary protocol to assist primary care physicians in the treatment of panic and generalized anxiety disorders. *General Hospital Psychiatry, 25*, 74–82.

Sable, J. A., & Jeste, D. V. (2001). Anxiety disorders in older adults. *Current Psychiatry Reports, 3*(4), 302–307.

Sadavoy, J., & LeClair, J. K. (1997). Treatment of anxiety disorders in late life. *Canadian Journal of Psychiatry—Revue Canadienne de Psychiatrie, 42*(Suppl. 1), 28S–34S.

Schimmel-Spreeuw, A., Linssen, A. C., & Heeren, T. J. (2000). Coping with depression and anxiety: Preliminary results of a standardized course for elderly depressed women. *International Psychogeriatrics, 12*(1), 77–86.

Sheikh, J. I., & Cassidy, E. L. (2000). Treatment of anxiety disorders in the elderly: Issues and strategies. *Journal of Anxiety Disorders, 14*(2), 173–190.

Sinoff, G., Ore, L., Zlotogorsky, D., & Tamir, A. (1999). Short Anxiety Screening Test—A brief instrument for detecting anxiety in the elderly. *International Journal of Geriatric Psychiatry, 14*(12), 1062–1071.

Small, G. W. (1997). Recognizing and treating anxiety in the elderly. *Journal of Clinical Psychiatry, 58*(Suppl. 3), 41–47; 48–50.

Stanley, M. A., & Beck, J. G. (2000). Anxiety disorders. *Clinical Psychology Review, 20*(6), 731–754.

Stanley, M. A., Beck, J. G., Novy, D. M., Averill, P. M., Swann, A. C., Diefenbach, G. J., et al. (2003). Cognitive-behavioral treatment of late-life generalized anxiety disorder. *Journal of Consulting & Clinical Psychology, 71*(2), 309–319.

Stoudemire, A. (1996). Epidemiology and psychopharmacology of anxiety in medical patients. *Journal of Clinical Psychiatry, 57*(Suppl. 7), 64–72, 73–65.

Teri, L., Ferretti, L. E., Gibbons, L. E., Logsdon, R. G., McCurry, S. M., Kukull, W. A., et al. (1999). Anxiety of Alzheimer's disease: Prevalence, and comorbidity. *Journals of Gerontology: Biological Sciences & Medical Sciences, 54*(7), M348–M352.

Wetherell, J. L., Gatz, M., & Craske, M. G. (2003). Treatment of generalized anxiety disorder in older adults. *Journal of Consulting & Clinical Psycholog, 71*(1), 31––40.

Whall, A. L., Black, M. E., Groh, C. J., Yankou, D. J., Kupferschmid, B. J., & Foster, N. L. (1997). The effect of natural environments upon agitation and aggression in late stage dementia patients. *American Journal of Alzheimer's Disease, 12*(5), 216–220.

Wilkinson. (1997). Cogntive therapy with older people. *Age and Ageing, 26*, 5–58.

Wright, J. H., Wright, A. S., Beck, A. T., & Salmon, P. (2004). *Good Days Ahead: The Interactive Program for Depression and Anxiety.* Retrieved January 5, 2004, from www.mindstree.com/depression&anxiety.

Wright, J. H., Wright, A. S., Salmon, P., Beck, A. T., Kuykendall, J., Goldsmith, L. J., et al. (2002). Development and initial testing of a multimedia program for computer-assisted cognitive therapy. *American Journal of Psychotherapy, 56*(1), 76–86.

Young, A. S., Klap, R., Sherbourne, C. D., & Wells, K. B. (2001). The quality of care for depressive and anxiety disorders in the United States. *Archives of General Psychiatry, 58*(1), 55–61.

CHAPTER 9

Psychosis in Older Adults

Janet C. Mentes, PhD, APRN, BC
Julia K. Bail, MS, APRN, BC

Mr. B., 65 years old, sits quietly smoking a cigarette in the corner of the waiting room. Occasionally he rocks back and forth in his seat as if he is restless. When you ask him how he is doing, he tells you in a soft voice about how he is controlled by "people from outer space," who read his thoughts and want him to behave in certain ways.

Mr. J., 79 years old, sits at the side of his bed in a local nursing home, eating his dinner. Suddenly, he becomes agitated and shouts out, "Nigel—please don't feed the elephants.... Nigel! Nigel!"

Both of these older men are exhibiting psychoses, caused by different etiologies. From an extensive history, we find that Mr. B. has been experiencing his symptoms since he was a young adult. His symptoms are attributable to chronic schizophrenia, paranoid type. On the other hand, Mr. J.'s history reveals that he had an abrupt change in mental status, indicative of a delirium with psychotic symptoms. On further evaluation, his delirium was found to be secondary to decreased cerebral oxygenation caused by internal bleeding.

INTRODUCTION

Historically, *psychosis* was an expansive term referring to a state of being cut off from reality. Psychotic behavior, or psychosis, signified that a person was unable to determine if what he or she was thinking and feeling about the real world was really true (Merriam-Webster, 1997). Currently, psychosis is recognized as a syndrome or constellation of psychiatric symptoms, which occurs in a number of physical and mental disease states. The predominant symptoms of psychosis include hallucinations, which are false sensory impressions affecting any of the five senses, and delusions, which are simply false beliefs (American Psychiatric Association [APA], 2000).

There are two distinct presentations of psychosis in older persons: chronic psychosis in older individuals who have had a lifelong schizophrenia, major depression, or bipolar disorder with psychosis, and older persons who develop psychotic symptoms for the first time in old age (See Table 9-1 for a comparison of psychotic features of various disease states). Psychosis that develops in older individuals can be the result of a primary

TABLE 9-1   Comparison of Signs and Symptoms Among Psychotic Disorders of Elders

Psychotic Disorder	Delusions	Hallucinations	Other
Alzheimer's disease	Simple, theft, infidelity, abandonment, house is not one's real house	Visual > auditory people from past, animals	Misidentification* Capgras syndrome**
Vascular dementia	Complex, persecutory, fear of infidelity	Visual	Capgras syndrome**, Presence of HTN, CAD, CVD
Lewy body disease	Not as evident	Visual, early in course of disease	Mild parkinsonism
Frontal lobe dementia	Bizarre, grandiose	Not as evident	Occurs in persons > 65 years
Parkinson's disease	Paranoid	Visual, small people, animals	Related to dopaminergic medications
Delirium	If present, simple	Visual, tactile, or olfactory	Abrupt onset, person appears physically ill
Substance abuse/use	Paranoid	Visual with illusions, tactile with withdrawal	
Delusional disorder	Nonbizarre, persecutory, focuses on one aspect of life, marital, occupational, interpersonal	Usually absent	Social function intact
Major depression with psychosis	Somatic, body parts missing or diseased, or guilt	Usually absent	Mood disturbance
Bipolar disorder	Grandiose, e.g., believe they are a celebrity	Auditory	Mood disturbance, mania
Early-onset schizophrenia	Bizarre, systematized persecutory	Auditory, e.g., persons making derogatory comments or commenting on behavior	Usual onset before 45 years
Late-onset schizophrenia	Persecutory, e.g., people spying on them or trying to poison them	Visual > auditory	Onset after 45 years
Charles Bonnet syndrome	None	Elaborate visual of people, animals, or geometric patterns	Person has visual deficits

Note. *Misidentification syndrome is when the person with dementia cannot recognize family members or even him- or herself.

Note. **Capgras syndrome is when the person with dementia feels that familiar people have been replaced by an identical imposter.

Desai & Grossberg (2003); Thorpe (1997)

psychiatric disorder or a secondary psychosis, which can be caused by a number of disease states and can often herald underlying neurologic disorders. Disease states associated with psychosis/psychotic symptoms in older persons include:

a) Schizophrenia, both early-onset (EOS) and late-onset (LOS)

b) Delusional disorder

c) Mood disorders with psychotic features, both major depression and bipolar disorder

d) Delirium

e) Psychosis manifested with other diseases: Parkinson's disease, Alzheimer's disease, and other dementias

f) Psychoses related to substance use, abuse, or polypharmacy

g) Benign hallucinatory states, Charles Bonnet syndrome

Schizophrenia

Schizophrenia is a severe mental disorder that is characterized by two or more of the following symptoms: delusions, hallucinations, disorganized thinking, disorganized behavior, affective flattening, poverty of speech, or apathy that cannot be attributed to other medical or psychiatric causes. These symptoms cause occupational and personal impairment (APA, 2000). Schizophrenia has been studied within three age groupings: early onset (EOS) before age 40 years, midlife onset (MOS) between 40–60 years of age, and late onset (LOS), over 60 years of age (Tune & Salzman, 2003). Some mental health professionals have hotly contested the validity of a diagnosis of late-onset schizophrenia because they believe LOS to be pathophysiologically different from EOS (Tune & Salzman). In relation to EOS, individuals with LOS have a greater prevalence of visual hallucinations (Howard, Castle, Wessely, & Murray, 1993), less prevalence of a formal thought disorder, and fewer

negative symptoms, such as flat affect, apathy, and poverty of speech; less family history of schizophrenia; a greater risk for developing tardive dyskinesia; and significant gender differences, with women more likely to have LOS than men (Tune & Salzman). Persons with LOS tend to live in the community and have been able to hold a job, maintain personal relationships, and marry (Castle, Wessely, Howard, & Murray, 1997).

Individuals with EOS who have entered old age present a slightly different picture. Schultze and colleagues (1997) conducted a cross-sectional study of persons aged 14–73 years with EOS. Older participants in the study had decreased hallucinations, delusions, and bizarre behavior as well as decreased inappropriate affect. In persons with EOS, positive symptoms waned and negative symptoms tended to persist into old age, unlike persons who have LOS. Further, persons with EOS are less likely to have had a successful career and to have married and had a family.

Delusional Disorder

Generally, delusional disorder increases in middle to old age (Thorpe, 1997) and is manifested by the presence of one or more nonbizarre delusions (APA, 2000). Delusional content is not pervasive and is related to everyday life, such as the belief that one's spouse is having an affair. Often overall functioning is not impaired or is limited to the area of life that is the focus of the delusion. As in the example above, the individual may have family problems but be able to function in an occupational setting.

Mood Disorder with Psychotic Features

Major depression and bipolar disorder can be accompanied by psychotic symptoms, both delusions and hallucinations. Mood symptoms are pervasive and psychotic symptoms can be mood congruent or mood incongruent. *Mood congruent* means that an individual who is depressed manifests delusions that reinforce this depression, such as delusions of guilt, or self nihilism, and an individual who is manic manifests grandiose delusions (Thorpe, 1997). *Mood incongruent* means that the psychotic symptoms are not related to the person's mood. Various sources report that psychotic symptoms are more prevalent in older depressed individuals (Gournellis, Lykouras, Fortos, Oulis, Roumbos, & Christodoulou, 2001). Late-onset bipolar disorder is likely to be accompanied by psychotic features and complicated with greater medical and neurological comorbidity. Some mania can be related to certain medical diseases and drugs. Right-sided cerebrovascular disease has been implicated in late-onset mania (Desai & Grossberg, 2003). The presence of psychotic symptoms in mood disorders makes treatment more challenging.

Delirium

Delirium is a syndrome of brain dysfunction that primarily affects one's ability to attend to meaningful stimuli and usually is accompanied by hallucinations and misinterpretation of environmental cues (Mentes, Culp, Maas, & Rantz, 1999; Thorpe, 1997). Hallucinations in delirium are typically visual and accompanied by illusions. Illusions are different than hallucinations in that an illusion is a misperception of a real sensory stimulus and a hallucination is a sensory experience with no real stimulus. Paranoid delusions may also be present. Studies show that delirium is present in 10–15% of older adults who enter the hospital and that an additional 5–30% become delirious during the hospital stay (Francis, 2000). Common causes of delirium can include infection, medication toxicity, recent hospitalization, recent surgery under general anesthesia, recent falls, trauma or pain, alcohol or drug

abuse, recent stroke or seizure, and nutritional deficiencies (Francis, 2000). Delirium is often mis- or undiagnosed in older persons by nurses and other care providers (Inouye, Foreman, Mion, Katz, & Cooney, 2001), leading to improper treatment and poor health outcomes, such as longer hospitalizations and decline in functional and cognitive abilities resulting in nursing home placement (Francis, 2000). The hallmark signs of delirium are its acute onset (hours to days) and fluctuating levels of consciousness.

Psychoses Manifested with Other Diseases

Many diseases may be accompanied by psychotic symptoms. Fifteen percent of individuals with untreated endocrine disorders, 20% of persons with systemic lupus erythematosus, and as many as 40% of persons with temporal lobe epilepsy are estimated to have psychotic symptomatology (APA, 2000). In addition, many elderly persons with Alzheimer's disease (AD), or other dementias (vascular dementia, Lewy body dementia, frontotemporal dementia), and Parkinson's disease (PD) also manifest psychotic symptoms at some time in the course of the disease.

Psychotic symptoms manifested in persons with dementia vary. Delusions manifested in persons with AD include persecutory delusions ("Someone has stolen my possessions") and auditory or visual hallucinations that are not usually frightening to the individual (Soares & Gershon, 1997). As the person becomes more cognitively impaired, the delusions become less elaborate. Hallucinations are reported to affect 21–41% of patients, with visual hallucinations being the most common (Paulsen et al., 2000). Visual hallucinations usually involve people from the past, intruders, or animals. Auditory hallucinations commonly accompany delusions and are usually persecutory (Desai & Grossberg, 2003).

Patients with vascular dementia (VaD) may also present with psychotic features. Delusions affect 9–40% of patients with VaD and are similar to those in AD patients. Hallucinations are usually visual and occur concurrently with delusions (Desai & Grossberg, 2003). Lewy body dementia (LBD) is characterized by fluctuations in cognitive impairment, intermittent parkinsonism, and recurrent visual hallucinations. The clinician should be suspicious about the possibility of LBD in a patient who presents with visual hallucinations early in the course of a dementia. Frontotemporal dementia is a disorder that is much less common than AD, LBD, or VaD, and is frequently misdiagnosed. It is characterized by language impairment, personality changes, and behavioral disturbances sometimes occurring for years before a diagnosis is made. The patient exhibits bizarre and grandiose delusions due to loss of frontal lobe function (Desai & Grossberg, 2003).

In PD, psychotic symptoms are most likely related to medications that are used to treat the PD or neuropathology that accompanies the progression of the disease. Common psychiatric symptoms in PD include visual and auditory hallucinations, delusions, agitation, delirium, sleep disturbances, and nightmares. Psychotic symptoms occur more commonly in the later stages of the disease and in PD patients with dementia. Approximately 20% of persons taking dopaminergic agents report visual hallucinations of people or animals (Thorpe, 1997).

It is important to remember that psychosis manifests primarily as delusions or hallucinations. Often, a whole range of problem behaviors in persons with dementia, such as wandering, escape behaviors, or excessive vocalizations, are misidentified and treated as psychotic behavior (Kidder, 2003). This can be problematic because these individuals are then medicated with powerful antipsychotic medications that do nothing to improve the problematic behaviors but can cause serious side effects.

Psychosis Related to Substance Use, Abuse, or Polypharmacy

Older individuals take many medications that can cause alterations in mental state, including psychotic symptoms. The biggest offenders are those drugs with anticholinergic properties, antiarrhythmics, H-2 blockers, benzodiazepines, tricyclic antidepressants, and antiparkinsonian drugs (Desai & Grossberg, 2003).

Abuse of alcohol or other drugs can occur in elderly individuals. Intoxication from or withdrawal of substances of abuse can trigger psychotic symptoms in older individuals. Psychotic symptoms are often very intense, accompanied by agitation and a fluctuating physical status. Therefore, it is important not to overlook substance abuse as a cause of psychotic behaviors in older persons.

Benign Hallucinatory State: Charles Bonnet Syndrome

Isolated visual hallucinations, in individuals with significant visual impairment, suggest Charles Bonnet syndrome (CBS) (Flaherty, Fulmer, & Mezey, 2003; Thorpe, 1997). Ten to thirteen percent of individuals with bilateral visual acuity worse than 20/60 are reported to have such visual hallucinations, which are extremely distressing to the individual. The visual hallucinations are sophisticated and consist of small children, animals, or a vivid movie-like scene. To be diagnosed with Charles Bonnet syndrome, the patient must meet the following criteria: visual hallucinations, partially intact sight, visual impairment, and lack of evidence of brain disease or other psychiatric disorder. The treatment of choice for CBS is information and support, but in cases where the hallucinations become significantly distressing, a cautious trial of low-dose atypical antipsychotic medication may be appropriate (Flaherty et al.).

Epidemiology of Psychotic Symptoms in Older Adults

The number of elderly persons with psychotic symptoms is not precise and has focused primarily on the presence of paranoid ideas. It is difficult to assess the presence of psychotic symptoms by self-report, as older individuals may have comorbid illnesses that prevent disclosure, and generally, individuals of all ages are less likely to report such symptoms. The prevalence of paranoid ideation in the general elderly population has been reported at 4–6% and this estimate may include persons with dementia (Henderson et al., 1998). One epidemiological study of psychotic symptoms in nondemented elderly persons over age 85 years reported the prevalence of any psychotic symptom at 10%, with 7% exhibiting hallucinations, 5.5% exhibiting delusions, and 7% exhibiting paranoid ideation (Ostling & Skoog, 2002). This investigation is most likely more accurate because data were collected through multiple sources including physical and psychiatric examinations, family interviews, and chart review.

When considering older nursing home residents, the increased prevalence of psychotic symptoms is related to the increased prevalence of dementia in this population. In an earlier study of psychiatric disorders in nursing home residents, Rovner and colleagues (1990) documented that 16% of 454 new admissions to a nursing home had either dementia (Alzheimer's disease, vascular or other dementias) with psychotic features or schizophrenia. In a study of 329 nursing home residents with AD who were followed for four years, over 50% exhibited psychotic symptoms (Paulsen, Salmon, Thal, et al., 2000).

Estimates of schizophrenia in the elderly population include those persons who have early-onset schizophrenia who have lived to old age and those persons who develop schizophrenia in old age. The prevalence of schizophrenia in persons 65 years and older ranges from 0.1–0.5% (Copeland et al., 1998).

Psychotic symptoms are not uncommon in older people living in the community, with one in ten community-dwelling persons without dementia having some psychotic symptom and as many as one in two persons with dementia exhibiting psychotic behaviors. These estimates are expected to increase over the next 20 years in tandem with the increasing aged population.

Risk Factors for Psychosis

Psychosis increases with age and is more prevalent in females versus males (Thorpe, 1997). Further there is evidence that sensory impairments, both visual and auditory deficits, are more common in older persons with psychotic symptoms. It has not been determined whether sensory impairment is a cause or a result of psychosis (Castle, Wessely, Howard, & Murray, 1997). Social isolation, lack of intimate contacts, such as a spouse or close friends, and premorbid paranoid personality traits have also been cited as risk factors for psychosis in old age (Thorpe, 1997). Cognitive impairment may be a contributing or risk factor for delirium that is associated with psychotic symptoms, and likewise, for the psychosis that often accompanies dementia.

ASSESSMENT

Most nurses find it challenging to identify, evaluate, and manage psychosis in older patients. Psychotic symptoms can occur as components of either medical or psychiatric illnesses. Medications are the most common cause of psychosis in the elderly patient with effects that are often reversible (Katz, Jeste, & Tariot, 2002). The clinician should approach the assessment and differential diagnosis of psychosis using a systematic approach (See Figure 9-1 for an assessment algorithm). Ostling and Skoog (2002) found psychotic symptoms to be associated with a poorer prognosis in patients and, thus, should be identified and treated as expeditiously as possible.

Determine Type of Psychosis

Psychotic disorders can be classified into either primary or secondary psychoses. Primary psychotic disorders include schizophrenia and related disorders, bipolar disorders, psychotic depression, and delusional disorder.

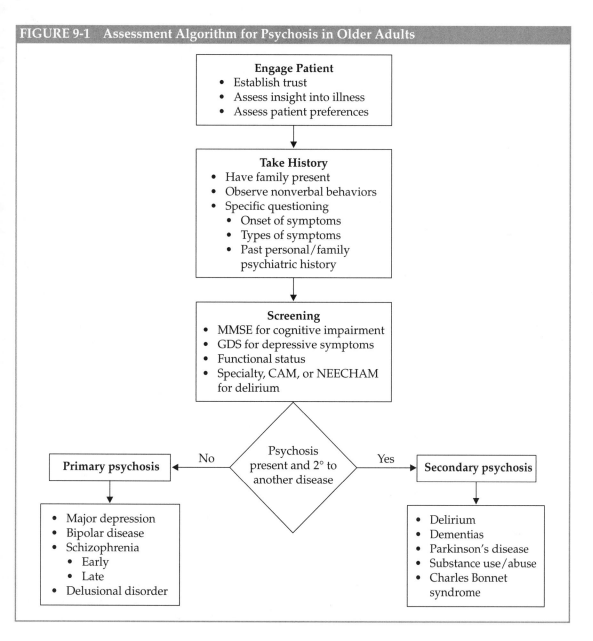

FIGURE 9-1   Assessment Algorithm for Psychosis in Older Adults

Engage Patient
- Establish trust
- Assess insight into illness
- Assess patient preferences

Take History
- Have family present
- Observe nonverbal behaviors
- Specific questioning
  - Onset of symptoms
  - Types of symptoms
  - Past personal/family psychiatric history

Screening
- MMSE for cognitive impairment
- GDS for depressive symptoms
- Functional status
- Specialty, CAM, or NEECHAM for delirium

Psychosis present and 2° to another disease

No → **Primary psychosis**

Yes → **Secondary psychosis**

Primary psychosis
- Major depression
- Bipolar disease
- Schizophrenia
  - Early
  - Late
- Delusional disorder

Secondary psychosis
- Delirium
- Dementias
- Parkinson's disease
- Substance use/abuse
- Charles Bonnet syndrome

The primary disorders comprise the bulk of chronic mental illness in geriatric patients. Secondary psychotic disorders include delirium, psychotic symptoms associated with dementia, and psychotic symptoms secondary to an identifiable medical condition or chemical agent, e.g., drug or alcohol toxicity (Desai & Grossberg, 2003). It is important to distinguish between these two types in order to determine prognosis and formulate an appropriate plan of care. The evaluation of a geriatric patient who presents with psychotic symptoms (hallucinations or delusions) should focus on determining whether the psychosis is primary or secondary, and then on eliminating any medical, toxic, or metabolic causes for the symptoms.

Onset of Psychosis

When evaluating psychosis, it is also of the utmost importance to determine when the psychotic symptoms began. An onset earlier in the patient's life, following a chronic course, would suggest a primary psychosis, whereas a more sudden onset in a patient without a previous psychiatric history suggests a secondary psychosis (Desai & Grossberg, 2003).

Obtain Accurate and Detailed Medical and Medication History

When assessing elderly patients for psychosis, it is crucial for the clinician to obtain a detailed and accurate history using information collected from the patient as well as from collateral sources, i.e., caregiver report, staff reports, and medical records. A good history and medication evaluation is crucial for differential diagnosis.

The Interview

The assessment of psychosis in geriatric patients ideally should begin with the interview. It is essential for the nurse to establish a therapeutic bond with the patient to assure a positive interview. Patience and active listening will help to facilitate this bond and will put the patient at ease. Informing the patient about the amount of time for, and content of, the interview is also important. Older patients may respond more slowly to questions and it is vital to give them ample time to answer before assuming there may be cognitive deficits. The interviewer should avoid any jargon, slang, or medical terminology and should speak slowly and in a low pitched voice. The best time for the interview depends on the patient and his or her needs and preferences. It is helpful to interview the patient when he or she is most awake and alert. Sensory deficits should be accounted for and corrected when possible. It is extremely worthwhile to have a family member or regular caregiver at the interview who is able to clarify responses given by the patient or when there is a question of reliability. The collateral informant becomes especially important when dealing with a psychotic patient who has previously been diagnosed with dementia. Multiple studies of demented patients have shown that caregiver reports yield higher rates of psychopathology than examination and evaluation by the clinician (Ostling & Skoog, 2002).

The nurse may use formal questions and screening tools, as well as behavioral observation, during the interview to help confirm a diagnosis of psychosis and begin to determine its etiology. Specific questions regarding psychotic symptoms should be used once the older patient is comfortable in the interview setting. The nurse can ask about hallucinations and delusional thinking directly; for example, "Do you see things that others do not see?" or "Do you hear voices when no one else is around?" Once the presence of psychotic symptoms is ascertained, a mental status assessment should be conducted, preferably toward the beginning of the interview. The determination of mental status will help guide the interview, as some of the necessary screening tools to determine the underlying etiology of the psychotic symptoms may be unreliable in patients with cognitive, attention, or orientation impairments. The most well-known and common screening tool is the Mini-Mental Status Examination (MMSE) (Folstein, Folstein, & McHugh, 1975). This is a relatively short, 30-item, reliable tool used to screen for cognitive and memory deficits (Kaye & Camicioli, 2000). If time does not permit, the interviewer may use components from the MMSE, such as the three-item recall and orientation questions. Additionally, there are a variety of brief screening tools for the evaluation of depression, dementia, and delirium that are easy to use during the interview process. The Geriatric Depression Scale (GDS) (Yesavage et al., 1983) is an example of a useful screening tool that can be used, as depression in old age is widespread and affects one in six patients in general medical practice and an even higher percentage in nursing homes and hospitals (Bosworth, Hays, George, & Steffens, 2002). Nurses are encouraged to establish a screening regimen (Figure 9-1) for psychotic patients that includes screening for dementia, delirium, and depression.

Behavioral observation may be the most effective way to assess the acutely psychotic patient because he or she most likely would not be able to sit through and complete an entire interview because of anxiety caused by delusions or hallucinations during the interview. A particularly helpful technique is to observe the patient at home or in his or her regular living environment to reduce the patient's anxiety level and to allow the nurse to observe for possible triggers of the psychotic behavior. If the psychotic patient is hospitalized, an in-room behavioral assessment may also be very useful. Assessment of functional status should also be included in the complete assessment of psychosis when possible. Mobility should be assessed along with functional level determined by an ADL/IADL

score as this information will aid the nurse in determining the patient's potential for independent living after treatment. The interview/behavioral assessment will often provide the nurse with enough valuable information to identify the patient's psychotic symptoms and can be a guide as to what the cause of the psychosis may be and how to proceed with evaluation and treatment.

TREATMENT

Treatment of older adults with psychotic symptoms should be based on a thorough assessment that has determined whether the psychosis is primary or secondary and the time of onset of first symptoms (early or late). In secondary psychosis—that is, psychosis caused by medical illness, dementia, substance use or abuse, or delirium—the most important intervention is to treat the underlying cause. In primary psychotic disorders, specifically schizophrenia, it is important to know the time of onset of first symptoms in order to plan appropriate care.

Establishing an Environment of Trust

Regardless of the treatment setting, a safe environment and trusting relationship must be established before further interventions are undertaken with older adults with psychosis (Blazer, 1998). These older adults are often isolated, lonely, and have sensory impairments that make negotiation of unfamiliar treatment environments difficult. In outpatient settings, consistency in care providers is essential for the development of a therapeutic alliance.

Strategies for developing a therapeutic alliance include interpersonal presence, effective listening skills, a nonjudgmental attitude, and shared problem solving. Initially, the nurse should listen to the older person's complaints without reinforcing the psychotic symptoms. It is important to understand the delusional or hallucinatory experience from the individual's perspective to better understand his or her level of distress and coping abilities. Often serious medical symptoms or side effects of medications are embedded in a person's delusional system, and if new or different delusions are dismissed as irrelevant, the person is subject to unnecessary suffering. The nurse can provide a safe, nonjudgmental environment where the psychotic individual can consistently know that someone will attempt to understand his or her distress and problem solve with him or her. Problem solving with the older individual returns personal control, minimizes paranoid ideas, and promotes adherence to other treatments such as pharmacotherapeutic and psychosocial interventions (Loffler, Kilian, Toumi, & Angermeyer, 2003). If the individual is incapacitated by psychosis, then the first effort should be to control the psychotic symptoms with pharmacotherapy. After stabilization of psychotic symptoms, a therapeutic alliance, and a comprehensive treatment plan should be developed that includes the therapeutic strategies discussed in this section.

Pharmacotherapy

Although there are other drugs that may be helpful in the treatment of psychosis, for the purposes of this chapter we will focus on the typical and atypical antipsychotic agents. Major uses for the antipsychotic drugs are in the treatment of schizophrenia, dementia with psychotic features, and delusional disorder. They may be used on a short-term basis in treating depression with psychotic features, mania, substance abuse induced psychosis, and aggression and behavioral problems common in older patients with dementia and delirium (Stuart & Laraia, 2001). The development of a pharmacotherapeutic treatment plan should include identification of target symptoms to be treated, drug selection and dose, observed side effects and their treatment as well as patient safety, education, and reas-

surance (Stuart & Laraia). When considering pharmacological treatment of psychotic disorders in older adults, it is important to remember that approximately 80% of older patients have at least one chronic serious physical illness and may be taking multiple medications. It is essential to try to minimize polypharmacy in these individuals for many reasons. Older adults also commonly have sensory deficits and cognitive impairment that can lead to nonadherence to complex medication regimens. The nurse's role in pharmacotherapy is to understand the action of antipsychotic agents, monitor the individual for side effects, and to provide information and support for continued adherence to the medication regimen.

The Typical Agents   The original drugs used to treat psychosis are known as the "typical" antipsychotics and are predominantly dopamine antagonists. Typical agents, such as haloperidol or fluphenazine, are rarely used as first-line agents today due to numerous shortcomings, such as: only providing partial relief of positive symptoms (hallucinations, delusions) with little to no effect on negative symptoms (flat affect, apathy), little effect or worsening of cognitive impairment, increased likelihood of uncomfortable side effects, and increased likelihood of noncompliance. The typical antipsychotics can be considered when a patient has not responded to treatment with atypical antipsychotics.

Atypical Agents   Atypical antipsychotics block dopamine receptor subtype 2 (D2) and serotonin receptor subtype 2 (5HT2) action by inhibiting the reception of the neurotransmitters, dopamine and serotonin, at specific postsynaptic sites. They are useful in treating the positive and negative symptoms of schizophrenia without causing significant extrapyramidal side effects (EPS). They have also been reported to help treat mood symptoms, hostility, violence, suicidality, and the cognitive impairment that is sometimes seen in schizophrenia.

The atypical agents offer a different pharmacological mechanism of action, an expanded spectrum of therapeutic efficacy, and less severe side effects. For these reasons, they are usually considered as first-line therapy for the treatment of elderly patients with psychosis.

Four agents are available in this class of drugs: clozapine, risperidone, olanzapine, and quetiapine. Clozapine was the first atypical agent approved for use in the treatment of schizophrenia and has been shown to have good efficacy but has major side-effect issues in the elderly population including agranulocytosis, which is considered a medical emergency, and limit the usability in a population of older adults. First-line choices for most older adults are risperidone or olanzapine. Each agent has special indications, for example risperidone is a good first choice because of good efficacy with aggressive behavior associated with psychosis and a better side-effect profile including less EPS and fewer falls and injuries (Katz, Jeste, & Tariot, 2002). Olanzapine is the current drug of choice for treating Parkinson's disease (PD) associated psychosis and psychosis and aggressiveness associated with Alzheimer's disease. Very low doses of clozapine also reduce drug-induced psychosis in elderly patients with PD without worsening PD associated motor symptoms (D'Souza, Barnett, Rangu, & Rowland, 2000). Refer to Tables 6-6 and 6-7 for doses, adverse effects, drug interactions, and geriatric considerations of atypical antipsychotic medications.

Promoting Adherence Psychotropic medications historically have a relatively poor rate of patient adherence. A review of research has shown that in persons receiving antipsychotics, only 58% took the medication as prescribed while persons receiving antidepressants took 65% of the recommended amount of medications (Cramer & Rosen-

check, 1998). Troubling side effects of some types of antipsychotic medications can cause nonadherence to the prescribed treatment. In fact, older persons with schizophrenia and other psychoses are at increased risk for such serious side effects as extrapyramidal side effects (EPS) and tardive dyskinesia. Persons with preexisiting cognitive impairment are at high risk for tardive dyskinesia (Katz, Jeste, & Tariot, 2002). Further threats to medication adherence in older persons include the increased prevalence of cognitive and sensory problems that can severely impair the ability to take medications correctly and regularly, as well as the likelihood that the older person is already on a complex medication regimen to manage other health problems. The addition of even one more medication can confuse the person and expose him or her to further drug-to-drug interactions. Another barrier for medication adherence in older persons living on a fixed income is the cost of the atypical agents, which can be considerable.

Nurses can promote medication adherence in older persons by carefully monitoring side effects, providing medications in a long-acting injectable form, and through helping individuals develop routines to promote medication adherence. Side effects can be assessed by observation and specific questions. Several instruments may be used to assess side effects including the Abnormal Involuntary Movement Scale (AIMS) (Guy, 1976) that assesses for the presence of tardive dyskinesia, and the Simpson–Angus Scale (Simpson & Angus, 1970) that assesses for the presence of EPS such as akinesias, dyskinesias and pseudo-Parkinson's syndrome. Use of depot administration of antipsychotic medications (every two to four weeks) in memory-impaired older individuals eliminates the need for the person to remember to take medications on a daily basis. Currently, only typical agents are available in long-acting injectable form (fluphenazine and haloperidol deconoate).

Nurses can also plan a medication regimen with the older person using simple, descriptive medication instructional materials describing the medication and the time it should be taken or using a pill sorter, which can be prefilled weekly for the older individual by the nurse or family members. Formal medication groups can also help maintain medication adherence (Larkin, 1982).

Primary Preventive Care

Older individuals with mental disorders are often not advised of preventive health screening options. Individuals with LOS, and other diseases with paranoid symptoms, have an increased prevalence of sensory deficits, both visual and auditory, which if corrected could improve their response to psychiatric treatment. In addition, as persons with EOS age, they are likely to develop conditions associated with aging, such as sensory deficits, arthritis, heart disease, diabetes, and respiratory disease. Older adults with schizophrenia should be offered preventive services such as an annual influenza vaccine, and a pneumonoccal vaccine, as well as screenings for hypertension and colorectal, prostate, breast, cervical, and skin cancer. Support and education about the necessity of these examinations are crucial because older persons with schizophrenia may be paranoid about the examination and the intrusiveness of some exams may make the individual uncomfortable. In addition, older individuals with schizophrenia should be taught health maintenance skills. The importance of diet and exercise to prevent medical problems, alleviate stress, and enhance coping skills is invaluable. Smoking cessation and moderate alcohol intake are other areas for consideration. All older persons with schizophrenia should have a primary care provider whom they trust, and the nurse can help identify a provider who is skilled in caring for persons with chronic mental illness and can reinforce

preventive health care practices with the older individual.

Crisis Intervention

At some time during the course of interviewing an older adult with psychosis, it may become evident to the nurse that there is a need for crisis intervention. Given the high prevalence of depression among older adults, it is imperative for the nurse to routinely inquire about suicide. This will help to properly identify older patients who are at risk of committing suicide. An older adult who is depressed with psychotic features may be at even higher risk for self-harm or suicide. Suicide rates in the United States are higher among older adults than any other age group. The highest rate occurs in people over 75, with men over 85 years of age having the highest rate overall (Menghini & Evans, 2000). More than 90% of adults who end their lives by suicide have an associated psychiatric condition. There are certain disorders that place individuals at higher risk for suicide. These include, but are not limited to, mood disorders, substance abuse, and schizophrenia. Patients with depression, in addition to their schizophrenia were at even higher risk for suicide (Gupta, Black, Arndt, Hubbard, & Andreasen, 1998). Suicide is the leading cause of premature death among patients with schizophrenia and the lifetime prevalence has been estimated at 10% (Meltzer, 1998). Among schizophrenic patients, 40% report suicidal thoughts, 20–40% make unsuccessful suicide attempts and 9–13% ultimately end their lives with suicide (Meltzer, 1998). The highest priority for nurses treating patients who are suicidal is the maintenance of patient safety. In cases of psychotic patients who are suicidal, hospitalization is clearly indicated.

Several studies have found that persons with schizophrenia are at higher risk for homicide than the general population and psychosis has been linked with increased violence. Schwartz, Reynold, Austin, and Petersen (2003) found that manic symptoms and psychotic symptoms had a significant correlation with homicidal ideation and intent. The investigators recommend that clinicians assess a male schizophrenic patient's overall lethality (homicidal ideation and intent) and evaluate it thoroughly in order to formulate an appropriate plan of care. It is clear that in the case of a psychotic homicidal patient, hospitalization most likely will be warranted.

Psychosocial Interventions

Evidenced-based practice for best psychosocial interventions for schizophrenia is in its infancy, but some recommendations do exist based on the Schizophrenia Patient Outcomes Research Team (PORT) work (Lehman & Steinwachs, 1998). The most significant finding from the PORT work is that the individual with schizophrenia needs comprehensive services at the individual, family, and community level plus pharmacotherapy. An array of services is preferable. Liberman (2003) refers to this as "wrap-around" services tailored to the specific person. Characteristics of successful services in each of these areas will be discussed and specific therapeutic modalities addressed. It is important to note that although most persons will have to be medicated with antipsychotics indefinitely, it is equally important for the nurse to establish a therapeutic relationship with the psychotic individual to engage him or her in the necessary array of therapies.

Individual-Focused Intervention Individual-focused interventions are those interventions that enhance or improve an individual's function, whether delivered individually or in a group format. Components of successful modalities include a combination of support, education, and cognitive–behavioral strategies to improve the individual's function, and

ability to self-manage his/her disease (Lehman & Steinwachs, 1998).

Disease management skill training is ideally accomplished in a group format where individuals can share their experiences. The content is broken into smaller learning modules including areas of medication management, communicating with the health care provider about symptoms, and how to deal with an increase in symptoms. The disease management modules are designed as a highly interactive learning activity where participants can use psychomotor skills, and coaching is available from the group leaders to master these skills (Liberman, 2003). Liberman strongly advocates for the use of a highly structured modular format for this educational intervention due to the age-related and disease-mediated cognitive changes seen in older persons. Psychoeducational groups that rely more on verbal memory and traditional methods of learning may not be successful with older persons with schizophrenia. Other open-ended formats, such as a weekly medication group that provides support combined with concrete problem-solving strategies around disease symptoms and medication side effects, are also effective (Larkin, 1982; Zygmunt, Olfson, Boyer, & Mechanic, 2002).

Community management skills focus on the successful adaptation of the individual to community living. Many of the older individuals who have lifelong schizophrenia may have spent long periods of time in state psychiatric hospitals and therefore require help to readjust to community living. Use of modular learning as described above can also be adapted to teaching community living skills. It is important to incorporate "hands on" learning experiences to teach home management skills, such as cooking and cleaning, and social skills, such as making conversation (Liberman, 2003).

Cognitive–Behavior Therapy (CBT) is a therapeutic approach widely employed across a wide variety of disorders including those individuals with schizophrenia who have refractory positive symptoms, specifically hallucinations and delusions (Tarrier et al., 1998). CBT techniques attempt to encourage the individual to reevaluate strongly held beliefs through "disputing and challenging, creating dissonance, using coping statements, generating alternative explanations for symptoms, cognitive restructuring of the meaning of symptoms, and behavioral experiments" (Liberman, 2003, p. 27–28). Older persons with schizophrenia can be coached to question their long-held delusions and reformulate another more reality-based explanation for the symptom. This is done in a supportive environment, encouraging the use of coping self-talk, opportunities to role-play new behaviors, and homework assignments. Liberman describes an easy mnemonic of the Three Cs—Catch the thought (identify irrational cognitions), Check it (assess any thought distortions), and Change it (develop alternative thoughts), to guide the initial sessions.

Family Intervention   Psychoeducation interventions designed to educate and support family members about schizophrenia and its treatment have a strong evidence base (Lehman & Steinwachs, 1998). However, traditional psychoeducation programs are designed for individuals who live with their families. Many older persons with schizophrenia live alone but maintain contact with their families (Lefley, 2003). Further, a majority of older persons with schizophrenia have lived with the disease for decades and family members have acquiesced or adapted to the notion of having a chronically ill member. Therefore, it is important to adapt the educational endeavors to include more age-appropriate content, such as the effect of age on schizophrenic symptoms and treatment, as well as helping families plan for the care of their relative after they die (Lefley). Culturally sensitive family patterns of caregiving must be addressed. For example, in African-American families, it may be likely that a sibling or younger family member will take responsibility for the individual with schizophrenia, (Lefley) and in Chinese and other Eastern Asian cultures, parents are cared for by their children in old age.

It would be important with older adults who have no family contact, but are living in assisted housing or long-term care facilities, to offer an adapted psychoeducation program to the formal caregivers. The program would focus on educating caregivers about the disease process, how to help the resident cope, and the importance of maintaining pharmacotherapy.

Community Interventions   Community interventions can be an array of services that provide the individual with safe, appropriate housing and support in navigating the health care and social welfare systems (Lehman & Steinwachs, 1998). Community services augment the therapeutic modalities discussed previously. Although research conducted in the area of community interventions demonstrates effectiveness, no study has been conducted solely with older individuals. Several of the studies demonstrating positive outcomes included persons over 50 years of age and may therefore hold promise for elderly persons with schizophrenia (Mohamed, Kasckow, Granholm, & Jeste, 2003).

Case management (CM) programs provide support for persons negotiating for services. Case managers do not provide direct service but contract with other providers for services and then oversee the integration of services. Clients come to the case manager, usually a member of the mental health team, who helps to link the client with needed services and may advocate for service improvements when gaps or deficiencies are identified. CM programs have primarily demonstrated effectiveness in improving psychological well-being of participants, through the integration of social skills training. Cost effectiveness in the form of decreased hospitalization and use of emergency services is less well demonstrated (Mohamed et al, 2003).

Supported housing is noninstitutional, permanent housing that offers supportive services based on the individual's functional ability and preference. Supported housing facilities often have a paraprofessional provider on site to provide for general housing needs of the tenants and to help provide the stable housing environment that a person with schizophrenia requires. Previously, the only community housing options available were transitional housing arrangements and individuals were ultimately expected to live independently. It is now recognized that older, isolated persons with schizophrenia have relatively few options for living arrangements: family, nursing home, public housing or some form of supported housing. Supported housing for older persons has not been well studied, although program evaluations demonstrate that supported housing helps decrease days of hospitalization, improve clients' homemaking skills, and increase self-esteem (McCarthy & Nelson, 1991).

Day treatment programs or partial hospital programs provide an alternative to extended hospitalization, through comprehensive services offered on an outpatient basis by a multidisciplinary team of psychiatric nurses, psychiatrists, social workers, and occupational therapists (Mohamed et al, 2003). Programs are scheduled five days per week, with some programs having structured, planned participation several days a week and other programs allowing the individual to build his or her own program, based on individual need. Many of the previously described modalities may be employed in a day treatment center such as medication management, group therapies focusing on disease management and social skills, and family education. Although it appears that persons with schizophrenia in day programs demonstrate better community adjustment at a cost effective

price, few studies using this treatment option have included persons older than 50 years of age (Mohamed et al).

Clubhouses are participant-run self-help clubs that are open seven days a week with supporting paraprofessional staff members. Persons who join the club are called "members," not "patients," to reinforce a healthy social role for members. In addition, members are expected to take an active role in the operation of the clubhouse and may transition from working at the clubhouse to outside employment. Social and supportive services are also available, particularly on evenings and weekends when members may feel most isolated. Again, it is unclear that this service has age-related benefits, because few studies have been conducted with older persons.

Community and Family Resources

Families of older persons with schizophrenia have the compounded difficulties of caring for a member who has a chronic disability as well as dealing with their own personal aging. Caregiver burden in these families is chronic and fluctuates depending on the symptoms and life stresses that their family member is experiencing. Although many older persons with schizophrenia live apart from their families, they still maintain contact with elderly parents, specifically their mothers (Lefley, 2003). In addition, there is evidence that families who are living apart from their relative with schizophrenia have some of the same stresses as families living with their relative (Laidlaw, Coverdale, Falloon, & Kydd, 2002). Two of the concerns expressed by parents of older persons with schizophrenia are: unmet service needs for their family member, specifically for permanent supported housing and recreation services, as well as services that help families plan for the future of their relative with schizophrenia (Smith, 2003).

Unfortunately, there are relatively few services explicitly for older persons with schizophrenia (Table 9-2). The National Alliance for the Mentally Ill (NAMI, www.nami.org) is the organization that provides the most comprehensive information about services for families and persons with schizophrenia and other mental illnesses. Most states have a local chapter of NAMI. The NAMI Web site provides educational resources as well as information about support groups, respite care, and maintaining a healthy lifestyle. One of the initiatives of this organization is to help older family members

plan for the legal, financial, housing, and health care needs of their relative with schizophrenia (Thompson, 2003). The Planned Lifetime Assistance Network (PLAN) programs were developed expressly to meet the needs of aging family members who want to plan for the future of their relative with schizophrenia or other disabling mental illnesses. These nonprofit programs affiliated with NAMI help families develop a future care plan, establish the resources for payment, and identify the person(s) or pro-

TABLE 9-2 Resources for Persons with Schizophrenia and Their Families		
Organization	**Contact Information**	**Mission/Purpose**
National Alliance for the Mentally Ill	Colonial Place Three 2107 Wilson Blvd. Suite 300 Arlington, VA 22201-3042 (703) 524-7600 (Main) (800) 950-NAMI (Member services) www.nami.org	Education, advocacy, support, and preventive care for persons with mental illness
National Mental Health Association	2001 N. Beauregard St. 12th floor Alexandria, VA 22311 (800) 969-6642 www.nmha.org	Education, advocacy, and support for persons with mental illness
Schizophrenia.com	Web community. No address www.schizophrenia.com	Education, support for persons with schizophrenia
Mental Health and Aging Advocacy Project	1211 Chestnut St. Philadelphia, PA 19107 (800) 688-4226 www.mhaging.org	Assists older persons and their families obtain mental health services appropriate for an older person
Compeer	259 Monroe Ave. Rochester, NY 14607 (800) 836-1475 www.compeer.org	Matches community volunteers in supportive friendship relationships with persons who have mental illness
Bazelon Center for Mental Health Law	1101 15th St. NW Suite 1212 Washington, DC 20005 (202) 467-5730 www.Bazelon.org	Legal advocacy to advance and preserve the rights of persons with mental illness and developmental disabilities
National Alliance for Research on Schizophrenia and Depression	60 Cutter Mill Rd. Suite 404 Great Neck, NY 11021 (800) 829-8289 www.narsad.org	Fund-raising for psychiatric brain research worldwide

grams responsible for carrying out the plan (NAMI, n.d.).

ETHICAL AND LEGAL ISSUES

Psychiatric Advance Directives

One of the prevailing ethical–legal concerns for persons with schizophrenia and other psychotic disorders is that of self-determination in psychiatric care decisions. Similar to advance directives for medical care, psychiatric advance directives (PAD) have been proposed to help persons with schizophrenia and other psychiatric disorders to predetermine the psychiatric care that they want should they become unable to make such decisions when they have a psychotic crisis (Srebnik, Russo, Sage, Peto, & Zick, 2003). PADs promote individual autonomy, enhance communication between families and mental health caregivers about treatment issues, decrease ineffective or unwanted treatments, and prevent crises that may result in involuntary commitment or use of seclusion or restraints. Several studies have indicated that between 40% and 75% of individuals with severe mental illness, such as schizophrenia, are interested in creating PADs (Srebnik et al., 2003). Further, a trusted caseworker or nurse may be the impetus for this interest. Although there are difficult implementation issues with PADs, patient advocacy groups and mental health professionals support the appropriate use of PADs for persons with severe mental illness. Materials to help with the preparation of a PAD can be obtained from the National Mental Health Association Web site or from the Bazelon Center for Mental Health Law Web site.

Social Stigmatization

Social stigma may be doubly damaging to older persons with chronic psychotic disorders such as schizophrenia. Ageism plus stigma from having a chronic mental illness can be overwhelming. Levy and associates (2002) have shown that ageism can affect cognition, physical abilities, and gait in older adults. When the stigma of mental illness is added, the individual feels dehumanized. Schulze and Angermeyer (2003) conducted focus groups of persons with schizophrenia, their relatives, and mental health workers, to better understand stigmatizing experiences from the individual's perspective. Stigma was reported at many levels including at the interpersonal and social levels (Schulze & Angermeyer). For example, interpersonal stigma was experienced as derogatory comments about people with mental illness, and social stigma was experienced as stereotyped public images characterizing all people with schizophrenia as violent and dangerous. This stigma forces individuals with schizophrenia to create a social distance between themselves and society, resulting in the individuals becoming nonadherent with treatment, socially isolated and underemployed, which significantly reduces quality of life. Programs to combat stigma associated with schizophrenia should have multiple foci, including encouraging the media to represent persons with schizophrenia in a more balanced manner, lobbying for better services for the mentally ill, and providing the individual with support to combat interpersonal stigma. The National Alliance for the Mentally Ill has several programs for combating stigma associated with mental illness. Their program entitled, "In Our Own Voice: Living with Mental Illness," helps individuals develop confidence through sharing their experience with mental illness with audiences of mental health professionals, students, and lay persons. NAMI also sponsors a monthly Stigmabuster newsletter, available on its Web site.

Role of the Geropsychiatric Nurse

Nurses are often the first health care professionals to identify psychosis in an older adult, primarily because of the close therapeutic relationship that is engendered between nurse and older patient. Nurses have an integral role in the assessment and treatment of older adults with psychoses resulting from the multiple etiologies discussed in this chapter. They may serve as case managers, coordinating all of the various aspects of treatment, both psychosocial and community services (Lancashire, Haddock, Tarrier, Baguley, Butterworth, & Brooker, 1997). Nurses who have been trained in cognitive–behavior therapeutic techniques may assist in helping persons with schizophrenia manage their symptoms and maintain their treatment regimen (Chan, 2003). Nurses conduct medication groups and other disease management, community

skills, and family psychoeducational groups (Lancashire et al., 1997; Larkin, 1982). Further, nurses are often the first providers to identify medication nonadherence or uncomfortable side effects, and can intervene before the individual becomes actively psychotic. Fluphenazine–haloperidol clinics, which provide injections of the long-acting form of these typical antipsychotic agents, are often managed by nurses.

Nurses are also in a pivotal position to help dispel misconceptions about psychotic disorders, specifically schizophrenia. Providing accurate public information about these disorders helps to decrease stigma, promotes an older individual's self-esteem, and improves his or her quality of life.

REFERENCES

American Psychiatric Association. (2000). *Diagnostic and Statistical Manual of Mental Disorders* (4th ed.). Washington, DC: Author.

Blazer, D. (1998). *Emotional Problems in Later Life. Interventions Strategies for Professional Caregivers* (2nd ed.). New York: Springer.

Bosworth, H., Hays, J., George, L. K., & Steffens, D. C. (2002). Psychosocial and clinical predictors of unipolar depression outcomes in older adults. *International Journal of Geriatric Psychiatry, 17,* 238–246.

Castle, D., Wessely, S., Howard, R., & Murray, R. (1997). Schizophrenia with onset at the extremes of adult life. *International Journal of Geriatric Psychiatry, 12,* 72–717.

Chan, S. (2003). Brief cognitive behavioral intervention delivered by nurses reduces overall symptoms in schizophrenia. *Evidence-based Mental Health, 6,* 26.

Copeland, J., Dewey, M., Scott, A., Gilmore, C., Larkin, B., Cleave, N., et al. (1998). Schizophrenia and delusional disorder in older age: Community prevalence, incidence, comorbidity and outcome. *Schizophrenia Bulletin, 24,* 153–161.

Cramer, J., & Rosencheck, R. (1998). Compliance with medication regimens for mental and physical disorders. *Psychiatric Services, 49,* 196–201.

Desai, A., & Grossberg, G. (2003). Differential diagnosis of psychotic disorders in the elderly. In C. Cohen (Ed.), *Schizophrenia Into Later Life. Treatment, Research, and Policy* (pp. 55–75). Washington, DC: American Psychiatric.

D'Souza, S., Barnett, S. K., Rangu, S., & Rowland, F. N. (2000). Treatment of psychosis in Parkinson's disease. *Journal of the American Medical Directors Association, 1,* 211–216.

Flaherty, E., Fulmer, T., & Mezey, M. (Eds.). (2003). Psychotic disorders. *Geriatric Nursing Review Syllabus: A Core Curriculum in Advanced Practice Geriatric Nursing* (pp. 224–227). New York: American Geriatrics Society.

Folstein M. F., Folstein, S., & McHugh, P. R. (1975). Mini-Mental State: A practical method for grading the cognitive state of the patients for the clinician. *Journal of Psychiatric Residency 12(3)* 189–198.

Francis, J. (2000). Delirium. In D. Osterweil, K. Brummel-Smith, & J. Morley, (Eds.), *Comprehensive Geriatric Assessment* (pp. 489–506). New York: Mc-Graw-Hill.

Gournellis, R., Lykouras, L., Fortos, A., Oulis, P., Roumbos, V., & Christodoulou, K. (2001). Psychotic (delusional) major depression in late life: A clinical study. *International Journal of Geriatric Psychiatry, 16,* 1085–1091.

Gupta, S., Black, D. W., Arndt, S., Hubbard, W. C., & Andreasen, N. C. (1998). Factors associated with suicide attempts among patients with schizophrenia. *Psychiatric Services 49*, 1353–1355.

Guy, W. (1976). *ECDEU Assessment Manual for Pharmacology* (Rev. ed.) Washington, DC: U.S. Department of Health, Education and Welfare.

Henderson, A., Korten, A., Levings, C., Jorm, A., Christensen, H., Jacomb, P., et al. (1998). Psychotic symptoms in the elderly: A prospective study in a population sample. *International Journal of Geriatric Psychiatry, 13*, 484–492.

Howard, R., Castle, D., Wessely, S., & Murray, R. (1993). A comparative study of 470 cases of early- and late-onset schizophrenia. *British Journal of Psychiatry, 163*, 352–357.

Inouye, S., Foreman, M., Mion, L., Katz, K., & Cooney, L. (2001). Nurses' recognition of delirium and its symptoms: Comparison of nurse and researcher ratings. *Archives of Internal Medicine, 161*, 2467–2473.

Katz, P. R., Jeste, D. V., & Tariot, P. N. (2002). Pharmacotherapy for the older patient with psychosis. *Journal of the American Medical Directors Association, 3*(Suppl. 4), H34–H41.

Kaye J., & Camicioli, R. (2000). Dementia. In D. Osterweil, K. Brummel-Smith, & J. Morley (Eds.), *Comprehensive Geriatric Assessment* (pp. 507–554). New York: McGraw Hill.

Kidder, S. (2003). Psychosis and the elderly—Whose delusion is it? *Geriatric Times, IV*(2), 25–26.

Laidlaw, T., Coverdale, J., Falloon, I., & Kydd, R. (2002). Caregivers' stresses when living together or apart from patients with chronic schizophrenia. *Community Mental Health Journal, 38*, 303–310.

Lancashire, S., Haddock, G., Tarrier, N., Baguley, I., Butterworth, C., & Brooker, C. (1997). Effects of training in psychosocial interventions for community psychiatric nurses in England. *Psychiatric Services, 48*, 39–41.

Larkin, A. (1982). What is a medication group? *Journal of Psychosocial Nursing and Mental Health Services, 20*(2), 35–37.

Lefley, H. (2003). Changing caregiving needs as persons with schizophrenia grow older. In C.

Cohen (Ed.), *Schizophrenia Into Later Life. Treatment, Research, and Policy* (pp. 251–268). Washington, DC: American Psychiatric.

Lehman, A., & Steinwachs, D. (1998). At issue: Translating research into practice: The schizophrenia patient outcomes research team (PORT) treatment recommendations. *Schizophrenia Bulletin, 24*, 1–21.

Levy, B., Slade, M., & Kasl, S. (2002). Longitudinal benefit of positive self-perceptions of aging on functional health. *Journal of Gerontology Psychological and Social Science, 57*, P409–P417.

Liberman, R. (2003). Biobehavioral treatment and rehabilitation for older adults with schizophrenia. In C. Cohen (Ed.), *Schizophrenia Into Later Life. Treatment, Research, and Policy* (pp. 223–250). Washington, DC: American Psychiatric.

Loffler, W., Kilian, R., Toumi, M., & Angermeyer, M. C. (2003). Schizophrenic patient's subjective reasons for compliance and noncompliance with neuroleptic treatment. *Pharmacopsychiatry, 36*, 105–112.

McCarthy, J., & Nelson, G. (1991). An evaluation of supportive housing for current and former psychiatric patients. *Hospital & Community Psychiatry, 42*, 1254–1256.

Meltzer, H. Y. (1998). Suicide in schizophrenia: Risk factors and clozapine treatment. *Journal of Clinical Psychology, 59*, (Suppl. 3), 15–20.

Menghini, V., & Evans, J. (2000). Suicide among nursing home residents: A population based study. *Journal of the American Medical Directors Association, 1*, 47–50.

Mentes, J., Culp, K., Maas, M., & Rantz, M. (1999). Acute confusion indicators: Risk factors and prevalence using MDS data. *Research in Nursing & Health, 22*, 95–105.

Merriam-Webster. (1997). *The Merriam-Webster Dictionary*. Springfield, MA: Merriam-Webster.

Mohamed, S., Kasckow, J., Granholm, E., & Jeste, D. (2003). Community-based treatment of schizophrenia and other severe mental illnesses. In C. Cohen (Ed.), *Schizophrenia Into Later Life. Treatment, Research, and Policy* (pp. 205–222). Washington, DC: American Psychiatric.

National Alliance for the Mentally Ill (n.d.). *PLAN (Planned lifetime assistance network)*. Retrieved

October 25, 2003, from http://www.nami.org/ Template.cfm?Section=Helpline1&template=/ ContentManagement/ContentDisplay.cfm& ContentID=4861.

Ostling, S., & Skoog, I. (2002). Psychotic symptoms and paranoid ideation in a nondemented population-based sample of the very old. *Archives of General Psychiatry, 59,* 53–59.

Paulsen, J., Salmon, D., Thal, I., Romero, R., Weisstein-Jenkins, C., Galasko, D., et al. (2000). Incidence of and risk factors for hallucinations and delusions in patients with probable AD. *Neurology, 54,* 1965–1971.

Rovner, B., German, P., Broadhead, J., Moriss, R., Brant, L., Blaustein, J., et al. (1990). The prevalence and management of dementia and other psychiatric disorders in nursing homes. *International Psychogeriatrics, 2,* 13—24.

Schultze, S., Miller, D., Oliver, S., Arndt, S., Flaum, M., & Andreasen, N. (1997). The life course of schizophrenia: Age and symptom dimensions. *Schizophrenia Research, 23,* 15–23.

Schulze, B., & Angermeyer, M. C. (2003). Subjective experiences of stigma. A focus group study of schizophrenic patients, their relatives and mental health professionals [Electronic version]. *Social Science & Medicine, 56,* 299–312.

Schwartz, R. C., Reynold, C. A., Austin, J. F., & Petersen, S. (2003) Homicidality in schizophrenia: A replication study. *American Journal of Orthopsychiatry, 73,*74–77.

Simpson, G. M., & Angus, J. W. (1970). A rating scale for extrapyramidal side effects. *Acta Psychiatrica Scandanavica, 212,* 11–18.

Smith, G. (2003). Patterns and predictors of service use and unmet needs among aging families of adults with severe mental illness. *Psychiatric Services, 54,* 871–877.

Soares, J., & Gershon, S. (1997). Therapeutic targets in late-life psychoses: A review of concepts and critical issues, *Schizophrenia Research, 27,* 227–239.

Srebnik, D., Russo, J., Sage, J., Peto, T., & Zick, E. (2003). Interest in psychiatric advance directives among high users of crisis services and hospitalization [Electronic version]. *Psychiatric Services, 52,* 981–986.

Stuart G., & Laraia, M. (2001). *Principles and Practice of Psychiatric Nursing.* St. Louis, MO: Mosby.

Tarrier, N., Yusupoff, L., Kinney, C., McCarthy, E., Gledhill, A., Haddock, G., et al. (1998). A randomized controlled trial of intensive cognitive behavior therapy for chronic schizophrenia. *British Medical Journal, 317,* 303–307.

Thompson, K. (2003). Stigma and public health policy for schizophrenia [Electronic version]. *Psychiatric Clinics of North America, 26,* 273–294.

Thorpe, L. (1997). The treatment of psychotic disorders in late life. *Canadian Journal of Psychiatry, 42* (Suppl 1), 19s–27s.

Tune, L., & Salzman, C. (2003). Schizophrenia in late life [Electronic version]. *Psychiatric Clinics of North America, 26,* 103–113.

Yesavage, J., Brink, T., Rose, T., Lum, O., Huang, V., Adey, M., et al. (1982–83). Development and validation of a geriatric depression screening scale. *Journal of Psychiatric Residency, 17*(1), 37–49.

Zygmunt, A., Olfson, M., Boyer, C., & Mechanic, D. (2002). Interventions to improve medication adherence in schizophrenia [Electronic version]. *American Journal of Psychiatry, 159,* 1653–1664.

CHAPTER 10

Substance Abuse in Older Adults

Betty D. Morgan, PhD, APRN, BC
Donna M. White, RN, PhD, CADAC-II, LADC-1
Ann X. Wallace, MSN, RN, APRN, BC, NP-C

INTRODUCTION

The extent of substance abuse in older adults in the United States is not clearly known despite recent research. Researchers have shown that substance abuse is common in this population. Alcohol is the most commonly abused drug, but abuse of narcotics and sedatives, as well as polysubstance abuse, also occurs (Fingerhood, 2000). Misdiagnosis is common due in part to complicated medical and psychosocial issues that are problematic in older adults.

This chapter will provide information on what is known about substance abuse in older adults, definition of terms, commonly used drugs, and a review of the literature on substance abuse in the older adult population. Additionally, information about assessment and screening tools that are appropriate for use in an older adult population will be included. Interviewing techniques and substance abuse treatment guidelines, along with special issues related to overall health care for older adults, will be provided. Finally caregiver stress will be addressed as it relates to family involvement with older adult substance abusers and as it relates to health care professionals caring for this population.

PREVALENCE OF SUBSTANCE ABUSE IN OLDER ADULTS

Since 1990, the National Survey on Drug Use and Health (NSDUH, formerly the NHSDA, National Household Survey on Drug Abuse), sponsored by the Substance Abuse and Mental Health Services Administration (SAMHSA), has conducted an annual survey of people in the United States over the age of 12 who are noninstitutionalized civilians. The 2002 survey included 2239 adults 65 or older (SAMHSA, 2003). However, the age categories in relation to specific substance abuse provide little explanation of older adult substance abuse as the categories used most frequently were ages 12–17, 18–25, and 26 and older. Two tables in the survey provide some detail on substance abuse in the age 65 or older category. In the group age 65 and older, 9.2% of the sample reported lifetime illicit drug use, 1.3% reported illicit drug use in the past year and 0.8% in the past month. Of those age 65 or older, 38.3% indicated any alcohol use in the past month, 7.5% indicated binge alcohol use in the past month, and 1.4% heavy alcohol use in the past month.

Using 1999 data, SAMHSA researchers attempted to project the number of substance abusers in 2020 among older adults using current prevalence rates and population projections. This projection estimated that in the population of persons aged 50 and older, the number of those who are alcohol or drug dependent will increase from 500,000 to 700,000 by the year 2020. The number of those who use illicit drugs or drink heavily is also expected to increase during this time period, from 930,000 to 1.1 million.

There are several potential problems with these projections. There is lack of a universally held definition of substance abuse, misdiagnosis and lack of reporting of substance abuse problems, and lack of information on recovery and/or death due to substance use or misuse. Perhaps most importantly, there is an expected increase in substance abuse in older adults due to the aging of the "baby boom" generation (those born between 1946 and 1964), who in their adolescence and early adulthood experimented and used substances in greater numbers than previous generations (SAMHSA, 2003).

The lack of clarity about the magnitude of the problem of substance abuse in older adults continues to be a public health issue. When money for public health issues is low and other illnesses have higher prevalence rates, this lack of detailed information about elder substance abuse will result in fewer dollars for treatment or research.

◼◼◼◼ DEFINITIONS

Substance abuse   The term *substance abuse* or *chemical dependency* is defined as "the use of a substance or substances in an uncontrolled, compulsive, and potentially harmful manner" (Savage, 1993, p. 265). Criteria for diagnosis of substance abuse include a maladaptive pattern of use of a substance during a 12-month period that results in impairment indicated by at least one of the following: (1) lack of fulfillment of role obligations such as job, school, or home; (2) risk of physical danger due to

use, such as use while operating machinery or a car; (3) legal problems, and (4) ongoing interpersonal problems as a result of or exacerbated by use of a substance (American Psychiatric Association [APA], 2000).

Dependency   Dependency can be physical and psychological. *Physical dependency* refers to the development of a withdrawal syndrome following abrupt cessation of the drug (Savage, 1993). Physical dependence may be accompanied by tolerance to the substance, which is a pharmacological property of opioid drugs and occurs when increased dosage is required to sustain the same effects of the drug (APA, 2000). Criteria for the diagnosis of substance dependence include a maladaptive pattern of use over a 12-month period that results in: (1) tolerance, (2) a withdrawal syndrome or use of a related substance to avoid withdrawal, (3) use of larger amounts of the substance or for a longer period of time than was planned, (4) attempts to cut down or control use, (5) spending a lot of time obtaining, using, or recovering from the substance, (6) change in social, occupational, or recreational activities due to substance use, and (7) continued use despite physical and psychological problems (APA, 2000).

Addiction   Addiction is characterized by the psychological dependence and "preoccupation with obtaining or using a substance, loss of control over the use of the substance, and continued use despite adverse consequences" (Savage, 1993, p. 266). The American Society of Pain Management Nurses (ASPMN) defines *addiction* based on definitions by the American Academy of Pain Management (AAPM), American Pain Society (APS), and the American Society of Addiction Medicine (ASAM) as: "A primary, chronic, neurobiologic disease with genetic, psychosocial, and environmental factors influencing its development and manifestations. It is characterized by behaviors that include one or more of the following: impaired control over drug use, compulsive use, continued use despite harm and craving" (ASPMN, 2003, p. 1).

DRUGS OF ABUSE

Alcohol   In terms of numbers affected and costs to society, alcohol abuse is the number one problem in North America. Ethanol is the chemical name for alcohol, which is metabolized primarily in the liver and in the stomach. Alcohol affects the central nervous system and initially acts as an anxiolytic; cognitive and motor skills are affected as alcohol concentrations increase. Higher concentrations of alcohol can lead to depression of vital centers of the brain and a slowed, "stuporous-to-unconscious mental state develops" (Allen, 2001, p. 385). Amnesia for the period of intoxication is common with ingestion of alcohol. All people with alcoholism have some loss of brain cells, and atrophy is seen on computed tomograms (CT) scans of the brain (Allen).

Cannabis or marijuana   Cannabis is the most commonly used illicit drug in the United States. The active ingredient is tetrahydrocannabinol (THC), which produces a calm, mildly euphoric state that can be accompanied by heightened sensations, distorted time perception, psychomotor retardation, and increased appetite. Marijuana is made from the leaves and flowers of the cannabis plant and is usually smoked. Data about the long-term effects of marijuana use are conflicting, with development of pulmonary problems as the clearest consequence of prolonged use (Allen, 2001). Marijuana is often used with other drugs to either extend or potentiate a high, prevent a crash, or lessen the anxiety associated with cocaine or other stimulants (D'Avonzo, 2001).

Stimulants   This category includes amphetamines (benzedrine), dextroamphetamines (dexedrine), cocaine, methamphetamines (Desoxyn), and methylphenidates (Ritalin). Amphetamines were used in the 1950s and 1960s for depression, fatigue, weight problems, and as bronchodilators (D'Avonzo). They are used in the treatment of narcolepsy, attention deficit disorder (ADD), and attention deficit hyperactivity disorder (ADHD) (D'Avonzo). Stimulants are also used to treat depression in the medically ill, particularly geriatric patients and people with HIV/AIDS (Keltner & Folks, 2001).

These drugs are used illicitly by the oral, intranasal, or intravenous routes. Stimulants produce heightened sensations including feelings of euphoria, increased energy, and decreased social inhibitions. Pleasurable activities, such as sex, seem more intense and are often accompanied by increased feelings of mastery, power, and self-confidence. Impairment in decision making and psychotic reactions can occur that can lead to hostile and violent behavior, especially when combined with alcohol (D'Avonzo, 2001).

Cocaine was introduced as an anesthetic in 1858. Cocaine is extracted from the coca plant and is available in several forms: white powder for intranasal use (snorting), dissolved and injected intravenously, smoked, or free-based in the form of "crack" (rocks of cocaine base). Freebasing involves removal of the water-soluble adulterants from the cocaine, thus producing a purified substance more palatable for smoking that also has better absorption (Holbrook, 1991). Cocaine can also be used orally in any of these forms. Intravenous, smoking, or freebasing provides an immediate high or rush. With respect to crime, morbidity, and mortality, cocaine and crack are the most costly illicit drugs to society (Allen, 2001).

Prescription Drugs

Adults over 65 years of age consume more prescription medications than any other age group. Prescription drug misuse or abuse among older adults usually involves benzo-diazepines and other sedative hypnotics. Benzodiazepines represent 17–23% of drugs prescribed to older adults (Center for Substance Abuse Treatment, SAMHSA, 1998). Benzodiazepine use in older adults is correlated with female gender, increased number of drugs used, college education, Caucasian ethnicity, and a history of depression (Finlayson, 1995).

Sedative–hypnotics   Many of the drugs in this class are commonly prescribed drugs that are used for a variety of medical problems. Barbiturates (Seconal, Nembutal, Amytal, Tuinal, and Phenobarbital), barbiturate-like drugs (Quaaludes), and benzodiazepines (Valium, Librium, Xanax, Klonopin, Halcion, and Ativan) are all widely abused drugs (Allen, 2001; D'Avonzo, 2001).

Barbiturates are used in headache preparations (Fiorinal, Fiorocet) and as anticonvulsants. Benzodiazepines are used to treat anxiety and panic disorders, sleep disorders, and are indicated as muscle relaxants and anticonvulsants. They cause significant central nervous system depression and reduce anxiety, cause a loss of inhibition, drowsiness, emotional instability, ataxia, decreased aggressiveness, or, on occasion, a paradoxical effect of increased aggression, memory loss, and lowered seizure threshold. Barbiturates can be lethal if taken in an overdose and, like benzodiazepines, produce physical and psychological dependence that has a severe, life-threatening withdrawal syndrome (Allen, 2001; D'Avonzo, 2001).

This group of drugs produces effects similar to alcohol and other sedative hypnotics. The withdrawal syndrome associated with sedative hypnotics is also consistent with the signs and symptoms seen in alcohol withdrawal. In particular, withdrawal from benzodiazepines produces autonomic and anxiety rebound, sensory excitement, motor and cog-

nitive excitation. These symptoms are dependent on the amount of the drug ingested and duration of time used (Boyd, 2002; Faltz & Skinner, 2002).

Narcotics or Opioids   *Opioid* refers to opiates and their derivatives, both natural and synthetic. This class of drugs includes legal and illicit drugs. Natural opiates include opium and morphine. Heroin is a semisynthetic narcotic and is an illicit drug in the United States. Synthetic opioids include drugs such as codeine sulfate, propoxyphene, meperidine, hydromorphone, fentanyl, dolophine, oxycodone, and morphine sulfate contin; these drugs are illegal except by prescription. They can be taken orally, smoked, snorted, injected into soft tissue (skin-popping) or used intravenously (Allen, 2001).

These drugs have both sedative hypnotic and analgesic effects. They can produce physical and psychological dependence. Use of these substances by older adults is often related to the management of chronic pain. Two to three percent of older adults use opioids by prescription. Opioids are ranked second only to benzodiazepines among abused prescription drugs in the older adult population and represent the second-most-commonly cited reason for admission for chemical dependence treatment by adults age 55 and older (SAMHSA, 2003). Aside from the legitimate use of opioids for pain, these drugs can be abused by people seeking the euphoric mood that may result from their use or abuse. Other common effects are relaxation and drowsiness ("nodding") and sleep. Heroin can be combined with cocaine in a mixture referred to as a "speedball which provides a potent effect of euphoria and analgesia" (Allen, 2001).

Nicotine   Nicotine is one of 4000 chemicals found in the smoke from tobacco in cigarettes, cigars, and pipes and is the component of tobacco that acts on the brain (National Institute on Drug Abuse [NIDA], 2003). It is a highly addictive substance and most smokers use tobacco regularly because they are addicted to nicotine.

Caffeine Although caffeine is abused or misued by all age groups, caffeine abuse will not be considered substance abuse for the sake of this chapter. Although caffeine misuse or overuse may have an effect on the physical condition of elders, it does not result in the same negative consequences encompassing all spheres of life as the other substances described in this section.

Other substances of abuse Substances such as hallucinogens, inhalants, anabolic steroids, and laxatives are abused in other age groups. Currently there are few data describing use of these drugs in older adults.

REVIEW OF THE LITERATURE

Research related to substance abuse in older adults has been developed in several areas: (1) definition and prevalence of the problem in the elder population, (2) identification of risk factors associated with substance abuse in elders, (3) morbidity and mortality rates with substance abuse in elders, (4) assessment and screening issues particular to the elder population, and (5) development of new techniques for treatment of substance abuse in elders (Fingerhood, 2000). Additionally, several studies have examined the issue of substance abuse in the older female (Eliason, 2001; CASA Report, 1998).

Most of the literature and research in the area of substance abuse in the older population has focused on the abuse of alcohol. As previously mentioned, with the aging of the baby boomer cohort, studies looking at the abuse of other substances, as well as alcohol, and polysubstance abuse will need to be developed. Although a thorough review

of the literature is beyond the scope of this chapter, several research studies will be highlighted.

SCREENING TOOLS FOR IDENTIFICATION OF SUBSTANCE ABUSE IN THE OLDER ADULT

There are a number of problems related to identifying substance abuse in the older adult. The use of screening instruments cannot be routinely generalized to older adults who have variant life issues and consequences from drug use and abuse. The vast amount of literature relies on measures primarily of alcohol and its impact. Other screening tools have been adjusted for applicability for the elderly individual. Although it is generally believed that the patient history and medical record provide a clear picture of substance use, too often patterns of use are overlooked by health care professionals or well-intended family members. Interviews and history taking are subject to inaccurate history of substance use and possible signs of dementia. Finlayson, Hurt, Davis and Morse (1988) reported that self-report methods are unreliable because of the aging person's memory deficits.

Following are the primary screening tools used when assessing the older adult for potential substance abuse and related life issues.

CAGE Questionnaire

The CAGE questionnaire was developed in the early 1970s by John Ewing, MD (1984) of the University of North Carolina at Chapel Hill. It is considered one of the most reliable and nonincriminating sets of questions to gauge an individual's use of a substance, primarily alcohol, and life effects. It consists of four questions that indicate covert problem drinking. It meets the requirements for brevity, ease of administration, sensitivity and validity (Mayfield, McLeod, & Hall, 1973). It is a screening technique that has become the gold standard for rapid assessment and usability. Because it has only four questions, it has long been considered the best screening tool to use for assessment of substance use and abuse potential.

Use of the tool, however reliable, continues to limit the scope of potential consequences of an older adult with an entrenched denial system. It offers a window through which a clinician can view the older adult's life concerns but can also shortsight the person's life consequences that relate to drug use and drinking patterns, loneliness, isolation, loss of family and friends, and health destruction. Another drawback to this tool is that the primary focus is on alcohol. Prescription drugs are not included as part of the screen, although this area of substance use and dependence can be significant for the older adult. Clinicians have attempted to make the tool more comprehensive by adapting the tool by replacing the word *alcohol* with the word *drugs* when asking the questions.

Fingerhood (2000) suggests additional questions be asked prior to the use of the CAGE questionnaire. He advocates the use of general assessment questions in an open-ended frame:

- Integrate alcohol use inquiry into the interview so that it follows inquiry about less sensitive habits:

  "We have talked about your usual diet and your smoking. Can you tell me how you use alcoholic beverages?"

- For patients who report present or past use of alcohol, screen for evidence of alcoholism:

  "Has your use of alcohol caused any kinds of problems for you?"

  or

  "Have you ever been concerned about your drinking?"

  (Fingerhood, p. 987).

By the use of these two lead questions, the nurse is now poised to utilize the CAGE questionnaire which can build on the information already provided.

1. "Have you ever felt you should Cut down on your drinking?

2. Have people Annoyed you by criticizing your drinking?

3. Have you ever felt bad or Guilty about your drinking?

4. Have you ever had a drink first thing in the morning to steady your nerves or get rid of a hangover (Eye-opener)?" (Ewing, 1984, p.1905)

In general, a score of two or more in response to the above four questions is considered a positive response and requires further assessment for substance use. A score of one or more on a CAGE questionnaire has a sensitivity and specificity of about 80% in adults older than 60 years and is considered a positive screen for substance use and potential abuse—requiring further assessment (Dekker, 2002). A CAGE-T, which has a question that involves trauma ("Have you ever been injured after drinking?"), may increase sensitivity in equivocal CAGE screenings of older adults. It is also considered less effective for screening of women problem drinkers.

MAST-G (Michigan Alcoholism Screening Test—Geriatric)

The Geriatric Michigan Alcoholism Screening Test is an adaptation of the original MAST series of 24 questions developed at the University of Michigan (Blow, Brower, Schulenberg et al., 1992). Respondents provide a yes or no answer to the questions. Five or more yes answers are considered a positive response to the screening tool and require further assessment for alcohol use or dependence. The sensitivity is 91–93% with a specificity of 65–84% (Blow et al.). The list that follows is the MAST-G series of questions:

1. After drinking, have you ever noticed an increase in your heart rate or beating in your chest?

2. When talking with others, do you ever underestimate how much you actually drink?

3. Does alcohol make you sleepy so often that you fall asleep in your chair?

4. After a few drinks, have you sometimes not eaten or been able to skip a meal because you didn't feel hungry?

5. Does having a few drinks help decrease your shakiness or tremors?

6. Does alcohol sometimes make it hard for you to remember parts of the day or night?

7. Do you have rules for yourself that you won't drink before a certain time of the day?

8. Have you lost interest in hobbies or activities you used to enjoy?

9. When you wake up in the morning, do you ever have trouble remembering part of the night before?

10. Does having a drink help you sleep?

11. Do you hide your alcohol bottles from family members?

12. After a social gathering, have you ever felt embarrassed because you drank too much?

13. Have you ever been concerned that drinking might be harmful to your health?

14. Do you like to end an evening with a nightcap?

15. Did you find your drinking increased after someone close to you died?

16. In general, would you prefer to have a few drinks at home rather than go out to social events?

17. Are you drinking more now than in the past?

18. Do you usually take a drink to relax or calm your nerves?

19. Do you drink to take your mind off your problems?

20. Have you ever increased your drinking after experiencing a loss in your life?

21. Do you sometimes drive when you have had too much to drink?

22. Has a doctor or nurse ever said he or she was worried or concerned about your drinking?

23. Have you ever made rules to manage your drinking?

24. When you feel lonely, does having a drink help?

A shortened version of the MAST-G encompasses a series of 10 selected questions from the full MAST-G. Questions number 2, 4, 5, 6, 18, 19, 20, 22, 23, 24 comprise the shortened version of the MAST-G. A scoring of two or more yes responses is indicative of an alcohol problem and requires further detailed assessment. The primary focus of this screening tool is alcohol; prescription (medication) drug abuse is not addressed in the screen.

IMADUS (Impressions of Medication, Alcohol, and Drug Use in Seniors)

This tool was developed by Gerald Shulman (2003), a noted addiction specialist in the field of elderly substance abuse, to address the limitations of the CAGE and MAST-G. This tool screens for problems with alcohol, prescription drugs, and over-the-counter medication and has a specific aim to reduce feelings of shame in the older adult being evaluated. Three or more positive answers indicate the need for further assessment.

1. Does your use of medication or alcohol make you feel so sleepy that you fall asleep in your chair?

2. Do you find yourself using alcohol to help you sleep?

3. Have you occasionally spent more time drinking or using other drugs than you intended?

4. Have you found yourself thinking a lot about taking your medication or drinking?

5. Do your social and recreational activities often involve drinking?

6. Have you given up activities because they did not involve drinking?

7. Does using medication or alcohol sometimes make it difficult for you to remember what you said or did?

8. Have you ever neglected doing something you should have done because of medications or drinking?

9. Have you ever used medication or alcohol to relieve emotional discomfort, such as sadness, anger, loneliness, or boredom?

10. Have you ever felt you needed medication or alcohol just to keep going?

11. Have you ever told anyone that you drank less than you actually did?

12. In the past 12 months, have you at any time used more medications or drunk more alcohol than you meant to?

13. Have you ever had an injury while drinking that required medical attention?

14. Have you used alcohol with prescribed or over-the-counter medications even after being instructed not to do so?

15. Have you ever found yourself short of money because of what you spent on alcohol?

16. Did your drinking change or increase after some event such as death of a loved one or retirement?

17. Has a relative, or friend, or doctor ever suggested changing the way you use your medications or cutting down on your drinking?

18. Have you ever felt that your medication use or drinking was a problem?

19. Do you ever wonder whether the use of medication or alcohol may be bad for your health, finances, or independence?

20. Has anyone (family, friends, or doctor) raised questions about or objected to your use of medications or alcohol?

(Shulman, p.18)
Reprinted with permission

ALCOHOL ABUSE AND THE OLDER ADULT

In a study as far back as 1982, Brody asserted that about 10–15% of elderly patients seeking medical help for any reason have an alcohol-related problem. The older adult who is using or abusing substances in any form poses a difficult challenge for geropsychiatric nurses. Only recently have primary providers begun to look at this emerging crisis. A review of current literature and methodology to examine this topic reflects a paucity of information. The unidentification of drug use in this particular age group is in response to many variables and societal attitudes. Discussion and review of the problem requires a frank conversation among health care providers at the national public policy level, the academic setting, and the clinical level.

Too often, attitudinal stereotyping of aging can influence a health care provider from assessing an aging person. The older adult can present a wide range of responses to questions about use of alcohol and/or other chemicals and too often the abuse potential can be overlooked. In addition, standardized screening tools do not differentiate between early- and late-onset elderly alcohol abuse, making treatment of this population more difficult. Close observation that comprehensively assesses the person's needs and issues will identify symptoms that may be subclinical or attributed to a comorbid diagnosis or another etiology.

Fingerhood (2000) describes older adults with two categories of alcoholism: early and late onset. In early onset alcohol abuse, the individual had alcoholism present earlier in life. According to earlier studies (Adams & Waskel, 1991; Atkinson, Tolson, & Turner, 1990) two thirds of older alcohol abusers fall into the early-onset group. This group is more likely to drink to intoxication, more likely to have been in alcohol treatment in the past, more likely to have legal, financial, or occupational problems, and less likely to have social supports. Often they are undiagnosed or have been diagnosed with substance abuse in various forms, but their longstanding substance use has been treated without success. In addition, untreated substance use in their lifetime may induce a chronic state of health problems with impaired cognition.

Late-onset alcohol abuse occurs after the age of 60. This group is more likely to enter treatment as a result of a crisis (e.g., driving under the influence), more likely to report feelings of depression or loneliness, more likely to deny an alcohol problem, and more likely to have identifiable supportive family or friends (Adams & Waskel, 1991; Atkinson et al. 1990; Fingerhood, 2000).

Shulman (2003) states that those individuals who develop late-onset alcoholism do so generally in response to the stress of aging. He defines situations that increase the likelihood of late-onset alcoholism as the following:

- Retirement with the loss of structure, support, and self-esteem provided by employment
- Loneliness and isolation that may be a result of widowhood
- Loss of sensory capabilities and/or reduced mobility exacerbating isolation and loneliness
- Geographical and emotional separation from family and friends with resultant loss of social and emotional support
- Reactive depression
- Combined use of multiple prescribed medications, over-the-counter drugs, and drinking, even in modest amounts

- Increased financial and health problems or concerns about these problems and the individual's ability to remain independent.
- Reduced ability of the aging body to handle alcohol

(Shulman, p.18)

HEALTH ASSESSMENT

Historically, substance abuse in older adults has been an underdiagnosed and undertreated problem. Not unlike many other disorders seen in the older adult population, the presentation of substance abuse is often nonspecific and atypical in nature. It can easily be mistaken for other geriatric illnesses or aging changes (DeHart & Hoffman, 1995; Lichtenberg, Gibbons, Nanna, & Blumenthal, 1993; Solomon, Manepalli, Ireland, & Mahon, 1993). Symptoms of substance abuse may appear as psychiatric or physical disorders. Assumptions regarding the prevalence of abuse, and the potential for recovery among older adults, may interfere with the provider's ability to correctly assess and plan for these individuals. Contrary to these assumptions, elders have a 75% recovery rate, the highest of any age group (Center for Substance Abuse Treatment, SAMHSA, 1998).

The use of health assessment and review of standard laboratory tests supplement standardized screens. Health assessment, performed by a skilled clinician–practitioner, can elicit much information regarding use of substances, even prior to review of laboratory data and clinical indices.

A review of systems approach offers a comprehensive view of overall health and the interplay of substances within the person's life patterns. In addition, a biopsychosocial review of the individual's life can illuminate substance use as it interfaces with the maturational changes of the aging adult. Very often, a person can have decades of substance use or abuse that can be confounded by the clinical presentation of dementia. In this case, it may be helpful to utilize a combination of tests and screening tools to make a more accurate clinical diagnosis. The geropsychiatric nurse is able to obtain an accurate assessment of the older adult with substance abuse and complicated maturational issues may be defined. Nurses can play a "vital role in identifying the range of alcohol-related problems" (Eliason, 1998, p. 23) in the older adults they work with.

Masters (2003) asserts that "the increases in affluence, education, and life expectancy achieved in the twentieth century have produced an aging population that has not only increased in numbers but also has more leisure time and disposable income, a more positive attitude toward alcohol, and higher rates of alcohol consumption than in previous generations" (p. 155). She further states that "longer life expectancy is associated with greater exposure to health risks and a concomitant increase in chronic disease and polypharmacy" (p. 155). Thus, a specific screening instrument for the older adult, combined with structured health assessment questions, will elicit the broadest base of information on which to base a comprehensive plan of care.

Strategies that may assist geropsychiatric nurses in assessment of this unique population include:

1. Health assessment techniques and tools geared toward the older adult

2. Strong knowledge base of alcohol and other substances and the physiological effects on the older adult

3. Routine utilization of geriatric standardized screening tools to examine for substance use or abuse in this population

4. Cultural awareness of substance use or abuse within a family or culture

5. Team approach for all providers to address the older adult's use of a substance

6. Humane planning for substance abuse education and treatment

7. Awareness of substance abuse programs that employ a geriatric track or utilize a case manager that is skilled in the care of this particular population

MEDICATION ASSESSMENT

A key role in geropsychiatric clinical nursing practice is the assessment of prescribed medications as well as active or suspected concomitant use of alcohol by the older adult. It is important to understand how the older adult conceptually values his or her prescribed medication. The individual's use of medication and understanding of the therapeutic effect can provide a clue as to the potential for substance use and misuse. A comprehensive review of all over-the-counter (OTC) and prescription medications is recommended. How the medications are taken can indicate the priority the aging adult places on a particular medication or practice. For example, a person may be unable to obtain antihypertensive medication but may view it as less important than having their prescribed benzodiazepine available, which they use for a sleep aid. The intended use of the benzodiazepine was as an antianxiety medication but the older adult begins the practice of self-medication for sleep and misuse of the drug begins. Development of tolerance to the therapeutic effect can ensue.

In addition, older adults can also believe particular medications assist them in their independence, which they value highly. Use of alcohol may steady their nerves, prescribed narcotics control painful conditions such as arthritis, mood stabilizers and antidepressants help to battle depression and loneliness, and sleeping pills assist with the common complaint of insomnia. The interplay among these drugs, compounded by the potentiation of additional medications, can wreak havoc in an aging body. In addition, older adults may not fully comprehend the criteria for use of the medication and the clinical reasoning as to why it was prescribed for them.

MEDICAL CONSEQUENCES OF SUBSTANCE ABUSE

Alcohol is the most commonly abused substance in any age group. Alcohol, or ethanol, is a central nervous system (CNS) depressant, and is classified as a sedative–hypnotic. At lower doses, the effect is psychologically calming while at higher doses it produces sleep induction. The CNS depression is not the only neuronal response. Some neurons, rather than decreasing their rate of firing, actually increase firing. This produces a removal of inhibitory response and may contribute to the disinhibition seen at lower doses, evidenced by excitement and aggression (Grilly, 2002). Alcohol causes a multiplicity of physical and psychological effects. Alcohol, when combined with other CNS depressants, can have a significant synergistic effect. Alcohol is capable of causing physical and psychological dependence. Physically, no body system is unaffected by alcohol, resulting in significant neurological, gastrointestinal, and cardiovascular effects. Psychologically, alcohol affects complex cognitive skills, fine and gross motor skills, visual accommodation, and unconditioned reflexes (Grilly).

Alcohol intake produces slowed mental functions, decreased coordination, slurred speech, ataxia, euphoric or labile mood, decreased blood pressure and pulse. Withdrawal symptoms usually develop within six to eight hours after cessation of alcohol ingestion. Withdrawal symptoms include increased blood pressure and pulse, nausea, vomiting, anxiety, tremor, and diaphoresis. Severe withdrawal signs and symptoms include hal-

lucinations, seizures, and delirium tremens (Lisanti, 2001; Saitz, 1998). The severity of withdrawal is highly individualized and can cover a wide range of clinical presentations. Varying opinions exist as to the effect of age on the severity of withdrawal. Kraemer, Mayo-Smith, and Calkins (1997) concluded that age did not significantly change the severity of withdrawal scores when quantitative self-report measures or instruments were used. However, the study cohort, age 60 and older, did demonstrate an increased risk for delirium and functional impairment. In spite of these findings, other sources include older age as a risk factor for increased severity of withdrawal. Additional risk factors for severity of withdrawal include past history of alcohol dependence and withdrawal, concomitant illness, and abnormal hepatic function (Saitz).

REVIEW OF SYSTEMS

The assessment includes a careful review of systems, the utilization of screening tools, corroboration of information from family and friends when appropriate, and complete physical examination and diagnostics. Changes that occur in gastrointestinal, cardiovascular, neurological, renal, musculoskeletal, and hematological systems are of particular significance when assessing the older substance abuser (Ebersole & Hess, 1998; Edlund & Spain, 2003).

Gastrointestinal

Gastrointestinal age-related changes include decreased gastrointestinal motility, prompting the use of OTC laxatives and antacids and decreased absorption of nutrients (Ebersole & Hess, 1998; Katzung, 2001). There is a decrease in gastric alcohol dehydrogenase, the enzyme that converts alcohol to acetaldehyde, in the first step of alcohol metabolism. This contributes to higher blood alcohol levels and increases the hepatic burden in older adults. Additionally, gastric ADH levels are lower for women at all ages (National Institute on Alcohol Abuse and Alcoholism [NIAAA], 1997; Smith, 1995). There is an age-related decrease in hepatic size and blood flow, which can be further affected by alcohol and drug use. This can produce slowed metabolic rate of certain drugs and increased risk of toxicity. Additionally, older adults demonstrate decreased ability to recover from hepatic damage (Ebersole & Hess).

Varieties of gastrointestinal disorders are related to the abuse of alcohol. Esophagitis, gastritis, and exacerbation of ulcer disease are related to frequent vomiting and increased gastric acid secretion. These disorders may be further complicated by the concurrent use of aspirin or nonsteroidal anti-inflammatory agents. The effect of alcohol on the small intestine produces a decrease in the absorption of nutrients including folic acid and vitamin B12. Alcohol-related pancreatitis produces a decrease in pancreatic enzymes with resulting malabsorption. Clinically, individuals with alcohol-related pancreatitis have nausea, vomiting, pain, weight loss, and diarrhea.

Effects on the liver include fatty infiltration, hepatitis, and cirrhosis. Fatty infiltration is usually asymptomatic while alcoholic hepatitis, an inflammatory process, produces a presentation similar to gallbladder disease, with hepatomegaly, fever, jaundice, leukocytosis, and pain. Elevations of hepatic enzymes aspartate aminotransferase (AST) and alanine aminotransferase (ALT), with AST higher than ALT, are often part of the clinical presentation of alcohol-induced hepatic disease (Martin, Schaffer & Campbell, 1999). Cirrhosis, a process of fibrosis, can cause portal hypertension, esophageal varices, edema, and ascites. Initial clinical presentation may include anorexia, fatigue, weakness, and weight loss. Jaundice, ascites, and edema are seen later in the course of the disease. Skin manifestations of liver disease can include spider nevi, palmar erythema, glossitis, and cheilosis. Hepatic encephalopathy may develop secondary to an accumulation of toxic substances, including ammonia. The early stages of encephalopathy resemble organic brain syndrome, progressing to delirium, somnolence, and coma. The amount and duration of alcohol intake that can precipitate these effects is individual-specific.

Cardiac

Cardiac age-related changes that are exacerbated by alcohol intake include a decrease in myocardial contractility, output, and coronary circulation. Alcohol can also contribute to an increase in blood pressure caused by an increase in peripheral vascular resistance (Ebersole & Hess, 1998; Smith, 1995).

Cardiomyopathy caused by alcohol may produce a clinical presentation of heart failure and arrhythmia with decreased exercise tolerance, tachycardia, dyspnea, edema, palpitations, and cough. Although treatment choices for cardiomyopathy are limited and the course is variable, the cessation of alcohol use can produce an improvement in cardiac function (Ebersole & Hess, 1998; Katzung, 2001; Massie & Amidon, 2003; Smith, 1995). Alcohol abuse can result in or present with hypertension, particularly in men and older adults, though advanced age alone is a risk factor for hypertension. Arrhythmias, including atrial fibrillation, premature ventricular beats, and sustained ventricular tachycardia, can be seen after episodes of heavy alcohol ingestion. Older adults with preexisting cardiac disease are at higher risk from alcohol ingestion. Risk of stroke is also increased with abuse of alcohol (Smith).

Neurological

Neurological age-related changes include slowed reaction time, forgetfulness, decreased short-term memory, slowed time for task completion, and altered kinesthetic sense (Ebersole & Hess, 1998; Edlund & Spain, 2003). All age-related neurological changes can be exacerbated by alcohol and other sedative hypnotics. Peripheral neuropathy is often caused by long-term exposure to alcohol. This type of neuropathy begins distally, usually noted in the feet before the hands, and progresses proximally. Pain, burning, tingling, and numbness are reported. This may progress to muscle weakness and wasting, producing a foot-drop gait.

Brain function changes that result from alcohol include impaired learning and decreased concentration, abstract thinking, judgment, short-term memory, and problem solving. These changes contribute to the behavioral manifestations noted with substance abuse. Advancing age is considered a risk factor for dementia related to alcohol (Smith, 1995). A recent review discusses the need to further understand the effects of alcohol on Alzheimer's disease, which is the most common cause of dementia. This review suggests that the use of alcohol can worsen the impairments produced by this form of dementia (Wiscott, Kopera-Frye, & Seifert, 2001).

The neurological effects of alcohol also include Wernicke's encephalopathy, an uncommon condition seen in long-term alcohol abuse produced by thiamine deficiency. This condition presents with paralysis of external eye muscles, ataxia, and confusion. Wernicke's encephalopathy is a reversible condition that can progress to Korsakoff's psychosis without treatment. Korsakoff's psychosis presents with confusion, memory loss, and confabulation. Unlike other forms of dementia, memory impairment is the predominant feature with sparing of other cognitive functions (Masters, 2001; Wilson, 1994).

Renal and Pharmacokinetics

Normal age-related renal changes include decreased renal blood flow producing a reduction in the glomerular filtration rate, measured by creatinine clearance. Excretion of drugs is predominantly a function of renal clearance. As function declines, drugs have a prolonged half-life. Distribution of drugs is affected by the decrease in muscle mass, total body water, and albumin, all of which accompany aging. This results in higher alcohol levels with less alcohol ingested and higher levels of protein-bound drugs (Masters, 2001). Age-related physiological changes, coupled with the significant consumption of prescription medications and drug interactions with alcohol, produce considerable risk to this population (Center for Substance Abuse Treatment, SAMHSA, 1998; NIAAA, 1995).

Musculoskeletal

Alcohol contributes to decreased bone density and accelerated bone loss. These effects contribute to poor mobility, falls, and fractures (Smith, 1995). Alcohol can also contribute to decreased muscle mass and cause both acute and chronic myopathy. Proximal muscle wasting and weakness that characterizes chronic myopathy increases the fall risk. Acute myopathy produces pain, tenderness, and edema in proximal muscle groups after excessive ingestion of alcohol. This acute process can elevate creatinine phosphokinase (CK); lactic acid dehydrogenase (LDH), and aspartate aminotransaminase (AST). This process may be significant enough to cause myoglobulinemia and acute tubular necrosis (Smith).

Hematological

All aspects of cell development are affected by alcohol. Erythropoietin production can be affected by hepatic and pancreatic disease, producing hypoproliferative disorders. Red blood cell maturation as well as survival is affected by alcohol and the decreased availability of folic acid. Additionally, hypersplenism seen in severe liver disease contributes to red blood cell destruction. A complete blood count with platelet count, red blood count indices, and white blood count differential should be used to diagnose these conditions. In addition to anemia, thrombocytopenia, and leukopenia, a macrocytic anemia, characterized by a decreased red blood count and an elevated mean corpuscular volume (MCV) and mean corpuscular hemoglobin (MCH), is often associated with alcohol abuse. This macrocytosis is secondary to low folic acid or vitamin B12 absorption (Linker, 2003; Smith, 1995).

Immune

Various aspects of the immune system are affected by alcohol, including lower polymorphonuclear leukocyte (PMN) counts, contributing to decreased ability to fight infection. Decreased lymphocytes also contribute to impaired cell-mediated immunity. Alcohol abuse may decrease total white blood cell and platelet counts. White blood cells' ability to fight infection may also be diminished. The risk of cancer is increased by the abuse of alcohol. Cancers of the liver, esophagus, larynx, and mouth are among the cancers increased by alcohol abuse. Also the effects of alcohol and smoking, behaviors that commonly coexist, contribute to oropharyngeal cancers (Masters, 2001; Smith, 1995).

Dermatological

Alcohol abuse is often associated with rosacea and rhinophyma. Rosacea presents as facial erythema, telangiectasias, and acne-like papules. Rhinophyma is a lobulated thickening of the lower portion of the nose. Psoriasis can be worsened by alcohol intake. Alcohol abuse has been associated with discoid eczema, usually seen on the lower extremities, as well as increased incidence of skin infections (Smith, 1995).

NURSING INTERVENTIONS TO ADDRESS SUBSTANCE ABUSE IN THE OLDER ADULT

Intervention capability, when working with an older adult who has substance abuse in his or her current lifestyle, requires a particular skill set that includes being adept at recognition, intervention, and referral. The intervention must be negotiated while supporting the integrity of the person as well as being respectful of their experiences and coping strategies, whether considered harmful or beneficial. Often older adults face discrimination and ageism regarding their own life choices and they may continue to shun health care providers and/or minimize their own use of substances for fear of reprisal, negative responses from family and caregivers, and an unwillingness to cease use altogether of the chemical of choice. Shame-based individuals will continue to remain reclusive about their use of substances (Shulman, 2003). Allowing the older adult a safe arena in which to discuss and respond to routine questions about substance use affords the beginning of a therapeutic relationship in which health promotion can be initiated to improve the quality of life.

Awareness by the nurse that alcohol-use disorders have been found to be a predictor of suicide risk in men and women should prompt an assessment for suicidal thoughts and plans (Waern, 2003). Older adults as a population are at risk for suicide, and this risk is increased with alcohol-use disorders. The deteriorating social function associated with alcohol disorders is thought to play an integral part in the loss of contact, changes in energy for life, and the effort required to sustain a sober lifestyle. Clearly, the geropsychiatric nurse attuned to the maturational needs and functional changes of the older person will have the capacity to address treatment in a humane and respectful manner.

Treatment for the older adult with a diagnosed substance-abuse disorder requires a unique blend of compassion and respect from staff who are specifically educated to treat this population. Clearly, geropsychiatric nurses attuned to the maturational needs and changes of the older person will have the capacity to address treatment in a humane and respectful manner.

A program of recovery for this population must address quality of life, as well as physical and mental capabilities. In addition, drug use and misuse and amounts of substances used must be clearly addressed in a caring and supportive manner. The confrontational model used in many substance-abuse treatment centers has little impact on a person who views him or herself at the final stage of life. Shulman (1998) describes traditional intervention strategies to be far less effective with this population. He states that the leverage conditions, such as loss of employment or criminal sanctions, do not have the same importance in this age group. In addition, Shulman further describes that families of the older adult may not respond to standard intervention methods because of the belief that they are being publicly humiliated by the substance abuse of their loved one. Often the goal of initial intervention is to improve the person's health status with the byproduct being enjoyment of life. If substance abuse is detected, a brief intervention can assist the individual to decrease his or her use of substances by utilizing a treatment plan. A series of brief intervention steps will facilitate change at this level.

Brief Intervention Steps

1. Give feedback on screening.
2. Discuss reasons for drinking.
3. Discuss consequences of drinking.

4. Discuss reasons to cut down or quit.
5. Develop strategies for achieving goal.
6. Develop an agreement in the form of a written contract.
7. Identify obstacles to achieving goal.
8. Discuss strategies to overcome obstacles.
9. Summarize session

(Fingerhood, 2000, p. 991).

Older adults who abuse substances and become chemically dependent will benefit from this structured approach. Utilizing these steps may help to modify heavy use of any substance and may be an effective methodology to create a treatment plan. Older persons who demonstrate mild symptoms of withdrawal may be monitored at home if family members are supportive and present to assist in the overall care. The elderly person who exhibits severe withdrawal, or who is medically compromised, requires an in-patient setting for safety and ongoing medical supervision of a potentially dangerous and unpredictable state. Use of pharmacological agents to withdraw a person requires a medical and nursing skill set and familiarity with the patterns of any acute abstinence syndrome (withdrawal). A focus on the psychosocial issues with older adults is an essential part of recovery in this age group (Liberto & Oslin, 1995). The management plan must also address the need for referral to specialists in the field of substance abuse and older adults, as well as collaborative approaches to the multidisciplinary care plans established.

The ultimate goal is to return older adults to the community with an enriched awareness of personal health in the domains of physical, mental, emotional, and spiritual connectedness in the twilight of their lifetime.

REFERENCES

Adams, S. L., & Waskel, S. A. (1991). Late onset of alcoholism among older mid-western men in treatment. *Psychology Reports, 68,* 432–434.

Allen, L. (2001). Drugs of abuse. In N. L. Keltner & D. G. Folks (Eds.), *Psychotropic Drugs* (3rd ed.) St. Louis, MO: Mosby.

American Psychiatric Association (2000). *Diagnostic and Statistical Manual of Mental Disorders* (4th ed.). Washington, DC: Author.

American Society of Pain Management Nurses (2003). *ASPMN Position Statement: Pain Management in Patients with Addictive Disease.* Pensacola, Florida: Author.

Atkinson, R. M., Tolson, R. L., & Turner, J. A. (1990). Late versus early onset drinking in older men. *Alcoholism: Clinical and Experimental Research, 14*(4), 574–579.

Blow, F. C., Brower, K. J., Schulenberg, J. E., et al. (1992). The Michigan Alcoholism Screening Test-Geriatric Version (MAST-G): A new elderly specific screening instrument. *Alcoholism: Clinical and Experimental Research, 16,* 372.

Boyd, M. A. (2002). *Psychiatric Nursing: Contemporary Practice* (2nd ed.). Philadelphia: Lippincott.

Brody , J. A. (1982). Aging and alcohol abuse. *Journal of the American Geriatrics Society, 30,* 123–126.

CASA Report (1998). *Under the Rug: Substance Abuse and the Mature Woman.* New York: National Center on Addiction and Substance Abuse at Columbia University.

Center for Substance Abuse Treatment, Substance Abuse and Mental Health Services Administration (1998). *Substance Abuse Among Older Adults: Treatment Improvement Protocol (TIP) Series 26.* Rockville, MD: Department of Health and Human Services, Public Health Service.

D'Avonzo, C. E. (2001). Common drugs of abuse. In M. A. Naegle & C. E. D'Avonzo (Eds.), *Addictions and Substance Abuse: Strategies for Advanced Practice Nurses* (pp. 333–354). Upper Saddle River, NJ: Prentice Hall Health.

DeHart, S. S., & Hoffman, N. G. (1995). Screening and diagnosis of alcohol abuse and dependence in older adults. *The International Journal of Addictions, 30*(13/14), 1717–1747.

Dekker, A. H. (2002, April). Alcoholism in the elderly. Program and abstracts presented at the 33rd Annual Meeting & Medical-Scientific Conference, American Society of Addiction Medicine, April 26, 2002.

Ebersole, P., & Hess, P. (1998). *Toward Healthy Aging: Human Needs and Nursing Response* (5th ed.). St. Louis, MO: Mosby.

Edlund, B. J., & Spain, M. (2003). Geriatric assessment. *Advance for Nurses, 3,* 18–22.

Eliason, M. J. (1998). Identification of alcohol-related problems in older women. *Journal of Gerontological Nursing, 24*(10), 8–15.

Eliason, M. J. (2001). Drug and alcohol intervention for older women: A pilot study. *Journal of Gerontological Nursing, 27*(12), 18–24.

Ewing, J. (1984). Detecting alcoholism: The CAGE questionnaire. *Journal of American Medical Association, 252*(14), 1905–1907.

Faltz, B. G., & Skinner, M. K. (2002). Substance abuse disorders. In M. A. Boyd (Ed.). *Psychiatric Nursing: Contemporary Practice* (2nd ed.). Philadelphia: J. B. Lippincott.

Fingerhood, M. (2000) Substance abuse in older people. *Journal of the American Geriatrics Society, 48*(8), 985–995.

Finlayson, R. E., Hurt R. D., Davis L. J., & Morse, R. M. (1988). Alcoholism in elderly persons: Study of the psychiatric and psychosocial features of 216 inpatients. *Mayo Clinic Proceedings, 63,* 761–768.

Finlayson, R. E. (1995). Misuse of prescription drugs. *The International Journal of Addictions, 30* (13/14), 1871–1901.

Grilly, D. M. (2002). *Drugs and Human Behavior* (4th ed.). Boston: Allyn & Bacon.

Holbrook, J. M. (1991). CNS stimulants. In E. G. Bennet & D. Woolf, *Substance Abuse: Pharmacological, Developmental and Clinical Perspectives* (2nd ed.). Albany, NY: Delmar.

Katzung, B. G. (2001). *Basic and Clinical Pharmacology* (8th ed.). New York: Lange Medical Books/ McGraw Hill.

Keltner, N. L., & Folks, D. G. (2001). *Psychotropic Drugs* (3rd ed.). St. Louis, MO: Mosby.

Kraemer, K. L., Mayo-Smith, M. F., & Calkins, D. R. (1997). Impact of age, severity, course, and complications of alcohol withdrawal. *Archives of Internal Medicine, 157,* 2234–2240.

Liberto J. G., & Oslin D. W. (1995). Early versus late onset of alcoholism in the elderly. *The International Journal of the Addictions, 30*(13/14), 1799–1818.

Lichtenberg. P. A., Gibbons, T .A., Nanna. M. J., & Blumenthal, F. (1993). The effects of age and gender on the prevalence and detection of alcohol abuse in elderly medical inpatients. *Clinical Gerontologist, 13*(3), 17–27.

Linker, C. A. (2003). Blood. In L. M. Tierney, S. J. McPhee, & M. A. Papadakis (Eds.). *Current Medical Diagnosis and Treatment 2003* (42nd ed., (pp. 469–521). New York: Lange Medical Books/McGraw Hill.

Lisanti, P. (2001). Adult health: Acute care. In M. A. Naegle & C. E. D'Avanzo (Eds.), *Addictions and substance abuse: Strategies for advanced practice nursing* (pp. 137–188). Upper Saddle River, NJ: Prentice Hall Health.

Martin, A. C., Schaffer, S. D., & Campbell, R. (1999). Managing alcohol-related problems in the primary care setting. *The Nurse Practitioner, 24*(8), 14–39.

Massie, B. M. & Amidon, T. M. (2003). Heart. In L. M. Tierney, S. J. McPhee & M. A. Papadakis (Eds.), *Current Medical Diagnosis and Treatment 2003* (42nd ed., pp. 312–408). New York: Lange Medical Books/McGraw-Hill.

Masters, J. (2003). Moderate alcohol consumption and unappreciated risk for alcohol-related harm among ethnically diverse, urban dwelling elders. *Geriatric Nursing, 24*(3), 155–161.

Masters, S. (2001). The alcohols. In B. G. Katzung (Ed.), *Basic and clinical pharmacology* (8th ed., pp. 1036–1044). New York: Lange Medical Books/McGraw Hill.

Mayfield D., McLeod G., & Hall, P. (1973). The CAGE questionnaire: Validation of a new alcoholism and screening instrument. *American Journal of Psychiatry, 131*(10), 1121–1123.

National Institute on Alcohol Abuse and Alcoholism (1995). *Alcohol Alert: Alcohol–Medication Interactions* (27 PH 355). Bethesda, MD: Author.

National Institute on Alcohol Abuse and Alcoholism. (1997). *Alcohol Alert: Alcohol Metabolism.* Bethesda, MD: Author.

National Institute on Drug Abuse (2003). Nicotine addiction. Retrieved December 14, 2004, from www.nida.nih.gov/researchreports/nicotine.

Saitz, R. (1998). Introduction to alcohol withdrawal. *Alcohol Health and Research World, 22*(1), 5–12.

SAMHSA, Office of Applied Studies. (2003). *The NHSDA Report: Substance Use Among Older Adults.* Rockville, MD: Author.

Savage, S. R. (1993). Addiction in the treatment of pain: Significance, recognition and management. *Journal of Pain and Symptom Management, 8*(5), 265–278.

Shulman, G. (1998). The challenge of assessment and treatment of the older alcoholic and substance abuser. A six-part Web site series—East Carolina University. Retrieved November 10, 2004, from www.counselors@addictioninfo.com.

Shulman, G. (2003*).* Senior moments: Assessing older adults. *Addiction Today, 15*(82), 17–19.

Smith, J. W. (1995). Medical manifestations of alcoholism in the elderly. *The International Journal of the Addictions, 30*(13/14), 1749–1798.

Solomon, K., Manepalli, J. M., Ireland, G. A., & Mahon, G. M. (1993). Alcoholism and prescription drug abuse in the elderly: St. Louis University grand rounds. *Journal of the American Geriatrics Society, 41*(1), 57–69.

Waern, M. (2003). Alcohol dependence and misuse in elderly suicides. *Alcohol and Alcoholism, 38,* 249–254.

Wilson, S. (1994). Can you spot an alcoholic patient? *RN, 57*(1), 46–50.

Wiscott, R., Kopera-Frye, K., & Seifert, L. (2001). Possible consequences of social drinking in the early stages of Alzheimer's disease. *Geriatric Nursing, 22*(2), 100–104.

Issues in Geropsychiatric and Mental Health of Older Adults

CHAPTER 11

Delirium

Karen Dick, PhD, APRN, BC, FAANP
Catherine R. Morency, MS, APRN, BC

CASE STUDY

Mrs. R. is an 80-year-old active woman with a history of hypertension and diabetes mellitus, controlled with oral medication. She lives alone in her own apartment and wears bilateral hearing aids. Yesterday she underwent a left cataract extraction in the day surgery department of a local hospital. She received a dose of a benzodiazepene before the procedure. She had significant back pain during the procedure from lying on the table and received two doses of Tylenol and codeine. She was sent home with instructions to return to see the eye surgeon the following day. On the morning of the appointment, her son arrives to pick her up. Mrs. R. answers the door in her nightgown. She seems surprised to see him. He notices from the pillbox that she has not taken her evening pills, nor her morning pills today. While he is talking to her, she drifts off to sleep. He assumes she has been up most of the night. She is unable to answer his questions and busies herself with a pile of newspapers by the door.

Imagine that you are the nurse for the eye surgeon. What are the risk factors for delirium in the above case? How would you go about evaluating contributing factors? What interventions would be appropriate? The above case represents a typical scenario that nurses frequently encounter in their daily practice.

INTRODUCTION

Delirium is a serious and significant health problem in the elderly population. It is a syndrome of disturbed consciousness, attention, cognition, and perception. Delirium represents complex interactions between medical conditions, cognitive function, and behavior and, for many elders, it is often the first and only indicator of underlying physical illness (Lyness, 1990). Delirium contributes to increased morbidity and mortality, longer hospital stays, functional impairment, and more permanent forms of cognitive impairment if it is not recognized and treated in a timely fashion (Levkoff, Besdine, & Wetle, 1986; Levkoff et al., 1992; Lipowski, 1983; Marcantonio et al., 2003; Murray et al., 1993). This syndrome can occur in elders at any point across the care continuum, from community, long-term care, to acute care settings. Delirium can be present in the emergency room on admission to the hospital, develop while the patient is hospitalized, and persist long after the patient is discharged to home or institutional settings. It is not clear why elders are at such high risk for this syndrome. Some believe that the brain is the "vulnerable" organ in an older adult and cumulative insults to the body may be reflected in changes in cognitive functioning from acute brain failure. But it is important for clinicians to know that delirium is reversible, if it is recognized as an *acute* change and precipitating causes are removed in a timely fashion.

The incidence estimates for delirium in hospitalized patients range widely because of both sampling and diagnostic criteria, and range from 14% to 56% (Inouye, 1994). Patients who have undergone hip fracture repair are particularly prone to delirium with incidence rates ranging from 35–65% (Marcantonio, Flacker, Wright, & Resnick, 2001). Delirium has also been described in patients at the end of life, particularly in patients with advanced cancers. Research has shown that the symptoms of delirium can last from weeks to months (Gruber-Baldini, et al., 2003; Murray, et al., 1993) and for some, a delirium can represent the beginning of a decline trajectory (Levkoff, et al., 1992). The costs to the health care system for care of patients with delirium have been estimated to be between $1 billion and $2 billion annually (Inouye, 1994). Patients with a preexisting dementia are at highest risk for delirium. Because delirium can be life threatening, it must be thought of as a medical emergency, which needs prompt recognition, treatment of potentially removable causes, and supportive care. Nurses are in key positions to recognize, identify, and manage patients with delirium in all health care settings. Nurses also play a critical role in identifying patients at risk for delirium and instituting measures to limit and even prevent an episode of delirium. The purpose of this chapter is to define delirium, identify individual patient risk factors, review how delirium is diagnosed, and outline treatment and nursing interventions.

■■■ TERMINOLOGY

Delirium has been described for thousands of years. Accounts of delirium in the medical literature have consisted primarily of case reports and clinical impressions (Levkoff, Cleary, Liptzin, & Evans, 1991). Even though the epidemiology of delirium has been studied for many decades, one of the greatest barriers to systematically integrating the research and writing to date has been the lack of a consistent nomenclature. More than 25 terms have been used to describe the confusional state from "acute brain syndrome" to "toxic befuddlement" (Francis & Kapoor, 1990). It has also been described as pseudosenility, pseudodementia, and acute confusional state. This syndrome is labeled in a number of ways depending on the clinical population and the background of the evaluator (Neelon, 1990). Acute confusion is the terminology that is used most commonly. Although delirium and acute confusion are used interchangeably, some do not believe that acute confusion and delirium are the same thing, and that delirium is a medical phenomenon. Rasin (1990) states "Nurses seem to use the term confusion as an abbreviated means to describe the constellation of clinical manifestations that fall within the medical diagnosis of dementia or delirium" (p. 910). Nurses also tend to identify both cognitive and behavioral manifestations of confusion, as well as a continuum from "slightly confused to highly confused" (Vermeersch, 1991). According to Foreman (1993), the term "acute confusion" requires no translation for the bedside practitioners, does not connote etiology, and represents more closely what is observed clinically by nurses (p. 6). But if confusion is defined as a loss of capacity to think with clarity and coherence, identifying confusion per se is just the labeling of a *symptom* and can represent different psychiatric syndromes (Johnson, 1990). That is why it is difficult to determine if the terminology and definitions that nurses use in fact represent the same or a different phenomenon when used by their physician counterparts. For the purpose of this chapter, delirium will be used, as it is the terminology most widely used by mental health providers when describing acute cognitive changes in older adults.

DEFINITION

The description that follows is the generally accepted definition of delirium as stated by the *Diagnostic and Statistical Manual* (4th ed., text revision) (American Psychiatric Association [APA], 2000). Again, it is important to remember that it serves as a method for making a clinical diagnosis. These diagnostic criteria for delirium are as follows:

1. Disturbance of consciousness (reduced clarity of awareness of the environment) with reduced ability to focus, sustain, or shift attention.

2. A change in cognition (such as memory deficit, disorientation, or language disturbance) or the development of a perceptual disturbance that is not better accounted for by a preexisting, established, or evolving dementia.

3. The disturbance develops over a short period of time (usually hours to days) and tends to fluctuate during the course of the day.

4. There is evidence from the history, physical examination, or laboratory findings that the disturbance is caused by the direct physiological consequences of a general medical condition (APA, 2000, p. 143).

A few points must be made. First, in regards to the change in cognition that is not accounted for by preexisting dementia, knowledge of the patient's baseline cognitive status needs to be determined. Often this is not immediately known and requires investigation of when the change in mental status actually occurred. This is critical to the diagnosis. Second, the DSM also describes other subcategories of delirium including substance-induced delirium, substance-withdrawal delirium, delirium attributed to multiple etiologies, and delirium not otherwise specified, but often the etiology of the delirium is not always known at the time of diagnosis. And third, the question of an incomplete manifestation of the delirium syndrome has been raised. Some believe that it is possible for patients to have some symptoms of delirium but not all; this is referred to as subsyndromal delirium (Cole, McCusker, Dendukuri, & Han, 2003). But how many of the DSM criteria must be met in order to make the diagnosis of delirium? There remains no clear consensus.

PATHOPHYSIOLOGY

Four mechanisms have been proposed to explain the physiologic precipitants that underlie the development of delirium (Johnson, 1990):

1. an insufficiency of cerebral metabolism as demonstrated by diffuse slowing on an electroencephalogram (EEG) in a patient with delirium,

2. a central abnormality caused by an imbalance of central cholinergic and adrenergic metabolisms,

3. activation of cytokines, and

4. a stress reaction as evidenced by abnormally high circulating corticosteriods.

There remains a lack of agreement as to the exact mechanism, but the acetylcholine theory has drawn more attention of late. Patients with Alzheimer's dementia have decreased acetylcholine due to loss of cholinergic neurons and are at high risk of delirium.

Anticholinergic drugs are known to precipitate delirium and certain metabolic abnormalities may decrease acetylcholine synthesis in the central nervous system and contribute to the development of delirium. There is also some evidence that even drugs used commonly in the elderly, such as digoxin, furosemide, prednisone, and theophylline, may have anticholinergic activity (Cole & McCusker, 2002). And finally, increased levels of anticholinergic activity have been shown to correlate with the severity of delirium in some hospitalized elderly patients (Mach, et al., 1995).

RISK FACTORS

Although there has been wide variability in reported risk factors associated with delirium,

individual, physiological, environmental, and pharmacological risk factors have been identified (Foreman, 1986; Foreman, 1989; Francis, Martin, & Kapoor, 1990; Inouye, Viscoli, Horwitz, Hurst, & Tinetti, 1993; Rockwood, 1993; Schor, et al., 1992) (see Table 11-1). It is most likely that predisposing factors interact with aggravating factors to influence the course. Research has suggested that between two and six factors may be contributing in any one case of delirium (Rudberg, Pompei, Foreman, Ross, & Cassel, 1997). It is believed that the risk of delirium increases as the number of risk factors increase. Patients with minimal risk factors may have a margin of safety before any dysfunction occurs as compared to those who might be near threshold where very little stress may precipitate cognitive dysfunction (Neelon, 1990). It may also be that

TABLE 11-1 Risk Factors for Delirium			
Individual	**Physiologic**	**Pharmacologic**	**Environment**
Advanced age	Postoperative state	Polypharmacy	Stress
Visual impairment	Infection	Withdrawal from	New or change in
Hearing impairment	Dehydration	alcohol or drugs	environment
Preexisting cognitive impairment	Hypoxia		Excessive or lack of
Preexisting brain disorders:	Anemia		sensory input;
stroke, Parkinson's	Malnutrition		isolation
Previous delirium episodes	B12, folate		Absence of clock,
Severe chronic illnesses	deficiencies		watch, reading
Immobility (including restraint	Hypovolemia		glasses
use)	Hypo- or		
Disordered sleep	hypernatremia		
Depression	Low-perfusion states		
Use of bladder catheters			

Note. Adapted from "Acute Confusional States in Hospitalized Elderly: A Research Dilemma," by M. Foreman, 1986, *Nursing Research, 35*(1), pp. 34–38; also from "Confusion in the Hospitalized Elderly," by M. Foreman, 1989, *Research in Nursing & Health, 12,* pp. 21–29; also from "A Prospective Study of Delirium in Hospitalized Elderly," by J. Francis, D. Martin, and W. Kapoor, 1990, *Journal of the American Medical Association, 263*(8), pp. 1097–1101; also from "A Predictive Model for Delirium in Hospitalized Elderly Medical Patients Based on Admission Characteristics," by S. Inouye, C. Viscoli, R. Horowitz, L. Hurst, and M. Tinetti, 1993, *Annals of Internal Medicine, 119,* pp. 474–481; also from "The Occurrence and Duration of Symptoms in Elderly Patients with Delirium," by K. Rockwood, 1993, *Journal of Gerontology, 48*(4) pp. M162–M166; also from "Risk Factors for Delirium in the Hospitalized Elderly," by J. Schor, S. Levkoff, L. Lipsitz, C. Reilly, P. Cleary, J. Rowe, et al., 1992, *Journal of the American Medical Association, 267*(6), pp. 827–831.

there are protective or mediating factors that influence the development of delirium. It is important for clinicians to not assume that there is just one single factor and stop in the search for any and all potentially contributing factors when assessing a patient's risk of delirium. In many circumstances, risk factors may not be modifiable, but clinicians may be alerted to patients at highest risk so that early surveillance and monitoring may allow for more timely interventions (Liptzin, 1995).

As for pharmacological factors, almost any drug can contribute to delirium with anticholinergics, benzodiazepines, and narcotics being the major offenders. Over-the-counter medications (OTC) must also be considered.

SUBTYPES AND PATTERNS

Clinical subtypes of delirium have been identified and these include hyperactive, hypoactive, and mixed variants (Lipowski, 1987; Liptzin & Levkoff, 1992). The hyperactive subtype is the classic picture of the patient who is agitated, restless, combative, and hyperalert. Patients may have fast or loud speech, be distractible, and have fast motor responses. These are the patients who pull out IV lines and catheters, try to climb over bedrails, and are at greatest risk for complications from injury and physical or chemical restraints. They also require increased nursing surveillance and care, often straining already depleted staffing resources. Surprisingly, these cases account for less than 25% of all cases but have the worst outcomes, including nursing home placement or death at one month (Marcantonio, Ta, Duthie, & Resnick, 2002).

The hypoactive subtype includes patients who have decreased alertness, sparse or slow speech, lethargy, slowed movements, and apathy. These patients may be somnolent or stuporous. Because these patients are quiet and do not present nursing staff with increased demands for care or surveillance, the chance that these patients will *not* be identified as delirious is high. But in one study of hip fracture patients that looked at both delirium severity and psychomotor types, patients with pure hypoactive delirium had better outcomes than patients with hyperactive delirium even after adjusting for severity (Marcantonio, Ta, Duthie, & Resnick, 2002). The mixed variant subtype includes symptoms of both hyper- and hypoactive subtypes with patients cycling between the two and accounts for more than 50% of cases. These patients often are not identified as being delirious until they become agitated and confused with more symptoms of the hyperactive state.

Neelon and colleagues (1989) have described three types of patterns of confusion development in hospitalized elderly. In the first pattern, patients with low cognitive reserve such as dementia are extremely susceptible to environmentally provoked states, including sensory deprivation or overload. In the second pattern, patients with low physiological reserve or instability are influenced by physiological factors including pain, hypoxia, and high illness levels. In the third pattern, patients with low biochemical reserve due to renal and hepatic impairment are vulnerable to toxic agents such as drugs, which are key in the development of delirium. The authors postulate that the risk for the development of acute confusion is a cumulative function of the patient's vulnerability, the timing and magnitude of the effect of multiple added stressors, and the support of biopyschosocial integrity (Neelon, 1990). The goal for nursing becomes one of identifying and treating the underlying causes in order to protect the vulnerable systems that have little reserve (Champagne & Wiese, 1992).

CLINICAL COURSE

There is no one classic trajectory of delirium, but features that are common to all delirium include sudden onset and fluctuating symptoms. This fluctuation in presentation is problematic, as patients may have periods of lucidity interspersed with inattention and high distractibility. Evaluating a patient's mental status once a day (picture morning rounds in the hospital) can totally miss the delirious state. Patients may also have motor restlessness, speech that is difficult to follow, and perceptual disturbances that range from misinterpretations of the environment to frank visual hallucinations. Memory, particularly in relation to recent events, is often impaired, and disorientation, most commonly to time (day of the week or time of the year) or place, is usually present. Patients may also exhibit affective signs of fear, anxiety, or anger. There may be a history of a fragmented and disordered sleep–wake cycle. Symptoms of anxiety, restlessness, and agitation may be worse in the late afternoon or evening; this presentation has been labeled "sundowning," but it is not clear if sundowning is a component of delirium or a separate clinical entity (Burney-Puckett, 1996). It is known that institutionalized patients with dementia are at greatest risk of sundowning. The temporal aspects of sundowning allow clinicians to predict vulnerable time periods and to utilize both nonpharmacologic and pharmacologic interventions to keep patients calm and safe.

THE PROBLEM OF RECOGNITION

Patients who become confused during the course of their hospitalization, or whose pre-existing cognitive impairment worsens, present nursing staff with the challenge of maintaining patient safety, well-being, and function (Miller, 1991). Misdiagnosis and subsequent failure to treat can have catastrophic consequences for the patient and have been associated with irreversible brain failure, institutionalization, increased patient care costs, and death (Francis & Kapoor, 1992;

Lipowski, 1989; Schor, et al., 1992). But nurses and physicians often fail to recognize and diagnose delirium and may attribute any form of cognitive impairment to normal aging (Lipowski, 1987).

In hospitalized elderly, a downward decline into acute confusion may be seen as a normal trajectory with no need for intervention (Csokasy, 1999). It has been suggested that between 37% and 72% of patients who become acutely confused are never recognized by physicians and nurses as being in an acute confusional state (Foreman, 1989). Patients may be incorrectly labeled as having a dementia, a psychiatric disorder, or unmanageable behavior (Lipowski, 1983; Wolanin & Phillips, 1981). Other explanations for underdiagnosis by nurses have included lack of knowledge (Brady, 1987), social factors and setting (Morgan, 1985), varied clinical reasoning styles (McCarthy, 1991), the presence of dementia (Fick & Foreman, 2000), degree of cooperation with care (Palmateer & McCartney, 1985), and individual factors in the nurse, patient, and environment which influence patient labeling (Ludwick, 1993). In a recent study of elderly patients admitted to an acute care hospital, four risk factors for underrecognition of delirium by nurses were identified: the presence of the hypoactive form, age 80 years or older, vision impairment, and dementia (Inouye, Foreman, Mion, Katz, & Cooney, 2001).

The multidimensional nature of delirium with its fluctuating course, variation in presentation from hyperactive and hypoactive subtypes, and lack of consensus as to its features, all contribute to its underrecognition. Because nurses have a full-time presence in acute care, intermediate, and long-term care settings, it is critical for nurses caring for elders to identify patients at risk, accurately assess patients with cognitive and behavioral changes, and institute appropriate interventions to support patient safety and recovery. To do this successfully requires ongoing education and training for nurses in all aspects of the delirium syndrome.

▬ EVALUATION

As there is no one single diagnostic test for delirium, the evaluation of the patient should focus on identifying that the disorder is in fact present and that any and all underlying contributing medical conditions and factors are treated or removed.

Identify the Presence of Delirium

The critical point is to understand the patient's baseline cognitive status and the timing and onset of the symptoms. How is what is being observed different from the patient's baseline? Does the patient have an underlying dementia or other brain diseases, such as Parkinson's disease or a history of stroke? When did the patient first demonstrate a change in cognition or behavior? Clinicians may have to obtain the history from family members, formal caregivers, or staff members if the patient comes from an institutional setting. Because the hallmark of delirium is inattention, utilizing mental status tests that require patient cooperation and attention may prove to be difficult. Standard mental status exams such as the MMSE (Folstein, Folstein, & McHugh, 1975) may be used to question the patient and at least obtain some screening information. But it is not uncommon to see patients with acute changes in mental status become more agitated with direct questioning. For patients who may be lethargic and slow to respond, direct questioning may not provide an accurate assessment.

While there are many tests of mental status, only a few are specific to diagnosing delirium (see Table 11-2). Tools most useful for nursing practice include those that are brief and easy to use without being burdensome to the patient. The most commonly used is the Confusion Assessment Method (CAM) developed by Inouye and colleagues (1990). The CAM is a simple tool that can be used quickly and accurately at the bedside by all clinicians to diagnose delirium. It has a sensitivity of 94–100% and a specificity of 90–95% (Inouye, et al., 1990) (see Table 11-3). The diagnosis of delirium requires the presence of features 1 and 2 and either 3 or 4. It can also help differentiate between delirium and dementia. The CAM-ICU is a version developed specifically for use in critical care settings and can be used with ventilated patients (Ely, et al., 2001).

While the CAM is useful for diagnosing the *presence* of delirium (patients either have it or they do not), another tool is available to quantify the severity or intensity of symptoms. The Memorial Delirium Assessment Scale (MDAS) was originally developed for use with cancer patients with delirium. It scores patients on a scale of 0–30 (30 being worst score) using a 10-item inventory that measures arousal, level of consciousness, psychomotor activity, memory, attention, orientation, and thinking (Breibart et al., 1997). The MDAS can be used in conjunction with the CAM for a complete assessment.

TABLE 11-2 Delirium Instruments	
Delirium Symptom Interview (DSI)	Albert et al., 1992
Delirium Rating Scale (DRS)	Trepacz, Baker, & Greenhouse, 1988
Confusion Assessment Method (CAM)	Inouye et al., 1990
Memorial Delirium Assessment Scale (MDAS)	Breibart et al., 1997
Delirium Observation Screening (DOS)	Schuurmans, Shortridge-Baggett, & Duursma, 2003
NEECHAM Confusion Scale	Neelon, Champagne, Carlson, Funk, 1996

TABLE 11-3 CAM (Confusion Assessment Method)	
1. Acute onset and fluctuating course	Usually obtained from a family member or nurse and shown by positive responses to the following questions: "Is there evidence of an acute change in mental status from the baseline?" and "Did the abnormal behavior fluctuate during the day, that is, tend to come and go, or increase and decrease in severity?"
2. Inattention	Shown by a positive response to the following: "Did the patient have difficulty focusing attention, for example, being easily distractible or having difficulty keeping track of what was being said?"
3. Disorganized thinking	Shown by a positive response to the following: "Was the patient's thinking disoriented or incoherent, such as rambling or irrelevant conversation, unclear or illogical flow of ideas, or unpredictable switching from subject to subject?"
4. Altered level of consciousness	Shown by any answer other than "alert" to the following: "Overall, how would you rate this patient's level of consciousness?" Normal = alert Hyperalert = vigilant Drowsy, easily aroused = lethargic Difficult to arouse = stupor Unarousable = coma

Note. From Inouye, et al. "Clarifying Confusion: The Confusion Assessment Method," by S. Inouye, C. van Dyck, C. Alessi, S. Balkin, H. Siegal, and R. Horowitz, 1990, *Annals of Internal Medicine, 13*(12), p. 946. Reproduced with permission from the American College of Physicians.

It is also important for clinicians to be able to differentiate features of delirium from dementia and from depression in elderly patients, as features of all three may coexist in an individual (see Table 11-4). It has been estimated that the prevalence of delirium superimposed on dementia ranges from 22–89% in both hospitalized and community-dwelling elders (Fick, Agostini, & Inouye, 2002). Patients with a hypoactive delirium may be identified as being depressed rather than delirious. When in doubt, always diagnose delirium because patients who go untreated are at greater risk than those patients who simply have a chronic cognitive impairment. In other words, always investigate a change in cognitive or behavioral signs and symptoms in elderly patients, and never assume they are "normal."

Identify and Treat Underlying Medical Conditions

The following mnemonic "DELIRIUM" is a helpful tool for identifying reversible causes of delirium (Beers & Berkow, 2000). Rarely is delirium only caused by one factor. It is important to review and treat *all* possible contributing factors.

D   Drugs
E   Electrolyte abnormalities, dehydration
L   Low-oxygen states (MI, stroke)
I   Infection
R   Reduced sensory input
I   Intracranial (CVA, TIA, seizure)
U   Urinary or fecal retention
M   Myocardial (CHF, MI, arrhythmia)
    (p. 351)

- **D**elirium—Review the record for the list of medications, with particular note of anything newly added or omitted which may lend a clue as to the cause of the change in mental status. Even if a person has been on a medication for years, this does not mean that it is not the cause for a delirium. A drug that was started when a person was 60 years of age is metabolized differently once that same person's liver and kidneys are 80 years old, and the situation may now be compounded by dehydration and sepsis. Is the patient undergoing withdrawal? Is the patient taking any over-the-counter medications? Drug levels may be useful in identifying toxic quantities.

- **E**lectrolyte abnormalities, dehydration— The usual evaluation includes blood work to identify imbalances in sodium, potassium, BUN, creatinine, calcium, and glucose. Is the patient dehydrated? A urine specific gravity and color test can indicate hydration status.

- **L**ow-oxygen states—An oxygenation saturation level can quickly rule out a low-oxygen state as a contributing factor.

- **I**nfection—A urinalysis and culture can rule in a urinary tract infection, which is a common cause of mental status changes. Patients recently discharged from an acute care setting are at risk for developing UTIs as an iatrogenic complication of hospitalization. Auscultate the patient's lungs; pneumonia in an older adult often presents without classic signs of fever and cough, and a change in mental status may be the only indication of an underlying pulmonary process. An elevated WBC can also indicate an acute infection.

- **R**educed sensory input—Is the patient without his or her glasses or hearing aids? Is the patient in an under- or overstimulating environment? Does the patient have access to orienting devices such as a watch, clock, and calendar? Has the patient re-

cently undergo multiple transfers across settings, from home to ER, to ICU, to general unit, to a skilled nursing facility?

- **I**ntracranial—Does the patient have a history of a recent fall that might indicate a slowly accumulating subdural hematoma? A screening neurological examination might reveal deficits that indicate vascular compromise. Determine if the patient has a history of seizures or other neurological conditions or impairments. Patients may undergo brain imaging, either CT or MRI, to rule out structural abnormalities.

- **U**rinary or fecal retention—An abdominal and rectal examination and review of the intake and output sheet will give a clue as to whether retention of urine or stool is a cause.

- **M**yocardial—Does the patient have a history of heart disease, including MI or arrhythmia? Again, in the older adult, an MI may present with only a change in mental status instead of the classic signs of substernal chest pain. A thorough cardiovascular assessment including an EKG can help determine cardiac abnormalities.

The family or staff should also be asked if the patient had ever experienced previous episodes of delirium and under what circumstances. In summary, a thorough evaluation of all potentially contributing factors is critical to a successful outcome.

SUPPORTING SAFETY AND RECOVERY

The goal of care for patients with a suspected delirium is to support and protect the patient while the underlying causes are identified and treated. There is no question that nursing care of the delirious, older patient can be both challenging and frustrating for even the most experienced nurse. No one thing works. Appropriate nursing care of delirious patients

TABLE 11-4   A Comparison of the Clinical Features of Delirium, Dementia, and Depression

Clinical Feature	Delirium	Dementia	Depression
Onset	Acute/subacute, depends on cause, often at twilight or in darkness	Chronic, generally insidious, depends on cause	Coincides with major life changes, often abrupt
Course	Short, diurnal fluctuations in symptoms, worse at night, in darkness, and on awakening	Long, no diurnal effects, symptoms progressive yet relatively stable over time	Diurnal effects, typically worse in the morning, situational fluctuations, but less than with delirium
Progression	Abrupt	Slow but uneven	Variable, rapid or slow but even
Duration	Hours to less than 1 month, seldom longer	Months to years	At least six weeks, can be several months to years
Awareness	Reduced	Clear	Clear
Alertness	Fluctuates, lethargic or hypervigilant	Generally normal	Normal
Attention	Impaired, fluctuates	Generally normal	Minimal impairment, but is easily distracted
Orientation	Generally impaired, severity varies	Generally normal	Selective disorientation
Memory	Recent and immediate impaired	Recent and remote impaired	Selective or "patchy" impairment, "islands" of intact memory
Thinking	Disorganized, distorted, fragmented, incoherent speech, either slow or accelerated	Difficulty with abstraction, thoughts impoverished, judgment impaired, words difficult to find	Intact but with themes of hopelessness, helplessness, or self-deprecation
Perception	Distorted, illusions, delusions, and hallucinations, difficulty distinguishing between reality and misperceptions	Misperceptions usually absent	Intact, delusions and hallucinations absent except in severe cases
Psychomotor behavior	Variable, hypokinetic, hyperkinetic, and mixed	Normal, may have apraxia	Variable, psychomotor retardation or agitation
Sleep–wake cycle	Disturbed, cycle reversed	Fragmented	Disturbed, usually early morning awakening
Associated features	Variable affective changes, symptoms of autonomic hyperarousal, exaggeration of personality type, associated with acute physical illness	Affect tends to be superficial, inappropriate and labile, attempts to conceal deficits in intellect, personality changes, aphasia, agnosia may be present, lacks insight	Affect depressed, dysphoric mood, exaggerated and detailed complaints, preoccupied with personal thoughts, insight present, verbal elaboration
Assessment	Distracted from task, numerous errors	Failings highlighted by family, frequent "near miss" answers, struggles with test, great effort to find an appropriate reply, frequent requests for feedback on performance	Failings highlighted by individual, frequently answers "don't know," little effort, frequently gives up, indifferent toward test, does not care or attempt to find answer

Note. From "Assessing Cognitive Function," by M. Foreman, K. Fletcher, L. Mion, and L. Simon, 1996, *Geriatric Nursing*, 17(5), p. 229. Copyright 1996 by Elsevier. Reprinted with permission.

generally includes psychosocial, behavioral, and environmental support. The number of research studies that have tested the effect of specific interventions on patient outcomes is quite limited. The lack of a strong relationship between specific nursing interventions and a change in a patient outcome (as in the reduction in the delirium state) compels us to challenge our assumptions about practices that have been defined as the "gold standard." Research has not been able to demonstrate which interventions work best in combination nor has it determined the timing or sequencing of these interventions. Interventions work best when they are *tailored* to the individual patient. In one study of experienced nursing care of delirious hospitalized elderly, nurses utilized a range of interventions that were tailored to the patient's degree of confusion (Dick, 1998). For example, reorienting, cueing, and explaining hospital routines were useful strategies when a patient was less confused or agitated. The same cognitive strategies were not useful in patients who were highly confused as they were found to agitate patients further. For these patients, environmental strategies of minimizing stimulation, dimming lights, and minimizing physical presence were more useful (See Figure 11-1).

Another finding from this study was that nurses did not always attempt to reorient the patients who were disoriented. If the patient was agitated, it made no sense to reply to the hospitalized patient who believes he is in his house and has to go upstairs, "Mr. Smith, you are not at home, you are in the hospital." Sometimes "going to where the patient is" is very useful and helps calm the patient, rather than arguing about the patient's perceptions, particularly if they are frightening or worrisome.

In practice, nurses often learn from trial and error. Most nurses have been taught the standard interventions, such as repeated orientation, promoting proper sleep habits, early mobilization, timely removal of catheters, avoiding restraints, and the use of glasses and

---

FIGURE 11-1   Nursing Strategies for Individualized Delirium Care Based on Degree of Confusion

High . . . . Low

←——————————————————————————————————→

Degree of patient's confusion/agitation

Environmental	Physical/Sensory	Cognitive
Close observation	Maximizing or minimizing touch	Orienting/Reorienting
Dimming lights, noise	Maximizing or minimizing physical presence	Cueing/Coaching
Minimizing stimulation/interventions	Assist with ADLs	Explanation/Reassurance
Restraints (use as last resort)	Ensuring sensory aids: glasses, hearing aids, watch, clock, calendar	Helping patient "make sense of it"

Note. From Dick, K. (1998). "Acute Confusion in the Elderly Hospitalized Patient: An Exploration of Experienced Nursing Care," (Doctoral dissertation, University of Rhode Island, 1998), *Dissertation Abstracts International,* 59, p. 4015. Reprinted with permission.

hearing aids. These are important components of care for the patient with delirium. But the question remains, what types of interventions work best with what kinds of delirium symptoms and when are they best carried out? For example, a family member may calm patients with a hyperactive delirium by being in constant attendance, and the reduction of environmental stimulation provided by being in a private room may be helpful. A patient with hypoactive delirium may do better with increased stimulation and staff contact. It is important to find out as much as possible about the patient's usual habits and patterns and, if possible, recreate them in an attempt to "restore normalcy." This may be hard to do in a busy hospital setting or when no information is available, but attempting to establish familiar routines can be very useful.

In a 1999 article by Inouye et al., standardized intervention protocols for the management of six risk factors for delirium were used as part of a multicomponent intervention study. The six standardized protocols were for the management of cognitive impairment, sleep deprivation, immobility, visual impairment, hearing impairment, and dehydration. This risk factor intervention strategy resulted in significant reductions in the number and duration of delirium episodes in hospitalized older patients. The intervention had no significant effect on the severity of delirium or on recurrence rates. This finding suggests that primary prevention of delirium is probably the most important treatment strategy.

Physical and chemical restraints should be avoided wherever possible and used only in situations where patients are at risk of injuring themselves or others, or when agitation and restlessness may interfere with necessary medical treatments. Small doses of haloperidol and droperidol may be useful in controlling agitation and psychosis, and dosing should be guided by the patient's initial response and by frequent reassessment. Benzodiazepines are useful in the treatment of alcohol and sedative withdrawal.

It can be very difficult for family members and friends to see their loved one agitated and disoriented. Patients and families need reassurance and explanation that the delirium is related to the medical condition and is not a sign that the patient is "crazy," is "losing his or her mind," or is becoming "senile." A thorough explanation of the condition and short-term course is helpful in allaying fears. Involve family members in the plan of care including providing one-on-one observation, stimulation, support, and the bringing in of familiar objects from home. Patients also need an opportunity to reflect on the experience and to express their feelings as symptoms subside. In summary, the goal of treatment is to promote recovery, prevent additional complications, maintain the patient's safety, and maximize function.

DOCUMENTATION

Nurses have information that needs to be communicated to the other caregivers who are only seeing the patient for a brief time during the day and not at all at night. Because the nature of delirium is that symptoms wax and wane, and as there are many components of delirium, documentation that is helpful in making an accurate diagnosis is essential. But nurses consistently underdocument cognitive symptoms. In a study of the medical and nursing records of 55 patients hospitalized with hip fracture who experienced delirium, documentation of essential symptoms including onset and course of the syndrome, as well as disturbances in consciousness, attention, and cognition were seldom or never found in the nursing records (Milisen et al., 2002).

It has been our experience that nurses tend to focus on orientation, which is just one marker of mental functioning. In our 1994 study of hospitalized elderly, we found that while nurses' assessment of level of orientation matched an independent rating by a standardized instrument for the detection of delirium symptoms 81% of the time, nurses did less well assessing and documenting alterations in other domains, including fluctuating behavior (56%), perceptual disturbances (41%), and increased or decreased psychomotor behavior (64%) (Morency, Levkoff, & Dick, 1994). Because many delirious patients may do well on the orientation portion of a cognitive status exam, only describing the patient's level of orientation is not useful or complete. Few nursing notes specifically mention fluctuating level of consciousness, which is the hallmark of delirium. Even the terminology used is confusing. For example, what is the difference between mental status and cognitive status? For clarification, *mental* status is a broader concept that includes intellectual functioning, as well as emotional, attitudinal, psychological, and personality aspects of an individual. In contrast, *cognitive* status refers more specifically only to the aspect of intellectual functioning. Nurses should use the term cognitive status to refer to what they are evaluating.

Does the lack of documentation about cognitive status mean that it was not assessed or that it was assessed and no problem was identified? Does "Appears alert and oriented x 3" mean that the nurse actually asked the orientation questions or that there was no discernable problem in general conversation? How many patients with intact social skills are called oriented, but actually are not? There also may be no relationship between level of orientation and patient safety. A patient who is identified as oriented may lack appropriate judgment and attempt to get out of bed while on bedrest, or interfere with medical treatments. Simply put, describing a patient as "oriented" is not particularly useful.

Consider the following nursing documentation of a patient whose admission note says "Appears alert and oriented x 3" with no other mention of cognitive status. There is nothing about any cognitive problems at home, although the patient was described as a "poor historian." The following day the note says "appears confused" but no clarification.

The third day the patient is described as "lethargic" and that night is "agitated." Although the warning signs were there and the patient was at risk for delirium, it is often not until the delirium is a full-blown problem that it is recognized in the nursing documentation. What kind of information in the documentation could have better addressed the issue of delirium? Why is it that if delirium is a medical emergency, nurses continue to be undereducated about its importance in the care of older adults?

Let us reexamine the nursing note from above. On admission, the patient is accompanied by his wife who appears to answer most of the history questions. The nurse can take this opportunity to either say to the wife "I'd like him to answer and then I'll ask you to fill in the information," or to ask the wife "Is your husband able to answer the questions?" If, for example, the wife answers, "Well, I handle all the medications," the nurse then can probe as to whether this is because of memory impairment or other cognitive deficit. Asking a simple question such as "Who pays the bills in your home?" gives a wealth of information. Paying the bills correctly and keeping the checkbook in balance requires a high level of cognitive functioning. This would provide good history in the nursing documentation as to whether there might be a preexisting dementia, which puts the person at risk for delirium. On the first day when the patient "appears confused," an alternative note might have read "patient asked me if he was in a bakery, speech slow and halting, repetitive, awake most of the night, restless but not attempting to get out of bed." This gives information about orientation, speech, sleep, and psychomotor activity. On the following day, instead of "lethargic," the note could read "falling asleep while I was talking to him" or "trouble following directions, appears not to be able to focus."

Delirium is not hard to miss in the subtype with psychomotor agitation where the patient is climbing out of bed or verbally loud, but as a person with psychomotor retardation demands less attention from the nursing staff, particularly given the shortage of time, this subtype is more morbid, as it is more difficult to identify. The person may simply appear sleepy or "spacey."

It is also important that nurses accurately describe and document patient's cognitive status during times of transition, as nurses may underestimate the impact of incompletely and inaccurately describing cognitive status. It is easy to label patients as "confused," "disoriented," or "crazy." It does not matter if the patient is being transferred from the ICU to a floor, from a hospital bed to a subacute bed, or from hospital to home: the documentation provided is critical to informing the receiving nursing staff. Often on discharge forms, it is common to see language such as "patient is confused." What does that really mean? What does the nurse in the nursing home do with that information?

Think about how much more helpful it would be to read something like, "Patient with a long history of dementia, previously cared for at home by husband, who became acutely confused during hospital stay but has returned to prehospitalization baseline per husband. She is oriented to place only, is now calm and cooperative, and able to answer some questions." Nurses must be aware of the negative consequences of prematurely labeling patients. This occurs when inaccurate and incomplete information is passed along, from setting to setting, and once labeled as "confused," patients may never be identified as having an acute problem. Again, it is much more useful to identify specific patient cognitive abilities and behaviors.

ETHICAL ISSUES

Delirium by its nature impairs capacity to make decisions. It seems that as long as the person with delirium is making a decision that the health care professionals agree with,

the person's ability to make decisions is not questioned. However, if a person with delirium is making a decision about treatment that the staff does not agree with or is refusing necessary treatment, it is more likely to see notes stating that the person is not able to make decisions because of impaired cognitive status. In a prospective study of 173 medical and surgical procedures in patients with delirium at a university hospital, investigators found no documented assessments of competency or decision capacity and found cognitive assessment in only 4% of cases (Auerswald, Charpentier, & Inouye, 1997). The fluctuating nature of delirium also becomes problematic: decisions involving informed consent are a good example. Are patients really able to make informed decisions with a mental status that waxes and wanes?

Patients who experience delirium may or may not be able to remember a delirious episode. Schofield (1997) found that those patients that had illusions (misinterpretation or inaccurate perception of sensory impressions) (Taber's Cyclopedic Medical Dictionary) or hallucinations (which has no source in fact) (Taber's Cyclopedic Medical Dictionary) were often able to describe their experiences in detail. The patients were more than willing to talk about their experiences. They ranged from being pleasant and entertaining to horrible and frightening. Patients were also able to remember short verbal commands from nurses. Some reported being reassured by explanations and comforting measures even though they were unable to communicate.

SUMMARY

Although more prevalent in older adults, delirium is a medical emergency and should not be considered a normal part of aging, or a normal occurrence associated with hospitalization. Confusion is a symptom that something is wrong. It is never normal. Nurses are key to timely and prompt recognition: there cannot be treatment without recognition. Now that we have defined delirium, identified individual risk factors, discussed recognition, diagnosis, and treatment, the questions about the initial case study of the woman with cataract surgery can be answered. We now recognize that she is disoriented, has an altered level of consciousness, cannot follow her normal routine, is sleep deprived, and inattentive. The risk factors for Mrs. R. included advanced age, visual and hearing impairment, medical conditions, and the use of pain medications. You would evaluate the contributing factors by going through the mnemonic of DELIRIUM, identifying contributors and then working in conjunction with her physician/APN to treat anything that can be treated or removed, remembering not to stop at one factor. Appropriate interventions include keeping her in a familiar environment but having a family member stay with her to ensure that she's wearing her hearing aids, ensure the proper administration of her medications, ensure that she's eating regular meals and monitoring her blood sugar, and encouraging normal sleep routines and patterns that reduce anxiety and promote familiarity. Nurses can make all the difference in patient outcomes, and nowhere is that more true than in a patient with delirium.

For a copy of the evidence-based protocol *Acute Confusion/Delirium* developed by the Gerontological Nursing Intervention Research Center (GNIRC) at the University of Iowa go to http://www.nursing.uiowa.edu/centers/gnirc/protocols.htm. Another valuable resource is the *Standard of Practice Protocol: Acute Confusion/Delirium* developed by the NICHE (Nurses Improving Care for Health System Elders) (1999).

REFERENCES

Albert, M., Levkoff, S., Reilly, C., Liptzin, B., Pilgrim, D., Cleary, P. et al. (1992). The delirium symptom interview: An interview for the detection of delirium symptoms in hospitalized patients. *Journal of Geriatric Psychiatry and Neurology, 5*(1), 14–21.

American Psychiatric Association (APA). (2000). *Diagnostic and statistical manual of mental disorders – Text revision* (4th ed.). Washington, DC: Author.

Auerswald, K., Charpentier, P., & Inouye, S. (1997). The informed consent process in older patients who developed delirium. *The American Journal of Medicine, 103*(5), 410–418.

Beers, M. H. (Ed.). (1989). *Taber's cyclopedic medical dictionary* (17th ed.). Philadelphia: F. A. Davis.

Beers, M. H. & Berkow, R. (Eds.) (2000). *The Merck manual of geriatrics* (3rd ed.) (p. 351) Whitehouse Station, NJ: Merck Research Laboratories.

Brady, P. (1987). Labeling of confusion in the elderly. *Journal of Gerontological Nursing, 13*(6), 29–32.

Breibart, W., Rosenfield, B., Roth, A., Smith, M., Cohen, K., & Passik, S. (1997). The Memorial Delirium Assessment Scale. *Journal of Pain and Symptom Management, 13*(3), 128–137.

Burney-Puckett, M. (1996). Sundown syndrome: Etiology and management. *Journal of Psychosocial Nursing and Mental Health Services, 34*(5), 40–43.

Champagne, M., & Wiese, R. (1992). Research on cognitive impairment: Implications for practice. In S. G. Funk, E. M. Tornquist, M. T. Champagne, & R. A. Wiese (Eds.), *Key aspects of elder care.* (pp. 340–346), New York: Springer.

Cole, M., & McCusker, J. (2002). Treatment of delirium in older medical inpatients: A challenge for geriatric specialists. *Journal of the American Geriatrics Society, 50*(12), 2101–2103.

Cole, M., McCusker, J., Dendukuri, N., & Han, L. (2003). The prognostic significance of subsyndromal delirium in elderly medical patients. *Journal of the American Geriatrics Society, 51*(6), 754–760.

Csokasy, J. (1999). Assessment of acute confusion: Use of the NEECHAM Confusion Scale. *Applied Nursing Research, 12*(1), 51–55.

Dick, K. (1998). Acute confusion in the elderly hospitalized patient : An exploration of experienced nursing care. (Doctoral dissertation, University of Rhode Island, 1998). *Dissertation Abstracts International, 59,* 4015.

Ely, E., Margolin, R., Francis, J., May, L., Truman, B., Dittus, R., et al. (2001). Evaluation of delirium in critically ill patients: Validation of the Confusion Assessment Method for the intensive care unit (CAM–ICU). *Critical Care Medicine, 29*(7), 1370–1379.

Fick, D., Agostini, J., & Inouye, S. (2002). Delirium superimposed on dementia: A systematic review. *Journal of the American Geriatrics Society, 50*(10), 1723–1732.

Fick, D., & Foreman, M. (2000). Consequences of not recognizing delirium superimposed on dementia in hospitalized elderly patients. *Journal of Gerontological Nursing, 26*(1), 30–40.

Folstein, M., Folstein, S., & McHugh, P. (1975). Mini-mental state—a practical method for grading cognitive state of patients for the clinician. *Journal of Psychiatric Research, 12,* 189–198.

Foreman, M. (1986). Acute confusional states in hospitalized elderly: A research dilemma. *Nursing Research, 35*(1), 34–38.

Foreman, M. (1989). Confusion in the hospitalized elderly. *Research in Nursing & Health, 12,* 21–29.

Foreman, M. (1993). Acute confusion in the elderly. *Annual Review of Nursing Research, 11,* 3–30.

Francis, J., & Kapoor, W. (1990). Delirium in hospitalized elderly. *Journal of General Internal Medicine, 5,* 65–79.

Francis, J., & Kapoor, W. (1992). Prognosis after hospital discharge of older medical patients with delirium. *Journal of the American Geriatrics Society, 40*(6), 601–606.

Francis, J., Martin, D., & Kapoor, W. (1990). A prospective study of delirium in hospitalized elderly. *Journal of the American Medical Association, 263*(8), 1097–1101.

Gruber-Baldini, A., Zimmerman, S., Morrison, R., Grattan, L., Hebel, J., Dolan, M., et al. (2003). Cognitive impairment in hip fracture patients: Timing of detection and longitudinal follow-up.

Journal of the American Geriatrics Society, 51(9), 1227–1236.

Inouye, S. (1994). The dilemma of delirium: Clinical and research controversies regarding diagnosis and evaluation of delirium in hospitalized elderly medical patients. *American Journal of Medicine, 97*(3), 278–288.

Inouye, S., Bogardus, S., Charpentier, P., Leo-Summers, L., Acampora, D., Holford, T., et al. (1999). A multicomponent intervention to prevent delirium in hospitalized older patients. *New England Journal of Medicine, 340*(9), 669–676.

Inouye, S., Foreman, M., Mion, L., Katz, K., & Cooney, L. (2001). Nurses recognition of delirium and its symptoms: Comparison of nurse and researcher ratings. *Archives of Internal Medicine, 16*(20), 2467–2473.

Inouye, S., van Dyck, C., Alessi, C., Balkin, S., Siegal, A., & Horwitz, R. (1990). Clarifying confusion: The confusion assessment method. *Annals of Internal Medicine, 13*(12), 941–948.

Inouye, S., Viscoli, C., Horwitz, R., Hurst, L., & Tinetti, M. (1993). A predictive model for delirium in hospitalized elderly medical patients based on admission characteristics. *Annals of Internal Medicine, 119,* 474–481.

Johnson, J. (1990). Delirium in the elderly. *Emergency Clinics of North America, 8*(2), 255–264.

Levkoff, S., Besdine, R., & Wetle, T. (1986). Acute confusional states in the hospitalized elderly. *Annual Review of Gerontology and Geriatrics, 6,* 1–26.

Levkoff, S., Cleary, P., Liptzin, B., & Evans, D. (1991). Epidemiology of delirium: An overview of research issues and findings. *International Psychogeriatrics, 3*(2), 149–167.

Levkoff, S., Evans, D., Liptzin, B., Cleary, P., Lipsitz, L., Wetle, T., et al. (1992). Delirium: The occurrence and persistence of symptoms among elderly hospitalized patients. *Archives of Internal Medicine, 152,* 334–340.

Lipowski, Z. (1983). Transient cognitive disorders in the elderly. *American Journal of Psychiatry, 140* (11), 1426–1436.

Lipowski, Z. (1987). Delirium (acute confusional states). *Journal of the American Medical Association, 258,* 1789–1792.

Lipowski, Z. (1989). Delirium in the elderly patient. *The New England Journal of Medicine, 320*(9), 578–582.

Liptzin, B. (1995). Delirium. *Archives of Family Medicine, 4*, 453–458.

Liptzin, B., & Levkoff, S. (1992). An empirical study of delirium subtypes. *British Journal of Psychiatry, 161*, 843–845.

Ludwick, R. (1993). Nurses' response to patient's confusion. (Doctoral dissertation, Kent State University, 1993). *Dissertation Abstracts International, 54*, 1548.

Lyness, J. (1990). Delirium: Masquerades and misdiagnosis in elderly inpatients. *Journal of the American Geriatrics Society, 38*(11), 1235–1238.

Mach, J., Dysken, M., Kuskowski, M., Richelson, E., Holden, L., & Jilk, K. (1995). Serum anticholinergic activity in hospitalized older persons with delirium: A preliminary study. *Journal of the American Geriatrics Society, 43*(5), 491–495.

Marcantonio, E., Flacker, J., Wright, R., & Resnick, N. (2001). Reducing delirium after hip fracture: A randomized trial. *Journal of the American Geriatrics Society, 49*(5), 516–522.

Marcantonio, E., Simon, S., Bergmann, M., Jones, R., Murphy, K., & Morris, J. (2003). Delirium symptoms in post acute care: Prevalent, persistent, and associated with poor functional recovery. *Journal of the American Geriatrics Society, 51*(5), 4–9.

Marcantonio, E., Ta, T., Duthie, E., & Resnick, N. (2002). Delirium severity and psychomotor types: Their relationship with outcomes after hip fracture repair. *Journal of the American Geriatrics Society, 50*(5), 850–857.

McCarthy, M. (1991). Interpretation of confusion in the aged: Conflicting models of clinical reasoning among nurses. (Doctoral dissertation, University of California at San Francisco, 1991), *Dissertation Abstracts International, 53*, O203.

Milisen, K., Foreman, M., Wouters, B., Driesen, R., Godderis, J., Abraham, I., et al. (2002). Documentation of delirium in elderly patients with hip fracture. *Journal of Gerontological Nursing, 28*(1), 23–29.

Miller, J. (1991). A clinical study to pilot test the environmental optimization interventions protocol. (Doctoral dissertation, Oregon Health Sciences University, 1991), *Dissertation Abstracts International, 53*, 0772.

Morgan, D. (1985). Nurses' perceptions of mental confusion in the elderly: Influence of resident and setting characteristics. *Journal of Health and Social Behavior, 26*, 102–112.

Morency, C., Levkoff, S., & Dick, K. (1994). Research considerations: Delirium in hospitalized elders. *Journal of Gerontological Nursing, 20*(8), 24–30.

Murray, A., Levkoff, S., Wetle, T., Beckett, L., Cleary, P., Schor, J., et al. (1993). Acute delirium and functional decline in the hospitalized elderly patient. *Journal of Gerontology, 48*(5), M181–M186.

Neelon, V. (1990). Postoperative confusion. *Critical Care Nursing Clinics of North America, 2*(4), 579–587.

Neelon, V., Funk, S., Carlson, J., & Champagne, M. (1989). The NEECHAM Confusion scale: Relationship to clinical indicators of acute confusion in hospitalized elders. *Gerontologist, 29*, 65A.

Neelon, V., Champagne, M., Carlson, J., & Funk, S. (1996). The NEECHAM Confusion scale: Construction, validation and testing. *Nursing Research, 45*(6), 324–330.

Nurses Improving Care for Health System Elders. (1999). Standard of practice protocol: Confusion/delirium. *Geriatric Nursing, 20*(3), 147–152.

Palmateer, L., & McCartney, J. (1985). Do nurses know when patients have cognitive impairments? *Journal of Gerontological Nursing, 11*(2), 6–16.

Rasin, J. (1990). Confusion. *Nursing Clinics of North America, 25*(4), 909–918.

Rockwood, K. (1993). The occurrence and duration of symptoms in elderly patients with delirium. *Journal of Gerontology, 48*(4), M162–M166.

Rudberg, M., Pompei, P., Foreman, M., Ross, R., & Cassel, C. (1997). The natural history of delirium in older hospitalized patients: A syndrome of heterogeneity. *Age and Ageing, 26*(3), 169–174.

Schofield, I. (1997). A small exploratory study of the reaction of older people to an episode of delirium. *Journal of Advanced Nursing, 25*, 942–952.

Schor, J., Levkoff, S., Lipsitz, L. Reilly, C., Cleary, P., Rowe, J., et al. (1992). Risk factors for delirium in the hospitalized elderly. *Journal of the American Medical Association, 267*(6), 827–831.

Schuurmans, M., Shortridge-Baggett, L., & Duursma, S. (2003). The Delirium Observation Scale: A screening instrument for delirium. *Research and Theory for Nursing Practice, 17*(1), 31–50.

Trepacz, P., Baker, R., & Greenhouse, J. (1988). A symptom rating scale for delirium. *Psychiatric Research, 23,* 89–97.

Vermeersch, P. (1991). Response to "The cognitive and behavioral nature of acute confusional states." *Scholarly Inquiry for Nursing Practice, 5*(1), 17–20.

Wolanin, M., & Phillips, L. (1981). *Confusion: Prevention and care.* St. Louis, MO: Mosby.

CHAPTER 12

Nursing Assessment of Clients with Dementias of Late Life: Screening, Diagnosis, and Communication

Kathleen Sherrell, RN, PsyD
Madelyn Iris, PhD

As a clinician, teacher, and researcher, I think of myself as somewhat of an expert in the field of dementia. However, when my mother—previously an intellectually brilliant person with a better than average memory—began to show signs of confusion, I denied that she could have dementia. At first, she lost some of her ability to concentrate. She had always been an avid reader, but was now losing her sight, so I sent her books on tape every month. Then I would call her long distance, planning to discuss the book over the phone. When she began to complain that the books were confusing or poorly written, I felt badly because I hadn't chosen the "right" books. Then Mother began to complain that my sister-in-law was being "mean" to her. This would have been totally out of character for my sister-in-law, but I believed my mother and became upset with my sister-in-law.

Eventually, I brought my mother to a medical center near my home for evaluation by a geriatric team. The neuropsychologist invited me to sit in on the exam. At first my mother seemed to pass all the tests with flying colors. She could repeat information back to the examiner, could repeat numbers backwards and forwards, and showed no signs of impairment. I felt relief. Then she was asked to name as many animals as she could within a short period of time. My mother's vocabulary had always been vast and comprehensive. Yet on this day, she was only able to name three common barnyard animals. Of course, fluency is a significant factor in assessing the cognitive domain of language, and animal naming is often used as a short test to screen for dementia.

That was the only sign of impairment revealed during the neuropsychological exam; nevertheless, she was given a diagnosis of probable Alzheimer's disease. The geriatrician told me that my mother's complaints were likely a sign of paranoia, a behavioral symptom of dementia. She said I should "start preparing for the next stage." Yet I still refused to believe my mother had dementia and that it was becoming worse. When I told my brother the diagnosis, he became angry with me, as if it were my fault since I had initiated the diagnostic process.

As time went on, the signs of dementia became more evident. When my mother had to be moved to nursing home, I finally had to accept the diagnosis. When the day came that she didn't know me, I was devastated once more, even though I had known that it was inevitable.

This is a brief version of the complex and difficult journey made by my mother, my siblings, and me. In our family as in many others, a diagnosis of *dementia has broad repercussions. There is a bene-fit in knowing the reason for the confusion, but this is often outweighed by the distressing knowledge that the condition is progressive and incurable. This calculation of benefit and cost makes the process of assessment and communicating the diagnosis a complex experience for all concerned. It cannot be adequately described by simple rules and standardized test results.*

Kathleen Sherrell

Nurses play an important role in the screening, diagnosing, and communicating of results when working with patients and families of older adults with dementia. This role has not been fully appreciated. The shortfall between the existing role of nursing and a fully realized role depends in large measure on the formalization of nursing knowledge and skills in these areas. This chapter provides a formulation of nursing knowledge and skills needed for nursing assessment of clients with dementias of late life. It encapsulates much of what we have learned as a nurse and psychologist who have worked with clients with dementias in a variety of settings, including clinics, nursing homes, research studies, and private practice.

The first section of this chapter deals with nurses' knowledge about dementia. It summarizes the relevant research on the neurobiological characteristics of dementia, as well as more recent research on treatable behavioral and psychological symptoms, and the existential experience of dementia.

The second section of the chapter focuses on the important role of nurses in the assessment process. This section includes a description of selected standardized instruments used in the assessment of dementia. The chapter describes the ideal interdisciplinary practice that is still in the future, but necessary, if nursing practice is to achieve an optimized role in dementia assessment. The role of nurses as a vital part of the assessment team is described.

Professionals need to know how difficult and confusing it is for a person or family members to initiate the search for a diagnosis of dementia. Diagnosis-seeking behavior is a qualitative aspect of assessment and has received less attention in past research than the quantitative use of evaluation tools to establish a diagnosis. Findings from research on diagnosis-seeking behavior in clients with Alzheimer's disease and their families are presented.

In the final section, the authors discuss techniques of communicating the diagnosis to the person with dementia and to the family. Communication about the dementia diagnosis is complex because of its devastating impact, because it is "incurable," and because, up until this point, families are often in denial about the possibility of receiving a diagnosis of dementia. We conclude with some recommendations for nursing practice and nursing research into the assessment of clients with Alzheimer's disease and other dementias.

ALZHEIMER'S DISEASE AND OTHER DEMENTIAS

In the past 20 years, there has been an exponential increase in knowledge about various kinds of dementia. While cognitive deficits caused by neurological degeneration remain the principal and most researched features of dementia, the disease is also characterized by clinically important behavioral and psychological symptoms. This section describes recent research advances in the assessment and treatment of behavioral and psychological symptoms and promotes a relatively new focus of research on the existential (or subjective and qualitative) experience of dementia. This recent research contributes to a unique nursing perspective on assessment of dementias.

With the aging of the world's population, research has shown a significant increase in the numbers of older adults with irreversible dementias. It is the most common disease of the aging brain and represents a growing public health problem as the world population grows and ages. According to statistics published by the Administration on Aging (2002), the older population (65+) numbered 35 million in 2000, an increase of 3.7 million, or 12%, since 1990. The number of Americans aged 45–65 who will reach 65 over the next two decades increased by 34% during this decade. Persons reaching age 65 have an average life expectancy of an additional 17.89 years. By the year 2030, the older population will more than double to about 70 million and the 85+ population is projected to increase from 4.2 million in 2000 to 8.9 million in 2030. Principal sources of data are the U.S. Bureau of the Census, the National Center on Health Statistics, and the Bureau of Labor Statistics. The subgroup of persons 85 years of age and above is growing six times faster than the rest of the U.S. population (Committee on a National Research Agenda on Aging, 1991; Schneider & Guralnick, 1990). These increases have major implications for the provision of health care generally and for dementia assessment in particular.

THE NEUROBIOLOGY OF DEMENTIA

Dementia has long been recognized as a syndrome of neurobiological etiology. The term dementia (from the Latin *demens*, meaning "without mind") has ancient origins. It was used in European vernaculars as early as the 17th and 18th centuries. Cognitive impairment was accepted as the defining feature of dementia by the late 1800s. When Alois Alzheimer published the first paper on the neuropathology of dementia in 1906, his description included the presence of neurofibrils and plaques in the brain. In the 1960s and 1970s, comprehensive neuropathological studies demonstrated that the brain changes described by Alzheimer were a common cause of cognitive decline in older adults. The elucidation of specific diseases under the rubric of dementia has continued into the 21st century.

Dementia, therefore, is not a disease but rather a syndrome, often of a chronic and progressive nature, in which there is a gradual or sometimes rapid decline of cognitive functions accompanied by deterioration in emotional control, language skills, and social behavior. Dementia occurs in Alzheimer's disease, cerebrovascular disorders, and other conditions primarily or secondarily affecting the brain. Most frequently, it affects older adults. Usually the course is progressive and irreversible and, despite significant advances, at present, treatments are only minimally effective in slowing the progression. One of the benefits of the diagnosis of dementia is to help distinguish this syndrome from a temporary disturbance in the level of consciousness called "delirium." Dementia can be differentiated from delirium because in the early stages of dementia there is no impairment of perception or consciousness. There is, however, loss of cognitive and intellectual abilities characterized by disorientation, loss of memory, impaired judgment, intellectual and social functioning, personality change, and shallow and labile affect. Along with these progressive cognitive disabilities, there is also a high prevalence of behavioral and psychological symptoms.

There has been a great deal of controversy regarding the use of the term "dementia" (Sachdev, 2000). Initially, it was used to describe a syndrome that was so general and all-inclusive that it might well be called a "garbage can diagnosis." More recent research has determined that there are at least 70 possible causes of dementia (Cohen et al.,

1993) and that each cause has a unique presentation of symptoms and laboratory results. However, these causes can also have great similarities in presentation, thus making definitive subtype diagnosis very difficult. Even though use of the term is confusing, a proposal to abandon the term is also problematic as the term dementia has wide acceptance beyond the medical community in general public health, legislation, community affairs, and lay usage. There is, moreover, a large and growing industry that is dependent on it. The most commonly used definitions of dementia, from the *Diagnostic and Statistical Manual* (4th ed.) and International Classification of Diseases and Related Health Problems, 10th rev. (ICD-10), emphasize memory impairment along with impairment in other cognitive domains. This "memory impairment" criterion is appropriate for Alzheimer's disease (AD), but it is restrictive when applied to dementia from other causes, such as vascular dementia (VaD) or frontotemporal dementia (FTD), in which memory impairment is not the most significant symptom. VaD can produce impairment in several cognitive domains while affecting memory only mildly or not at all, and in FTD, frontal-executive and language disturbance may be quite prominent early in the course of the disease.

Despite the above-mentioned problems with the term, "dementia" is still the most universal term used to describe the cognitive changes affecting intellectual and physical function and occurring mostly in older adults. The major development leading to expanded research on dementia has been the increase in prevalence of Alzheimer's disease (AD) caused by the aging of our growing population. At present, AD has become the prototypical dementia. Even though more than 70 conditions can cause dementia in older adults (Cohen et al., 1993), Alzheimer's disease is by far the most common. AD accounts for more than 50% of dementia cases, followed

by vascular dementia (15–20%). Because Alzheimer's disease and vascular dementia (VaD) are the two most common causes of dementia, together accounting for nearly two thirds of all dementia cases, this chapter will focus primarily on assessment of dementia from these two causes. Considerable overlap is present between the two, including progressive cognitive, functional, and behavioral decline; neuronal loss; shared risk factors, and neurochemical deficits (Brashear, 2003; Erkinjuntti et al., 2002; Kalaria & Ballard, 1999). The course of the disease in VaD is said to be more fluctuating, with a more stepwise progression. Also, higher rates of depressive symptoms have been described in vascular dementia as compared to Alzheimer's disease (Evans, 1990).

BEHAVIORAL AND PSYCHOLOGICAL SYMPTOMS OF DEMENTIA

There are two major groups of symptoms that characterize the dementias: symptoms of cognitive dysfunction and behavioral and psychological symptoms. In most cases, the two groups of symptoms co-occur. For example, in this chapter's introductory vignette, two of the early symptoms were difficulty in concentration, which is a cognitive symptom, and paranoia, which is a behavioral symptom.

As stated earlier, treatments for cognitive dysfunctions have been limited and not very effective. Instead, the greatest opportunities for intervention and alleviation of patient suffering, family burden, and societal costs lie within the domain of behavioral and psychological symptoms. Prior to the assessment of behavioral and psychological symptoms, these symptoms were usually dismissed under the label of agitation. Typically, a patient who was old and "senile" would also be "agitated." Fortunately, times have changed (Tune, 2003). Clinicians now agree that it is often possible to successfully treat dementia-associated symptoms such as agitation and paranoia even though it is not possible to reverse or stop the progress of the dementia itself.

In 1996, the International Psychogeriatric Association (IPA) convened an international consensus conference to develop an operational definition of behavioral and psychological symptoms of dementia (BPSD). In the past, these symptoms had not received as much attention as had cognitive symptoms. The IPA grouped these symptoms into two major clusters: (1) symptoms usually and mainly assessed on the basis of interviews with patients and relatives, which may include anxiety, depressed mood, hallucinations, and delusions; and (2) symptoms usually identified on the basis of observation of patient behavior, which may include aggression, screaming, restlessness, agitation, wandering, culturally inappropriate behaviors, sexual disinhibition, hoarding, cursing, and shadowing (Finkel et al., 1998). Although there have been many research studies focusing on BPSD, researchers have not been able to differentiate these behaviors and psychological symptoms sufficiently among the different types of dementia. Despite symptoms that are common to individuals with dementia, there is growing awareness that dementias are experienced by each individual in a particularly unique and subjective manner.

Moreover, the uniqueness of each family's experience of coping with the effects of dementia on their loved ones cannot be minimized. Downs (1997) contributed to the nursing perspective on dementia because she built on the profession's historical focus on holistic care. Downs writes of the "emergence of the person in dementia." She describes the need for attention to the person with dementia, especially the individual's sense of self, their unique perspective, and

their individual rights. In Downs' view, it is both possible and necessary to obtain the views of people with dementia. Therefore, research and practice must focus on the sufferer. She distinguishes this approach from the medical model in dementia research, which focuses almost exclusively on the symptoms of the disease. Downs also distinguishes this "emergence of the person" perspective from past research that focused on psychosocial aspects of dementia, but concentrated on family caregivers more than on the person with the disease.

Measures of the Behavioral and Psychological Symptoms of Dementia

Several reliable, valid, and clinically useful measures of BPSD are available for nurses to use in the assessment process:

1. The Neuropsychiatric Inventory (NPI) (Cummings et al., 1994) evaluates a wide range of psychopathology; it records severity and frequency separately. Administration time is 10 minutes. The scoring is from 1 to 144. It has been translated into a number of languages and is widely used in drug trials.

2. The Behavioral Pathologic Rating Scale for Alzheimer's Disease (BEHAVE-AD) (Reisberg et al., 1987) was designed to be used in prospective studies of symptoms in pharmacological trials and takes 20 minutes to administer.

3. The Cohen-Mansfield Agitation Inventory (CMAI) (Cohen-Mansfield, Marx, & Rosenthal, 1989) rates agitated behaviors in patients with cognitive impairment. It takes between 10 and 15 minutes to complete and can be used by formal caregivers in a clinical setting after training.

4. The Cornell Scale for Depression in Dementia (Alexopoulos, Abrams, Young, & Shamoian, 1988) is a 19-item scale specifically designed for the assessment of

depression in dementia and is administered by a clinician, taking 20 minutes with the caregiver and 10 minutes with patient.

THE ROLE OF NURSES IN THE DEMENTIA ASSESSMENT PROCESS

Nurses are a vital part of the interdisciplinary team needed for the assessment and diagnosis of dementia. This assessment team includes the disciplines of neurology, internal medicine, geriatrics, psychiatry, social work, neuropsychology, and nursing. The importance of nurses in this process is based on: (1) the large increase in numbers of people with dementia; (2) the lack of adequate numbers of geriatricians, psychiatrists, and neurologists to address these cases; and (3) the clear demonstration in research that nurses' diagnoses using standardized tools are as accurate as other professional groups (Trapp-Moen, Tyrey, Cook, Heyman, & Fillenbaum, 2001). Another important factor is that the approaches used by other disciplines are frequently less adequate than nursing approaches in assessing the functional, social, and family dimensions of dementia. The medical disciplines involved in the diagnosis of dementia have well-established procedures for assessment and diagnosis, but they are sometimes too narrowly focused to pick up on the true scope of the problems. Nurses have been shown to be very effective in diagnosing dementia. A study of nurse assessment procedures (Dennis, Furness, Lindesay, & Wright, 1998) showed that nurses performed well in detecting dementia when compared to diagnoses made by other medical professionals. Other researchers have provided evidence that community psychiatric nurses are able to effectively differentiate dementia from other psychiatric disorders (Collighan, Macdonald, Herzberg, Philpot, & Lindesay, 1993; Seymour, Saunders, Wattis, & Daly, 1994)

Assessment tools specifically designed for nursing are scarce. Abraham et al. (1990) describe the Psychogeriatric Nursing Assessment Protocol (PNAP) for use in multidisciplinary geriatric–neuropsychiatric outpatient clinics. It was designed to complement other general physical assessments used by nurses, and filled a gap in the tool kit for the assessment and diagnosis of behaviorally disordered older adults. This tool was further developed for assessment of patients with Alzheimer's disease (Abraham et al., 1994). The complexity of health problems in older adults requires in-depth investigation into each medical problem and its possible relationship to cognitive and behavioral symptoms. Because multiple medical problems are commonly present in the elderly, they are likely to be taking multiple medications, and some of these can affect the central nervous system and cause symptoms of altered cognitive function. The Abraham protocol is accompanied by a rating form that permits quantification of essential data for purposes of clinical summary, epidemiological inquiry, research, and evaluations.

Dementia is a syndrome that, like fever, requires a systematic evaluation to identify its many causes (Mega, 2002). The Consortium to Establish a Registry for Alzheimer's Disease (CERAD) was established in 1986 by the National Institute on Aging to develop standardized assessments for patients with Alzheimer's disease (Fillenbaum et al., 1997). Since that time, CERAD has developed and evaluated clinical and neuropsychological test batteries, a neuroimaging protocol, and an assessment of the neuropathological findings at autopsy of the brains of Alzheimer's disease patients. The two basic assessments used for evaluating dementia are the CERAD Neuropsychological Battery, which is designed to determine the type and severity of cognitive impairment, and the CERAD Clinical Battery, which assesses the presence, type, and severity of dementia (Morriss, Rovner, Folstein, &

German, 1990). The Clinical Battery includes: (1) a detailed standardized inquiry using a nonpatient informant to determine changes in the patient's cognitive performance, including memory, orientation, verbal ability, calculation, concentration, judgment, and problem-solving; (2) evaluation of activities involving community, home, and hobbies; (3) activities of daily living; (4) instrumental activities of daily living; and (5) the CERAD Clock Drawing Test, which assesses spatial orientation, dysphasia for numbers, and aspects of executive functioning.

Instruments Used for Nursing Assessment

There are many instruments used by nurses for the assessment of dementia.

The Mini Mental Status Examination (MMSE) The MMSE is the most widely used screening instrument (Folstein, Folstein, & McHugh, 1975). It was developed as a short, easy-to-administer measure of mental status and as a screening tool for dementia. It has been used extensively in research involving dementia patients and found to be an acceptable measure of mental status. The MMSE yields a total score of 30, with a score of 24 established as the cutoff point for dementia. It consists of 11 questions or commands, such as "What is the year?" or "Write a sentence" and assesses seven categories of cognitive function including orientation to time and place, registration of three words, attention and calculations, recall of three words, language, and visual construction. The MMSE takes 5–10 minutes and does not require extensive training to administer. Folstein determined that a score of 23 points or less with an individual with more than eight years of education can be a diagnostic indication of cognitive impairment. There is a need for further evaluation to establish a more definitive diagnosis (Folstein, 1983).

The Cognitive Abilities Screening Instrument (CASI) The CASI was developed and pilot tested in Japan and the United States (Teng et al., 1994) to determine cross-cultural applicability and usefulness in screening for dementia, monitoring disease progression, and providing a profile of cognitive impairment. The CASI contains 25 items that are grouped into cognitive domains according to the items' face validity. The CASI has a total score ranging from 0–100, with a suggested cutoff score of 74 for classifying dementia. It provides quantitative assessment in nine domains: attention, concentration, orientation, long-term memory, short-term memory, language, visual construction, fluency, and abstraction and judgment. Typical administration time is 20–30 minutes. Scores from the MMSE can be estimated from the responses to selected CASI items. In a study by White et al. (1996), the CASI was used to evaluate 4000 men who participated in the Honolulu–Asia Aging Study of Dementia. The CASI scores declined significantly with increasing dementia severity, as measured by family informants and other standardized cognitive tests including the MMSE. Sherrell, Buckwalter, Bode, and Strozdas (1999) conducted a study in which they compared the MMSE and CASI. It was found that the CASI demonstrated greater specificity in determining level of cognitive function than did the MMSE.

Short Portable Mental Status Questionnaire (SPMSQ) The SPMSQ is a short, reliable instrument to detect the presence and degree of intellectual impairment. It is easily administered by a nurse in the office, community, or hospital. It has been standardized and validated (Pfeiffer, 1975).

Older Americans Resources and Services (OARS) This methodology was designed to assess functional capacity in five dimensions (social resources, economic resources, mental health, physical health, and activities of daily living) and to measure need for and use of 24 types of generic services (Fillenbaum & Smyer, 1981; George & Fillenbaum, 1985).

The Ten Point Clock Test This test is used by many clinicians in the assessment of cognitive impairment and is useful in distinguishing disease process and normal aging. The test is a screen for visuoconstructional difficulties, as constructional apraxia is a common neuropsychological disturbance in dementia and often occurs early in the course of the disease. One system for scoring clock drawing was developed by Manos and Wu (1994) (Table 12-1). Manos and Wu's (1994) research on the Ten Point Clock Test was conducted by

TABLE 12-1 Ten Point Clock Test

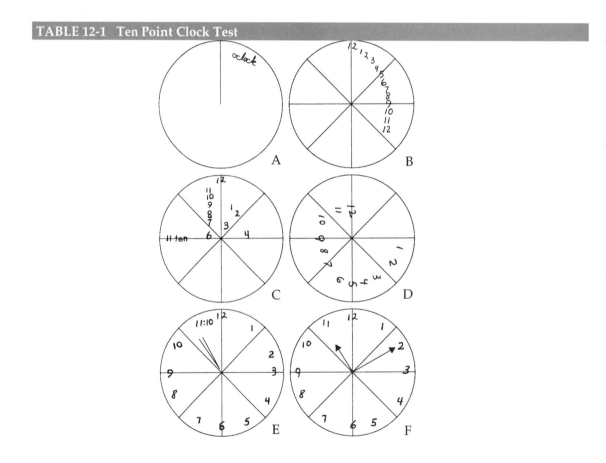

Scoring: (A) Score = 0. (B) The number 1 is in the correct position; score = 1. (C) Numbers 1 and 11 are in the correct positions. Score = 2. (D) Numbers 7, 8, 10, and 11 are in the correct positions; score = 4. (E) Numbers 1, 2, 4, 5, 7, 8, 10, and 11 are in the correct positions; score = 8. No points for hands of equal length regardless of position. (F) Numbers 1, 2, 4, 5, 7, 8, 10, and 11 are in correct position for 8 points. The little hand is on the 11 (1 point) and the big hand is on the 2 (1 point); score = 10 points.

Note. From "The Ten Point Clock Test: A Quick Screen and Grading Method for Cognitive Impairment in Medical and Surgical Patients," by P. Manos and R. Wu, 1994, *International Journal of Psychiatry in Medicine*, 24(3) pp. 229–244. Reprinted with permission.

nurses on hospital patients and clinic outpatients, with and without dementia. The purpose was to evaluate the clinical utility of the test in screening for and grading cognitive deficits in medical and surgical patients. Clock scores correlated with neuropsychological test scores and with the MMSE. The objective of the case study was to evaluate the clinical utility of the ten point clock test in screening for cognitive deficits. Clock scores correlated with neuropsychological test scores and with the mini-mental state examination. The mean clock score of elderly outpatient controls was 8.5 which was significantly different from the mean of 5.5 scored by patients with dementia. The study, therefore, found the ten point clock test to be valid in identifying dementia. The results also correlated well with nurses' bedside assessments of observable, functional deficits in their patients. The test was easy to administer, and found to be reliable, valid, and useful as a quick screening and grading method for cognitive deficits in medical and surgical patients (p. 229). Moretti, Torre, Antonella, Cozzato, and Bova (2002) used the Ten Point Clock Test and also found it to be reliable and easy to complete. The test detects cognitive impairment even in mild deterioration, which is defined by the MMSE as a score of around 23.

Scoring the Ten Point Clock Test A circle, approximately 5 in. in diameter is traced, using a template (see Table 12-1). The patient is asked to "Put the numbers in the face of the clock," and when the task is completed to "Make the clock say ten minutes after eleven."

To score the test, the number 12 is rotated to the top of the page. A line is drawn through the center of the number twelve and the middle of the circle, dividing the circle in half. (In the rare instances when the 12 is missing, its expected position is assumed to be counter-clockwise from the number 1, at a distance equivalent to the distance between the number 1 and the number 2). A second line is drawn at right angles to the first through the center of the circle, dividing it into quarters. Two more lines are drawn through the center of the circle, dividing it into eighths. One point is given for each of the following numbers that falls in its proper eighth of the circle relative to the 12: 1, 2, 4, 5, 7, 8, 10, and 11. (At least half of the spatial volume occupied by the number must be in the correct eighth of the circle.) One point is given each to a short hand pointing at the number 11, and a long hand pointing at the number 2. No points are given for the hands if they are approximately equal in length or for a long hand on the 11 and a short hand on the 2, or for hands of any length pointing at other numbers. A short hand on the number 11 and a long hand on the number 3 would be worth one point—for the short hand. Numbers drawn outside the circle are scored by simply extending the dividing lines. Marks in place of numbers do not count.

Activities of Daily Living (ADL) This is a measure of daily function that is important in understanding the degree of disability and level of dependence experienced by people with dementia. The Barthel Activities Instrument (BAI) has had widespread use in research including use with elderly patients. It is easy to use and shows little variation between objective performance of tasks and reports gathered from witnesses. The BAI only includes self-care tasks, however.

The Instrumental Activities of Daily Living Scale (IADL) This scale measures seven areas of more complex activities required for optimal independent functioning (Lawton & Brody, 1969). The scoring indicates whether the patient is completely independent, requires assistance, or is dependent for the performance of each activity. It covers such skills as using the telephone, traveling, shopping, preparing meals, doing housework, taking medicine, and managing money.

Therapeutic Environment

The standardized instruments just listed are important tools for assessment. However, researchers and clinicians have also described the importance of establishing a therapeutic environment for the assessment process. This has been a forte of nurses over the years. One of the first theoretical nursing models was based on interpersonal relations (Peplau, 1952). Fifty years ago, Peplau described nursing as "a significant, therapeutic, interpersonal process." More recently, Abraham et al. (1992) emphasized the need for a "therapeutic climate" as a background for the implementation of the PNAP. He and his colleagues provide pointers for nurses to follow. Eight of these pointers are particularly relevant in assessing dementia patients:

1. Accommodate physical impairment. This includes being aware of any vision or hearing problems, or any physical symptoms that infringe on the therapeutic effectiveness of the assessment. "An uncomfortable patient is an uncooperative patient" (Abraham et al., 1992, p.17).

2. Create a warm and inviting atmosphere. The patient needs to feel safe, cared about, and heard. Distractions in the environment and confusing messages do not create this feeling of safety that is needed for accurate assessment of a dementia patient.

3. Integrate verbal and nonverbal communication. This is particularly important for elderly people who may have lost some of their verbal language abilities. In this case, nonverbal messages take on even more importance than usual. Simple "yes" and "no" questions tend to mask problems when talking to elderly persons and should be avoided. Well-known interviewing skills of active listening, clarifying, and reflecting are also of paramount importance when interviewing elderly persons in general, and particularly those with some dementia.

4. Use all the senses. Listening to the sound of the person's voice and physical presentation (condition of the skin, mobility, characteristics of speech), and using the sense of touch to assess strength (e.g., when shaking hands) are all aspects of an intuitive assessment ability that goes beyond the scores of any instrument.

5. Interview several people. Abraham et al. (1992) advise interviewing family members and friends if possible and then following this with a group interview. Obtaining information from others can help clear up any conflicting stories as well as provide observations of communication patterns within the family and family dynamics.

6. Assess the entire time. Beginning with the initial phone call, the assessment includes all aspects of each contact, for instance sitting in the waiting room, walking to the office, and so on.

7. Facilitate storytelling. Stories of the person's past provide a basis to judge what the present dementia symptoms may mean to the patient. Asking them to "tell me a story about a typical day for you" provides information on many levels about their ability to function independently.

8. Clarify, verify, and revisit. Because there are usually language and comprehension problems for persons with dementia, there is a need to clarify confusing or incomplete information (Abraham et al., 1992).

As they seek to establish a therapeutic environment as described above, nurses need to know the symptoms of dementia that can result from a loss in each cognitive domain and respond with effective strategies for communication. Problems that may hinder communication and some strategies for compensating for them are well described by Weintraub (1998):

1. Attention—This involves the loss of ability to sustain attention and the ability to grasp

a normal amount of information from a conversation. Strategies include breaking information down into small portions and repeating instructions as the task is being done.

2. Learning and memory—This involves the loss of ability to learn new information and retain it over time. Strategies include repeating instructions and immediately asking the patient leading questions about the information.

3. Language—This involves the loss of ability to convey messages effectively and to understand what others are saying. Strategies include speaking in simple sentences, and devising a system for emergency situations bypassing the need to use the telephone.

4. Visual perception—This involves the loss of ability to look at something and recognize it, find objects in a cluttered array, judge distance and spatial relations, and navigate around the home. Strategies include keeping personal items, objects, and clothing in the same location and simplifying the visual environment.

5. Emotional regulation—This involves loss of the ability to control emotions and even to express emotions (apathy). Strategies include not challenging the patient's responses, but accepting them and using techniques to "defuse" potentially volatile interactions, such as changing the topic.

Therefore, principles of communication are important aspects of both assessment and communicating the diagnosis. One of the problems encountered in our work with older adults with dementia is that the need for diagnosis can become more important than the process of assessment. For example, the family of one older adult requested evaluation of the older adult in order for him to be placed in a drug research program, for which the inclusion criterion was a diagnosis of Alzheimer's disease. During the evaluation it became clear that he could relate the story of his past, which included having been orphaned at an early age and placed with several abusive foster parents, coming to a large city, finding work, eventually marrying, buying a home, and raising his children who were now successful adults. However, he could not state what day of the week it was, or the year, or his present address nor could he count backwards from 20 by 2 (serial 2s). The diagnosis seeking in this case was focused more on the criterion for being in the drug study than on the meaning for him of now having his car taken away from him and of becoming dependent after a life of amazing survival. This is not to dismiss the need for quantitative measures for evaluation. We would only urge that professionals be more mindful of the stories that elderly people have to tell about their lives to understand more clearly what the losses caused by dementia may mean to them in the present. In the context of the assessment process, this telling of stories is important in getting to know the person versus the symptoms of his or her disease. Also, telling stories depends on long-term memory, which generally remains intact after other cognitive functions are impaired. Therefore, it is ego saving to focus on that remaining strength as much or more than on the deficits of short-term memory loss.

THE PROCESS OF DIAGNOSIS SEEKING IN DEMENTIA

This section focuses on the complexity of the entire decision-making process in establishing a diagnosis of dementia. Denial on the part of family members often delays bringing the problem to the attention of a medical professional. Denial can come in many forms. For several reasons, both patients and family members have a difficult time recognizing the changes in memory and behavior that are early signs of developing dementia. First, early changes are similar to changes associated with normal aging or with other preexisting health conditions, such as alcoholism or mental illness or even personal idiosyncrasies. Second, these changes often come and go, and this inconsistency can make it more difficult to take the changes seriously enough to seek evaluation and help. Third, the inconsistency of symptoms in the early stages may not have a significant impact on daily life activities for many months or even years. The recognition and, more importantly, the transformation in interpretation of these changes from usual aging to symptoms of a memory problem are fuzzy and ambiguous. To move from noticing changes in memory and behavior to labeling such changes as memory loss or cognitive impairment is a complicated process (Berman, Iris, Robinson, & Morhardt, 2002; Iris et al., 2001, 2002). Changes may be recognized, but they are not always seen as problems that need medical intervention. In addition, many physicians see early or mild changes in memory or behavior as part of normal aging and may respond by dismissing them as a concern. While some family members may reject this conclusion, most feel comforted and reassured and thus the length of time to diagnosis increases.

The story of Mrs. B. and her family illustrates the complex path from first recognition of changes to the point in time of actually obtaining a diagnosis (see Case Study). The case study of Mrs. B. is drawn from data produced as part of a study of family decision making with regard to seeking a diagnosis for cognitive and behavioral changes observed in older family members. The Pathways study, funded by the Alzheimer's Association, focused on how family members moved from first observing change in their older relative to eventually seeking a medical evaluation (Iris et al., 2002).

In the first phase of this study, the researchers conducted open-ended interviews with 47 family members who played a major role in the process of seeking a diagnosis. Participants were recruited from various sites, including community-based adult day care centers, a geriatrician's private practice, a university-based Alzheimer's disease center, and a medical center's geriatric assessment center. Just over 60% of participants were African-American and 39% were non-Hispanic Whites. Approximately 75% were women, and over half were daughters of the patients (51.5%), followed by wives (15.2%). The remainder were sons, husbands, or other family members such as siblings or nieces. Areas of inquiry included questions about the circumstances surrounding the diagnosis-seeking behavior, by using key events as triggers for recall. Findings from the first phase showed that there are four critical time points in this process: (1) first notice of change, (2) identification of the change as a problem, (3) first time the problem is brought to the health care provider's attention by the family member, and (4) time of diagnosis.

Forty-four family members participated in the second phase, of whom 53% were African-American and 45% were non-Hispanic white. Forty-one of these participants were women. The study demonstrated that the time span from first notice of change to the time of diagnosis can be a period of months or even years. Identification of change as a problem warranting medical attention is difficult, as symptoms of cognitive impairment are often seen as natural concomitants of normal aging. In addition, family members are often reluctant to step in and take charge of an older family member's medical care out of respect for the older person's autonomy and independence. Once the changes are seen as a problem, however, families usually act rather quickly to get medical attention and the lag time between points two and three is comparatively short.

When cognitive changes come to the attention of health care professionals, however, there are many intervening factors that may delay obtaining a diagnosis. First and foremost, many physicians are not well educated about the dementia process in older people, and they too frequently dismiss the changes as "normal aging." In fact, in the Pathways study, it was unusual for a primary care physician to refer the patient for more specialized assessment such as neuropsychological testing. Second, changes in health insurance plans frequently led to disruptions

Case Study: Story of Mrs. B.

Mrs. B. is an 80-year-old African-American woman, married to Mr. B. for over 40 years. They have three daughters; SB, VB, and RB, all live nearby and take an active role in caring for their mother. Mr. B. first realized that Mrs. B was changing when he noticed that she was not paying many of the household bills. When Mrs. B. started sleeping all day and not paying attention to her hygiene and dress, Mr. B. realized there was a real problem. After Mrs. B. started exhibiting minor paranoid behaviors, her daughters stepped in and became more active observers of their mother as well. Mrs. B. also noticed changes in herself. She commented repeatedly that she couldn't remember things, and she started to worry about having Alzheimer's disease. These subtle or insidious changes occurred, on and off, over a period of three years. As SB commented, "It changes when people get older . . . you do not necessarily think there is anything wrong with them, you think they are getting older, she is losing her memory...and that sort of thing." This illustrates the persistent idea that memory loss is a normal part of aging, and it is difficult for patients and families to separate out signs of a memory problem from the signs of usual aging. The subtleties of these changes made it difficult for family members to definitively label such changes as problems. Although they observed many changes in her behavior, Mrs. B.'s daughters were so concerned about not alarming their parents that they put off seeking medical attention for her for some time. Because Mrs. B.'s symptoms were intermittent, and at times she appeared fine, it was easy to deny the problem. As VB said, "Things you should have been noticing, or things that you knew in your heart were not quite right, you could easily say, 'Well, it is just forgetfulness and it will go away.' So that delayed trying to get any kind of evaluation . . . you do not want to face the possibility that your mother has Alzheimer's."

VB started accompanying her parents to their medical appointments, thinking that her mother's problems might be side effects of medications. Initially, the physician displayed some signs of resentment at her questions and her new role vis-à-vis her mother's medical care. The physician described Mrs. B. as having a "light case of Alzheimer's" but stated he was "speculating." However, when he recommended that Mrs. B. start taking Aricept, VB backed off, not wanting to see Mrs. B. carry a diagnosis of Alzheimer's. In response, the physician delayed treatment. RB stated, "We just did not want to deal with it...it was just a matter of getting the proper help. We knew it had to happen. It is very difficult. It is like facing death."

It was approximately three years before the family took further action. The sisters went to a community forum and heard about some of the non-AD causes of memory loss from a female geriatrician. This prompted them to pursue another evaluation for Mrs. B. SB stated, "She did make me less afraid and more hopeful, and so we decided immediately that she was the doctor for us."

Mrs. B.'s daughters also raised two issues that may hinder seeking a diagnosis: cultural sensitivity and stigma. First, the physician at the forum was also African-American and the daughters felt she would understand their culture and the intensity of their family relationships. In particular, they described the stigma of having AD and how

continues

Case Study: Story of Mrs. B.   *(continued)*

much they wanted to avoid exposing their mother to this. Second, the physician's approach was to conduct a comprehensive physical, neurological, and neuropsychological evaluation, which reassured them that their mother's diagnosis was soundly based and not simply a quick response.

This family's journey through the diagnosis-seeking pathway took over three years. During the years from the time they first noticed changes to the time they received a final diagnosis, Mrs. B. and her family experienced a range of emotions, including fear, anxiety, and denial, as well as a need to protect themselves from the social stigma they associated with AD. The fluctuating nature and character of Mrs. B.'s symptoms contributed to their resistance to accept the first physician's opinion, and his lack of thoroughness in conduct-

ing an evaluation further fostered their denial. In retrospect, Mrs. B.'s daughters see that their hesitations and fears furthered their mother's anxieties and kept her from receiving timely care and treatment. As SB said, "I think when you do not go (for a diagnosis) and you stay in denial, you also deny the patient the opportunity for treatment that can make them better." VB added, "When I look back, I regret the time that it took for a diagnosis because I think mother was so relieved for herself, once she could just stop trying to pretend, even trying to pretend that nothing was wrong. Because I think she tried for so long to hide it and I think she was scared and so alone." Although difficult to accept, receiving a diagnosis eased Mrs. B.'s pain and gave the family a way to confront their own fears and losses.

---

in patient–physician relationships. Family members often had to start the process all over again when a new physician was introduced into the picture. The number of physicians involved in the process of obtaining a diagnosis ranged from one or two to as many as six. Mrs. B.'s story captures some of these issues, and typifies how a family moves forward through the decision-making pathway.

■ COMMUNICATING THE DIAGNOSIS

Informing patients and families about a diagnosis of Alzheimer's disease is a complex ethical and practical issue. One challenge for the physician and nurse is deciding how much information to give patients and families about the results of the assessment. Providing too much information can overwhelm some patients and families and give them the impression that the condition is more severe than indicated by test results. Others, in contrast, may want to know every detail. Provid-

ing them with insufficient information could lead them to conclude that the assessment was incomplete and perhaps to doubt the results. Also at issue are the patient's moral and legal rights to receive the diagnosis.

The following are examples of people with dementia and family caregivers describing the manner in which they were given (or not given) information. The verbatim quotes are from patients in an early dementia support group. These quotes show that sensitivity is sometimes missing. The group members frequently describe the kind of "marginalized" position they experience after they have been diagnosed with dementia.

- "My cardiologist told me I had Alzheimer's disease and therefore shouldn't drive. He painted a vivid picture of little children being mowed down by me. It could have been done in a more helpful way."

- "Initially my doctor met with me along with my wife and sons. He ignored me and explained everything to them and I was slipping into the background."

- (A family member) "My father's doctor is an internist and he doesn't really concern himself with his memory."

The most recent AMA guidelines on diagnosis of dementia advise giving the diagnosis directly to the patient if at all possible. Yet researchers suggest that the AMA guidelines do not adequately address the clinical complexities of patient disclosure in dementia.

Do patients want to know? Studies of older adult community-based samples revealed that a majority of elderly persons would want to be told that they had dementia (Erde, Nadal, & Scholl, 1988; Holroyd, Turnbull, & Wolf, 2002). Turnbull, Wolf, and Holroyd (2003) found that of 200 subjects over the age of 65, those with prior involvement with persons with Alzheimer's disease were less likely to state that the diagnosis should be given to the patient. In a study by Marzanski (2000), patients already diagnosed with dementia were asked about their preferences regarding "knowing the truth" about their diagnosis of dementia. Of the 50% of participants with satisfactory insight, 70% clearly declared they would like to know more about their illness.

Do families want patients to know? Interestingly, in some studies, the majority of dementia sufferers' relatives (57–83%) did not want the patient to be told of his or her diagnosis, but 70% of the relatives would want to be told the truth if they had the disorder themselves (Barnes, 1997; Maguire et al., 1996). In Marzanski's (2000) study, three families believed the patient suffered as a result of the assessment. Some family members described the patient as someone with AD to other relatives but did not want the patient informed. In Holroyd, Turnbull, and Wolf's (2002) study, 60 family members of dementia patients attending support groups were asked to answer a questionnaire regarding their experience and attitudes regarding patients being told their dementia diagnosis. Ninety-three percent of family caregivers reported that they had been told the patient's diagnosis by a physician. Only 49% of patients had been told their diagnosis. Only 23% of patients had been told of any symptoms to expect with the illness, while 77% of family members were told.

At the moment, the most prominent advocates of truth-telling seem to believe that the nature and degree of the disease may limit the right to information. Johnson, Bouman, and Pinner (2000) studied a group of geriatricians and psychiatrists working with older adults with dementia in the United Kingdom and found that only 40% disclosed the diagnosis to their patients. Although aware of the benefits, they hesitated because of the uncertainty of the diagnosis, the patient's lack of insight, and the potential detrimental effects. The Alzheimer Association of Canada has published an information sheet available online at http://www.Alzheimer.ca that recommends establishing a plan for disclosure that takes into account patients' and family members' expectations of what the assessment will reveal. A study by Smith and Beattie (2001) underlines the need to further investigate the psychosocial factors that are involved in the lay interpretation of diagnostic information and the uncertainty associated with the assessment of dementia disorders.

Clinicians will doubtless continue to use their clinical judgment to determine whether the diagnosis should be disclosed to the patient. Just as with most issues surrounding dementia, the question of whether to tell the truth or not about the diagnosis does not have a clear and definitive answer. It must be a decision based on clinical wisdom of the sort that has the best interest of the patient as its core value. Many patients in early stages of dementia who not only want to know their diagnosis, but want to know as much as possible about prognosis, research, and advocacy. To quote a member of an early-stage AD support group, "I want the information firsthand. I don't want someone else giving me 'trickle-down' facts." On the other hand, many patients maintain their denial of the diagnosis into the middle stages of the disease and up to the time when they no longer are capable of having insight. It seems to be their wish to translate the symptoms into "What do you expect from a person my age?" or "Why should I know the date? I don't have to go to work anymore!"

SUMMARY

Nurses, especially those with specialized education in geropsychiatric nursing, can function as brokers or bridges between physicians and families and patients, guiding interaction and facilitating communication, especially in a care manager role. An active nursing role in patient and family education about chronic disease management and care is currently a missing component of a comprehensive and holistic professional response to dementia. The realization of nurses' important role in the screening and diagnosis of dementias of late life relies on a solid base of knowledge about dementias, skills in the nursing assessment of such conditions, and the ability to use communication techniques to process the diagnosis with patients and their families. This chapter has provided an overview of these issues.

Solid background information is available about the neurobiology of Alzheimer's disease and other dementias. The epidemiological data show that there is a great increase in the number of elderly persons with dementia. This will continue to rise exponentially as the baby boomer cohort enters the vulnerable age in which dementia is more prevalent. Neurobiological research has demonstrated that dementia can result from as many as 70 different disease entities. Thus, it is not a disease itself but rather a syndrome. Even though each cause brings unique symptoms, the general cognitive decline seen in dementia cuts across diagnostic categories. Alzheimer's dis-

ease is a prototype of the dementia syndrome and the increase in AD has given impetus to the increased focus in both the clinical and research arena.

Neuropsychiatric features of dementia include a wide range of behavioral and psychological symptoms. Dementia is incurable and inexorably progressive, but the behavioral and psychological symptoms frequently associated with it are treatable. The chapter lists several instruments that nurses can use to assess cognitive changes in dementia, as well as instruments to assess behavioral and psychological symptoms.

No task in our experience is as professionally challenging as assessment of elderly persons with dementia. The complexity of dementia identification, assessment, and care points to the need for nurses to play a central role in all of these stages as part of an interdisciplinary team. Research demonstrates that nurses who have been specifically trained can assess and assist in the diagnosis of dementia. Beyond using standardized instruments for assessment and diagnosis, nurses can direct the team's attention to social, cultural, biological, and psychological factors and coordinate appropriate responses. Nurses also can make a specific contribution, as part of the interdisciplinary team, by focusing on daily functioning, adaptation, and health status.

A future challenge for nursing requires the synthesis of the traditional nursing theoretical orientation to holistic care with recent research advances on the individual subjective experience of dementia. Nurses have historically been in the forefront of planning patient care from a holistic theoretical framework. In clinical settings, nurses also contribute their expertise in the complexity of family dynamics and can relate to the assault on the personhood of the patient with dementia.

Much work remains to be done to integrate the nursing field's traditional focus on caring relationships and holistic care into nursing research on dementia. This chapter describes one such research project, which analyzed seeking of the diagnosis using interview data from family members of persons with dementia. The project found that several factors—including lack of information, confusion regarding what is normal aging and what is dementia, denial, and the inadequacies of the medical model—contribute to the delay in obtaining a diagnosis and therefore delay any treatment that may be available.

Finally, this chapter speaks to the difficulties associated with communicating the diagnosis of dementia to the affected person and to family members. There are no clear guidelines for how much information to give, who should receive the information about the diagnosis, and what the follow-up to diagnostic interventions should be. According to Amy Levine, a nurse clinician working in a memory clinic, "You don't want to send people home without necessary information, but it is also important not to bombard them with too much information" (personal communication, November 2003). Acute clinical judgment (as well as humane sensitivity) is required to balance the need for information with the need for maintaining a level of hope. Decisions about who, what, and when to tell must be based on clinical wisdom and commitment to the best interest of the patient. While our nursing experience and available research tells us that patients with Alzheimer's disease or other dementias need and want this type of care, it is still far from reality for many patients. Much work deserves to be done to bring nursing care of dementia patients to this universal standard.

REFERENCES

Abraham, I. L., Fox, J. M., Harrington, D. P., Snustad, D. G., Steiner, D. A., Abraham, L. H., et al. (1990). A psychogeriatric nursing assessment protocol (PNAP) for use in multidisciplinary practice. *Archives of Psychiatric Nursing, 4*(4), 242–259.

Abraham, I. L., Holroyd, S., Snustad, D. G., Manning, C. A., Brashear, H. R., Diamond, P. T., et al. (1994). Multidisciplinary assessment of patients with Alzheimer's disease. *Nursing Clinics of North America, 29*(1), 113–128.

Abraham, I. L., Smullen, D. E., & Thompson-Heisterman, A. A., (1992). Assessing geropsychiatric patients. *Journal of Psychosocial Nursing, 30*(9), 13–19.

A Profile of Older Americans: 2002, from the Administration on Aging (2002). Retrieved December 5, 2004, from http://www.aoa.gov/prof/Statistics/profile/highlights.asp

Alexopoulos, G. S., Abrams, R. C., Young, R. C., & Shamoian, C. A. (1988). Cornell scale for depression in dementia. *Biological Psychiatry, 23*(3), 271–284.

Barnes, R. C. (1997). Telling the diagnosis to patients with Alzheimer's disease: Relatives should act as proxy for patient. *British Medical Journal, 314*(7077), 375–376.

Berman, R., Iris, M., Robinson, C., & Morhardt, D. (2002, October). *Physician feedback in assessing memory changes in older adults: Implications for early diagnosis of dementia.* Poster session during Best Practices Poster Day at the Cognitive Neurology and Alzheimer's Disease Center, Feinberg School of Medicine, Northwestern University, Chicago.

Brashear, H. R. (2003). Galantamine in the treatment of vascular dementia. *International Psychogeriatrics, 15*(Suppl. 1), 187–194.

Chiu, E. (2003). Vascular burden and BPSD: A reconceptualization. *International Psychogeriatrics, 15*(Suppl. 1), 183–186.

Cohen, D., Eisdorfer, C., Gorelick, P., Pavesa, G., Luchins, D. J., Freels, S., et al. (1993). Psychopathology associated with Alzheimer's disease and related disorders. *Journal of Gerontology, 48*(6), M255–M260.

Cohen-Mansfield, J., Marx, M. S., & Rosenthal, A. S. (1989). A description of agitation in a nursing home. *Journal of Gerontology, 44*(3), M77–M84.

Collighan, G., Macdonald, A., Herzberg, J., Philpot, M., & Lindesay, J. (1993). An evaluation of the multidisciplinary approach to psychiatric diagnosis in elderly people. *British Medical Journal, 306*(6881), 821–824.

Committee on a National Research Agenda on Aging. (1991). *Extending life, enhancing life. A national research agenda on aging.* Washington, DC: National Academy Press.

Cummings, J. L., Mega, M., Gray, K., Rosenberg-Thompson, S., Carusi, D., & Gorbein, J. (1994). The Neuropsychiatric Inventory: Comprehensive assessment of psychopathology in dementia. *Neurology, 44*(12), 2308–2314.

Dennis, M., Furness, L., Lindesay, J., & Wright, N., (1998). Assessment of patients with memory problems using a nurse-administered instrument to detect early dementia and dementia subtypes. *International Journal of Geriatric Psychiatry, 13*(6), 405–409.

Downs, M. (1997). The emergence of the person in dementia research. *Ageing & Society, 17*(5), 597–607.

Erde, E., Nadal, E., & Scholl, T. (1988). On truth-telling the diagnosis of Alzheimer's disease. *Journal of Family Practice, 26*(4), 401–406.

Erkinjuntti, T., Kurz, A., Gauthier, S., Bullock, R., Lilienfeld, S., & Damaraju, C. V. (2002). Efficacy of galantamine in probable vascular dementia and Alzheimer's disease combined with cerebrovascular disease: A randomised trial. *Lancet, 359*(9314), 1283–1290.

Evans, D. A. (1990). Estimated prevalence of Alzheimer's disease in the United States. *Milbank Quarterly, 68*(2), 267–289.

Fillenbaum, G. G., & Smyer, M. A., (1981). The development, validity, and reliability of the OARS multidimensional functional assessment questionnaire. *Journal of Gerontology, 36*(4), 428–434.

Fillenbaum, G. G., Beekly, D., Edland, S., Hughes, J., Heyman, A., & Van belle, G. (1997). Consortium to establish a registry for Alzheimer's Disease (CERAD): Development, database structure, and selected findings. *Topics in Health Information Management, 18*(1), 47–58.

Finkel, S. I., Costa e Silva, J., Cohen, G. D., Miller, S., & Sartorius, N. (1998). Behavioral and psychological symptoms of dementia: A consensus statement on current knowledge and implications for research and treatment. *American Journal of Geriatric Psychiatry, 6*(2), 97–100.

Folstein, M. F. (1983). The Mini-Mental State Exam. In T. Crook, S. H. Ferris, & R. Bartus (Eds.). *Assessment in Geriatric Psychopharmacology* (pp. 47–51). New Canaan, CT: Mark Powley.

Folstein, M. F., Folstein, S., & McHugh, P. (1975). Mini-mental state: A practical method for grading the cognitive state of patients for the clinician. *Journal of Psychiatric Research, 12,* 185–198.

George, L. K., & Fillenbaum, G. G. (1985). OARS methodology. A decade of experience in geriatric assessment. *Journal of the American Geriatrics Society, 33*(9), 607–615.

Holroyd, S., Turnbull, Q., & Wolf, A. M. (2002). What are patients and their families told about the diagnosis of dementia? Results of a family survey. *International Journal of Geriatric Psychiatry, 17*(3), 218–221.

Iris, M., Berman, R., & Morhardt, D. (2001, November). The centrality of circumstance: Decision-making, diagnosis-seeking, and dementia. Paper presented at the American Anthropological Association Annual Meeting, Washington, DC.

Iris, M., Berman, R., Robinson, C., Engstrom-Goehry, V., Morhardt, D., & Schrauf, R. (2002, October). *Pathways to Alzheimer's disease: Identifying factors that promote or inhibit early detection.* Poster session during Best Practices Poster Day at the Cognitive Neurology and Alzheimer's Disease Center, Feinberg School of Medicine, Northwestern University, Chicago.

Johnson H., Bouman, W., & Pinner, G., (2000) On telling the truth in Alzheimer's disease: A pilot study of current practice and attitudes. *International Journal of Psychogeriatrics, 12*(2), 221–229.

Kalaria, R. N., & Ballard, C. (1999). Overlap between pathology of Alzheimer's disease and vascular dementia. *Alzheimer's Disease & Associated Disorders, 13*(Suppl. 3), S115–S123.

Lawton, M., & Brody, E. (1969). Assessment of older people: Self-maintaining and instrumental activities of daily living. *The Gerontologist, 9*(3), 179–186.

Maguire, C. P., Kirby, M., Coen, R., Coakley, D., Lawlor, B. A., & O'Neill, D. (1996). Family members' attitudes towards telling the patient with Alzheimer's disease their diagnosis. *British Medical Journal, 313,* 529–530.

Manos, P., & Wu, R. (1994). The ten point clock test: A quick screen and grading method for cognitive impairment in medical and surgical patients. *International Journal of Psychiatry in Medicine, 24*(3), 229–244.

Marzanski, M. (2000). On telling the truth to patients with dementia. *Western Journal of Medicine, 173*(5), 318–323.

Mega, M. S. (2002). Differential diagnosis of dementia: Clinical examination and laboratory assessment. *Clinical Cornerstone, 4*(6), 53–65.

Moretti, R., Torre, P., Antonella, R., Cozzato, G., & Bova, A. (2002). Ten Point Clock Test: A correlation analysis with other neuropsychological tests in dementia. *International Journal of Geriatric Psychiatry, 17*(4) 347–353.

Morriss, R. K., Rovner, B. W., Folstein, M. F., & German, P. S. (1990). Delusions in newly admitted residents of nursing homes. *American Journal of Psychiatry, 147*(3), 299–302.

Peplau, H. (1952). *Interpersonal relations in nursing.* New York: Putnam.

Pfeiffer, E. (1975). A short portable mental status questionnaire (SPMSQ) for the assessment of organic brain deficit in elderly patients. *Journal of the American Geriatrics Society, 23*(10), 433–441.

Reisberg, B., Borenstein, J., Salob, S. P., Ferris, S. H., Franssen, E., & Georgotas, A. (1987). Behavioral symptoms in Alzheimer's disease: Phenomenology and treatment. *Journal of Clinical Psychiatry, 48*(Suppl.), 9–15.

Sachdev, P. (2000). Is it time to retire the term "dementia"? *Journal of Neuropsychiatry & Clinical Neuroscience, 12*(2), 276–279.

Schneider, E. L., & Guralnick, J. M. (1990). The aging of America: Impact on health care costs. *Journal of the American Medical Association, 263* (17), 2335–2340.

Seymour, J., Saunders, P., Wattis, J. P., & Daly, L. (1994). Evaluation of early dementia by a trained nurse. *International Journal of Geriatric Psychiatry, 9*(1), 37–42.

Sherrell, K., Buckwalter, K. C., Bode, R., & Strozdas, L. (1999). Use of the Cognitive Abilities Screening Instrument (CASI) to assess elderly persons with schizophrenia in long-term care settings. *Issues in Mental Health Nursing, 20*(6), 541–558.

Smith, A. P., & Beattie, B. L. (2001). Disclosing a diagnosis of Alzheimer's disease: Patient and family experiences. *Canadian Journal of Neurological Sciences, 28*(Suppl. 1), S67–S71.

Teng, E. L., Hasegawa, K., Homma, A., Imai, Y., Larson, E., Graves, A., et al. (1994). The Cognitive Abilities Screening Instrument (CASI): A practical test for cross-cultural epidemiological studies of dementia. *International Psychogeriatrics, 6*(1), 45–58.

Trapp-Moen, B., Tyrey, M., Cook, G., Heyman, A., & Fillenbaum, G. G. (2001). In-home assessment of dementia by nurses: Experience using the CERAD evaluations. *Gerontologist, 41*(3), 406–409.

Tune, L. E. (2003). Great progress in diagnosis and treatment of dementia. *American Journal of Geriatric Psychiatry, 11*(4), 388–390.

Turnbull, Q., Wolf, A., & Holroyd, S. (2003). Attitudes of elderly subjects toward "truth telling" for the diagnosis of Alzheimer's disease. *Journal of Geriatric Psychiatry and Neurology, 16*(2), 90–93.

Weintraub, S. (1998). *Individual differences in dementia symptoms: Their causes and management.* Paper presented to the National Association of Professional Geriatric Care Managers, Chicago. October 24, 1998.

White, L., Petrovitch, H., Ross, G., Masaki, K., Abbott, R., Teng, E., et al. (1996). Prevalence of dementia in older Japanese-American men in Hawaii: The Honolulu–Asia Aging Study. *Journal of the American Medical Association, 276,* 955–960.

CHAPTER 13

Nursing Management of Clients Experiencing Dementias of Late Life: Care Environments, Clients, and Caregivers

Ruth Remington, PhD, APRN, BC
Linda A. Gerdner, PhD, RN
Kathleen C. Buckwalter, PhD, RN, FAAN

INTRODUCTION

As people age, they are at greater risk for developing a dementing illness, which is a pathological condition that impairs cognitive function. Dementia is not a single disease, but rather a group of symptoms that negatively impact the person's functional ability. Among these symptoms, cognitive impairment is one of the most devastating losses that older adults and their caregivers face. Although memory loss may be the earliest and most common indication, dementia also causes changes in personality, behavior, sensorimotor function, and language. A challenge in working with older adults with dementia is to provide care that maintains physical and functional well-being while upholding dignity.

Nurses practicing in most settings can expect, at some time, to care for older adults with cognitive impairment. This chapter explores different environments where the geropsychiatric nurse plays a pivotal role in the promotion of health for people with dementia and their formal and informal caregivers. Most of the care for these persons is provided by nurses or the nursing assistants they supervise. A goal for nursing care is to promote maximum function, dignity, and quality of life for the person with dementia. An overview of nursing interventions is presented with a focus on care environments, clients, and their caregivers.

CARE ENVIRONMENTS

Regardless of the care environment, persons with dementia pose numerous challenges to the caregiver. Family caregivers often face caregiving responsibilities for aging parents and young children simultaneously, while trying to maintain employment and other social roles. Community resources that can enhance and support caregiving roles are discussed below.

Adult Day Care

Many times family caregivers become so consumed with the care recipient's needs that they neglect their own. Respite may provide the caregiver with needed temporary relief. Adult day care centers provide health, social, and recreational services to older adults who need supervision for a portion of the day. Meals, rest periods, and therapeutic activities are scheduled with an effort to maximize the functional ability of the individual. Adult day care programs are sponsored by both public and private organizations, with variable schedules, fees, and program foci (Ebersole & Hess, 2001; Miller, 2004). The National Adult Day Services Association in Washington, DC, can provide information on local programs. See its website at http://helpguide.org/elder/adult_day_services.htm.

Home Health Care

Visiting nurse associations provide multidisciplinary health care services for persons who need intermittent skilled care at home. Nonskilled, personal care services are offered but not usually covered by insurance. Individual and environmental assessments, treatment for clients, and education for caregivers provided by these agencies can be instrumental in helping to defer institutionalization (Ebersole & Hess, 2001; Miller, 2004).

Assisted Living

Assisted living facilities are residences in which special services are offered to maximize the functional ability of the individual who needs some help with activities of daily living, but not the intensity of care provided by a long-term care facility (LTCF). Services can include meals, housecleaning, and personal care. Architectural features are adapted to the older or disabled adult. A growing number of facilities have dedicated units for the care of the adult with dementia.

Long-Term-Care Facilities

Persons are usually cared for in the home by family members until caregiving demands exceed the ability to cope or a caregiver is no longer available due to illness or death. It is at this time that a decision may be made for placement in an LTCF. The average length of time and the degree of importance with which the caregiving role is viewed may have an important impact on the family member's

response to institutionalization and should be examined (Davis & Buckwalter, 2001). Over time, caregiving may become the dominant role of the family member, who may experience ambivalent or adverse feelings, such as guilt and depression, when these responsibilities are relinquished to paid staff in an LTCF.

Special care units (SCUs), devoted to the care of persons with dementia, are flourishing. The education of caregivers regarding elements of "special" care needs to be increased, and nurses are in an excellent position to undertake this challenge. Family consumers should be encouraged to obtain comparison information about the characteristics of the SCUs in their geographic area. It is also important for them to know that their personal preference and values are relevant in selecting a unit. Pertinent issues for family consumers and their advocates to explore can include features that distinguish the special care unit from an integrated unit. Architectural features, staff training, and activity programs should be adapted to the physical and cognitive deficits of the older adult with dementia. Family members need to know how the unit is secured, what plan is in place for fire or other emergency, and whether the resident is permitted off the unit with supervision (Gerdner & Buckwalter, 1996).

Hospice Care

Core nursing responsibilities related to end-of-life care when the client with dementia is dying include being: (1) a skilled clinician who understands symptom management and can provide comfort care, (2) an advocate to assure that all members of the health care team are available to the client and his or her family members, and (3) a guide to assist the client and family through the dying experience (Norlander, 2001). Norlander has outlined five principles for comprehensive end-of-life nursing care that are applicable to a wide range of client populations, including those with dementia. These principles include: (1) client and family treatment preferences will be discussed among all team members and respected; (2) undesirable symptoms will be relieved; (3) emotional, spiritual, and personal suffering will be addressed; (4) clients and families will be prepared emotionally for death; and (5) grieving will be acknowledged. For many years, persons with dementia were disproportionately excluded from hospice or palliative care because it was difficult for clinicians to determine if death was imminent within the 6-month period covered by insurers. More recently, hospice care has moved into nursing homes and SCUs to better accommodate persons with dementia and their families. For example, palliative care is especially challenging for persons with dementia, who may be unable to articulate their need for additional pain medication. Community-based nurses with advanced education in geropsychiatric nursing can play an important role in encouraging early-stage clients with dementia and their families to participate in advance care planning (advance directives) and to make their end-of-life care treatment preferences clearly known while they are still cognitively intact enough to participate in the decision making process. Sensitivity to the psychological conflicts associated with end-of-life decision making can assist the geropsychiatric nurse in supporting the individual and family through this process.

Advance Directives Most persons with dementia will benefit from the two types of advance directives that exist: (1) a living will or health care directive, and (2) durable health care power of attorney, health care agent, or health care proxy. These are legally binding documents that direct health care and decision making when clients are no longer able to make their own decisions (Norlander, 2001). Norlander and McSteen (2000) have outlined six key elements of advance care planning discussion, including: (1) client goals and values,

(2) client experience with death, (3) client understanding of illness, (4) family support and understanding of client goals and values, (5) communication with physician, and (6) identification of resources. Meaningful client input into advance care planning requires a certain level of cognitive ability. Therefore, it is essential that this process take place early enough in the course of the dementing illness for the person's wishes to be known so that their wishes can be honored at the end of life.

▬ FRAMEWORKS FOR INTERVENTIONS

The Progressively Lowered Stress Threshold (PLST) model, proposed by Hall and Buckwalter (1987), provides a conceptual framework for care of persons with dementia. The model posits that the ability to tolerate stress declines with the progression of the disease. This includes both internal (i.e., pain, fatigue) and external stressors (i.e., overwhelming environmental stimuli). Maximum function can be maintained through a supportive environment in which stress-producing triggers are identified and reduced or eliminated. A plan of care based on the PLST model encompasses interventions that are client-centered, environment-centered, and caregiver-centered, to support the client in functioning within the limits of the dementing illness.

A source of stress and frustration for the older adult with dementia is the inability to plan. The nurse can assist the individual to compensate by providing a consistent routine and limiting the choices that the client is expected to make. Functional losses are due to progressive, irreversible cortical deterioration; therefore, the client should not be encouraged or expected to regain lost skills. Asking the client to "try harder" will only result in increasing frustration. Providing adequate rest is necessary to prevent increased stress levels because of the lowered tolerance to stress and diminished energy reserves. This can be accomplished by alternating stimulating activities with rest periods. Caregivers and families require ongoing education and support regarding the disease process, care routines, and problem-solving strategies (Hall & Buckwalter, 1987). The PLST model has been used to plan, implement, and evaluate care for persons with dementia across institutional and community-based settings (Smith et al., in press).

The Need-Driven Dementia-Compromised Behavior Model (NDB) (Algase et al., 1996) offers another perspective, which essentially reframes disruptive behaviors as an expression of unmet needs of the person with dementia. These unmet needs may be emotional, social, physical, or psychological in nature, but because the person with dementia may have lost language skills necessary to communicate their needs, they do so behaviorally. By assessing and organizing personal and environmental factors, the nurse can identify individuals at risk for dysfunctional behavior and individualized interventions can evolve (Algase et al.)

The cognitive developmental approach is used to characterize cognitive impairment in dementia. This approach proposes that cognitive skills and functional abilities are lost in reverse order from which they were originally acquired. The stages of dementia, from diagnosis to death, are equated to the reverse order of Piaget's developmental levels of children for the purpose of individualizing assessment and intervention (Matteson, Linton, & Barnes, 1996).

The neurodevelopmental sequencing model recommends that interventions should be chosen to match the functional skills of the older adult with dementia to ensure success. Three levels of functional ability direct interventions. For ambulatory individuals, active sports and games and cognitive stimulation with a motor component are examples of interventions. Activities for the wheelchair-bound individual would include exercises and sensory stimulation, and for the non-

ambulatory individual, range-of-motion exercises, massage, and sensory integration activities are appropriate (Buettner & Kolanowski, 2003).

■ INTERVENTIONS DIRECTED TOWARD THE PERSON

Group Activity

Structured group activities have been shown to reduce agitation in the nursing home environment. In one study, disruptive residents were taken to a 2-hour supervised session, which included orientation activities, movement therapy, or relaxation activities, such as therapeutic touch and music. In addition to the participants becoming calmer, other residents and staff on the unit reported that respite from the disruptive residents facilitated their relaxation. Nursing staff also reported increased job satisfaction (Smith-Jones & Francis, 1992). In a systematic review of psychosocial interventions in early dementia, Bates and colleagues (2004) found that reality orientation was effective in improving cognitive ability in persons in the early stages of dementia. Although there was a small decline in improvement at the end of the intervention period, the effect was sustained up to three months. No evidence was found, however, to demonstrate the effectiveness of group counseling sessions on well-being or procedural memory stimulation sessions on functional performance and cognitive ability (Bates, Boote, & Beverly, 2004).

Reminiscence

Reminiscence therapy is not simply recalling the past. It is a structured process of reflection on significant life events (Hsieh & Wang, 2003). The ability to retrieve events from long-term memory can persist long after the capacity to recall newly learned information diminishes (Pittiglio, 2000). Reminiscence therapy was effective in stimulating communication, promoting self-esteem (Woodrow,

1998), and decreasing depression in older adults with and without dementia (Hsieh & Wang; Pittiglio, 2000). Hsieh and Wang note that although studies of reminiscence therapy do not consistently produce statistically significant results, any intervention that has the potential to decrease depression has clinical significance and should be considered.

In addition to having positive effects on nursing home residents, biographical storytelling resulted in improved staff attitudes toward older adults in their care. Staff reported that they understood the older adults better and were able to form closer relationships. Increased involvement with the residents and their families occurred while gathering biographical data. The intervention demonstrated the potential for increased job satisfaction (Clark, Hanson, & Ross, 2003). Activities that elicit pleasant memories may produce a soothing effect on the client who is agitated. This process may be enhanced by stimulation of multiple senses (vision, smell, taste, touch, hearing). Examples of sensory cues include the introduction and discussion of photo albums, personal memorabilia, providing a favorite food item, playing a musical instrument, or listening to music.

An individual or group reminiscence therapy session can begin with techniques to trigger memory recall, such as the use of pictures, photographs, music, foods, tools, or memorabilia. Open-ended questions help to focus the individual on the past, e.g., "Can you tell me what it was like growing up in Springfield?" These questions stimulate conversation and build rapport. Family and friends can assist in identifying significant historical events (Pittiglio, 2000).

Remotivation

Providing opportunities for clients to experience a sense of control can stimulate them to become remotivated to interact with the environment (Ryden, 1992). Examples include consistency in the daily routine and offering simple choices in terms of food and clothing whenever possible, e.g., "Would you like to wear the red dress or the blue dress?"

Art

Art may be an alternate form of communication for persons with dementia when the disease process makes language difficult or impossible. Creative art activities can also offer the person a sense of control by manipulating art materials and making decisions within a limited sphere (Harlan, 1993). In addition, sensory stimulation is provided through the exploration of various art mediums, colors, and forms. Art forms provide for an expression of self, and incorporating the personal identity of the older adult with dementia links art to reminiscence (Kahn-Denis, 1997).

A three-dimensional art form designed for older adults with dementia can provide a vehicle for sensory stimulation. For example, art that depicts familiar activities such as fishing, baking, or gardening can encourage reminiscence. Related items, such as a potholder or baseball glove, incorporated into the art, add dimension and stimulation of tactile and visual sensation. The addition of aromatic oils adds olfactory stimulation (Sanzotta, 1996).

Indications for Pharmacological Therapies

Currently there are no pharmacological agents that can cure or stop the progression of dementia. Five agents have been developed that can temporarily improve cognitive function for many with mild to moderate Alzheimer's disease (Table 13-1). Four of these drugs—tacrine (Cognex), donepezil (Aricept), rivastigmine (Exelon), and galantamine (Reminyl)—act to increase the amount of acetylcholine in the central nervous system, by inhibiting the enzyme cholinesterase. Acetylcholine is a memory- and cognition-regulating neurotransmitter. Prolonging the

TABLE 13-1	Selected Drugs for Alzheimer's Disease		
Drug (trade name)	Total daily dose	Pharmacokinetics	Adverse effects
donepezil (Aricept)	5 to 10 mg qd	Partially metabolized by the liver and partially excreted by kidneys Half-life: 70 h	Headache, fatigue, insomnia, diarrhea, nausea, anorexia, weight loss, frequent urination
galantamine (Reminyl)	4 to 12 mg bid	Mostly metabolized by the liver Half-life: 7 h	Fatigue, bradycardia, anorexia, diarrhea, weight loss
rivastigmine (Exelon)	1.5 to 6 mg bid	Metabolized by the liver, excreted by the kidneys Half-life: 1.5 h	Weakness, dizziness, anorexia, nausea, vomiting, weight loss
tacrine (Cognex)	10 to 40 mg qid	Highly metabolized by the liver Half-life 2 to 4 h	GI bleeding, anorexia, diarrhea, drug-induced hepatitis, nausea, vomiting, bradycardia
memantine (Namenda)	5 to 10 mg bid	Excreted in urine	Dizziness, headache, constipation

Note. Adapted from *Drug Therapy in Nursing,* by D. S. Aschenbrenner, L. W. Cleveland, and S. J. Venable, 2002, New York: Lippincott (pp. 292–296); also from *Nursing for Wellness in Older Adults: Theory and Practice,* by C. A. Miller, 2004, New York: Lippincott (pp. 566–569).

activity of acetylcholine on the cholinergic receptors and in the synapses permits more effective transmission (Aschenbrenner, Cleveland, & Venable, 2002). Although currently approved only for Alzheimer's-type dementia, it has been suggested that these drugs may be equally effective for people with vascular or Lewy body dementias. Tacrine, the first of the cholinesterase inhibitors approved, is rarely used today because the other drugs in the class have fewer adverse effects (Miller, 2004). Nausea, vomiting, diarrhea, anorexia, and weight loss are common side effects of these medications. Less frequent cholinergic effects include urinary retention, sleep disturbance, seizures, and bronchospasm.

Memantine (Namenda) is the first drug shown to be effective in clients with moderate to severe Alzheimer's disease. Approved by the FDA in 2003, memantine acts by blocking selective receptors that are stimulated by glutamate. Glutamate, a neurotransmitter involved in memory, is produced in excessive amounts in people with Alzheimer's disease. It has been proposed that memantine may reduce neuronal cell destruction (Garnett, 2003; Libow, 2003). Other drugs that are being investigated to manage symptoms of dementia include antioxidants (e.g., ginkgo biloba, vitamin E), nonsteroidal anti-inflammatory drugs (NSAIDs), and statins (Miller, 2004).

Monitoring Medication Side Effects

Safe administration and ongoing assessment of the client with a dementing illness who is receiving these drugs is an important nursing function related to pharmacologic interventions. It is important that nurses insure that clients have actually swallowed their medication, as well as closely monitor their response (Buckwalter, Stolley, & Farran, 1999). Clients and families should be instructed to take medications as prescribed, as higher doses may not increase cognitive benefits, but may increase side effects. To maximize absorption of the drug, galantamine (Reminyl) and rivastigmine (Exelon) should be administered with food while donepezil (Aricept) and memantine (Namenda) can be administered without regard to food (Deglin & Vallerand, 2003).

Complementary and Alternative Therapies

Medicinal Herbs and Nutritional Supplements   Herbs have been recognized for their healing properties since ancient times. Increasingly, herbal remedies and dietary supplements are being suggested as treatments for Alzheimer's disease and other dementias. Although research is being conducted on the safety and effectiveness of these products, many of the claims are anecdotal. In the United States, medicinal herbs are classified as dietary supplements, and not subject to the rigorous scientific research required by the Food and Drug Administration for sale as a prescription drug. Manufacturers may make claims about the effects of the herbs, but are not permitted, by law, to claim that the herbs can prevent or cure disease.

Some herbal supplements may be effective interventions for managing symptoms related to dementia; however, older persons considering their use should be cautioned that the purity and potency of the supplement is not standardized. The chemical composition of the product may be affected by growing and harvesting conditions, and storage. The amount of active ingredient in the product may vary from one brand to another. Most importantly, medicinal herbs can have serious adverse interactions with some prescription medications, or increase the risk for bleeding, and should only be taken with the supervision of a health professional.

Researchers have shown interest in ginkgo biloba. Preliminary reports suggest that it improves memory and cognitive function in older adults with dementia; however, results are not consistent. Ginkgo biloba has antioxidant, anti-inflammatory, and vasodilating properties. Few side effects are reported, but it does inhibit platelet aggregation and can increase the risk of bleeding, especially if the person is taking anticoagulants. Other herbal and dietary supplements promoted as treatments for dementia include vitamin E and coenzyme Q10, because of their antioxidant properties. Studies of these supplements have shown inconsistent results (Keegan, 2001; Miller, 2004; Spoelhof & Foerst, 2002).

Therapeutic Use of Touch   Hands-on, touch modalities have been practiced by nurses throughout history. Therapeutic back massage promotes relaxation, as well as stimulates the circulation. Touch, in the form of massage, can be viewed as a form of nonverbal communication for the person with dementia whose ability to communicate verbally is declining. Gentle hand massage has been shown to reduce agitation in nursing home residents with dementia (Remington, 2002; Snyder, Egan, & Burns, 1995). These techniques require little training and can be performed by professional and lay caregivers alike.

Activity Kits   Therapeutic activity kits contain items that can be used to provide diversional activity. Items chosen for the kit are individualized with the help of family members, and include articles that can provide cognitive and sensory stimulation. Examples of items that can be included in the activity kit include audiotapes of family members and familiar music, photo albums, videotapes, art therapy, textured cloth for tactile stimulation and folding activity (Conedera & Mitchell, 2004).

Buettner (1999) conducted a two-part study to test a multilevel sensorimotor intervention for nursing home residents with dementia called "simple pleasures." During Part One, trained families and volunteers created 30 therapeutic sensorimotor recreational items that were age- and stage-appropriate for persons with dementia. In Part Two, the interventions were tested. For example, an activity apron was created and used for residents with repetitive motor patterns whereas picture dominos were used for residents who were lethargic and isolated. Family members used these items to interact with their loved ones during visits and reported an increase in the quality of their visits. In addition, residents exhibited less agitation with use of the "simple pleasures" intervention.

Doll Therapy The therapeutic use of dolls can elicit pleasure and provide a sensory stimulus, reassurance, and comfort in the older adult with dementia and can stimulate verbal and nonverbal communication (Ehrenfeld & Bergman, 1995). Dolls and stuffed animals used for this purpose should be constructed safely with nontoxic dyes and nondetachable parts that the client could swallow. Caregivers must be careful to avoid speaking to the older adult in a childlike manner when dolls are being used therapeutically.

Video Respite Carefully selected videotapes can engage the older adult while providing a brief period of respite for the caregiver. Video Respite refers to the creation of videotapes that utilize music, light, movement, and pleasant memories to maintain the interest of the older adult. There are two methods used for creating these tapes. The first involves taping a family member who articulates scripts with individualized content. However, the time and energy involved in creating these tapes may add to existing caregiver burden. Consequently, generic videotapes have been created to reach a wide audience. Professional actors or actresses appear on the tapes by presenting simple, slow-paced conversation. Messages relate to experiences, people, and objects that are likely to be ingrained in long-term memory. Early research findings revealed that most persons with dementia can watch and participate with the tapes, and staff on SCUs reported the tapes were calming for residents (Lund, Hill, Caserta, & Wright, 1995). More recent investigations of the intervention have shown that there are more positive verbal and nonverbal responses when the tapes are viewed alone, rather than in a group setting (Caserta & Lund, 2002). Research has shown that there is no relationship between cognitive ability and the ability to participate with and respond to the tapes (Caserta & Lund, 2002; Malone-Beach, Royer, & Jenkins, 1999). Hall and Hare (1997) evaluated the effectiveness of one selected videotape ("Remembering When") in the series of 10 Video Respite tapes. Although findings did not reveal a significant reduction in agitated behaviors, there was a significant increase in positive behaviors.

Simulated Presence Therapy Simulated presence therapy uses a similar concept, by capturing a personalized conversation on audiotape about personal memories and family anecdotes. Soundless spaces are incorporated into the tape to encourage the cognitively impaired person to respond and engage in the conversation. Studies have shown significant improvement in problem behaviors and social isolation following the use of presence therapy (Miller et al.; 2001; Woods & Ashley, 1995).

INTERVENTIONS DIRECTED TOWARD THE ENVIRONMENT

Environmental Modification

Whether the person is living at home or in a long-term-care facility, it is often necessary to modify the environment to compensate for the person's impaired functional and cognitive status. Safety becomes a primary concern.

Potentially harmful items, such as sharp objects and toxic fluids, should be removed from the client's environment. Misinterpretation of environmental stimuli can be confusing and frightening. Mirrors and photographs may need to be covered or removed and television and radio programming should be monitored for appropriateness. In the living area, clutter, highly polished floors, or scatter rugs can lead to falls in patients who may already suffer from an unsteady gait. To the extent possible, keep belongings, frequently used items, and furniture in the same place, so the person with dementia does not have to relearn their whereabouts and may rely more on habit and routine to negotiate the environment.

Home

Maintaining comfort in the home, while creating a safe environment for the older adult with dementia, is a challenge for caregivers. In addition to removing potentially dangerous objects from the client's environment, some relatively simple alterations to the home can have considerable benefits. Using contrasting colors for the walls and woodwork make it easier for the older adult to more clearly distinguish doorways. Patterned wallpaper, curtains, and upholstery can cause confusion, and should be replaced with solid colors wherever possible. Furniture should be in a contrasting color to the floor to make it easier to distinguish. The older adult with dementia may no longer have the skills to properly use rockers, recliners, and furniture on wheels. These types of furnishings may also present a hazard when leaned against to steady oneself. Carpeting, heavy curtains, and upholstered furniture help to absorb sound and can minimize confusion.

Grab bars installed in the bathtub and beside the toilet provide a measure of safety for all members of the household. A hand-held shower can make bathing less frighten-ing. Antiscalding devices installed in bathtub faucets and showers can prevent sudden changes in water temperature and accidental burns. Further, lowering the temperature on the hot water heater can prevent burns. Replacing the bathroom door and glass shower doors with shower curtains will continue to offer privacy but prevent the person from getting stuck or locked in the bathroom. If the color of the toilet and floor are similar, changing the toilet seat to a contrasting color will help the person distinguish the seat.

In the kitchen, removing extra pots, dishes, and utensils will help to minimize an overwhelming number of choices. Childproof locks can be installed on cabinet doors and oven doors to restrict access. Control knobs for the stove and oven should be removed to prevent injury. Labels or pictures of objects can help the older adult to identify correct cabinets or drawers.

Cognitive impairment limits the person's ability to differentiate between safe and unsafe acts. Age-related sensory impairments can further contribute to accidents or injury. Environmental camouflage or visual barriers, such as two-dimensional grid patterns on the floor in front of exits or cloth panels over doorknobs, have been shown to be effective in discouraging entrance into areas that are potentially unsafe (Dickinson, McLain, & Marshal-Baker, 1995). Other strategies that have been used with mixed results include placing stop signs before restricted areas, or painting a dark stripe on the floor in front of the "off limits" areas. Paint and wallpaper can be used to disguise or camouflage exits, closets, thermostats, and other potential architectural hazards.

Modifications made to the living environment are done primarily to maintain the safety of the individual. The challenge in planning modifications is in maintaining the independence and dignity of the older adult while doing so. The approach will likely need to be adapted as the disease progresses.

Snoezelen

Snoezelen was developed in the Netherlands by Ad Verheul and Jan Hulsegge, to facilitate relaxation for persons with sensory, physical and learning disabilities. The word is a contraction of the Dutch words for *sniffing* and *dozing*. It is used to describe the combination of aroma and relaxation therapy used in this protocol. A multisensory environment is created through the use of a breeze machine, fiber optic lights, columns of bubble tubes that change colors, soft images projected on the walls, and gentle music to enhance feelings of relaxation. The literature to support the use of Snoezelen in persons with dementia remains largely anecdotal (Savage, 1996).

Music

Nursing research on the use of music has utilized two types of music: calming and individualized. Calming or relaxing music is chosen for the qualities of the music that are soothing, such as slow tempo, soft dynamic levels, and repetitive themes. In order to re-duce the cognitive effort necessary to process the music, lyrics and well-known tunes are avoided. It has been suggested that calming music mediates the release of stress hormones, altering the stress response, resulting in functionally adaptive behaviors. Calming music can be expected to reduce agitation for several persons simultaneously, such as in a group dining room (Ragneskog, Kihlgren, Karlsson, & Norberg, 1993; Remington, 2002; Tabloski, McKinnon-Howe, & Remington, 1995).

Alternatively, the presentation of carefully selected music, based on personal preference, provides an opportunity to stimulate remote memory. This changes the focus of attention and provides an interpretable stimulus, overriding stimuli in the environment that are meaningless or confusing. The elicitation of memories associated with positive feelings (happiness, love, etc.) has a soothing effect on the person with dementia, which in turn prevents or alleviates agitation (Box 13-1). There is a positive correlation between the degree of significance music had in the per-

---

Box 13-1   Research with Individualized Music

Theoretical Basis: Mid-Range Theory of Individualized Music for Agitation (Gerdner, 1997)

Theory Testing Through Research: Gerdner (2000) used an experimental repeated measures pretest–posttest crossover design to compare the immediate and residual effects of individualized music to classical "relaxation" music relative to baseline on the frequency of agitated behaviors in 39 elderly persons with dementia residing in six LTCFs in Iowa. The selection of individualized music was based on information obtained from a close family member. Findings showed a significant reduction in agitation during and following individualized music compared to classical music.

Evidence-Based Protocol: Individualized music (Gerdner, 2001) or access information at http://www.guideline.gov/summary.aspx? doc_id+3073.

Feasibility: This intervention is relatively inexpensive and required minimal time expenditure. Following instruction by nursing staff, music may be implemented by nursing assistants and family members.

Translating Research into Practice: Gerdner (in press) evaluates the effectiveness of individualized music when implemented by trained staff and family members. Music was administered daily for 30 minutes at a prescribed time and "as needed" by CNAs. Family members were also encouraged to play music for their loved one during visits. A statistically significant reduction in agitation was found during the presentation of music. Music also promoted meaningful interaction between the residents, staff, family, and others.

son's life before the onset of cognitive impairment and the effectiveness of the intervention (Gerdner, 1997).

![img] ## INTERVENTIONS DIRECTED TOWARD THE CAREGIVER

Family Caregivers

Family members often care for persons with dementia in the home during the early to middle stages of cognitive impairment. Indeed, 70% of persons with dementia are cared for in their own home or a family member's home (Grant, Patterson, Hauger, & Irvin, 1992; Rabins, Fitting, Eastham, & Zabora, 1990) (Box 13-2). Caring for a relative with chronic confusion is among the most difficult of family responsibilities, triggering significant emotional, physical, and financial stress. The stress associated with caring for someone with Alzheimer's disease and related disorders (ADRD) has been linked to a number of adverse outcomes, including depression, high psychotropic drug use, decline in physical health, and compromised immune response (Gallagher-Thompson & Powers, 1997; Garand et al., 2002; Meshefedjian, McCusker, Bellavance, & Baumgarten, 1998;

Mort, Gaspar, Juffer, & Kovarna, 1996; Schulz, O'Brien, Bookwala, & Fleissner, 1995). Nurses are in an excellent position to provide training to empower family members with the knowledge and skills necessary in handling these problematic behaviors, while maintaining their own well-being.

Education and Support in Caregiving Responsibilities

The Progressively Lowered Stress Threshold (PLST) model, as previously discussed, was used as the basis for a psychoeducational intervention to train in-home caregivers of family members with dementia. The PLST intervention was individualized for each caregiving dyad and focused on psychological support while providing instruction in behavioral techniques aimed at diminishing dysfunctional behaviors in the care recipient. Instruction focused on reducing environmental stressors, compensating for executive dysfunction and communication deficits, providing unconditional positive regard, and planning care based on a lowered stress threshold. An ongoing nursing relationship is pivotal in guiding family caregivers to establish a routine that maximizes abilities and

---

Box 13-2   Dementia Portrayed in Popular Literature and Films

Personal stories can help to facilitate an understanding of Alzheimer's disease from the perspective of the family member and the afflicted person. Professional and lay caregivers can learn from the experiences of those telling their story. Below are some of the many examples of these accounts that are available at larger bookstores.

- Bob Artley and Yasmin Khan (1993). *Ginny: A Love Remembered.* Ames, Iowa: Iowa State Press.
- Daniel A. Pollen (1993). *Hannah's Heirs: The Quest for the Genetic Origins of Alzheimer's Disease.* Oxford: Oxford University Press.
- Esther Strauss Smoller and Kathleen O'Brien (1997). *I Can't Remember: Family Stories of*

Alzheimer's Disease. Philadelphia, PA: Temple University Press.

- Joyce Dyer (1996). *In a Tangled Wood: An Alzheimer's Journey.* Dallas, TX: Southern Methodist University Press.
- Diana Friel McGowin (1994). *Living in the Labyrinth: A Personal Journey Through the Maze of Alzheimer's.* New York: Delta.

Movies and contemporary films can depict a lifelike example of living with an older adult with dementia. Two recent motion pictures include:

- *Iris* (2002), Buena Vista Home Video
- *The Notebook,* (2004), New Line Cinema

minimizes stress for both the care recipient and the caregiver.

Referral to Support Groups for Care and Assistance

Family caregiving can become an all-consuming job for which caregivers often receive inadequate support and training (Kelley, Buckwalter, & Maas, 1999). Support groups provide an avenue to meet other family caregivers to share feelings and concerns, as well as provide emotional support and decrease the caregiver burden. Many support groups also provide learning opportunities via formal community experts and the informal expertise of other caregivers. Caregivers frequently identify lack of respite care and geographic location as barriers to attending support group meetings. As a means of overcoming these barriers, nurse researchers are exploring the effectiveness of alternative methods, such as Internet support via home computers (White & Dorman, 2000) and telephone support (Davis, 1998).

Nursing Home Placement

When the family member is no longer able to care for his or her loved one at home, nursing home placement may be warranted. However, relocation to a nursing home does not necessarily mean an end to the stress experienced by family caregivers (Collins et al., 1994). Following placement, family members must develop a different caregiving role. Most families do not know how to make the transition from direct care tasks to a more indirect, supportive, interpersonal role, nor are they likely to receive assistance from nursing home staff in how to go about making changes in their caregiver role. In some cases, families may encounter resistance and resentment from staff who view them as disruptive "outsiders" or "visitors" when they try to carry out decision making and protective care in the facility, resulting in staff–family role conflict

(Maas, Buckwalter, Swanson, Specht, Hardy, & Tripp-Reimer 1994).

Staff Training and Management

Care of persons with dementia and the accompanying problematic behaviors has been reported as a major stressor to nursing staff (Hallberg & Norberg, 1993; Ragneskog, Kihlgren, Karlsson, & Norberg, 1993) and can potentially lead to burnout. Certified nursing assistants (CNAs) provide the majority of direct care to residents in long-term-care facilities. Research has shown that training alone is not sufficient to ensure the retention of knowledge and skills over time. To address this concern, Stevens and colleagues (1998) developed an integrated in-service and staff management system that resulted in maintenance of skill performance over time. Staff nurses are trained to provide the supervision and mentoring of CNAs, while CNAs are trained to self-monitor performance. Staff members support this form of management because it is easy to use.

Researchers in Sweden developed a 2-day training session for staff nurses regarding individualized care of persons with dementia. Nurses were subsequently supervised in the application of this knowledge. In evaluating the effectiveness, nurses were encouraged to express personal feelings regarding the challenges they encountered, and problem-solving measures were undertaken. Following a 1-year period, nurses reported a higher degree of support and trust. They also experienced a significant reduction in the frequency and intensity of burnout, and exhibited a more cooperative interaction with the clients (Berg, Hansson, & Hallberg, 1994; Edberg, Hallberg, & Gustafson, 1996; Hallberg & Norberg, 1993).

Staff–Family Partnership in Care

When planning care and developing a training program, it is important to recognize that family caregivers are a rich source of information regarding the resident's personal history, individualized routines, and personal preferences. Family may be able to share personal caregiving tips that they have found to be effective through years of trial and error. This knowledge can serve a foundation for personalized and individualized care. Consequently, family members should be an important part of the dementia care team. Stressors for both the nursing staff and family can be eased by working together in a team approach. However, the degree of involvement will vary depending on the family member's desires and abilities.

The Family Involvement in Care (FIC) protocol was developed by Maas and colleagues (1994) to diminish these potential conflicts, decrease family and staff stress, and increase satisfaction with caregiving roles. The FIC intervention is a step-by-step method designed to help nursing home staff and family members work together by achieving a negotiated partnership, in which control is shared and the particular expertise of each is used to the best advantage. The partnership emphasizes cooperation between staff and families and includes specific and clearly outlined roles for the family caregiver in the institutional setting (e.g., will co-lead reminiscence group every Wednesday afternoon). Key elements of the FIC protocol include: (1) orientation of the family to the facility and the partnership role, (2) negotiation and formation of a partnership contract, (3) education of family members for involvement in care, and (4) follow-up family member and staff evaluation and renegotiation of the partnership contract as needed.

DEMENTIA CARE RESOURCES

Theory can be used as a framework to plan, implement, and evaluate care. As research provides a growing foundation of knowledge, care is increasingly anchored in evidence-based protocols. Electronic Dementia Guide for Excellence (the EDGE Project) was developed by Ann Marie Bradley, Judah Ronch, and Elizabeth Pohlmann and funded by the New York State Department of Health. The project was developed to identify and disseminate intervention protocols generated from research specific to care of persons with dementia. Guidelines include staff training and evaluation of these interventions. The EDGE project can be accessed via the Internet at http://dementiasolutions.com/edge/index.htm

The John A. Hartford Institute for Geriatric Nursing is another resource for nurses that can be accessed through the Internet. Its programs identify and develop best nursing practice to older adults, and are updated frequently. Abundant resources related to geriatric nursing practice, education and research are available at www.hartfordign.org.

SUMMARY

Dementia is characterized by a progressive cognitive and functional decline, affecting the physical and mental health of the older adult. The geropsychiatric nurse working with the older adult with dementia needs to utilize knowledge and skills from a variety of nursing specialties. Clearly, the geropsychiatric nurse must be an expert in gerontological and psychiatric nursing. Understanding issues related to the aging process, complicated by cognitive losses, is key in formulating effective treatment plans. Knowledge of the community and community resources enable the nurse to help families enhance their caregiving role. Treatment plans that address the person, the environment, and the caregiver have the potential to maintain the dignity and quality of life for the person, family, and caregivers.

REFERENCES

Algase, D. L., Beck, C., Kolanowski, A., Whall, A., Berent, S., Richards, K., et al. (1996). Need-driven dementia-compromised behavior: An alternative view of disruptive behavior. *American Journal of Alzheimer's Disease, 1*(6), 10–19.

Aschenbrenner, D. S., Cleveland, L. W., & Venable, S. J. (2002). *Drug therapy in nursing.* New York: JB Lippincott.

Bates, J., Boote, J., & Beverly, C. (2004). Psychosocial interventions for people with a milder dementing illness: A systematic review. *Journal of Advanced Nursing, 45,* 644–658.

Berg, A., Hansson, U. W., & Hallberg, I. R. (1994). Nurses' creativity, tedium and burnout during 1 year of clinical supervision and implementation of individually planned nursing care: Comparisions between a ward for severely demented patients and a similar control ward. *Journal of Advanced Nursing, 20,* 742–749.

Buckwalter, K. C., Stolley, J. M., & Farran, C. J. (1999). Managing cognitive impairment in the elderly: Conceptual, intervention and methodological issues [Electronic version]. *The Online Journal of Knowledge Synthesis for Nursing, 6*(10), 10.

Buettner, L. L. (1999). Simple pleasures: A multi-level sensorimotor intervention for nursing home residents with dementia. *American Journal of Alzheimer's Disease, 14*(1), 41–52.

Buettner, L. & Kolanowski, A. (2003). Practice guidelines for recreation therapy in the care of people with dementia. *Geriatric Nursing, 24*(1), 18–25.

Caserta, M., & Lund, D. (2002). Video respite on an Alzheimer's care center: Group versus solitary viewing. *Activities, Adaptation and Aging, 27*(1), 13–26.

Clark, A., Hanson, E. J., & Ross, H. (2003). Seeing the person behind the patient: Enhancing the care of older people using a biographical approach. *Journal of Clinical Nursing, 12,* 697–706.

Collins, C. Stommel, M., Wang, S., & Given, C. W. (1994). Caregiving transitions: Changes in depression among family caregivers of relatives with dementia. *Nursing Research, 43*(4), 220–225.

Conedera, F. & Mitchell, L. (2004). Therapeutic activity kits. *Try This: Best Practices in Nursing Care for Hospitalized Older Adults 1*(4). Retrieved July 28, 2004, from http://www.hartfordign.org/publication/trythis/theraAct.pdf

Davis, L. L. (1998). Telephone-based interventions with family caregivers: A feasibility study. *Journal of Family Nursing, 4*(3), 255–270.

Davis, L. L., & Buckwalter, K. C. (2001). Family caregiving after nursing home admission. *Journal of Mental Health and Aging, 7*(3), 361–379.

Deglin, J. H. & Vallerand, A. H. (2003). *Davis's drug guide for nurses.* Philadelphia: F.A. Davis.

Dickinson, J. I., McLain, J. K., & Marshal-Baker, A. (1995). The effects of visual barriers on existing behavior in a dementia care unit. *Gerontologist, 35*(1), 127–130.

Ebersole, P., & Hess, P. (2001). *Geriatric nursing & healthy aging.* Philadelphia: Mosby.

Edberg, A., Hallberg, I. R., & Gustafson, L. (1996). Effects of clinical supervision on nurse-patient cooperation quality. *Clinical Nursing Research, 5*(2), 127–149.

Ehrenfeld, M., & Bergman, R. (1995). The therapeutic use of dolls. *Perspectives in Psychiatric Care, 31*(4), 21–22.

Gallagher-Thompson, D., & Powers, D. V. (1997). Primary stressors and depressive symptoms in caregivers of dementia patients. *Aging & Mental Health, 1*(3), 248–255.

Garand, L., Buckwalter, K. C., Lubaroff, D., Tripp-Reimer, T., Frantz, R. A., & Ansley, T. N. (2002). A pilot study of immune and mood outcomes of a community-based intervention for dementia caregivers: The PLST Intervention. *Archives of Psychiatric Nursing, 16*(4), 156–67.

Garnett, W. E. (2003). Memantine for Alzheimer's disease. *Long-Term Care Interface, 4*(12), 14–15.

Gerdner, L. A. (1997). An individualized music intervention for agitation. *Journal of the American Psychiatric Nurses Association, 3*(6), 177–184.

Gerdner, L. A. (2000). Effects of individualized vs. classical "relaxation" music on the frequency of agitation in elderly persons with Alzheimer's disease and related disorders. *International Psychogeriatrics, 12*(1), 49–65.

Gerdner, L. A. (2001). Evidence-based protocol: Individualized music intervention. In M. Titler (Series Ed.) *Series on Evidence-Based Practice for*

Older Adults. Iowa City, IA: The University of Iowa College of Nursing Gerontological Nursing Interventions Research Center, Research Dissemination Core.

Gerdner, L. A. (in press). Translating research into practice: Implementation and evaluation of the evidence-based protocol of individualized music by trained staff and family. *Journal of Gerontological Nursing*.

Gerdner, L. A., & Buckwalter, K. C. (1996). Review of state policies regarding special care units: Implications for family consumers and health care professionals. *American Journal of Alzheimer's Disease and Other Dementias, 11*(2), 16–27.

Grant, I., Patterson, T., Hauger, R., & Irwin, M. (1992). Current research on dementia and Alzheimer's disease. *Archives of Psychiatry, 4* (Suppl.), 77–80.

Hall, G. R., & Buckwalter, K. C. (1987). Progressively lowered stress threshold: A conceptual model for care of adults with Alzheimer's disease. *Archives of Psychiatric Nursing, 1*, 399–406.

Hall, L., & Hare, J. (1997). Video respite for cognitively impaired persons in nursing homes. *American Journal of Alzheimer's Disease, 12*(3), 117–121.

Hallberg, I. R., & Norberg, A. (1993). Strain among nurses and their emotional reactions during 1 year of systematic clinical supervision combined with the implementation of individualized care in dementia nursing. *Journal of Advanced Nursing, 18*, 1860–1875.

Harlan, J. E. (1993). The therapeutic value of art for persons with Alzheimer's disease and related disorders. *Loss, Grief, & Care: A Journal of Professional Practice, 6*, 99–106.

Hsieh, H., & Wang, J. (2003). Effect of reminiscence therapy on depression in older adults: A systematic review. *International Journal of Nursing Studies, 40*, 335–345.

Kahn-Denis, K. B. (1997). Art therapy with geriatric dementia clients. *Journal of the American Art Therapy Association, 14*, 194–199.

Keegan, L. (2001). *Healing with complementary & alternative therapies*. Albany, NY: Delmar.

Kelley, L. S., Buckwalter, K. C., & Maas, M. L. (1999). Access to health care resources for family caregivers of elderly persons with dementia. *Nursing Outlook, 47*(10), 8–14.

Kelly, A. W., Buckwalter, K. C., Hall, G., Weaver, A. L., & Butcher, H. K. (2002). The caregivers' story: Home caregiving for persons with dementia. *Home Health Care Management & Practice, 14*(2), 99–109.

Libow, L. S. (2003). Memantine: A new hope for treating patients with dementia in nursing homes. *Long-Term Care Interface, 4*(9), 8–9.

Lund, D. A., Hill, R. D., Caserta, M. S., & Wright, S. D. (1995). Video respite: An innovative resource for family, professional caregivers, and persons with dementia. *The Gerontologist, 35*, 683–687.

Maas, M., Buckwalter, K., Swanson, E., Specht, J., Hardy, M., & Tripp-Reimer, T. (1994). The caring partnership: Staff and families of persons institutionalized with Alzheimer's disease. *American Journal of Alzheimer's Disease and Related Disorders & Research*, Nov/Dec, 21–30.

Malone-Beach, E. E., Royer, M., & Jenkins, C. C. (1999). Is cognitive impairment a guide to use of video respite? Lessons from a special care unit. *Journal of Gerontological Nursing, 25*(5), 17–21.

Matteson, M.A., Linton, A., & Barnes, S. J. (1996). Cognitive developmental approach to dementia. *Image—The Journal of Nursing Scholarship, 28*, 233–240.

Meshefedjian, G., McCusker, J., Bellavance, F., & Baumgarten, M. (1998). Factors associated with symptoms of depression among informal caregivers of demented elders in the community. *Gerontologist, 38*(2), 247–253.

Miller, CA. (2004). *Nursing for wellness in older adults: Theory and practice*. New York: Lippincott.

Miller, S., Vermeersch, P., Bohan, K., Renbarger, K., Kruep, A., & Sacre, S. (2001). Audio presence intervention for decreasing agitation in people with dementia. *Geriatric Nursing, 22*(2), 66–70.

Mort, J. R., Gaspar, P. M., Juffer, D. I., & Kovarna, M. B. (1996). Comparison of psychotropic agent use among rural elderly caregivers and non-caregivers. *Annals of Pharmacotherapy, 30*(6), 583–585.

Norlander, L. (2001). *To comfort always: A nurse's guide to end of life care*. Washington, DC: American Nurses Association.

Norlander, L., & McSteen, K. (2000). The kitchen table discussion: A creative way to discuss end-of-life issues. *Home Healthcare Nurse, 18*(8), 532–540.

Pittiglio, L. (2000). Use of reminiscence therapy in patients with Alzheimer's disease. *Lippincott's Case Management, 5,* 216–220.

Rabins, P., Fitting, M., Eastham, J., & Zabora, J. (1990). Emotional adaptation over time in caregivers for chronically ill elderly people. *Age & Ageing, 19,* 185–190.

Ragneskog, H., Kihlgren, M., Karlsson, L., & Norberg, A. (1993). Nursing home staff opinions of work with demented patients and effects of training in integrated-promoting care. *Vard I Norden Nursing Science & Research in the Nordic Countries, 13*(1), 5–10.

Remington, R. (2002). Calming music and hand massage with agitated elderly. *Nursing Research, 51,* 317–323.

Ryden, M. B. (1992). Alternatives to restraints and psychotropics in the care of aggressive, cognitively impaired elderly persons. In K. C. Buckwalter (Ed.), *Geriatric mental health nursing: current and future challenges* (pp. 84–93). Thorofare, NJ: Slack.

Sanzotta, M. D. (1996). Journal lab: The magic of three-dimensional interactive art. *Journal of Long-Term Care Administration, 23,* 41–42.

Savage, P. (1996). Snoezelen for confused older people: Some concerns. *Elder Care, 8*(6), 20–21.

Schulz, R., O'Brien, A. T., Bookwala, J., & Fleissner, K. (1995). Psychiatric and physical morbidity effects of dementia caregiving: Prevalence, correlates, and causes. *The Gerontologist, 35*(6), 771–791.

Smith-Jones, S. M., & Francis, G. M. (1992). Disruptive institutionalized elderly: A cost effective intervention. *Journal of Psychosocial Nursing and Mental Health Services, 30,* 17–20.

Smith, M., Gerdner, L. A., Hall, G., & Buckwalter, K. C. (in press). The history, development, and future of the Progressively Lowered Stress Threshold Model: A conceptual model for dementia care. *Journal of the American Geriatrics Society.*

Snyder, M., Egan, E. C., & Burns, K. R. (1995). Efficacy of hand massage in decreasing agitation behaviors associated with care activities in persons with dementia. *Geriatric Nursing, 16,* 60–63.

Spoelhof, G. D., & Foerst, L. F. (2002). Herbs to magnets: Managing alternative therapies in the nursing home. *Annals of Long-Term Care, 12*(12), 51–57.

Stevens, A. B., Burgio, L. D., Bailey, E., Burgio, K. L., Paul, P., Capilouto, E., et al. (1998). Teaching and maintaining behavior management skills with nursing assistants in a nursing home. *The Gerontologist, 38*(3), 379–384.

Tabloski, P. A., McKinnon-Howe, L., & Remington, R. (1995). Effects of calming music on level of agitation in cognitively impaired nursing home residents. *The American Journal of Alzheimer's Disease and Related Disorders & Research, 10*(1), 10–15.

White, M. H., & Dorman, S. M. (2000). Online support for caregivers: Analysis of an internet Alzheimer's mailgroup. *Computers in Nursing, 18*(4), 168–179.

Woodrow, P. (1998). Interventions for confusion and dementia: Reminiscence. *British Journal of Nursing, 7,* 1145–1149.

Woods, P., & Ashley, J. (1995). Simulated presence therapy: Using selected memories to manage problem behaviors in Alzheimer's disease. *Geriatric Nursing, 16*(1), 9–14.

CHAPTER 14

Addressing Problem Behaviors Common to Late-Life Dementias

Ruth Remington, PhD, APRN, BC
May Futrell, PhD, FAAN, FGSA

INTRODUCTION

Problem behaviors associated with late-life dementias are disturbing for the older person and tax the ability of their caregivers. Behaviors such as agitation, wandering, feeding difficulties, sleep disturbances, and inappropriate sexual advances often hasten nursing home placement. These behaviors can also be an indication of stressors that the person with dementia is not able to communicate to caregivers. The individual becomes less able to tolerate stress because of the progressive loss of brain cells. Physical stressors or environmental stimuli may provoke a stressful response in the individual, resulting in problem behaviors. Ineffective management of these behaviors, by both formal and informal caregivers, subjects the individual to additional stress and escalation of the behaviors.

Identification of antecedents to problem behaviors and prompt intervention can help the individual to continue to communicate and function effectively. Caregivers and families can be taught to recognize behaviors that may indicate increasing stress and respond in a way that preserves the dignity and function of the person with dementia.

PAIN

Pain is a frequently cited antecedent to agitated behavior, which further imperils the quality of life of the individual with dementia (Cohen-Mansfield, 1995). The presence of agitation increases the likelihood that the person will receive medications to control behavior. This becomes particularly problematic if the agitation is related to pain, which would be better managed with analgesics or nonpharmacological measures. A negative correlation was found between pain reports and the severity of dementia, suggesting that the more severe the dementia, the less the person was able to verbalize pain as a word or number (Buffum, Miaskowski, Sands, & Brod, 2001).

Pain is a relatively common problem for older adults who often have one or more medical conditions that are likely to be painful, such as degenerative joint disease, back pain, or angina (Buffum et al., 2001). In older adults, and particularly those with dementia, pain is frequently undetected, untreated, or undertreated. Individuals with dementia have fewer analgesics prescribed and are administered less pain medication by nurses than cognitively intact older adults, even though the number of diagnoses of painful conditions is similar in both groups. Inadequate pain management threatens the functional ability and quality of life for these persons (Epps, 2001; Kaasalainen et al., 1998; McCaffery & Pasero, 1999).

Barriers to Effective Pain Management

Dementia presents many barriers to effective pain assessment. The literature is not clear as to whether individuals with dementia actually experience less pain, or have a decreased ability to express pain and/or appropriately respond to commonly used assessment instruments. One view is that individuals with dementia experience less pain as a result of the neuropathology of the disease (Miller, Nelson, & Mezey, 2000). Alternatively, because dementia of the Alzheimer's type affects the neocortex, sparing the somatosensory cortex, pain perception is likely to be preserved. The emotional responses to pain may be influenced by the changes in the prefrontal cortex and limbic structures, possibly resulting in disinhibition or indifference to pain. The expression of pain may be further compromised because of expressive aphasia and memory impairment associated with dementia (Farrell, Katz, & Helme, 1996).

Nursing research suggests that individuals with dementia do experience pain, with between 62% and 80% having at least one pain complaint at any given time (Ferrell, Ferrell, & Rivera, 1995; Parmelee, Smith, & Katz, 1993). Older adults may deny the presence of pain, but may admit to hurt, discomfort, soreness, or aching (American Geriatrics Society [AGS], 2002). Studies have shown that cognitively impaired persons complain of pain less frequently than cognitively intact persons; however, their complaints are reliable indicators of pain (Krulewitch et al., 2000). In those who can reliably report the existence of pain, many are unable to initiate a request for pain medication on an "as needed" basis (Miller, Nelson, & Mezey, 2000).

Lack of knowledge and skill on the part of professional caregivers presents an obstacle to pain assessment and management. Exacerbation of the behavioral symptoms associated with dementia has been linked to the presence of pain. Some of the reasons nurses cited for undermedicating demented individuals include fear of respiratory depression, of addiction, or of being associated with attempted euthanasia, and excessive concern about side effects (Miller, Nelson, & Mezey, 2000).

Indicators of Pain

Self-report is the most accurate indicator for assessing pain. Because the cognitively impaired person may be unable to communicate his or her distress in a way that caregivers can understand, it may be necessary to use other measures to determine the presence and intensity of pain (Bowser, 2002; Buffum et al., 2001).

In the noncommunicative adult, inference can be made about the pain associated with procedures and obvious pathologic conditions, such as open wounds or inflamed joints. This strategy has limited utility for general use with the older adult with dementia, as many of the chronic conditions that cause pain in this group are not visible.

Unusual, new, or escalating behavior in a person with dementia should indicate the need to assess for evidence of pain. Vocal behaviors that may suggest pain include crying, screaming, negative vocalizations, and moaning. Physical behaviors shown to be associated with pain include aggression (Feldt, Warne, & Ryden, 1998), and resistiveness to care (Mahoney et al., 1999). Additionally, facial grimacing, guarding, rubbing, frowning, and fidgeting may be a sign of pain in the cognitively impaired older adult (Epps, 2001; Hurley, Volicer, Hanrahan, Houde, & Volicer, 1992).

Less effective indicators are reports of pain from individuals who are close to the person with dementia, such as family members or professional caregivers (McCaffrey & Pasero, 1999). There are times, however, that this is the only information available, and must be considered. Studies have indicated that health professionals underestimate the amount and severity of pain in individuals with dementia. However, caregivers can be educated to identify signs that a person may be experiencing pain (Miller, Nelson, & Mezey, 2000). Family members may be a source of historical information about the person's past responses to painful situations. Surrogate reports should only be used if the person is unable to communicate his or her pain to caregivers (AGS, 2002).

The least sensitive indicators of pain in the noncommunicative person are physiologic measures, such as changes in temperature, pulse, respiratory rate, or blood pressure. While an increase in blood pressure and heart rate has been associated with pain, these measures are also associated with many other physical and emotional states (McCaffrey & Pasero, 1999).

Pain Assessment Tools

There is a lack of consensus in the literature with regard to the most effective way to assess for the presence of pain in the cognitively impaired elder. Although self-report is the most accurate indicator of pain, several researchers suggest that it is often not reliable for the individual with dementia. Results from these studies show that no single assessment tool is uniformly effective in this group, and that the measure selected should be matched to the person's cognitive abilities and language skills.

One of the most commonly used pain rating scales is the numerical rating scale (NRS). In the verbally administered 0 to 10 scale, the person assigns a number to indicate the amount of pain experienced, from 0, indicating no pain, to 10, indicating the worst pain imaginable. Using the same word anchors as the NRS, the Visual Analog Scale (VAS) is a visual representation of the range of pain from "none" to "worst." The person is asked to make a mark along a 10 cm vertical or horizontal line to indicate pain intensity (McCaffery & Pasero, 1999).

Faces rating scales, originally developed for use with children, are another commonly used pain rating scale. The scale is composed of a series of faces, ranging from a smile, depicting no pain, to a sad face, indicating excruciating pain. Faces rating scales have been translated and validated in several languages (McCaffery & Pasero, 1999). Simple line drawings of faces have also been used to assess mood states in older adults with dementia. The Dementia Mood Picture Test consists of a series of six faces depicting different moods; good mood, bad mood, happy, sad, angry, and worried. Word descriptors are presented beneath the picture in two-inch letters. Each mood is scored 0 for "yes," 1 for "no," and 2 for "very much" to represent how positive a mood the person indicated (Tappan & Barry, 1995). When using drawings of faces with older adults with dementia, the evaluator should be alert to interpretations of both pain and mood associated with these instruments.

Word descriptor scales consist of a list of easily understood adjectives depicting pain intensity. The Simple Descriptor Scale (SDS) utilizes the terms *no pain, mild, moderate,* and *severe,* and is scored by assigning a number between 0 and 3 (McCaffery & Pasero, 1999). Six descriptors used in the McGill Word Scale are *none, mild, discomforting, distressing, horrible,* and *excruciating* (Wynne, Ling, & Remsburg, 2000). The Pain Intensity Scale (PIS) is composed of six questions. For five of the questions, the subject is asked to respond with one of the following five answers; *not at all, a little, moderately, quite a bit,* or *extremely,* and is scored from 1 to 5 for each question. The last question asks for the number of days in the week that pain is present (Krulewitch et al., 2000).

The above scales are the most commonly used pain scales in the United States and all have demonstrated validity. They are easily administered, scored, and recorded, and well liked by patients. It is important, however, that one scale is used consistently with each patient to minimize confusion (McCaffery & Pasero, 1999).

Proxy pain ratings should never replace self-report of pain; however, observation of behaviors may help the nurse identify pain in a noncommunicative patient. Both vocal behaviors, such as crying, groaning, and screaming, and motor behaviors such as facial grimacing, rubbing, and fidgeting, have been associated with painful states. The Discomfort Scale for Patients with Dementia of the Alzheimer's Type (DS-DAT) is an objective scale, based on observed behaviors, developed to measure discomfort in persons with advanced dementia. The scale consists of nine vocal and motor behaviors indicating discomfort. Each behavior is given a score between 0 and 3 to indicate the frequency, intensity, and duration of the behavior. The total score is determined by summing the scores for each behavior, resulting in a total score of between 0 and 27 (Hurley et al., 1992). Psychometric evaluation conducted by nurse experts demonstrated reliability and validity of the instrument.

The Pain Assessment in Advanced Dementia (PAINAD) scale is a five-item observational tool developed to measure the frequency, duration, and intensity of behaviors that indicate pain in cognitively impaired older adults. The scale consists of five behaviors indicative of pain that were obtained from existing pain scales and the literature. Each of the five behaviors is scored from 0 to 2 to indicate the frequency, duration, and intensity of the behavior. Total score for the instru-

ment is between 0 and 10 (Warden, Hurley, & Volicer, 2003).

AGITATION

Agitation is a common management problem in persons with late-life dementia. Up to 50% of community-dwelling older people (Carlson, Fleming, Smith, & Evans, 1995) and 93% of nursing home residents exhibit agitated behaviors, with the highest percentage being in persons with dementia (Beck & Shue, 1994). The presence of agitated behaviors is distressing to the older person and presents considerable challenges to caregivers. Agitated behaviors, coupled with the loss of communication skills, may put the person with dementia at risk for inadequate assessment and treatment. For example, a hearing impairment may increase the person's disorientation, which results in agitation. Additionally, the agitated person is less likely to be offered, or participate in, audiometric testing to identify hearing loss.

The concept of agitation and its expression has not been consistently described in the literature. *Agitation* has been defined as "inappropriate verbal, vocal, or motor activity that is not explained by needs" (Cohen-Mansfield & Billig, 1986); "an unpleasant state of excitement" that persists after interventions are carried out to reduce stimuli and manage resistiveness, physical discomfort, and stress (Hurley et al., 1999); and an excess of one or more behaviors occurring in a state of altered consciousness (Corrigan, Bogner, & Tabloski, 1996).

There is disparity among researchers as to the behavioral components of agitation. Some consider agitation to be specific behaviors such as hitting, repetitive movement, and negative vocalizations (Cohen-Mansfield, 1986), whereas others group clusters of behaviors including memory problems, delusions and hallucinations (Teri et al., 1992), and resistance to care (Vance et al., 2003). Still others describe agitation as behavioral excess rather than a specific behavior (Corrigan, Bogner, & Tabloski, 1996). Terms associated with agitation include *disruptive behavior, problem behavior, troublesome behavior, behavior disturbance, dysfunctional behavior,* and *behavior symptoms associated with dementia* (AGS & AAGP, 2003).

Agitated behaviors can be physically aggressive (e.g., hitting, kicking, grabbing, cursing), physically nonaggressive (e.g., pacing, repetitous mannerisms, handling things inappropriately), or verbal (e.g., complaining, screaming, or repetitious sentences). These behaviors are inappropriate or performed with excessive frequency. The severity of the behaviors is related to the degree of physical danger the behavior poses to the person or caregiver, or the disruptiveness to the person, caregiver, and the environment (Cohen-Mansfield & Billig, 1986).

The pathophysiological basis for agitation is not well understood. It has been suggested that neurotransmitter dysregulations are implicated in the development of agitation. The restlessness associated with agitation is thought to be the result of abnormalities in the striatum, cortex, and thalamus, and mediated in part by gamma-amino-butyric acid (GABA). Persons with dementia are reported to have a higher sensitivity to norepinephrine, a reduced serotonergic function, and GABA deficits (Lindenmayer, 2000; Neugroschi, 2002). Agitation associated with aggression may be related to an increase in noradrenergic activity and a decrease in serotonergic activity.

The presence of agitated behaviors is predictive of caregiver burden, and increases the likelihood that the individual will enter a nursing home. Once in the nursing home, agitation affects the cost of care by increasing the need for staff and special environmental design (Cohen-Mansfield, 1995). Agitation places the health of the individual at further risk. Agitated nursing home residents are more likely to fall than nonagitated residents,

and the physically compromised older person with severe agitation is at higher risk for hip fractures, subdural hematoma, or cardiovascular collapse from exhaustion (Beresin, 1988; Cohen-Mansfield & Werner, 1995). Agitation results in individuals being more likely to be physically or chemically restrained. Research has repeatedly shown that, in addition to loss of dignity and potential for injury, agitated persons who are restrained exhibit the same or more agitation, confusion, incontinence and falls than those who are not restrained. Reduction in restraint use has actually been shown to result in fewer falls and injuries (Meyer, Kraenzle, Gerrman, & Morley, 1994; Tinetti, Liu, Marottoli, & Gentner, 1991; Weinrich, Egbert, Eleazer, & Haddock, 1995).

Chemical restraint, or pharmacological agents, are effective in managing agitated behaviors; however, age-related changes subject the agitated individual to longer duration of action of the drug, and increased incidence of adverse drug reactions. These medications introduce the potential for gait impairment, falls, anorexia, sedation, hypotension, diminished cognitive function, and may even paradoxically exacerbate the agitation (Chutka, 1997; Gardner & Garrett, 1997).

Antecedents

Examining events or phenomena that precede the occurrence of agitation is the first step in planning interventions to manage agitated behavior (Gerdner & Buckwalter, 1994). Prior to the work of Cohen-Mansfield and colleagues, information regarding the antecedents of agitation was mostly anecdotal (Cohen-Mansfield, 1986; Cohen-Mansfield & Billig, 1986). More recently, empirical studies have identified factors that precede the manifestation of agitation.

Cognitive Impairment Both acute and chronic cognitive impairment in the older adult may present with agitation. Delirium can cause confusion and agitation that can be difficult to differentiate from dementia. Delirium is an acute, reversible form of cognitive impairment, affecting up to 60% of hospitalized older adults (Ely et al., 2001). Nurses identified delirium in only 31% of hospitalized patients (Inouye, Foreman, Mion, Katz, & Cooney, 2001). When the underlying cause for the delirium is identified and treated, the patient may return to his baseline behavior.

Cognitive impairment has been shown to be strongly related to manifestations of agitation. The type of agitated behavior is influenced by the degree of cognitive impairment. The amount of physically nonaggressive agitation increases as the dementia progresses. Physically aggressive behaviors are likely to accelerate in the later stages of dementia, whereas verbally agitated behaviors are more frequent in the early to middle stages of dementia. In general, increases in the frequency of agitation are associated with increasing cognitive impairment until the development of profound neurological impairment, when the total number of all behaviors, including agitation, tends to decrease.

Changes in the brain that cause impairments in memory, judgment, language, and impulse control predispose a person with dementia to agitation. As language skills are lost, behavior becomes the main form of communication. It has been suggested that agitation may be the person's attempt to communicate needs or feelings that cannot be verbalized in a way that caregivers can understand (Sutor, Rummans, & Smith, 2001). The loss of functioning brain cells associated with dementia causes the person to become less able to receive and process sensory stimuli. As the level of dementia increases, the threshold between baseline and agitated behavior declines, placing the person at a greater risk for agitated behaviors. Agitated behaviors constitute a greater proportion of the individual's behaviors over the course of the disease (Hall & Buckwalter, 1987).

Sensory Impairment Sensory impairment has been implicated in the development of agitation. Hearing and vision impairments are common among older adults; however, most can compensate for the losses. For the person with dementia, this can cause misinterpretation of environmental cues. Hearing and vision impairment were shown to be strong predictors of agitation. It has been suggested that persons with dementia become disoriented by the lack of clear auditory and visual information and are likely to speak more loudly. This, coupled with communication losses, can cause these vocalizations to be considered noisy and disruptive by others in the environment (Algase et al., 1996; Vance et al., 2003). When asked to identify apparent reasons for agitation, nurses reported deafness as a disability predisposing older persons to agitation (Cohen-Mansfield, 1986). Interventions as simple as providing clean eyeglasses and hearing aids with fresh batteries can reduce the effects of sensory impairment on behavior (Gerdner & Buckwalter, 1994).

Sensory components of activities of daily living (ADL) have been linked with agitation in persons with dementia. Increased agitation during bathing was postulated to be due to frustration and a sense of loss of control (Sutor et al., 2001; Cohen-Mansfield, 1986; Mahoney et al., 1999). During meals, increased agitation was attributed to noise (Goddaer & Abraham, 1994). Aggressive agitated behaviors increased while nursing home residents were touched, in response to a hypothesized violation of personal space (Marx, Werner, & Cohen-Mansfield, 1989).

Physiological Agitation may be precipitated by physiological processes, such as infections, cardiovascular insufficiency, hypoxia, alcohol use, dehydration, fatigue, and constipation. Pain is an often-overlooked antecedent to agitated behaviors and is discussed earlier in this chapter. The worsening of a chronic medical condition may lead to agitated behaviors, just as an increase in agitation may signify a change in the medical condition. Prompt assessment, careful monitoring, and treatment of underlying conditions can alleviate the behavior problem.

Information processing and rhythm generation has been linked to the hypothalamic suprachiasmatic nucleus. The decrease in function of this center that occurs with aging is more pronounced in persons with dementia. The resulting altered circadian rhythm has been associated with an increase in agitation. This may explain an increase in agitation in the late afternoon, called sundown syndrome as reported by many (Algase et al., 1996; Evans, 1987). Others have found that agitation was more frequent during the day shift than evening or night shifts (Cohen-Mansfield, Marx, & Rosenthal, 1989). Another rhythm, the lunar phase, has been associated with increases in agitation. There have been anecdotal accounts from caregivers of increased agitation occurring during the full moon. This has not been supported by research (Cohen-Mansfield, Marx, & Werner, 1989).

Personality/Psychiatric   Agitation is a common manifestation of depression, some psychoses, and anxiety. Unresolved past issues, premorbid personality, and coping style have been proposed as influencing the expression of agitation (Cohen-Mansfield & Billig 1986; Hall, 1994). Delusions and hallucinations are fairly common as causes of agitated behaviors, occurring in 14% to 19% of people with dementia (Neugroschi, 2002).

Pharmacological Effects   Drug toxicity is one of the most common precipitants of agitation. Both prescription and over-the-counter drugs frequently used among older adults for their therapeutic effect are often implicated. Corticosteroids, anticholinergics, levodopa, sedative–hypnotics, and barbiturates are some of the drugs of concern. Withdrawal from central nervous system depressants pro-

duces agitation as well. The risks associated with psychotropic medications have come under scrutiny in recent years, yet these medications are often used to manage agitation. Side effects include gait impairment, falls, difficulty swallowing, diminished cognitive function, and paradoxical increases in agitation. The risks associated with the use of these drugs are great and the benefits unpredictable (Gerdner & Buckwalter, 1994; Tabloski, McKinnon-Howe, & Remington, 1995).

Environment   Environmental conditions clearly can influence the specific agitated behaviors manifested. Verbal agitation occurring mainly in the evening and when the person is alone suggests that the agitation may be a response to boredom or loneliness. Aggressive behavior occurs most often at night, when it is cold, and when the person is in close contact with others, and can be viewed as a response to a real or perceived threat. Other environmental conditions associated with an increase in agitation include the use of physical restraints, inactivity, and high levels of noise. Decreased staffing or unlicensed caregivers in nursing homes have also been found to be related to an increased prevalence of agitation. Conversely, structured activity, music, and opportunity for social interaction can decrease agitated behaviors (Algase et al., 1996; Cohen-Mansfield & Werner, 1995).

Interventions to Manage Agitation

Interventions shown to decrease agitation include behavioral approaches, environmental modifications, and pharmacological approaches. None of these approaches is universally successful in reducing agitation, and successful management may necessitate use of more than one strategy. The treatment plan needs to be individualized according to ongoing assessment data.

Behavioral Approach Behavioral treatment of agitation centers on identifying and modifying the physiologic, psychosocial, and environmental factors that are antecedents of the agitated behaviors. Comprehensive assessment is key to developing an individualized treatment plan. It is important to determine the type of agitated behavior exhibited, as well as its frequency, duration, and severity. Any temporal pattern of agitation should be noted. Certain activities, such as bathing, can precipitate agitation. Intervening before the agitation escalates will enhance the efficacy of the plan.

Basic Needs Before behavioral interventions can be effective, it is essential to ensure that the individual's basic needs are met. Causes of physical illness and delirium, such as urinary tract infection, should be identified and treated. Other physiological sources of agitation, including pain or discomfort, need to use the toilet, and restrictive clothing, should be assessed and managed.

Meeting nutritional needs can be a challenge. Agitated persons may not be able to sit long enough to complete a meal. Additionally, because of the presence of apraxia (inability to perform purposeful acts) and agnosia (inability to recognize familiar objects), which are often associated with dementia, the person may be unable to feed him- or herself adequately. Limiting or eliminating alcohol and caffeine, as well as offering smaller meals, finger foods, and nutritious snacks between meals, can improve intake. Regular vision and hearing evaluations and ensuring that eyeglasses and hearing aids are in use, especially at mealtimes, can decrease confusion and agitation.

Communication As dementia progresses, language and reasoning skills deteriorate. The person with dementia experiences trouble expressing thoughts in a manner that can be understood by caregivers. Problem behaviors can be viewed as a way of communicating. For example, aggression may express a response to a perceived threat in the environment, whereas repetitious mannerisms are likely to communicate boredom (Cohen-Mansfield & Werner, 1995). Speaking to the person in a calm manner, using a low tone and with a slow rate can convey a sense of trust. A conscious effort to utilize good verbal and nonverbal communication skills is needed. Eye contact should be established by standing or sitting at eye level. Explaining what you intend to do before approaching the person using simple instructions, rather than commands, is important. The person with dementia has an impaired ability to learn or reason. Reorienting a confused person to the environment or trying to teach new information can be frustrating for the older person as well as the caregiver. An alternative strategy is to redirect the person to a meaningful, "failure-free" activity that he or she can accomplish.

Autonomy and Sense of Control Memory deficits can impair understanding, making tasks and directions seem too difficult or overwhelming to understand. Dividing tasks into small manageable steps and allowing adequate time for completion increases the likelihood of success. Caregivers should be instructed to be patient and avoid criticism and reprimands. It is important to give the individual opportunities to exercise some control when possible. Offering choices with what to eat or what to wear allows the person control in a supervised setting. Eating dessert before the meal or wearing mismatched clothing is less distressful for both the individual and caregivers than escalating agitation in response to frustration.

The application of physical restraints severely limits the agitated person's autonomy. Restraints restrict mobility and usually increase agitation and distress, and should only be used in rare instances to protect the safety of the individual. An alternative to restraints is to remove potentially dangerous objects from the person's environment and provide space for safe pacing.

Environmental Modifications Environmental factors can influence the development of agitation. Environmental stimuli can be overwhelming or misinterpreted. Voices coming from radios or overhead pagers can lead to confusion and suspicion. Television can be interpreted as reality and perceived as frightening. Caregivers should be instructed to ensure that the surroundings are consistent, predictable, and familiar to help reduce confusion, fear, and agitation.

Clocks and calendars facilitate orientation to time. Simple cues such as signs or pictures can prevent a sense of feeling lost. A picture of a toilet on the bathroom door or a picture of the person in his or her bedroom can help to direct them. Because of the loss of short-term memory, the person may not see him- or herself as an old person, and pictures taken when they were younger tend to be more easily identifiable by older adults with dementia. Similarly, if the image of the person viewed in a mirror is distressing to the older person, mirrors may need to be covered or removed.

Activities for the agitated person should be kept simple. Failure-free activities, such as folding napkins, feeding the birds, or counting a pile of coins, can help the older adult have a sense of accomplishment and self-worth. Agitation may be triggered if the instructions are confusing or the environment is too noisy. Care should be taken to avoid unnecessary competing stimuli that may be overwhelming or difficult for the person to interpret. Equally important is preventing understimulation, which can lead to boredom, frustration, and further agitation.

There is a growing body of research on the therapeutic effects of music as an environmental modification for agitated persons with dementia. Nursing research on the use of music has utilized two types of music: calming and individualized. Calming or relaxing music is chosen for the qualities of the music that are soothing, such as slow tempo, soft dynamic levels, and repetitive themes. In order to reduce the cognitive effort necessary to process the music, lyrics and well-known tunes are avoided. Calming music can be expected to reduce agitation for several persons simultaneously, such as in a group dining room (Remington, 2002; Tabloski, McKinnon-Howe, & Remington, 1995). Individualized or familiar music is selected based on the individual's preference and is intended to evoke an emotional response. The reduction in agitation shown with individualized music is attributed to the memories associated with the familiar music and lyrics (Gerdner, 2000).

Simple interventions to modify the environment have been shown to reduce agitation. Caregiver singing during bathing resulted in increased cooperation with care and the need for fewer instructions from caregivers (Gotell, Brown, & Ekman, 2002). Audio presence, or simulated presence therapy, is a personalized tape recording of a family member discussing memories or pleasurable topics. Significant improvement in problem behaviors and social isolation was reported following the use of presence therapy (Miller et al., 2001; Woods & Ashley, 1995). Brief interventions of hand massage or slow-stroke back massage reduced the frequency of agitated behaviors (Remington, 2002; Rowe & Alfred, 1999; Snyder, Egan, & Burns, 1995).

Pharmacological Approach Pharmacological agents should only be used if the agitated behaviors interfere with daily functioning. Age-related changes in the older adult increase the incidence of adverse drug reactions. Additionally, the use of these pharmacological agents may actually exacerbate the agitation, resulting in even more medication being prescribed. Medications used to treat

Research

This study investigated calming music and hand massage as nonpharmacological interventions to reduce agitation in nursing home residents with dementia. Using a four-group repeated measures experimental design, agitation was measured during four 10-minute observation periods: (1) before the intervention, (2) during the intervention, (3) immediately after the intervention, and (4) at one hour. The experimental intervention consisted of a 10-minute exposure to either calming music, hand massage, both calming music and hand massage simultaneously, or no intervention (control group).

Each of the experimental interventions reduced the frequency of agitated behaviors more than no intervention. The benefit was sustained over the hour and actually increased over time.

Each of the interventions produced similar results and there was no additive benefit to the combination of calming music and hand massage.

The findings of this study show that either calming music or hand massage is effective in reducing agitated behaviors. Both of these interventions are easily administered, require little training, and incur little cost. The use of nonpharmacological interventions alone or to supplement an individualized plan of care for the agitated individual has the potential to reduce the use of physical and chemical restraints and to improve the quality of life for the older adult with dementia.

Note. Adapted from "Calming Music and Hand Massage with Agitated Elderly," by R. Remington, 2002, *Nursing Research, 51*, pp. 317–323.

underlying medical conditions can also increase agitated behavior as a side effect of the medication or the resultant change in the person's health status. If behavioral symptoms are not severe, behavioral interventions should be utilized first. If pharmacological agents are necessary, the lowest effective dose should be used. Gradual dosage reductions should be attempted several times per year in an attempt to withdraw the medication.

Antipsychotic Medications   Delusions and hallucinations are common in dementia and often respond well to low doses of antipsychotics. Several studies have reported the effectiveness of haloperidol (Haldol), risperidone (Risperdal), and olanzapine (Zyprexa) in managing physical aggression, verbal outbursts, and difficulty sleeping in patients with dementia. The most common side effects with these drugs include extrapyramidal symptoms (EPS), orthostatic hypotension, sedation, and tardive dyskinesia. Haloperidol is associated with a higher rate of EPS than risperi-

done and olanzapine (Table 14-1) (Bower, McCullough, & Pille, 2002; Neugroschi, 2002). Where feasible, caregivers should encourage individuals taking antipsychotics to make slow position changes to minimize postural hypotension. Alcohol should be avoided. Parkinsonian symptoms (difficulty swallowing, tremor, rigidity, shuffling gait) should be promptly reported to the prescriber so that a dosage adjustment can be made. Signs of tardive dyskinesia include uncontrolled rhythmic movements of face and extremities, lip smacking, and tongue thrusting, and are indications that the drug be discontinued.

Antidepressants   In patients with coexisting depression and associated agitation, antidepressants can be used to manage disruptive behaviors. Depression, which occurs in up to 57% of persons with dementia, often leads to anxiety and an inability to initiate meaningful activity, worsening the behavioral problems of dementia (Volicer, Hurley, & Mahoney, 1995). The literature reports that most antidepres-

TABLE 14-1 Selected Pharmacological Therapy for Problem Behaviors Common to Late-Life Dementias

Class	Drug	Starting Dose	Total Daily Dose	Adverse Effects
Antipsychotic				
	haloperidol (Haldol)	0.25–0.5 mg qd or bid	1 to 3 mg	Sedation, EPS, akathesia, tardive dyskinesia, acute dystonia
	risperidone (Risperdal)	0.25 mg qd-bid	1 to 3 mg	Sedation, hypotension, tardive dyskinesia, hyperglycemia, EPS
	olanzapine (Zyprexa)	2.5 mg qhs	5 to 10 mg	Sedation, weight gain, hypotension, tardive dyskinesia, hyperglycemia, EPS
Antidepressant				
	trazodone (Desyrel)	25–50 mg qhs or bid	50 to 250 mg	Sedation, hypotension
Mood stabilizer				
	carbamazepine (Tegretol)	200 mg qhs	300 to 400 mg	Sedation, GI distress, agranulocytosis, aplastic anemia
	gabapentin (Neurontin)	100 mg qd or bid	300 to 2400 mg	Sedation, tremor, ataxia
	valproic acid (Depakote, Depakene)	125 mg qhs	250 to 1000 mg	Nausea, sedation, tremor, ataxia

Note. Adapted from "Agitation: How to Manage Behavior Disturbances in the Older Patient with Dementia," by J. Neugroschi, 2002, *Geriatrics, 57*(4), pp. 33–40; also from "Assessment and Management of Behavioral Disturbances in Nursing Home Patients with Dementia," by B. Sutor, T. A. Rummans, and G. E. Smith, 2001, *Mayo Clinic Proceedings, 76*, pp. 540–550.

sants have similar efficacy; however, the selective serotonin reuptake inhibitors (SSRIs) have a better side-effect profile in older adults. Trazodone, a heterocyclic antidepressant with serotonin reuptake inhibition, can induce sedation and should be considered in persons who have disturbed sleep (Gardner & Garrett, 1997; Neugroschi, 2002).

Mood Stabilizers Anticonvulsant medications have been shown to be effective for the treatment of agitation and aggression. Drugs such as carbamazepine (Tegretol), valproic acid (Depakote), and gabapentin (Neurontin) are believed to control aggression by affecting neurohormonal mediators. The most common side effects are sedation and gastrointestinal disturbance. Serum drug levels, hepatic function tests, and CBC should be monitored for carbamazepine and valproic acid (Bower, McCullough, & Pille, 2002; Gardner & Garrett, 1997; Neugroschi, 2002).

Wandering

Wandering is a behavioral problem associated with early to mid-stage Alzheimer's disease. Individuals at risk for this behavior include community-residing or institutionalized older adults with dementia. *Wandering* is defined by the North American Nursing Diagnosis Association (NANDA) *Nursing Diagnoses* (2001) as "meandering, aimless, or repetitive locomotion that exposes the individual to harm, frequently incongruent with boundaries, limits, or obstacles" (pp. 206–207). According to Peatfield, Futrell, and Cox (2002), "there is no single cause for wandering and no single solution" (p. 45). There are, however, common wandering behaviors and situations that can provoke these behaviors as described in Table 14-2. Consideration of physiological

---

TABLE 14-2   Common Wandering Behaviors and Situations That Can Provoke Wandering

Wandering Behaviors
- Exit seeking
- Purposeless walking
- Pacing
- Persistent locomotion
- Getting lost
- Searching
- Following caregiver
- Hyperactivity
- Repetitive visits to the same place
- Walking to unauthorized places
- Nighttime walking aimlessly

Situations That Can Provoke Wandering
- Cognitive impairment
- Nocturnal confusion
- Full bladder
- Medication effects
- Unfamiliar surroundings
- Emotional frustration
- Hunger or thirst
- Pain
- Constipation
- Over- or understimulation
- Lifestyle prior to illness (e.g., night shift worker)

---

changes, psychological needs, and the environment is important when planning an intervention to lessen the problem behavior.

The first step in management of wandering includes assessment of the individual and the behavior. Futrell and Melillo (2002a; 2002b) suggest assessment for cognitive decline, depression, anxiety, agitation, wandering patterns, and neurocognitive deficits, as well as premorbid lifestyle. The frequency with which memory and behavior problems occur and the degree to which the problem upsets the caregiver is of importance. Nursing staff should try to determine whether the wandering is an attempt by the resident to acquire additional attention, sensory stimulation, or access desired items.

Assessment tools and instruments that can be used to assess the risk of wandering include: Mini-Mental Status Exam (Folstein, Folstein, & McHugh, 1975), Algase Wandering Scale (Algase, Beatie, & Yao, 2001), Short Geriatric Depression Scale (Sheikh & Yesavage, 1986), Cohen-Mansfield Agitation Inventory: Long Form (Cohen-Mansfield 1999; Cohen-Mansfield, Marx, & Rosenthal, 1989), and Memory and Behavior Problems Checklist, 1990 R (Zarit & Zarit, 1983, 1990).

Management of wandering behavior is difficult. An individualized approach to the problem is necessary. Music therapy, social interaction, structured physical activity, environmental adaptation and technological devices are interventions that appear to lessen problem behaviors (Peatfield et al., 2002). The need for formal caregivers to transmit knowledge related to these strategies to families and to offer families psychosocial support is recommended (Peatfield et al.). It is also suggested that staff in institutions and families who are caring for individuals with wandering problems need to learn how to communicate with patients who have this behavior.

Interventions to address wandering behavior can be grouped into four categories: (1) environmental modifications, (2) interventions addressing technology and safety, (3) physical and psychosocial interventions, and (4) caregiving support and education (Table 14-3) (Futrell & Melillo, 2002a, 2002b). Safety of the individual who wanders requires environmental modifications at home or in the institution. A secure area where wandering can take place is necessary. In the institutional setting, one caregiver can watch problem wanderers in a secured area, thus

---

TABLE 14-3   Interventions to Address Wandering

Environmental Modifications
- Provide a secure place to wander such as a wandering lounge—a large, safe walking area.
- Enhance the environment by increasing visual appeal, such as tactile boards or three-dimensional wall art.
- Place gridlines in front of doors to decrease exit seeking.
- Make exits less visible and accessible by covering panic bars with cloth.
- Allow walking where doors are not in the path.
- Utilize safety locks, complex and less accessible door latches.
- Maintain safety by removing clutter and disabling appliances.
- Provide stimulation clues such as pictures and signs.
- Use a combination of large-print signs and portrait-like photographs to aid in way finding.
- Use a multifaceted approach to environmental modifications, as it is more effective than singular modifications.

Technology & Safety
- Use technological devices to locate and monitor wandering.
- Use a verbal alarm system as it is more effective than an aversive alarm system.
- Use mobile locator devices for quickly locating wanderers.

Physical & Psychological Interventions
- Assess for and treat depression.
- Decrease wandering during structured activities by using social interaction of staff and/or visitors or music.
- Music sessions are more effective than reading sessions in decreasing wandering behavior.
- Prevent risky situations by adequate supervision.
- Walking should not be unnecessarily limited.
- Decrease wandering by eliminating stressor from the environment, such as cold at night, changes in daily routines, and extra people at holidays.
- Decrease wandering by providing regular exercise.

Caregiving Support & Education
- Educate caregivers to assist in their ability to care for the wanderer.
- A facility-based approach could include identification of the problem, a wandering prevention program, interactions with staff, and staff mobilization around the problem.

Note. Adapted from "Evidence-based "Protocol: Wandering," by M. Futrell and K. D. Melillo, 2002, In M. G. Titler (Series Ed.), *Series on Evidence-based Practice for Older Adults.* Iowa City, IA: The University of Iowa College of Nursing Gerontological Nursing Interventions Research Center, Research Dissemination Core; also from "Evidence-based Protocol: Wandering," by M. Futrell and K. D. Melillo, 2002, *Journal of Gerontological Nursing, 28*(11), pp. 14–22.

allowing other caregivers time for patient care. Technology devices that monitor wandering and locate wanderers are available. These devices may alleviate stress for family caregivers in the home environment. Use of door latches, safety locks, and other environmental modifications may also promote safety. Increasing the visual appeal of environmental surroundings with art gives the bored individual a more stimulating experience. It is not clear what part boredom plays in wandering behavior. On the other hand, overstimulation seems to cause patients to wander as much as boredom. Identifying patterns of wandering may be helpful in care planning.

Social interaction of staff and visitors with individuals who wander during mealtimes can decrease wandering and ensure eating. Structured activities, exercise, and the use of music also decreases wandering. Wandering during the night may also occur. This problem is often caused by medications or too much sleeping during the day. It is useful to ask if the individual's lifestyle was that of a day or night person. For instance, did they work the night shift? The type of job or the sleeping patterns that existed prior to the onset of dementia is information useful for individualized care planning. Observation of the individual alerts the caregiver to specific stressors that trigger the problem behavior. Interventions should be evaluated and discontinued if the problem wandering does not decrease.

The Need-Driven Dementia–Compromised Behavior Model offers caregivers structure for planning care that is individualized (Algase et al., 1996). According to Ann Whall, this is "a middle-range theoretical model that addresses what has been called 'disruptive behavior' or 'disturbed behavior' (DB) in individuals with dementia" (Whall, 2002, p. 5). She further suggests the model "posits that behavior, such as wandering, aggression, and problematic vocalizations, is an attempt to convey some meaning" (p. 5). Knowing that

this wandering behavior may represent meaning to the individual would prompt the nurse to assess for and address contributing factors.

In summary, wandering becomes a problem when it disrupts the individual's sleep, eating, safety, or the caregiver's ability to provide care. Assessment of premorbid factors, the disease process, behaviors typical of the disease, medications and their side effects are important when individualizing interventions for wandering behavior. Other factors, such as the environment and the knowledge and skill of the caregiver, should be considered when planning care for older adults with dementia who are at risk for wandering behaviors.

OTHER PROBLEM BEHAVIORS

Sleep Disturbances

Sleep–wake cycle disturbances are common in older adults with cognitive impairment. Nighttime awakening and excessive napping often become problems for those caring for older adults with dementia. Medications and their side effects may cause drowsiness and vivid dreams. Too much caffeine and a warm room may prevent the patient from sleeping and may cause night wandering. It may become necessary to assist the patient with bedtime routines and to consider the individual's previous wake cycle when considering interventions related to sleep. Hunger or the need to urinate may cause sleep disturbance. Brief naps, especially in the morning, may refresh the older individual if sleep has been disturbed. Naps longer than 1 hour or naps late in the day may interfere with night sleep, however.

Eating Disorders

Eating disorders appear in the ambulatory (early) stage of dementia. They can become acute and need immediate attention. Individuals may either lose interest in eating or eat constantly. Eating too little or too much may be a result of boredom, overstimulation, or the disease process. Individuals may not be able to feed themselves or prepare the food, or they may forget to eat, which may lead to inadequate food intake and poor nutrition.

Weight changes are common in dementia. As the disease progresses, supervision of eating may help to prevent malnutrition. Visitors, family, and volunteers can assist during mealtime in the home or institutional setting. This assistance may make eating less chaotic, while providing a social dimension. For patients who overeat, restricting access to food and providing structure and supervision may help.

Norberg and Athlin (1989) suggest interventions should target the appropriate eating/feeding problem: (1) problems associated with the ability to eat and drink, (2) problems associated with the social dimension of eating, and (3) problems associated with the environmental aspect. Similarly, Watson and Deary (1994) identified three components of feeding difficulty in individuals with dementia. The components were named: (1) patient obstinacy or passivity, which reflects the lack of cooperation with feeding; (2) nursing intervention, or the amount of help or supervision required with feeding; and (3) indicators of feeding difficulty, such as food spillage and leaving food on the plate at the end of the meal. Understanding the basis of the eating disorder will help caregivers to select specific interventions that have a high likelihood of success.

With these suggested components in mind, mealtimes for those with dementia may need to be longer. Older adults with dementia take longer to chew and swallow. Finger foods, proper body positioning, and frequent small meals in the same place and at the same time each day may appeal to some individuals. In late stages, the individual may need to be reminded to open his or her mouth and chew (Cacchione, 2000). Caregivers should consider the use of music at mealtimes, social inter-

action with family and other patients, and colorful surroundings. When music was played during meals, nursing home residents with dementia have been shown to spend more time with dinner and eat more. Relaxing music played during the main meal of the day reduced the overall level of agitation among nursing home residents (Goddaer & Abraham, 1994). Soothing music had a more positive effect than rock music or tunes from the 1920s and 1930s (Ragneskog, Kihlgren, Karlsson, & Norberg, 1996).

Kinahan (1999) suggests "persons with dementia often consume more at breakfast or lunch than at the evening meal" (p. 34). She further states, "this coincides with the sundowning phenomenon seen at the end of the day, which is displayed as restlessness, insecurity, and agitation" (p. 245). Caregivers who are aware of this behavior can make an effort to encourage intake earlier in the day.

Providing a consistent caregiver may improve communication between an individual with dementia and the caregiver during feeding. McGillivray and Marland (1999) recommend primary nursing to provide consistency of caregivers to improve communication of an individualized plan of care. Training and supervision of assistive personnel will enhance their understanding of the patient's disability by helping them to carry out feeding in a sensitive and therapeutic manner.

Sexual Disturbances

Inappropriate sexual behavior is not uncommon among dementia patients. Research is needed to better understand this behavior. Touching the genitals or undressing are not necessarily sexual. The caregiver needs to determine if the patient is responding to physical discomfort such as sore areas due to incontinence pads. A firm but calm response needs to be given if unwanted advances are made. The older adult should be gently redirected. If the person exposes genitals, he or she should be taken back to his or her room for privacy. Cover the lap with a pillow and attempt to distract him or her.

According to Lyketsos, Steele, and Steinberg (1999), "men may develop hypersexuality, manifested by inappropriate propositioning, inappropriate touching, or public displays of masturbation. In women, repeated touching and rubbing of the genital area may be the result of vaginal infection, uterine prolapse, or similar physical problems" (p. 223). In men with dangerously hypersexual or aggressive behavior, medication may be used to reduce the sexual drive.

Increased sexual demands of a married partner with dementia may result in a pathologic bond if the spouse is the caregiver. Brown, Lyon, and Sellers (1988) discuss the need to educate the spouse to the disease process and "teach how to dissuade or distract the sexually persistent patient, using medications when advisable" (p. 38).

SUMMARY

Problem behaviors of the dementia patient present major challenges to caregivers. The cause or causes of these behavioral disturbances are often not clearly identified. Caregivers need to be alert to a variety of stressors that may precipitate problem behaviors. Physical stressors might be a urinary tract infect-

ion and/or pain. Mental health disturbances such as depression and anxiety can also be stressors, leading to problem behaviors. The environment where care is given and the individuals providing care may provoke a stressful response. No single stressor is universally responsible for problem behaviors.

Thorough assessment is a first step in planning interventions for compassionate care. Assessing the individual's behavior and reasons for the onset or continuation of the behavior is accomplished with assistance from the caregiver and the family. Careful attention to the environment, the medical and mental health condition of the individual, and medications being given for this and other conditions is important during the assessment process.

Information regarding the caregiver relationship with the older adult with dementia and knowledge of the physical and mental status of the older person are important before recommending a management plan. Once an individualized plan has been developed, education and support of caregivers is essential. A "fallback" plan should be available for emergencies, and caregivers need to be informed that treatment may take longer and need more than one attempt in order to be successful. Supporting the caregiver is an important role of the geropsychiatric nurse.

REFERENCES

Algase, D. L., Beattie, E., & Yao, L. (2001). The Algase wandering scale: Initial psychometrics of a new caregiver reporting tool. *American Journal of Alzheimer's Disease and Other Dementias, 16*(3), 141–152.

Algase, D. L., Beck, C., Kolanowski, A. Whall, A., Berent, S., Richards, K., et al. (1996). Need-driven dementia-comprised behavior: An alternative view of disruptive behavior. *American Journal of Alzheimer's Disease, 11*(6), 10–19.

American Geriatrics Society (AGS). Panel on persistent pain in older persons (2002).The management of persistent pain in older persons. *Journal*

of the American Geriatrics Society (suppl), 50, S205–S224.

American Geriatrics Society and American Association for Geriatric Psychiatry. (2003). Consensus statement on improving the quality of mental health care in U.S. nursing homes: Management of depression and behavior symptoms associated with dementia. *Journal of the American Geriatrics Society, 51,* 1287–1298.

Beck, C. K., & Shue, V. M. (1994). Interventions for treating disruptive behavior in demented elderly people. *Nursing Clinics of North America, 29*(1), 143–155.

Beresin, E. V. (1988). Delirium in the elderly. *Journal of Geriatric Psychiatry and Neurology, 1,* 127–143.

Bower, F. L., McCullough, C. S., & Pille, B. L. (2002). Synthesis of research findings regarding Alzheimer's disease: Part II, care of people with AD. *Online Journal of Knowledge Synthesis for Nursing, 9*(4), 1–38.

Bowser, A. (2002). Management of pain in patients with cognitive impairment requires a thoughtful approach. *Central Nervous System Education for the Long-term Care Professional, 1*(2), 1, 12.

Brown, J., Lyon, P., & Sellers, T. D. (1988) Caring for the family caregivers. In L.Volicer, K. Fabiszeuski, Y. Rheaume, & K. Lasch (Eds.), *Clinical management of Alzheimer's disease* (pp. 29–41). Rockville, MD: Aspen.

Buffum, M. D., Miaskowski, C., Sands, L., & Brod, M. (2001). A pilot study of the relationship between discomfort and agitation in patients with dementia. *Geriatric Nursing, 22*(2), 80–85.

Cacchione, P. (2000) Cognitive and neurologic function. In A. Lueckenotte (Ed.), *Gerontologic nursing* (pp. 615–654). St. Louis, MO: Mosby.

Carlson, D. L., Fleming, K., Smith, G. E., & Evans, J. M. (1995). Management of dementia-related behavioral disturbances: A non-pharmacologic approach. *Mayo Clinic Proceedings, 70,* 1108–1115.

Chutka, D. S. (1997). Medication use in nursing home residents. *Nursing Home Medicine, 5,* 180–187.

Cohen-Mansfield, J. (1986). Agitated behaviors in the elderly II. Preliminary results in the cognitively deteriorated. *Journal of the American Geriatrics Society, 34,* 722–727.

Cohen-Mansfield, J. (1995). Assessment of disruptive behavior/agitation in the elderly: Function, methods, and difficulties. *Journal of Geriatric Psychiatry and Neurology, 8*(1), 52–60.

Cohen-Mansfield, J. (1999). Assessment measurement of inappropriate behavior associated with dementia. *Journal of Gerontological Nursing, 25*(2), 42–51.

Cohen-Mansfield, J., & Billig, N. (1986). Agitated behaviors in the elderly I. A conceptual review. *Journal of the American Geriatrics Society, 34*(10), 711–721.

Cohen-Mansfield, J., Marx, M. S., & Rosenthal, A. S. (1989). A description of agitation in a nursing home. *Journal of Gerontology: Medical Sciences, 44*(3), M77–M84.

Cohen-Mansfield, J., Marx, M. S., & Werner, P. (1989). Full moon: Does it influence agitation in nursing home residents? *Journal of Clinical Psychology, 45*(4), 611–613.

Cohen-Mansfield, J., & Werner, P. (1995). Environmental influences on agitation: An integrative summary of an observational study. *The American Journal of Alzheimer's Care and Related Disorders & Research, 10*(1) 32–39.

Corrigan, J. D., Bogner, J. A., & Tabloski, P. A. (1996). Comparisons of agitation associated with Alzheimer's disease and acquired brain injury. *American Journal of Alzheimer's Disease, 11*(6), 20–24.

Ely, E. W., Margolin, R., Francis, J., May, L., Truman, B., Dittus, R., et al. (2001). Evaluation of delirium in critically ill patients: Validation of the Confusion Assessment Method for the Intensive Care Unit (CAM-ICU). *Critical Care Medicine, 29,* 1370–1379.

Epps, C. D. (2001). Recognizing pain in the institutionalized elder with dementia. *Geriatric Nursing, 22*(2), 71–77.

Evans, L. K. (1987). Sundown syndrome in institutionalized elderly. *Journal of the American Geriatrics Society, 35*(2), 101–108.

Farrell, M. J., Katz, B., & Helme, R. D. (1996). The impact of dementia on the pain experience. *Pain, 67,* 7–15.

Feldt, K. S., Warne, M. A., & Ryden, M. B. (1998). Examining pain in aggressive cognitively impaired older adults. *Journal of Gerontological Nursing, 24*(11),14–22.

Ferrell, B. A., Ferrell, B. R., & Rivera, L. (1995). Pain in cognitively impaired nursing home patients. *Journal of Pain and Symptom Management, 10,* 591–598.

Folstein, M., Folstein, S., & McHugh, P. (1975). Mini mental state exam: A practical guide for grading the cognitive state of patients for clinicians. *Journal of Psychiatric Research, 12*(3), 189.

Futrell, M., & Melillo, K. D. (2002a). Evidence-based protocol: Wandering. In M. G. Titler (Series Ed.), *Series on evidence-based practice for older adults.* Iowa City, IA: The University of Iowa College of Nursing Gerontological Nursing Interventions Research Center, Research Dissemination Core.

Futrell, M., & Melillo, K. D. (2002b). Evidence-based protocol: Wandering. *Journal of Gerontological Nursing, 28*(11), 14–22.

Gardner, M. E. & Garrett, R. W. (1997). Review of drug therapy for aggressive behaviors associated with dementia. *Nursing Home Medicine, 5*(6), 199–208.

Gerdner, L. A. (2000). Effects of individualized versus classical "relaxation" music on the frequency of agitation in elderly persons with Alzheimer's disease and related disorders. *International Psychogeriatrics, 12*(1), 49–65.

Gerdner, L. A. & Buckwalter, K. C. (1994). A nursing challenge: Assessment and management of agitation in Alzheimer's patients. *Journal of Gerontological Nursing, 20*(4), 11–20.

Goddaer, J., & Abraham, I. L. (1994). Effects of relaxing music on agitation during meals among nursing home residents with severe cognitive impairment. *Archives of Psychiatric Nursing, 8,* 150–158.

Gotell, E., Brown, S., & Ekman, S. L. (2002). Caregiver singing and background music in dementia care. *Western Journal of Nursing Research, 24*(2), 195–216.

Hall, G. R. (1994). Caring for people with Alzheimer's disease using the conceptual model of Progressively Lowered Stress Threshold in the clinical setting. *Nursing Clinics of North America, 29,* 129–141.

Hall, G. R., & Buckwalter, K. C. (1987). Progressively lowered stress threshold: A conceptual model for care of adults with Alzheimer's disease. *Archives of Psychiatric Nursing, 1,* 399–406.

Hurley, A. C., Volicer, L., Camberg, C., Ashley, J., Woods, P., Odenheimer, G., et al. (1999). Measurement of observed agitation in patients with dementia of the Alzheimer's type. *Journal of Mental Health and Aging, 5*(2), 117–133.

Hurley, A. C., Volicer, B. J., Hanrahan, P. A,. Houde, S., & Volicer, L. (1992). Assessment of discomfort in advanced Alzheimer's patients. *Research in Nursing & Health, 15,* 369–377.

Inouye, S. K., Foreman, M. D., Mion, L. C., Katz, K. H., & Cooney, L. M. (2001). Nurses' recognition of delirium and its symptoms. *Archives of Internal Medicine, 161,* 2467–2473.

Kaasalainen, S., Middleton, J., Knezacek, S., Hartley, T., Stewart, N., Ife, C., et al. (1998). Pain & cognitive status in the institutionalized elderly: Perceptions and interventions. *Journal of Gerontological Nursing, 24*(8), 24–31.

Kinahan, M. J. (1999) Nutritional issues. In S. Molony, C. Waszynski, & C. Lyder, (Eds.), *Gerontological nursing: An advanced practice approach* (pp. 221–257). Stamford: CT: Appleton & Lange.

Krulewitch, H., London, M. R., Skakel, V. J., Lundstedt, G. J., Thomason, H., & Brummel-Smith, K. (2000). Assessment of pain in cognitively impaired older adults: A comparison of pain assessment tools and their use by nonprofessional caregivers. *Journal of the American Geriatrics Society, 48,* 1607–1611.

Lindenmayer, J. (2000). The pathophysiology of agitation. *Journal of Clinical Psychiatry, 61.* 5–10.

Lyketsos, C., Steele, C., & Steinberg, M. (1999) Behavioral disturbances in dementia. In J. Gallo et al. (Eds.), *Reichel's care of the elderly: Clinical aspects of aging* (pp. 214–228). Philadelphia: Lippincott Williams & Wilkins.

Mahoney, E. K., Hurley, A. C., Volicer, L., Bell, M., Gianotis, P., Hartshorm M., et al. (1999). Development and testing of the resistiveness to care scale. *Research in Nursing & Health, 22,* 27–38.

Marx, M. S., Werner, P., & Cohen-Mansfield, J. (1989). Agitation and touch in the nursing home. *Psychological Reports, 64,* 1019–1026.

McCaffery, M., & Pasero, C. (1999). *Pain: Clinical manual.* Boston: Mosby.

McGillivray, T., & Marland, G. R. (1999). Assisting demented patients with feeding: Problems in a ward environment. A review of the literature. *Journal of Advanced Nursing, 29,* 608–614.

Meyer, R. M., Kraenzle, R. N., Gerrman, J., & Morely, M. B. (1994). The effect of reduction in restraint use on falls and injuries in two nursing homes. *Nursing Home Medicine, 2*(6), 23–26.

Miller, L. L., Nelson, L. L., & Mezey, M. (2000). Comfort and pain relief in dementia: Awakening a new beneficence. *Journal of Gerontological Nursing, 26*(9), 32–40.

Miller, S., Vermeersch, P. E., Bohan, K., Renbarger, K., Kruep, A., & Sacre, S. (2001). Audio presence intervention for decreasing agitation in people with dementia. *Geriatric Nursing 22*(2), 66–77.

Neugroschi, J. (2002). Agitation: How to manage behavior disturbances in the older patient with dementia. *Geriatrics, 57*(4), 33–40.

Norberg, A., & Athlin, E. (1989). Eating problems in severely demented patients: Issues and ethical dilemmas. *Nursing Clinics of North America, 24,* 781–789.

North American Nursing Diagnosis Association. (2001). *Nursing diagnosis: Definitions and classifications, 2001-2002.* Philadelphia: Author.

Parmelee, P. A., Smith, B., & Katz, L. R. (1993). Pain complaints and cognitive status among elderly institution residents. *Journal of the American Geriatrics Society, 41,* 517–522.

Peatfield, J., Futrell, M., & Cox, C. (2002). Wandering: An integrative review. *Journal of Gerontological Nursing, 28*(4), 44–50.

Ragneskog, H., Kihlgren, M., Karlsson, I., & Norberg, A. (1996). Dinner music for demented patients: Analysis of video-recorded observations. *Clinical Nursing Research, 5,* 262–282.

Remington, R. (2002). Calming music and hand massage with agitated elderly. *Nursing Research, 51,* 317–323.

Rowe, M., & Alfred, D. (1999). The effectiveness of slow-stroke massage in diffusing agitated behaviors in individuals with Alzheimer's disease. *Journal of Gerontological Nursing, 25*(6), 22–34.

Sheikh, J. I., & Yesavage, J. A. (1986). Geriatric Depression Scale (GDS): Recent evidence and development of a shorter version. *Clinical Gerontologist, 5,* 165–173.

Snyder, M., Egan, E. C., & Burns, R. (1995). Efficacy of hand massage in decreasing agitation behaviors associated with care activities in persons with dementia. *Geriatric Nursing, 16*(2), 60–63.

Sutor, B., Rummans, T. A., & Smith, G. E. (2001). Assessment and management of behavioral disturbances in nursing home patients with dementia. *Mayo Clinic Proceedings, 76,* 540–550.

Tabloski, P. A., McKinnon-Howe, L., & Remington, R. (1995). Effects of calming music on the level of agitation in cognitively impaired nursing home residents. *The American Journal of Alzheimer's Care and Related Disorders & Research, 10*(1), 10–15.

Tappan, R. M. & Barry, C. (1995). Assessment of affect in advanced Alzheimer's disease: The Dementia Mood Picture Test. *Journal of Gerontologic Nursing, 21*(3), 44–46.

Teri, L., Traux, P., Logsdon, R., Uomoto, J., Zarit, S., & Vitaliano, P. P. (1992). Assessment of behavioral problems in dementia: The revised memory and behavior problems checklist. *Psychology and Aging, 7,* 622–631.

Tinetti, M. E., Liu, W., Marottoli, R. A., & Gentner, S. F. (1991). Mechanical restraint use among residents of skilled nursing facilities: Prevalence, patterns, and predictors. *Journal of the American Medical Association, 265,* 468–471.

Vance, D. E., Burgio, L. D., Roth, D. L., Stevens, A. B., Fairchild, D., & Yurick, A. (2003). Predictors of agitation in nursing home residents. *The Journals of Gerontology: Medical Sciences, 58B*(2), M129–M137.

Volicer, L., Hurley, A. C. & Mahoney, E. (1995). Management of behavioral symptoms of dementia. *Nursing Home Medicine, 3,* 300–306.

Warden, V., Hurley, A. C., & Volicer, L. (2003). Development and psychometric evaluation of the Pain Assessment in Advanced Dementia (PAINAD) Scale. *Journal of the American Medical Directors Association, 4*(1), 9–15.

Watson, R. & Deary, I. J. (1994). Measuring feeding difficulty in patients with dementia: Multivariate analysis of feeding problems, nursing intervention and indicators of feeding difficulty. *Journal of Advanced Nursing, 20,* 283–287.

Weinrich, S., Egbert, C., Eleazer, G. P., & Haddock, K. S. (1995). Agitation: Measurement, management and intervention research. *Archives of Psychiatric Nursing 5,* 251–260.

Whall, A. L. (2002). Developing needed interventions for the Need-Driven Dementia-Compromised Behavior Model. *Journal of Gerontological Nursing, 28*(10), 5.

Woods, P., & Ashley, J. (1995). Simulated presence therapy: Using selected memories to manage problem behaviors in Alzheimer's disease patients. *Geriatric Nursing, 16*(1), 9–14.

Wynne, C. F., Ling, S. M., & Remsburg, R. (2000). Comparison of pain assessment instruments in cognitively intact and cognitively impaired nursing home residents. *Geriatric Nursing 21*(1), 20–23.

Zarit, S. H., & Zarit, S. M. (1983). Cognitive impairment. In P. M. Lewinsohn & L. Teri (Eds.), *Clinical geropsychology: New directions in assessment and treatment.* New York: Pergaman Press.

Zarit, S. H., & Zarit, S. M. (1990). Cognitive impairment. In P. M. Lewinsohn & L. Teri (Eds.), *Clinical geropsychology: New directions in assessment and treatment.* New York: Pergaman Press.

CHAPTER 15

Family Caregiving

Susan Crocker Houde, PhD, APRN, BC

INTRODUCTION

Informal caregiving refers to the unpaid care provided by family, friends, and other relatives to functionally impaired individuals in the community. If informal caregivers were reimbursed for the care they provide, the costs to society would be substantial. It has been estimated that the economic value of informal caregiving in the United States for the year 1997 was $196 billion (Arno, Levine, & Memmott, 1999). Most informal care to older adults in the home is provided by family members. Many of the older adult care recipients have dementia and have difficulty functioning independently in the community. Approximately 12% of caregivers are 65 and older, and many of the older caregivers are wives providing care to functionally impaired husbands (Pandya & Coleman, 2000). Women are estimated to provide 73% of the informal care in the United States. If a wife is not present, a daughter is often the primary caregiver. Many of the daughter caregivers are in their mid-40s, provide care an average of 18 hours per week, are in the work force, and are married (Pandya & Coleman, 2000). Employment may make it difficult for daughters to provide the needed care,

so others in the informal network may provide assistance to help meet the needs of the functionally impaired older adult (Doty, Jackson, & Crown, 1998). Other relatives who may provide informal care in the home include daughters-in-law, sons, husbands, siblings, and nieces. If a relative is not available, friends and neighbors may serve as informal caregivers.

Female caregivers have been found to spend more time than males providing informal care to functionally impaired older adults (Yee & Schulz, 2000). There are differences in the type of care provided by male and female caregivers. Females are more likely to provide hands-on care than males, such as assistance with activities of daily living (ADLs), including bathing, dressing, toileting, bowel and bladder care, eating, and ambulation (Cancian & Oliker, 2000). Males are more likely to provide care with instrumental activities of daily living (IADLs), including money management, home repairs, and transportation, although they also provide emotional and social support as well as assistance with ADLs (Kaye, 1997). The responsibilities of caregivers may be many and varied, including preventing wandering and falls, providing care related to health problems, incontinence care, and medication management. Providing social support is also an important role of the caregiver.

▮ EMOTIONAL RESPONSES TO CAREGIVING

Well-Being and Positive Responses to Caregiving

Caregiving of functionally impaired older adults with dementia has been reported to result in a variety of emotional responses. Much has been written about the increase in stress and burden that may be experienced by caregivers because of the added responsibility of caring for a family member. For many, however, caregiving is viewed as a positive experience. A number of factors have been identified as being associated with a positive caregiving relationship, including a sense of fulfillment or reward by the caregiver, feelings of caring, and companionship with the care recipient (Cohen, Colantonio, & Vernich, 2002). Caregivers have reported an improved

relationship with the family member receiving the care, an increased sense of competence in providing the care, personal growth, and an improved understanding of the aging process (Amirkhanyan & Wolf, 2003). Caregivers who report a higher level of satisfaction with caregiving experiences and those with a high level of mastery or emotional support have been found to report lower levels of depression regardless of the level of caregiving stress (Martire, Parris Stephens, & Atienza, 1997; Yates, Tennstedt, & Chang, 1999). Negative effects of caregiving, such as burden, have been found to be offset by the positive rewards of caregiving, resulting in fewer symptoms of depression (Amirkhanyan & Wolf, 2003; Cohen, Colantonio, & Vernich).

The well-being of caregivers has been explored in the literature. It is considered to be a complex and multidimensional concept (Berg-Weger & Tebb, 1998). An instrument, the Caregiver Well-Being Scale, has been developed to measure the resources and strengths of caregivers (Table 15-1) (Tebb, 1995). The scale is useful as a means for the

TABLE 15-1 Caregiver Well-Being Scale				
Below are listed a number of basic needs. For each need listed, think about your life over the past three months. During this period of time, indicate to what extent you think each need has been met by circling the appropriate number on the scale provided below.				
1. Never or almost never 4. Often, frequently 2. Seldom, occasionally 5. Almost always 3. Sometimes				
1. Having enough money	1	2	3	4	5
2. Eating a well-balanced diet	1	2	3	4	5
3. Getting enough sleep	1	2	3	4	5
4. Attending to your medical and dental needs	1	2	3	4	5
5. Having time for recreation	1	2	3	4	5
6. Feeling loved	1	2	3	4	5
7. Expressing love	1	2	3	4	5
8. Expressing anger	1	2	3	4	5
9. Expressing laughter and joy	1	2	3	4	5
10. Expressing sadness	1	2	3	4	5
11. Enjoying sexual intimacy	1	2	3	4	5

12.	Learning new skills	1	2	3	4	5
13.	Feeling worthwhile	1	2	3	4	5
14.	Feeling appreciated by others	1	2	3	4	5
15	Feeling good about family	1	2	3	4	5
16.	Feeling good about yourself	1	2	3	4	5
17.	Feeling secure about the future	1	2	3	4	5
18.	Having close friendships	1	2	3	4	5
19.	Having a home	1	2	3	4	5
20.	Making plans about the future	1	2	3	4	5
21.	Having people who think highly of you	1	2	3	4	5
22.	Having meaning in your life	1	2	3	4	5

Activities of Living

Below are listed a number of activities of living that each of us do or someone does for us. For each activity listed, think over the past three months. During this period of time, indicate to what extent you think each activity of living has been met by circling the appropriate number on the scale provided below. You do not have to be the one doing the activity. You are being asked to rate the extent to which each activity has been taken care of in a timely way.

1. Never or almost never   4. Often, frequently
2. Seldom, occasionally   5. Almost always
3. Sometimes

1.	Buying food	1	2	3	4	5
2.	Preparing meals	1	2	3	4	5
3.	Getting the house clean	1	2	3	4	5
4.	Getting the yard work done	1	2	3	4	5
5.	Getting home maintenance done	1	2	3	4	5
6.	Having adequate transportation	1	2	3	4	5
7.	Purchasing clothing	1	2	3	4	5
8.	Washing and caring for clothing	1	2	3	4	5
9.	Relaxing	1	2	3	4	5
10.	Exercising	1	2	3	4	5
11.	Enjoying a hobby	1	2	3	4	5
12.	Starting a new interest or hobby	1	2	3	4	5
13.	Attending social events	1	2	3	4	5
14.	Taking time for reflective thinking	1	2	3	4	5
15.	Having time for inspirational or spiritual interests	1	2	3	4	5
16.	Noticing the wonderment of things around you	1	2	3	4	5
17.	Asking for support from your friends and family	1	2	3	4	5
18.	Getting support from your friends and family	1	2	3	4	5
19.	Laughing	1	2	3	4	5
20.	Treating or rewarding yourself	1	2	3	4	5
21.	Maintaining employment or career	1	2	3	4	5
22.	Taking time for personal hygiene and appearance	1	2	3	4	5
23.	Taking time to have fun with family and friends	1	2	3	4	5

geropsychiatric nurse to identify assets, supports, and resources that may be helpful in counseling of family caregivers with the goal of promoting well-being (Berg-Weger, Rubio, & Tebb, 2001). The instrument may facilitate communication with caregivers about priorities and changes that they can make in their daily life that could increase their sense of well-being. It may be used for both screening and intervention planning, and may assist in the identification of caregiver coping strategies using a strength-based perspective (Berg-Weger, Rubio, & Tebb).

The Caregiver Well-Being Scale consists of 45 items and has two subscales. The scales address basic human needs and activities of living (Tebb, 1995). The basic needs subscale consists of items related to four areas that include attendance to physical needs, expression of feelings, self-esteem and esteem for others, and security. The activities of living subscale includes items related to household maintenance, leisure activities, time for self, family support, and maintenance of functions outside the home (Rubio, Berg-Weger, & Tebb, 1999). The coefficient alpha of the scale was high at .94, and it has demonstrated high criterion and construct validity.

Stress and Burden in Caregivers

Caregiving of a family member with dementia can be a stressful experience for the caregiver (Gaugler, Lietsch, Zarit, & Pearlin, 2000). The emotional response to caregiving may be related to one's relationship with the care recipient, the caregiver's usual response to stress, and other life circumstances and experiences of the caregiver (Bumagin & Hirn, 2001). Competing role responsibilities have also been considered a factor in contributing to stress in the caregiver. Care recipients who are excessively demanding of the caregiver also create stress for the caregiver (Zarit & Zarit, 1998). Factors that have been identified

as being associated with vulnerability to stresses among caregivers include being a caregiver at age 65 or older, caregiving of a family member with a high level of need, declining physical health of the caregiver, and a low educational level of the caregiver (Navaie-Waliser et al., 2002).

Caring for a spouse with dementia can be especially difficult emotionally for a caregiver, because of changes in the relationship that occur as a result of the disease process. Intimacy and companionship that previously were important in their relationship may no longer be possible. In advanced stages of the disease, the spouse with dementia may not be able to recognize the spouse who provides the care. A decrease in trust by the spouse with dementia may also result, and this can contribute to great difficulty in the provision of care. This, too, contributes to the emotional stress of the spousal caregiver (Ebersole, 2004). Wives report decreased marital satisfaction, decreased leisure time activity participation, and a decreased perception of the quality of family relationships as a result of caregiving (Seltzer & Li, 2000). It has also been found that wives may be more likely to report negative effects of caregiving than husbands. This variation may be related to gender differences in attention to emotions, coping styles, and caregiving tasks (Rose-Rego, Strauss, & Smyth, 1998).

There is concern that some of the gender differences seen in the reported levels of stress among family caregivers may be that male caregivers are minimizing the level of stress they are experiencing (Kaye, 1997). There are also differences in the levels of stress reported among adult-child caregivers. Daughters who provide care report higher levels of emotional strain than sons (Mui, 1995). Other gender differences have been reported. Female caregivers report not having as much time for themselves, including less time for doing the things they enjoy doing, such as hobbies and travel. Females also report feeling more physical strain and physical or mental health problems as a result of caregiving responsibilities (National Academy on an Aging Society, 2000).

Social isolation has also been identified as a factor that may contribute to stress and burden in family caregivers of older adults with dementia. Family caregivers often report giving up leisure time activities, taking time off from work, and spending less time with family members as a result of their caregiving activities (Ory, Hoffman, Yee, Tennstedt, & Schulz, 1999). In fact, spousal caregivers often become socially isolated from their family members (Ory, Yee, Tennstedt, & Schulz, 2000). Loneliness may result because of the increased responsibility of caregiving, the social isolation that may occur, and the loss of companionship of the spouse with dementia (Bergman-Evans, 1994).

It is not uncommon for caregivers to feel they have a lack of support from others as they provide care (Ory, Yee, Tennstedt, & Schulz, 2000). This lack of support may lead to a sense of burden. Burden has been shown to result in a decrease in life satisfaction, lower energy levels, or depression in caregivers (Bumagin & Hirn, 2001). Emotional response to caregiving may depend on the losses experienced by the caregiver as a result of providing the care. Losses may include the lack of personal time, the need to readjust employment, economic costs, and sleep difficulties. It becomes increasingly difficult for caregivers of older adults with dementia as functional ability decreases and disruptive behavior increases.

Cultural differences have been found in the emotional responses to caregiving. White caregivers have reported more stress and fewer rewards from caregiving than African-American caregivers (White, Townsend, & Stephens, 2000). Several reasons have been proposed as to the causes for these differences in the responses to caregiving, including differences in cultural meaning, the role of religion in assisting in coping with caregiving stress, and cultural differences in support systems (Hooyman & Kiyak, 2002).

Psychiatric Health Effects

In a review of the caregiving literature, Schulz et al. (1995) found that there was a strong link between dementia caregiving and psychiatric health effects. Depression symptoms and the use of psychotropic drugs were higher among caregivers than noncaregivers. Caregivers who provide care to family members who display disturbing behaviors are reported to experience higher levels of burden, which are associated with increased depression (Clyburn, Stones, Hadjistavropoulos, & Tuokko, 2000; Hinton, Haan, Geller, & Mungas, 2003). Higher levels of anxiety have also been found in caregivers (Yee & Schulz, 2000). Problem behaviors, as well as a decline in the health of a loved one, were found to be factors contributing to the negative psychiatric health effects in caregivers.

There are differences in gender in relation to the presence of depression symptoms among family caregivers. Females have been found to report symptoms of depression more frequently than males and should be considered at risk for depression (Yee & Schulz, 2000). Research-based estimates project that 50% of female caregivers are at risk for clinical depression, and this increase seems to be attributable to the caregiving experience (Yee & Schulz). Male caregivers have been found to get assistance with caregiving, and be more active in preventive health behaviors (Yee & Schulz). These differences may contribute to the lower levels of depression seen in males. Interventions that are targeted to women may be helpful in decreasing the high incidence of psychiatric symptoms in this population. Specific interventions for caregivers will be discussed later in this chapter.

Physical Health Effects

Twenty-two percent of family caregivers of individuals with dementia have been found to experience emotional or physical problems (Ory, Hoffman, Yee, Tennstedt, & Schulz, 1999). Caregiving may provide an adverse effect on one's physical health, and African-American caregivers have been found to be in poorer health than white caregivers (Wallsten, 2000). Caregivers have also reported more problems with health symptoms and difficulty performing ADLs compared to non-caregivers (Wallsten). Depression has been shown to predict declining physical health in caregivers (Pruchno, Kleban, Michaels, & Dempsey, 1990). Adherence to a regular program of physical activity to promote health is also considered problematic for many caregivers (King & Brassington, 1997).

Grief and the Family Caregiver

The concepts of loss, sorrow, and grief in caregivers of family members with dementia have been explored. Losses that are both psychological and social occur among caregivers prior to the physical loss of a loved one with dementia (Kuhn, 2001). Losses for spousal caregivers may include leisure time, companionship, financial well-being, and sexual intimacy, and losses for other family caregivers may be related to career and time for other family members (Kuhn). The losses associated with family caregiving may result in feelings of sorrow and grief for the caregiver. Chronic sorrow has been defined as the feelings of grief that occur as the result of the loss of the normal lifestyle of individuals with chronic health problems and their caregivers (Burke & Eakes, 1999). Grief is considered to be the behavioral, social, physical, and psychological response to loss (Kuhn).

Living with loss has been identified as an important theme among caregivers of family members with dementia (Moyle, Edwards, & Clinton, 2002). Geropsychiatric nurses have an important role in supporting family members with the anticipatory grieving of losses. Assisting caregivers with a redefinition of their relationship with the family member is important as losses from dementia progress. The sense of helplessness that occurs and results in decreased control can also be difficult for caregivers (Kuhn, 2001).

In a study that addressed the characteristics of grief among spouse and adult-child caregivers at each stage of dementia, Meuser and Marwit (2001) found that there were differences in the grief responses between these two groups of family caregivers. Early in the disease, spouse caregivers were more open and realistic about their partner's condition and burdens that may occur in the future, while adult-child caregivers minimized their feelings and did not accept early signs of dementia. Spouse caregivers expressed concern about the loss of companionship with their spouse, while adult-child caregivers were concerned about the loss of their own freedom and support from their siblings. Later in the disease, adult-child caregivers expressed a mix of anger, frustration, and resentment concerning mounting personal losses and a sense of having placed their lives on hold. Guilt over escapist thoughts (e. g., wishing the parent would die) and adequacy of care was also evident in some adult-child caregivers. These emotions were not found in spousal caregivers. Spouse caregivers were found to accept caregiving responsibilities with dignity and affection, but experienced the highest level of grief upon nursing home placement. Frustration and anger often accompanied nursing home placement for spouses, as they no longer identified themselves as a couple. On the other hand, adult-child caregivers experienced a decrease in anger during this phase of caregiving, and reported more reflection and concern for their parent.

Because of the differences found in grief responses between adult-child and spouse caregivers at different stages of the disease,

Meuser and Marwit (2001) proposed that interventions for caregivers be individualized and consideration be given to the stage of the disease and the relationship of the caregiver to the older adult with dementia. Anger management strategies, education, counseling, and opportunities for reflection may be beneficial interventions for family caregivers during various phases of the grief process, but because adult-child and spouse caregivers may experience the grief process differently depending on the progression of the disease, careful assessment of the grief response in the individual caregiver and appropriate targeting of the intervention are important.

The Marwit–Meuser Caregiver Grief Inventory (MM-CGI) is an instrument that may be helpful to the geropsychiatric nurse in assessing the grief response of the caregiver providing care to a family member with progressive dementia (Marwit & Meuser, 2002). (Table 15-2). Because the MM-CGI is a newly developed instrument, psychometric testing continues to confirm the validity and reliability of the instrument. Testing has established that the instrument has a high internal consistency (Cronbach's alpha=.96), and adequate test–retest reliability and concurrent validity. The instrument consists of 50 items, and the construct validity has been supported by a

TABLE 15-2   MM Caregiver Grief Inventory

Instructions: This inventory is designed to measure the grief experience of <u>current</u> family caregivers of persons living with progressive dementia (e.g., Alzheimer's disease). Read each statement carefully, then decide how much you agree or disagree with what is said. Circle a number 1-5 to the right using the answer key below (For example 5 = Strongly Agree). It is important that you respond to all items so that the scores are accurate. Scoring rules are listed at the end.

ANSWER KEY

1 = Strongly Disagree // 2 = Disagree // 3 = Somewhat Agree // 4 = Agree // **5 = Strongly Agree**

1	I've had to give up a great deal to be a caregiver.	1	2	3	4	5	A
2	I miss so many of the activities we used to share.	1	2	3	4	5	B
3	I feel I am losing my freedom.	1	2	3	4	5	A
4	My physical health has declined from the stress of being a caregiver.	1	2	3	4	5	A
5	I have nobody to communicate with.	1	2	3	4	5	C
6	I don't know what is happening. I feel confused and unsure.	1	2	3	4	5	C
7	I carry a lot of stress as a caregiver.	1	2	3	4	5	A
8	I receive enough emotional support from others.	1	2	3	4	5	Cr
9	I have this empty, sick feeling knowing that my loved one is "gone".	1	2	3	4	5	B
10	I feel anxious and scared.	1	2	3	4	5	C
11	My personal life has changed a great deal.	1	2	3	4	5	A
12	I spend a lot of time worrying about the bad things to come.	1	2	3	4	5	C
13	Dementia is like a double loss…I've lost the closeness with my loved one and connectedness with my family.	1	2	3	4	5	C
14	I feel terrific sadness	1	2	3	4	5	B
15	This situation is totally unacceptable in my heart.	1	2	3	4	5	B
16	My friends simply don't understand what I'm going through.	1	2	3	4	5	C
17	I feel this constant sense of responsibility and it just never leaves.	1	2	3	4	5	A

continues

TABLE 15-2   (continued)

18	I long for what was, what we had and shared in the past.	1	2	3	4	5	B
19	I could deal with other serious disabilities better than with this.	1	2	3	4	5	B
20	I can't feel free in this situation.	1	2	3	4	5	A
21	I'm having trouble sleeping.	1	2	3	4	5	A
22	I'm at peace with myself and my situation in life.	1	2	3	4	5	Cr
23	It's a life phase and I know we'll get through it.	1	2	3	4	5	Cr
24	My extended family has no idea what I go through in caring for him/her.	1	2	3	4	5	C
25	I feel so frustrated that I often tune him/her out.	1	2	3	4	5	A
26	I am always worrying.	1	2	3	4	5	C
27	I'm angry at the disease for robbing me of so much.	1	2	3	4	5	B
28	This is requiring more emotional energy and determination than I ever expected.	1	2	3	4	5	A
29	I will be tied up with this for who knows how long.	1	2	3	4	5	A
30	It hurts to put her/him to bed at night and realize that she/he is "gone."	1	2	3	4	5	B
31	I feel very sad about what this disease has done.	1	2	3	4	5	B
32	I feel severe depression.	1	2	3	4	5	C

ANSWER KEY
1 = Strongly Disagree   //   2 = Disagree   //   3 = Somewhat Agree   //   4 = Agree   //   5 = Strongly Agree

33	I lay awake most nights worrying about what's happening and how I'll manage tomorrow.	1	2	3	4	5	C
34	The people closest to me do not understand what I'm going through.	1	2	3	4	5	C
35	His/her death will bring me renewed personal freedom to live my life.	1	2	3	4	5	A
36	I feel powerless.	1	2	3	4	5	B
37	It's frightening because you know doctors can't cure this disease, so things only get worse.	1	2	3	4	5	B
38	I've lost other people close to me, but the losses I'm experiencing now are much more troubling.	1	2	3	4	5	B
39	Independence is what I've lost…I don't have the freedom to go and do what I want.	1	2	3	4	5	A
40	I've had to make some drastic changes in my life as a result of becoming a caregiver.	1	2	3	4	5	A
41	I wish I had an hour or two to myself each day to pursue personal interests.	1	2	3	4	5	A
42	I'm stuck in this caregiving world and there's nothing I can do about it.	1	2	3	4	5	A
43	I can't contain my sadness about all that's happening.	1	2	3	4	5	B
44	What upsets me most is what I've had to give up.	1	2	3	4	5	A
45	I'm managing pretty well overall.	1	2	3	4	5	Cr
46	I think I'm denying the full implications of this for my life.	1	2	3	4	5	C
47	I get excellent support from members of my family.	1	2	3	4	5	Cr
48	I've had a hard time accepting what is happening.	1	2	3	4	5	B
49	The demands on me are growing faster than I ever expected.	1	2	3	4	5	A
50	I wish this was all a dream and I could wake up back in my old life.	1	2	3	4	5	B

FAIR USE OF THE MM-CGI: The inventory was developed and pilot tested on two samples of dementia caregivers: 87 caregivers (45 adult child, 42 spouse) in the development phase and 166 (83 of each type) for pilot testing. Funding support came from the Alzheimer's Association (Grant 1999-PRG-1730). A 3-factor solution materialized (KMO = .889) and these factors are listed below. The authors consider this instrument to be part of the public domain. The authors would appreciate hearing feedback on how the scale is used. Researchers who wish to administer the inventory and/or modify it as part of a formal study are asked to notify the authors of their plans (Tom Meuser, Ph.D., meusert@abraxas.wustl.edu; 314-286-2992).

Meuser, T.M., & Marwit, S.J. (2001). A comprehensive, stage-sensitive model of grief in dementia caregiving. *The Gerontologist,* Vol 41(5), 658–770. Marwit, S.J., & Meuser, T.M. (2002). Development and Initial Validation of an Inventory to Assess Grief in Caregivers of Person with Alzheimer's Disease. *The Gerontologist,* 42(6), 751–765.

Self-Scoring Procedure: Add the numbers you circled to derive the following sub-scale and total grief scores. Use the letters to the right of each score to guide you. <u>C Items with "r" afterwards must first be reversed scored (1 ($\rightarrow$) 5, 2 ($\rightarrow$) 4, 3 ($\rightarrow$) 3, 4 ($\rightarrow$) 2, 5 ($\rightarrow$) 1) before adding to calculate your scores.</u>

Personal Sacrifice Burden (*A Items*) = _____
(18 items, M = 54.3, SD = 14, 1, Alpha = .93, Split-Half = 91)

Heartfelt Sadness & Longing (*B Items*) = _____
(15 Items, M = 48.2, SD = 11.1, Alpha = .90, Split-Half = .86)

Worry & Felt Isolation (*C Items*) = _____
(17 Items, M= 40.6, SD = 11.9, Alpha = .91, Split-Half = .91)

Total Grief Level (*Sum A + B + C*) = _____
(50 Items, M = 144, SD = 31.6, Alpha = .96, Split-Half = .87)

Plot your scores using the grid to the right. Make an "X" in the shaded section nearest to your numeric score for each sub-scale. This is your grief profile. Discuss the profile with your support group leader or counselor.

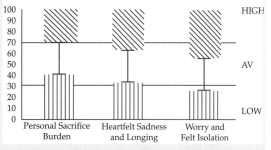

MM-CGI Personal Grief Profile

What do these scores mean?

Scores in the top area are higher than average based validation sample statistics (1 SD above the Mean). High scores may indicate a need for formal intervention or support assistance to enhance coping. Low scores in the bottom lined section (1 SD below the Mean) may indicate denial or a downplaying of distress. Low scores may also indicate positive adaptation if the individual is not showing other signs of suppressed grief. Average scores in the center indicate common reactions. These are general guide for discussion and support only – more research is needed on more specific interpretation issues.

Note. From "A Comprehensive, Stage-Sensitive Model of Grief in Dementia Caregiving," by T. M. Meuser and S. J. Marwit, 2001, *The Gerontologist,* 41(5), pp. 658–770; Also from "Development and Initial Validation of an Inventory to Assess Grief in Caregivers of Person with Alzheimer's Disease," by S. J. Marwit and T. M. Meuser, 2002, *The Gerontologist,* 42(6), 751–765. Reprinted with permission of the authors and publisher.

factor analysis that identified three factors explaining the items in the instrument.

The items that relate to the first factor are referred to as Personal Sacrifice Burden items. They focus on personal losses in the caregiver's life that occurred as a result of care-

giving, such as loss of sleep and personal freedom. The second factor items are referred to as Heartfelt Sadness and Longing and relate to intrapersonal emotional reactions to caregiving that seem to be associated with grief. These items measure emotional reactions to the losses associated with a family member with dementia. The responses are personally based responses. The third factor items, the Worry and Felt Isolation items, are related to social support and losing the sense of connection with others (Marwit & Meuser, 2002). The factors are important because those items in Factor 1 and Factor 3 address areas of perceived loss and social isolation. Caregivers identifying problems in these areas may respond to cognitive–behavioral interventions. Caregivers with problems identified in Factor 2 may respond to interventions that are supportive, such as empathetic listening because the items measure personal affective concerns (Marwit & Meuser).

CAREGIVER ASSESSMENT AND THE GEROPSYCHIATRIC NURSE

It is important for the geropsychiatric nurse to assess the caregiver when the older adult with dementia is assessed. The development of a caregiver and care recipient management plan may be effective in managing problems that affect both parties and may help to alleviate caregiver stress (Schulz, O'Brien, Bookwala, & Fleissner, 1995). The Modified Caregiver Strain Index (Modified CSI) (Thornton & Travis, 2003), which is a modification of the Caregiver Strain Index (Robinson, 1983), may be helpful in evaluating caregiver stress. The instrument serves as an assessment tool for geropsychiatric nurses to identify areas of strain that may indicate a need for intervention (Table 15-3). The internal reliability coefficient of the Modified CSI was .90 and the test–retest reliability was strong at .88 (Thornton & Travis). The Caregiver Well-Being Scale and the MM Caregiver Grief Inventory, described previously in this chapter, are also helpful assessment tools, as they can assist nurses in targeting interactions so that issues for the caregiver can be explored and interventions that can address problem areas can be discussed. Each of the assessment

instruments may be useful in the tailoring of counseling interventions by geropsychiatric nurses.

The assessment of caregiver need by the geropsychiatric nurse should also include how caregivers are coping with changes in their role as a caregiver. An instrument developed by Melillo and Futrell (1995) may be helpful in assessing the needs of family caregivers of older adults with dementia. This instrument provides a guideline for a comprehensive assessment of the caregiver including information about the caregiver's health status, employment, resources available, and relationship with the care recipient, as well as information about the type and amount of care provided. The instrument includes indicators about the type of education and referrals needed by the caregiver and provides space for the development of an assessment and care plan. The instrument may be helpful to nurses in assessing the need for professional caregivers in the home who may provide assistance to the family caregiver.

One of the roles of the nurse may also include helping to coordinate formal services if needed. By evaluating caregivers on an ongoing basis, the nurse can assist the caregiver in better meeting his or her needs. The nurse may facilitate the use of respite care and provide encouragement to utilize available social support, including caregiver group support (Ebersole, 2004). Nursing assessment of the caregiver can assist the nurse in recommending health promotion and preventive self-care activities that are individualized for each caregiver. Encouraging the caregiver to address his or her own health concerns as well as participating in health promotion and preventive health behaviors is important for the maintenance of the caregiver's support of the functionally impaired older adult in the home setting.

Targeting interventions to promote self-care activities in caregivers is an important nursing role. Interventions focused on increasing

TABLE 15-3   The *Modified* Caregiver Strain Index

DIRECTIONS: *Here is a list of things that other caregivers have found to be difficult. Please put a check mark in the columns that apply to you. We have included some examples that are common caregiver experiences to help you think about each item. Your situation may be slightly different, but the item could still apply.*

	Yes, On a Regular Basis = 2	Yes, Sometimes = 1	No = 0
My sleep is disturbed (*For example:* the person I care for is in and out of bed or wanders around at night)	____	____	____
Caregiving is inconvenient (*For example:* helping takes so much time or it's a long drive over to help)	____	____	____
Caregiving is a physical strain (*For example:* lifting in and out of a chair; effort or concentration is required)	____	____	____
Caregiving is confining (*For example:* helping restricts free time or *I* cannot go visiting)	____	____	____
There have been family adjustments (*For example:* helping has disrupted *my* routine; there has been no privacy)	____	____	____
There have been changes in personal plans (*For example:* I had to turn down a job; I could not go on vacation)	____	____	____
There have been other demands on my time (*For example:* other family members *need me*)	____	____	____
There have been emotional adjustments (*For example:* severe arguments *about caregiving*)	____	____	____
Some behavior is upsetting (*For example:* incontinence; *the person cared for* has trouble remembering things; or *the person I care for* accuses people of taking things)	____	____	____
It is upsetting to find *the person I care for* has changed so much from his/her former self (*For example:* he/she is a different person than he/she used to be)	____	____	____
There have been work adjustments (*For example:* I have to take time off *for caregiving duties*)	____	____	____
Caregiving is a financial strain	____	____	____
I feel completely overwhelmed (*For example:* I worry about *the person I care for*; I have concerns about how I will manage)	____	____	____
(Sum responses for 'yes, on a regular basis' (2 pts each) and 'yes, sometimes' (1 pt each) **Total Score =**	____		

Thornton, M., & Travis, S. S. (2003). Analysis of the reliability of the Modified Caregiver Strain Index. *Journal of Gerontology: Social Sciences, 58B*(2), S127–S132.

Words appearing in *italics* represent modifications from the original Caregiver Strain Index from Robinson, B. (1983).Validation of a caregiver strain index. *Journal of Gerontology, 38,* 344-348. Copyright by The Gerontological Society of America. Reprinted with permission.

physical activity and exercise may be especially important in the prevention of chronic health problems in the older adult population and may assist the caregiver in maintaining optimal health (Matthews, Dunbar-Jacob, Sereika, Schulz, & McDowell, 2004).

Research has been reported that explores issues related to self-care and the family caregiver. Burton and colleagues (1997) found that caregivers who provide a high intensity of care were more likely to get inadequate rest and exercise, as well as forget to take prescription medication compared to noncaregivers. Acton (2002) also found that caregivers had more barriers to health promotion behaviors and practiced fewer self-care behaviors than noncaregivers. Caregivers who provide more ADL care, provide more hours of care, report more symptoms of depression, have less social support, and report less self-efficacy have been found to be at a higher risk for a decrease in self-care activities (Gallant & Connell, 1997). Evidence is conflicting about the effect of caregiving on the caregivers' participation in self-care activities, however. Some researchers have found no evidence that caregivers had poorer self-care practices than noncaregivers. In fact, it has been proposed that caregivers may take better care of themselves because of the need to be able to provide care to the dependent family member. Findings have also supported that health-promoting behaviors may have a positive effect on caregiver stress (Acton).

INTERVENTIONS TO SUPPORT CAREGIVERS

Because of the high levels of burden, depression, and anxiety found in female caregivers, interventions to support women who provide care are very important. Male caregivers are also in need of support when providing care to family members, but it is not clear whether the interventions that are effective for female caregivers are effective in meeting the needs

of male caregivers (Houde, 2002). Support groups may be helpful in assisting women to learn methods that are effective in providing care, as well as sharing concerns related to caregiving. Educational programs that address and promote preventive health behaviors may also be beneficial in preventing psychiatric symptoms by encouraging women to participate in self-care activities (Yee & Schulz, 2000). Skills training, individual and family psychotherapy, counseling, and respite care are also interventions that have been used as supportive interventions for family caregivers (Farran, 2001).

Technology is increasingly being used as a support for caregivers of older adults with dementia. Many organizations have developed resources for caregivers that are available for caregivers through the Internet. The U.S. Administration on Aging (AOA) provides information for caregivers through its Web site, www.aoa.gov. The Caregivers' Resource Room provides information about the AOA National Family Caregiver Support Program. This site provides important information links for both caregivers and professionals about issues of importance to caregivers. Other Web sites are available to assist caregivers with informational needs related to caregiving (Table 15-4). There are also Web sites available that allow caregivers the opportunity to communicate with each other and offer support and suggestions. Chat rooms are available online where caregivers can communicate with others that are also providing care in the home. Using computer technology in the home can assist caregivers who have difficulty networking with other informal caregivers and who have inadequate support in the community to feel a sense of support without needing to leave the home environment. Computer use may help to prevent the sense of social isolation that occurs with many older caregivers who are unable to leave the home environment because of caregiving responsibilities.

TABLE 15-4   Web Sites to Assist Caregivers

National Family Caregivers Association   www.nfcacares.org
- Provides current information about family caregiving for caregivers
- Provides tips for caregivers, including self advocacy
- News releases related to caregiving
- Publications to assist caregivers

Alzheimer's Association   www.alz.org
- Detailed information about Alzheimer's disease, including warning signs, diagnosis, treatment, and stages
- Research information
- Many brochures available online in different languages
- Information about educational programs and local chapters
- Specific information for both family caregivers and professionals

National Alliance for Caregiving   www.caregiving.org
- Information for both family caregivers and professionals
- Many resources available with links to multiple Web sites
- Tips for caregivers
- Information about international caregiving legislation

Family Caregiver Alliance   www.caregiver.org
- Monographs related to caregiving
- Information about public policy and caregiving with policy briefs
- Newsletters for caregivers
- Fact sheets of interest to caregivers
- Online discussion groups for caregivers
- Caregiving information and advice

A number of research studies have been developed to evaluate the use of interventions to support caregivers in the home. Resources for Enhancing Alzheimer's Caregiver Health (REACH), is a large multisite program, sponsored by the National Institute on Aging and the National Institute on Nursing Research. The purpose of this program is to evaluate the effectiveness of interventions to support family caregivers of those with Alzheimer's disease. A number of different interventions have been evaluated including psychoeducational and skill-based training, technology support systems, group support and family therapy, individual information and support,

and environmental interventions (Schulz et al., 2003).

Interventions evaluated in the REACH study were a structural ecosystem (SET) and computer–telephone integrated system (CTIS) that when used together were shown to decrease the level of depression in both white non-Hispanics and Cuban-American caregivers (Eisdorfer et al., 2003). The purpose of SET was to identify problems of caregivers and the resources available for the caregivers. Restructuring interactions linked to caregiver burden was an important goal. The CTIS supplemented SET by linking caregivers with family members and other resources. Results showed that SET and CTIS together had a positive impact on caregivers, but that the individual interventions alone did not have a significant impact on depression (Eisdorfer et al.).

The Environmental Skill-Building Program (ESP) is another program evaluated under the REACH project (Gitlin et al., 2003). This program educated caregivers about the effect of the environment on behaviors and how to modify the environment to decrease problem behaviors. Strategies to maintain control and manage problems on a daily basis were also addressed. Results of this demonstration program showed a decrease in perceived burden and an improvement in the sense of well-being among caregivers (Gitlin et al.).

In a comparison of a Behavior Care intervention and Enhanced Care intervention, it was found that those caregivers who participated in the Behavior Care intervention had greater levels of distress and an increased risk of depression compared to those who participated in the Enhanced Care intervention (Burns, Nichols, Martindale-Adams, Graney, & Lummus, 2003). The Behavior Care intervention focused on the management of behavior problems in the care recipient only, while the Enhanced Care intervention also focused on the well-being of the caregiver. In the Behavior Care intervention, the caregiver's level of knowledge related to problem behaviors was assessed, and solutions to behavior problems and behavior management strategies were discussed. In the Enhanced Care intervention, not only were behavioral problems addressed, but cognitive-behavioral skills training, such as relaxation training and coping strategies, were included as important components in the program (Burns et al.)

Many of the intervention programs that have been evaluated in the literature have been interventions that do not address the individualized needs of caregivers. It has been suggested that an individualized approach to targeting interventions to meet caregiver

needs be adopted as the needs of caregivers are varied (Schulz et al., 2003). While some caregivers may respond positively to group interventions, other caregivers may respond more favorably to individual counseling. An intervention using a multicomponent approach that is tailored using an individual risk profile is being evaluated in the follow-up study to REACH, named REACH II. This intervention focuses on several areas related to caregiver health outcomes, including self-care, emotional well-being, problem behaviors, social support, and safety (Schulz et al.).

Interventions more readily available in the community that are effective in addressing caregiver needs include support groups, and respite or day-care programs. Support groups provide caregivers with emotional support by meeting with a group of other caregivers who may be experiencing similar stresses related to caregiving. Support groups allow caregivers to exchange suggestions of strategies that have been helpful in the caring of their family member with dementia. Many support groups are coordinated by community agencies, local hospitals, or the Alzheimer's Association. Some support groups are helpful in that they teach caregivers skills that are important in caring for functionally impaired older adults in the home. Feeling that they have the skills necessary to provide care may help caregivers to minimize the stress associated with the need to provide care. Men, who have been shown to discontinue caregiving sooner than women, may benefit from educational programs that teach skills including direct personal care, such as bathing, dressing, and feeding, as well as housekeeping skills. Studies have reported that male caregivers appreciate programs that provide advice and information about caregiving and female caregivers have been shown to benefit from support groups that offer emotional support (Kaye, 1997).

An intervention that combined structured individual and family counseling, weekly support groups, and the availability of counselors by telephone was shown to decrease symptoms of depression in caregivers, as well as a delay in nursing home placement of care recipients with dementia (Mittelman, Roth, Haley, & Zarit, 2004). The counseling intervention was tailored to individual caregiver needs, and included strategies for managing problem behaviors, communication and conflict resolution skills, improving support, and education and resource information about Alzheimer's disease.

Day-care centers provide respite for caregivers of older adults with dementia, and are especially helpful for caregivers who are employed and care for someone who cannot be left home alone during the day. Respite programs are programs that provide relief from care for the caregiver by providing care to the functionally impaired older adult. There are day-care centers that specialize in the care of older adults with dementia. These centers can provide socialization for the older adult as well as decreased levels of stress in the family member providing the informal care in the home (Zarit, Stephens, Townsend, and Greene, 1998). Lower levels of stress and higher levels of psychological well-being have been found in those caregivers who use a day-care program regularly when compared to those who do not (Zarit et al.).

There are also respite services available in some communities that provide care to older adults with dementia for more extended periods of time than day-care centers. This service would provide care for weekends or weeks, allowing caregivers longer periods of time without providing care, so that they may vacation or have time to pursue individual interests. Respite services may help a caregiver to decrease the social isolation that sometimes occurs when caring for a family member with dementia. Knowing that their family member is being cared for in a safe environment enables the caregiver time to pursue his or her own interests and to social-

ize, which might not be possible without respite services. Despite potential benefits to the caregiver, these support services have been underutilized by family caregivers (McCabe, Sand, Yeaworth, & Nieveen, 1995). Reasons for poor utilization include a lack of knowledge and education related to needs (McCabe et al.), guilt (Rosenheimer & Francis, 1992), and concern regarding care provided by respite and community service programs (Collins, Stommel, King, & Given, 1991). An important role for the geropsychiatric nurse is to be able to inform the caregiver of services available in the community that may provide respite and support, as well as educate the caregiver related to their individual needs and the quality of services available. Exploring the services offered though churches, hospitals, nursing homes, and community service organizations, so that this information can be shared with caregivers, may help to empower caregivers to seek out services that will help them to fulfill the caregiving role and meet their own self-care needs.

By providing assistance in the identification of available resources, the geropsychiatric nurse may be able to help prevent stress and burnout in family caregivers, which in turn may help to prevent institutionalization of the older adult with dementia. Helping caregivers to work through ambivalence about nursing home placement is also an important role. Hospice care for family members with end-stage dementia should also be explored with the caregiver (Kuhn, 2001). Hospice care can provide support to caregivers and palliative care to individuals with dementia in the final stages of life.

There is a need to provide emotional support to families providing care. Because assuming a new role of caregiver may be difficult for both parties involved, it is important for the nurse to be available for reinforcement and encouragement. Encouraging the family member with dementia to maintain independence for as long as possible may also be an important role of the nurse (Ebersole, 2004). Establishing helping relationships and facilitating the grieving process for losses resulting from dementia requires empathy, knowledge, and skill, as well as the establishment of trust (Kuhn, 2001). The sharing of feelings related to the provision of care should be encouraged. Caregivers may need permission to discuss the losses associated with caregiving and should be provided with education about dementia and the grief process. They may also need help recognizing that grief is a normal response to losses experienced in the caregiving role.

Assisting caregivers to discuss needs with other family members and friends may help to mobilize support for the person assuming the primary responsibility for care. Church members often serve as sources of support for caregivers when they are aware of the need for support. Helping caregivers overcome the hesitancy to ask for help is an important role for nurses. Neighbors may also be a source of emotional support and provide a means for a caregiver to get respite. The use of all available resources and assistance should be encouraged.

The geropsychiatric nurse should allow caregivers the opportunity to verbalize anger toward the care recipient. Caregivers may feel anger, guilt, or helplessness because of personal losses resulting from caring for a family member with dementia. These feelings may be inappropriately directed toward the im-paired family member. Feelings of anger may be conscious or unconscious, but need to be addressed (Kuhn, 2001). The expression of negative feelings may assist the caregiver in diffusing anger and providing care in a more positive manner. It may also assist the nurse in identifying the need for resources that will help to maintain the caregiving relationship. Because of the stress associated with caregiving and the multiple demands often experienced by caregivers, expressions of anger toward the care recipient may be an early indicator of the potential for abuse. Identifying unresolved anger and ineffective coping may be a first step in the prevention of an abusive caregiving relationship.

SUMMARY

Nurses with knowledge and skills in geropsychiatric nursing can play a major role in the assessment and support of family caregivers of functionally impaired older adults in the home. The negative psychological effects of caregiving, which may include stress, burden, and grief reactions, can be adequately assessed by the geropsychiatric nurse, and appropriate interventions may be implemented effectively. Nursing intervention strategies, including counseling, emotional support, and mobilizing resources within the community, may help to promote well-being and a positive caregiving relationship for both the caregiver and functionally impaired family member.

REFERENCES

Acton, G. (2002). Health-promoting self-care in family caregivers. *Western Journal of Nursing Research, 24*(1), 73–86.

Amirkhanyan, A. A., & Wolf, D. A. (2003). Caregiver stress and noncaregiver stress: Exploring the pathways of psychiatric morbidity. *The Gerontologist, 43*(6), 817–827.

Arno, P. S., Levine, C., & Memmott, M. M. (1999). The economic value of informal caregiving. *Health Affairs, 18,* 182–188.

Bergman-Evans, B. (1994). Alzheimer's and related disorders: Loneliness, depression, and social support of spousal caregivers. *Journal of Gerontological Nursing, 20*(3), 6–16.

Berg-Weger, M., Rubio, D., & Tebb, S. (2001). The Caregiver Well-Being Scale revisited. *Health and Social Work, 25*(4), 255–263.

Berg-Weger, M., & Tebb, S. (1998). Caregiver well-being: A strengths-based case management approach. *Journal of Case Management, 7*(2), 67–73.

Bumagin, V. E., & Hirn, K. F. (2001). *Caregiving: A guide to those who give care and those who receive it*. New York: Springer.

Burke, M., & Eakes, G. (1999). Milestones of chronic sorrow: Perspectives of chronically ill and bereaved. *Journal of Family Nursing, 5*(4), 374–388.

Burns, R., Nichols, L. O., Martindale-Adams, J., Graney, M. J., & Lummus, A. (2003). Primary care interventions for dementia caregivers: 2–year outcomes from the REACH study. *The Gerontologist, 43*(4), 547–555.

Burton, L., Newsom, J., Schulz, R., Hirsch, C., & German, P. (1997). Preventive health behaviors among spousal caregivers. *Preventive Medicine, 26*, 162–169.

Cancian, F., & Oliker, S. (2000). *Caring and gender*. Thousand Oaks, CA: Pine Forge.

Clyburn, L. D., Stones, M. J., Hadjistavropoulos, T., & Tuokko, H. (2000). Predicting caregiver burden and depression in Alzheimer's disease. *Journal of Gerontology: Social Sciences, 55B*(1), S2–S13.

Cohen, C., Colantonio, A., & Vernich, L. (2002). Positive aspects of caregiving: Rounding out the caregiving experience. *International Journal of Geriatric Psychiatry, 17*(2), 184–188.

Collins, C., Stommel, M., King, S., & Given, C. W. (1991). Assessment of the attitudes of family caregivers toward community services. *The Gerontologist, 31*(6), 756–761.

Doty, P., Jackson, M., & Crown, W. (1998). The impact of female caregivers' employment status on patterns of formal and informal eldercare. *Gerontologist, 38*(3), 331–341.

Ebersole, P. (2004). Relationships roles and transitions. In P. Ebersole, P. Hess, & A. S. Luggen (Eds). *Toward healthy aging: Human needs and nursing response* (pp. 490–517). St. Louis, MO: Mosby.

Eisdorfer, C., Czaja, S. J., Loewenstein, D. A., Rubert, M. P., Argüelles, S., Mitrani, V. B., & Szapocznik, J. U. (2003). The effect of family therapy and technology-based intervention on caregiver depression. *The Gerontologist, 43*(4), 521–531.

Farran, C. J. (2001). Family caregiver intervention research: Where have we been? Where are we going? *Journal of Gerontological Nursing, 27*(7), 38–45.

Gallant, M. P., & Connell, C. M. (1997). Predictors of decreased self-care among spouse caregivers of older adults with dementing illnesses. *Journal of Aging and Health, 9*(3), 373–395.

Gaugler, J. E., Leitsch, S. A., Zarit, S. H., & Pearlin, L. I. (2000). Caregiver involvement following institutionalization: Effects of preplacement stress. *Research on Aging, 22*(4), 337–359.

Gitlin, L. N., Winter, L., Corcoran, M., Dennis, M. P., Schinfeld, S., & Hauck, W. W. (2003). Effects of the home environmental skill-building program on the caregiver-care-recipient dyad: 6–month outcomes from the Philadelphia REACH initiative. *The Gerontologist, 43*(4), 532–546.

Hinton, L., Haan, M., Geller, S., & Mungas, D. (2003). Neuropsychiatric symptoms in Latino elders with dementia or cognitive impairment without dementia and factors that modify their association with caregiver depression. *The Gerontologist, 43*(5), 669–677.

Hooyman, N., & Kiyak, H. A. (2002). *Social gerontology: A multidisciplinary approach*. Boston: Allyn and Bacon.

Houde, S. (2002). Methodological issues in male caregiver research: An integrative review of the literature. *Journal of Advanced Nursing, 40*(6), 626–640.

Kaye, L. (1997). Informal caregiving by older men. In J. Kosberg & L. Kaye, (Eds.). *Elderly men: Special problems and professional challenges* (pp. 231–249). New York: Springer.

King, A., & Brassington, G. (1997). Enhancing physical and psychological functioning in older family caregivers: The role of regular physical activity. *Annals of Behavioral Medicine, 16*(2), 91–100.

Kuhn, D. (2001). Living with loss in Alzheimer's Disease. *Alzheimer's Care Quarterly, 2*(1), 12–22.

Martire, L. M., Parris Stephens, M. A., & Atienza, A. A. (1997). The interplay of work and caregiving: Relationships between role satisfaction, role involvement, and caregivers' well-being. *Journal of Gerontology: Social Sciences, 52B*, S279–S289.

Marwit, S. J., & Meuser, T. M. (2002). Development and initial validation of an inventory to assess grief in caregivers of persons with Alzheimer's disease. *The Gerontologist, 42*(6), 751–765.

Matthews, J., Dunbar-Jacob, J., Sereika, S., Schulz, R., & McDowell, B. (2004). Preventive health practices: Comparison of family caregivers 50 and older. *Journal of Gerontological Nursing, 30* (2), 46–54.

McCabe, B. W., Sand, B. J., Yeaworth, R. C., & Nieveen, J. L. (1995). Availability and utilization of services by Alzheimer's disease caregivers. *Journal of Gerontological Nursing, 21*(1), 14–22.

Melillo, K. D., & Futrell, M. (1995). A guide for assessing caregiver needs: Determining a health history database for family caregivers. *Nurse Practitioner, 20*(5), 40–46.

Meuser, T. M., & Marwit, S. J. (2001). A comprehensive, stage-sensitive model of grief in dementia caregiving, *The Gerontologist, 41*(5), 658–670.

Mittelman, M. S., Roth, D. L., Haley, W. E., & Zarit, S. H. (2004). Effects of a caregiver intervention on negative caregiver appraisals of behavior problems in patients with Alzheimer's disease: Results of a randomized trial. *Journals of Gerontology: Psychological Sciences, 59B*(1), P27–P34.

Moyle, W., Edwards, H., & Clinton, M. (2002). Living with loss: Dementia and the family caregiver. *Australian Journal of Advanced Nursing, 19*(3), 25–31.

Mui, A. (1995). Caring for frail elderly parents: A comparison of adult sons and daughters. *The Gerontologist, 35*(1), 86–93.

National Academy on an Aging Society (2000). *Helping the elderly with activity limitations: Caregiving, #7*: Washington, DC: Author.

Navaie-Waliser, M., Feldman, P., Gould, D., Levine, C., Kuerbis, A., & Donelan, K. (2002). When the caregiver needs care: The plight of vulnerable caregivers. *American Journal of Public Health, 92*(3), 409–413.

Ory, M., Hoffman, R. R., Yee, J. L., Tennstedt, S., & Schulz, R. (1999). Prevalence and impact of caregiving: A detailed comparison between dementia and nondementia caregivers. *The Gerontologist, 39*(2), 177–185.

Ory, M., Yee, J., Tennstedt, S., & Schulz, R. (2000). The extent and impact of dementia care: Unique challenges experienced by family caregivers. In R. Schulz (Ed.), *Handbook on dementia caregiving* (pp. 1–32). New York: Springer

Pandya, S. M., & Coleman, B. (2000). Caregiving and long-term care. Retrieved April 13, 2004, from http://research.aarp.org/health/fs82_caregiving.html

Pruchno, R. A., Kleban, M.H., Michaels, E., & Dempsey, N. P. (1990). Mental and physical health of caregiving spouses: Development of a causal model. *Journal of Gerontology: Psychological Sciences, 45*(5), P192–P199.

Robinson, B. (1983). Validation of a caregiver strain index. *Journal of Gerontology, 38,* 344–348.

Rosenheimer, L., & Francis, E. (1992). Feasible without subsidy? Overnight respite for Alzheimer's. *Journal of Gerontological Nursing, 18*(4), 21–29.

Rose-Rego, S., Strauss, M., & Smyth, K. (1998). Differences in the perceived well-being of wives and husbands caring for persons with Alzheimer's Disease. *Gerontologist, 38*(2), 224–230.

Rubio, D. M., Berg-Weger, M., & Tebb, S. S. (1999). Assessing the validity and reliability of well-being and stress in family caregivers. *Social Work Research, 23*(1), 54–64.

Schulz, R., O'Brien, A. T., Bookwala, J., & Fleissner, K. (1995). Psychiatric and physical morbidity effects of dementia caregiving: Prevalence, correlates, and causes. *The Gerontologist, 35*(6), 771–791.

Schulz, R., Burgio, L., Burns, R., Eisdorfer, C., Gallagher-Thompson, D., Gitlin, L. N., et al. (2003). Resources for Enhancing Alzheimers's Caregiver Health (REACH): Overview, site-specific outcomes, and future directions. *The Gerontologist, 43*(4), 514–520.

Seltzer, M., & Li, L. (2000). The dynamics of caregiving: Transitions during a three-year prospective study. *The Gerontologist, 40,* 165–178.

Tebb, S. (1995). An aid to empowerment: A caregiver well-being scale. *Health and Social Work, 20*(2), 87–92.

Thornton, M., & Travis, S. S. (2003). Analysis of the reliability of the Modified Caregiver Strain Index. *Journal of Gerontology: Social Sciences, 58B*(2), S127–S132.

Wallsten, S. S. (2000). Effects of caregiving, gender, and race on the health, mutuality, and social supports of older couples. *Journal of Aging and Health, 12,* 90–111.

White, T. M., Townsend, A. L., & Stephens, M. A. P. (2000). Comparison of African American and white women in the parent care role. *Gerontologist, 40*(6), 718–728.

Yates, M., Tennstedt, S., & Chang, B. (1999). Contributors to and mediators of psychological well-being for informal caregivers. *Journals of Gerontology: Psychological Sciences and Social Sciences, 54B*(1), P12–P22.

Yee, J., & Schulz, R. (2000). Gender differences in psychiatric morbidity among family caregivers: A review and analysis. *Gerontologist, 40*(2), 147–164.

Zarit, S. H., Stephens, M. A. P., Townsend, A., & Greene, R. (1998). Stress reduction for family caregivers: Effect of adult day care use. *Journals of Gerontology: Psychological Sciences and Social Sciences, 53B*, S267–S277.

Zarit, S. H., & Zarit, J. M. (1998). *Mental disorders in older adults: Fundamentals of assessment and treatment.* New York: Guilford Press.

CHAPTER 16

Sleep Disorders of Late Life

Barbara Resnick, PhD, CRNP, FAAN, FAANP
Marianne Shaughnessy, PhD, CRNP
Marjorie Simpson, MS, CRNP, doctoral student

INTRODUCTION

Approximately one out of three adults experiences difficulty with sleep and nearly half of older adults report at least transient sleep difficulties. Moreover, older adults consume 40% of all prescription sleep medications and use these drugs regularly (Sleep in America, 1995). Some 12% to 25% of those over age 65 actually report chronic insomnia; however, less than 15% of these individuals receive treatment (Ancoli-Israel & Roth, 1999). Lack of sleep can have a significant impact on quality of life. Insufficient sleep can exacerbate underlying illness, alter both mood and behavior, particularly in those with cognitive impairment, and result in accidents (e.g., driving mishaps, falls, or household accidents). Unfortunately, the evaluation of sleep patterns is often ignored in older adults, especially when there are other acute or chronic illnesses being addressed during a typical office visit. In order to help older adults obtain and maintain optimal health, sleep and sleep patterns should be evaluated and aggressively managed.

PHYSIOLOGY OF SLEEP

An intrinsic body clock residing within the hypothalamus regulates a complex series of rhythms, including sleep and wakefulness. Hormones and neurotransmitters control circadian oscillation and regulate timing of sleep, in conjunction with external cues (the light–dark cycle). The light–dark cycle is the primary synchronizer of endogenous circadian rhythms. Body temperature fluctuations, and the release of cortisol and growth hormone, are also associated with the sleep–wake cycle. Melatonin, the hormone of darkness, is produced by the pineal gland and inhibits the major neurotransmitters associated with arousal: histamine, norepinephrine, dopamine, and serotonin. Most adults in nontropical areas are comfortable with 6.5 to 8.0 hours of sleep daily, taken in a single period (Vgontzas & Kales, 1999).

Normal sleep consists of four to six behaviorally and electroencephalographically defined cycles (Vgontzas & Kales, 1999) (Table 16-1). Generally, adults pass through five phases of sleep: NREM (nonrapid eye

TABLE 16-1 Sleep Cycles	
Sleep Cycle	
Stage 1	Light sleep in which the individual drifts in and out of sleep and can be awakened easily.
	Eyes move very slowly and muscle activity slows.
	May experience sudden muscle contractions called hypnic myoclonia, often preceded by a sensation of starting to fall.
Stage 2	Eye movements stop and brain waves become slower, with occasional bursts of rapid waves called sleep spindles.
Stage 3	Extremely slow brain waves called delta waves begin to appear, interspersed with smaller, faster waves.
	Deep sleep—difficult to wake the individual.
Stage 4	The brain produces delta waves almost exclusively.
	Deep sleep—difficult to wake the individual.
	No eye movement or muscle activity.
	If awakened the individual may feel groggy and disoriented for several minutes.
Stage 5	Stage 5 is REM sleep.
	Breathing becomes more rapid, irregular, and shallow; eyes jerk rapidly in various directions, and the limb muscles become temporarily paralyzed.
	Heart rate increases, blood pressure rises, and males develop penile erections.
	If the individual awakens during REM sleep, he or she may recall dreams.
	The first REM sleep period usually occurs about 70 to 90 minutes after falling asleep.

movement) stages 1, 2, 3, 4, and REM (rapid eye movement) sleep. NREM sleep begins with stage 1, the transitional period of drifting to sleep when one can be easily aroused. Stage 2 is light sleep, and stages 3 and 4 are progressively deeper and more restorative periods, when the pulse, respirations, and metabolism slow. REM sleep follows the four stages of NREM sleep. REM is the deepest level of sleep and is characterized by an active EEG pattern and vital signs similar to that exhibited in a wakeful state, but with profound muscular relaxation (Hoffman, 2003). REM is the stage of sleep where dream activity occurs, and large muscle inactivity prevents us from acting out dreams during this stage. During any given night, these stages progress in a cycle from stages 1 through 4, with possible drift back to stages 3 and 2 before the REM stage, then the cycle starts over again with stage 2. The cycle is usually about 90 minutes, and repeats itself throughout the night. Awaken-

ings disrupt the cycle with a return to stage 1 (Hoffman). The first sleep cycles each night contain relatively short REM periods and long periods of deep sleep. As the night progresses, REM sleep periods increase in length while deep sleep decreases. By morning, people spend nearly all their sleep time in stages 1, 2, and REM.

With aging, however, typical changes in sleep patterns occur. Overall, sleep tends to be less efficient with advanced age, although sleep requirements remain unchanged (generally 5 to 9 hours in most individuals). The first stage of deterioration of sleep due to aging actually occurs between young adulthood (ages 16 to 25) and midlife (35–50) and is associated with a decline in growth hormone (Van Cauter, 2000). The second stage of deterioration of sleep occurs after age 50, during the transition from midlife to late life. It includes decreased total sleep, declining by about 27 minutes per decade, more frequent nocturnal awakening, a progressive decline in deeper stages of sleep (stages 3 and 4), more frequent and longer nighttime awakenings, and a significant reduction in REM sleep (Floyd, 2002). The loss of REM sleep appears to be associated with elevated evening levels of the stress-related hormone cortisol (Van Cauter). Further, older adults experience a decrease in body temperature and melatonin production. Consequently these individuals tend to wake early in the morning when their body temperature is at the lowest point.

COMMON SLEEP DISTURBANCES IN OLDER ADULTS

Older adults may complain of sleep problems due to underlying physiological or psychological problems such as pain, anxiety, depression, shortness of breath, gastritis, or unrealistic sleep expectations (i.e., belief in the need to sleep for a straight 8 hours). In addition, there are a number of specific sleep disorders that are known to present more frequently in older individuals.

Obstructive Sleep Apnea

The most common sleep-related problem is disturbed breathing, brought on by obstructive sleep apnea (OSA). The development of OSA seems to be age-dependent and male dominant. The incidence is also higher in those individuals who are obese and have enlarged neck circumferences. Recent evidence suggests that diabetics may also be more likely to have this disorder (Barthlen, 2002; Schneider, 2002). Patients with sleep apnea snore very loudly and stop breathing for 10–30 seconds repeatedly through the night due to a relaxation and collapse of the upper airway during sleep. The arterial desaturation stimulates surges in sympathetic activity, including increased heart rate, blood pressure, and muscle contraction of the chest, abdomen,

and diaphragm. As those muscles are repeatedly and more forcefully stimulated, patients awaken and begin breathing again. Initially thought to be of significant consequence primarily to sleep-deprived partners, recent evidence suggests that patients with OSA have significantly higher risk of cardiovascular complications such as hypertension, congestive heart failure, acute coronary syndromes, and stroke (Lattimore, Celermajer, & Wilcox, 2003).

Treatment for Obstructive Sleep Apnea All patients with suspected OSA should be evaluated at a sleep center to identify the cause and scope of problem. The treatment of choice for OSA is a continuous positive airway pressure device (CPAP). A small air compressor delivers pressurized air to the upper airway, forcing it to stay open via a face-fitting mask. Alternatives are: (1) dental devices, such as splints or mandibular advancement devices (MAD), which move the jaw forward and are more effective in mild to moderate forms of OSA; or (2) surgical removal of soft tissues around the uvula and soft palate to enlarge the airway. This is rarely done, as most patients are able to tolerate a CPAP device (Dattilo & Drooger, 2004).

Restless Legs Syndrome (RLS)

Approximately 9.8% of all older adults experience RLS (Rothdach, Trenkwalder, Haberstock, Keil, & Gerger, 2000), although this increases to 20% of those 80 years of age or older (Barthlen, 2002). Patients with restless legs syndrome have uncomfortable sensations in the lower extremities, which they attempt to relieve by moving their legs during sleep, or rising and walking around. These sensations have been described as pulling or crawling. There are many possible causes of restless legs syndrome in the adult population, although there is no definitive explanation. Strong associations with RLS include kidney failure, several nerve disorders, vitamin deficiencies, pregnancy, iron deficiency, and some medications (such as antidepressants). About 50% of those who have restless leg syndrome have relatives with the same condition. It is more common in middle aged or older adults. Patients with RLS experience delayed sleep or awakenings during the night. Almost 20% of patients with RLS also experience Periodic Limb Movement Disorder (PLMD) (Rothdach et al., 2000).

Periodic Limb Movement Disorder (PLMD)

PLMD is characterized by episodes of repetitive limb movements caused by muscle contractions during sleep. Patients with PLMD kick or jerk their legs every 20–40 seconds, usually during non-REM sleep stage 1 or 2. Those who have this problem may not awaken, or complain of any other symptoms besides daytime fatigue. Unfortunately, many cases go undetected if a sleep partner does not notice the leg movements.

Appropriate pharmacologic treatment options for RLS or PLMD include the use of primary agents such as dopamine precursors, dopamine-receptor agonists, opioids, benzodiazepines, and anticonvulsants (Minnick, 2003). While management of RLS varies based on individual response to medications, research indicates that gabapentin showed marked reduction in leg movements with no evidence of drug side effects (Garcia-Borreguero et al., 2002).

Insomnia

Insomnia is the single most common sleep complaint and occurs more frequently with increasing age and in women (Vgontzas & Kales, 1999). Short-term insomnia may result from stressful life events, or with the recent onset of a medical disorder. Patients with

mental health problems, such as undiagnosed depression or anxiety, may initially present with complaints of sleep disorders. Those with underlying shortness of breath, paroxysmal nocturnal dyspnea, and gastroesophageal reflux disease are likely to suffer from insomnia as these medical problems are exacerbated with a recumbent posture and may interfere with falling or staying asleep.

▬ ASSESSMENT OF SLEEP DISORDERS IN LATE LIFE

The initial approach that sleep specialists and researchers use to accurately diagnose sleep disorders includes a medical history, physical examination, and multiple questionnaires or sleep diaries (Table 16-2). For older adults with cognitive impairment, or those in institutional settings, information should be obtained from families or other caregivers. When assessing a patient, it may be helpful to ask the patient if he or she specifically has any of the following problems: (1) not being able to fall asleep (sleep latency), (2) not being

TABLE 16-2   Information to Obtain in Sleep Diaries
Routine sleep patterns: normal bedtime and arising time
Habits before bed: i.e., nighttime rituals and any food, drink, medications
—Use of alcohol: amount and timing
—Use of caffeine: amount and timing
Bedtime activities: i.e., activities once in the bed
Nocturnal awakenings
Quality of sleep (subject can use 0 to 10 scale)
Daytime sleepiness
Daytime napping
Environment at hour of sleep: light, noise, temperature
Associated symptoms at hour of sleep: pain, anxiety, fear, shortness of breath

able to stay asleep (sleep efficiency), (3) early morning awakening, and/or (4) not feeling refreshed, or "waking up tired." A complete description of the history of the problem should follow. Insomnia can be a sleep disorder or a symptom of another health problem, and providers should pay careful attention to sleep complaints in the context of physical and emotional disorders. Patients with mental health problems, such as undiagnosed depression or anxiety, may present with complaints of sleep disorders. See Table 16-3 for guidelines for taking a sleep history.

Diagnostic evaluations to measure sleep patterns may include tests such as the electroencephalogram (EEG), electrooculogram (EOG), and electromyogram (EMG). This type of testing requires significant involvement of the patient and would likely not be appropriate for the individual with cognitive impairment. An EEG records brain wave activity. Sensors, placed on both temples, are wired to a polygraph machine that displays brain activity. An EOG is a device that traces eye movements, which are particularly active during REM sleep. Muscle tension is measured using an EMG, typically with electrodes placed under the chin and on the legs.

A polysomnogram (PSG) is a comprehensive and noninvasive test that records vital signs and physiology during a night of sleep. The study includes results from the EEG,

EOG, and EMG. It also measures respiratory airflow, blood oxygen saturation, pulse rate, heart rate, body position, and respiratory effort. The information is recorded and gathered throughout the night, and is used mainly to establish the underlying cause of the sleep disturbance.

■ THERAPEUTIC NURSING INTERVENTIONS TO ADDRESS SLEEP DISORDERS

Behavioral Interventions

Cognitive–behavioral therapy is used to clarify the misconceptions about sleep and sleep disorders and change the behaviors that interfere with the onset, duration, and quality of sleep. In addition to counseling and providing information about sleep and sleep disorders, educating patients about establishing a routine sleep–wake schedule and avoiding sleep-incompatible behaviors in the bed or bedroom, such as watching television in bed, can enhance sleep quality (Edinger, Wohlgemuth, Radtke, Mahr, & Quillian, 2001). These behavioral approaches are also referred to as good sleep hygiene techniques and are described in Table 16-4.

Sleep Hygiene

The bedroom environment is one of the most important factors that can influence or interfere with sleep. The environment should be quiet and dark with a comfortable temperature. Older adults should be instructed to use the bed *only* for sleep or sexual activity and avoid other activities such as watching television, listening to the radio, or reading in bed. Additionally, older adults should be instructed to get out of bed and engage in a relaxing activity such as reading if sleep onset does not occur within 15 minutes. Bedtime snacks and eating before bed are a common

TABLE 16-3	Guidelines for Taking a Sleep History

Define the specific sleep problem.
Assess the onset and clinical course of the condition.
Evaluate 24-hour sleep–wakefulness patterns.
Question the bed partner.
Determine the presence of other sleep disorders.
Obtain a family history of sleep disorders.

TABLE 16-4   Lifestyle Modifications and Sleep Hygiene to Facilitate Sleep
• Try to go to bed and get up at the same time every day.
• Try not to take naps longer than about 20 minutes.
• Don't have caffeinated drinks after lunch.
• Don't play the radio or television when going to sleep.
• Don't drink alcohol in the evening.
• Don't eat a heavy meal within 3 hours of going to bed; have a light snack if hungry at this time.
• Don't lie in bed for a long time trying to go to sleep. After 30 minutes of trying to sleep, get up and do something quiet for a while, like reading or listening to quiet music. Then try again to fall asleep in bed (no radio, television, or reading).
• Keep room temperature sufficiently warm.
• Relieve pain using medication or positioning.
• Exercise every day for at least 20 to 30 minutes but avoid aerobic activity within 4 hours of going to bed.
• Utilize relaxation techniques such as massage, aromatherapy, or deep breathing
• Light therapy, which involves sitting in front of a light box that emits a bright fluorescent light (usually 10,000 lux), for up to two hours a day.
• Progressive muscle relaxation: Patient tenses and relaxes various muscle groups.

nighttime ritual. Eating large meals in the evening before bedtime, however, can interfere with sleep onset. Food stimulates gastric acid production and lying down after a large meal can result in symptoms associated with gastric reflux, such as heartburn. Instruct patients to eat evening meals at least three hours before bedtime and eat only a light snack before bed if they are hungry.

Relaxation Techniques

One of the most effective sleep-inducing techniques is relaxation. Minor daily stressors can have an impact on presleep arousal and subsequently reduce sleep onset, duration, and quality (Morin, Rodrigue & Ivers, 2003). Relaxation techniques such as progressive muscle relaxation and guided imagery improve sleep quality by reducing presleep arousal (Richardson, 2003). With progressive muscle relaxation, patients are instructed to tense and then relax major muscle groups starting with the head and neck and working their way down to

their feet (Cochran, 2003). Other methods of relaxation can include relaxing in a warm bath or shower, or meditating before bedtime.

Exercise

Inadequate levels of physical activity put older adults at significant risk for acute and chronic insomnia (Morgan, 2003). Regular exercise that includes aerobic activity, strength training, and stretching can improve sleep onset latency, total sleep duration, and global sleep quality (Montgomery & Dennis, 2003a). Regular exercise can also improve physiologic factors that interfere with sleep onset, duration, and quality such as chronic back pain (Van Tulder, Malmivaara, Esmall, & Koes, 2003) or depression (Penninx et al., 2002). To improve sleep, older adults should engage in 30–40 minutes of moderate intensity endurance, resistance, and stretching activities at least four days a week (King, Oman, Brassington, Bliwise, & Haskell, 1997). Exercise programs, such as those provided by the

National Institute of Aging (2001), provide older adults with a comprehensive program that is easy to follow.

Light Therapy

Light therapy to improve sleep onset and quality involves having the patient sit in front of a light box that emits a bright fluorescent light (usually 10,000 lux) for up to two hours a day. While research to support the effectiveness of light therapy in older adults is inconclusive, the therapy has been effective in other populations and can be considered as a treatment option in older adults (Montgomery & Dennis, 2003b).

Massage Therapy

Massage therapy utilizes manual soft tissue manipulation, and includes holding, causing movement, or applying pressure to the body with the purpose of improving health and well-being (American Massage Therapy Association, 1999). Massage therapy is believed to work by increasing the synthesis of endogenous opioids that inhibit pain by activating the descending pain inhibitory system and thereby reducing pain (Lund et al, 2002). Massage therapy is believed to reduce muscle tension and the overall stress that can interfere with the onset of sleep. In addition, massage therapy has been shown to improve sleep by reducing chronic lower back pain (Williamson, Fletcher, & Dawson, 2003; Wolsko, Eisenberg, Davis, Kessler, & Phillips, 2003). Family members and caregivers should be instructed in massage techniques to use at bedtime to enhance the quality of sleep.

Dietary Supplements

Herbal or natural products, which are categorized as dietary supplements by the Food and Drug Administration (FDA), are commonly used by older adults to facilitate sleep (Williamson, Fletcher, & Dawson, 2003). Although some research has supported the efficacy of herbal preparations, clinical trials on these products are limited and frequently show publication bias. In addition, the lack of quality control and standardization of herbal products limits confidence in their usefulness. Testing of herbal preparations has shown that many of these products have no trace of the compounds listed on the labels, and contamination with pesticides, herbicides, and other substances is prevalent (Ernst, 2002). In addition, herbal products can affect cytochrome P-450 (CYP) isozymes and either enhance or inhibit the metabolism of many medications (Scott & Elmer, 2002). Therefore, these products should be used with caution in older adults. Table 16-5 lists the herbal products that are commonly used to treat sleep disorders.

ENVIRONMENTAL APPROACHES IN INSTITUTIONAL SETTINGS

Institutionalized older adults are required to adopt the schedule and nighttime routine set by the facility and the nursing staff. Decisions that individuals usually make independently, such as when to go to bed, when to rise, and when to eat, are too often made by the staff. This change in routine can have a serious impact on the sleep–wake cycle of older adults and result in impaired overall quality of sleep. Creating an environment in institutions where the residents have the freedom to decide their own wake time, bedtime, and nap time can have a positive effect on sleep satisfaction (Matthews, Farrell, & Blackmore, 1996). In addition, adjusting nighttime routines in institutions to reduce the number of times residents are awakened for care-related activities can increase the total sleep time and

TABLE 16-5   Herbal Products to Treat Sleep Disorders

Agent	Indications	Adverse Effects	Usual Dose	Drug Interactions	Efficacy
Melatonin	To induce sleep	Excessive drowsiness	1–3 mg	Fluvoxamine reduces the metabolism of melatonin by inhibiting CYP1A2 or CYP2C9. Reduces the antihypertensive effect of slow-release nifedipine.	May be effective in treating jet lag and other sleep disorders.
Kava	Anxiolytic; used in South Pacific as a recreational drink	Liver damage; long-term use at high doses is associated with dry skin, yellow discoloration of skin, ataxia, hair loss, partial hearing loss, decreased appetite, and weight loss.	10 mg to 200 mg	Effects are enhanced when taken with alcohol or other medications that act on the central nervous system.	Short-term use is effective in reducing anxiety. Causes muscle relaxation and anticonvulsant action and may improve sleep onset.
Chamomile	Induces sleep	Rare and usually allergic in nature	Two to four dried flowers qd-tid	May inhibit CYP 3A4 and decrease the metabolism of calcium-channel blockers, cisapride, lovastatin, and simvastatin.	May have a mild hypnotic effect.
Passion flower	Used as a sedative–hypnotic to induce sleep		0.25 g to 1 g of dried herb as a tea; 0.5 ml to 1 ml liquid extract tid		
Ginseng	Used as sedative, hypnotic, and antidepressant activity.	Insomnia, diarrhea, vaginal bleeding, severe headache, schizophrenia, and Stevens–Johnson syndrome	200 mg; in extract form is mostly used in a multi-supplement; generally 200 mg bid to tid is recommended. Pure ginseng supplements normally contain up to 1,000 mg per capsule/dose.	Decreases effects of warfarin	No evidence from clinical trials to support the use of ginseng for neuropsychological symptoms
Lemon balm (Melissa officinalis L)	Anxiolytic, hypnotic, and analgesic effects.	No serious side effects have been reported from ingestion.	1 g to 4 g daily	May potentiate the effects of other central nervous system depressants. May interact with thyroid medication.	May be an effective anxiolytic.
Skull cap	Used as a sedative and anti-convulsant	Giddiness, confusion, sedation, seizures, and possibly hepatotoxicity	1 g to 2 g of dried herb; 2 ml to 4 ml of liquid extract qd to tid		Effectiveness may depend of the species or part of the plant that is used.

Note. Adapted from "The Risk-Benefit Profile of Commonly Used Herbal Therapies: Gingko, St. John's Wort, Ginseng, Echinacea, Saw Palmetto, and Kava," by E. Ernst, 2002, *Annals of Internal Medicine, 136*(1), pp. 42–53; and from "Update on Natural Product-Drug Interactions," by G. Scott and G. Elmer, 2002, *American Journal of Health Systems Pharmacy, 59*(5), pp. 339–347; and from "Herbal Remedies in Psychiatric Practice," by A. Wong, M. Smith, and H. Boon, 1998, *Archives of General Psychiatry, 55*(11), pp. 1033–44.

the amount of uninterrupted sleep (O'Rourke, Klaasen, & Sloan, 2001).

INDICATIONS FOR PHARMACOLOGICAL THERAPIES

When behavioral interventions alone are not effective and impaired sleep is impacting quality of life, pharmacological therapies may be indicated. Table 16-6 provides an overview of treatment options. Medication management of insomnia should supplement, not replace, behavioral interventions and complementary therapies. Identification and treatment of an underlying cause of insomnia, such as RLS, PLMD, or pain, should be attempted first. In the event no underlying cause is identified, behavioral, complementary, and pharmaceutical therapies should be attempted.

TABLE 16-6 **Pharmacological Management of Insomnia for Older Adults: Appropriate Dosage Recommendations**

Drug Group	Dosing recommendations (mg/d)	Half-life	Side Effects by Drug Categories
Nonbenzodiazepine/ Nonbarbiturates			Dizziness Weakness
Chloral hydrate	250 mg	4 to 8 hours	Gastrointestinal irritation
Ethchlorvynol (Placidyl®)	200 mg	10 to 20 hours	Blurred vision Tolerance develops
Zolpidem (Ambien®)	5 mg	1.5 to 4.5 hours	Headache
Zaleplon (Sonata®)	5 mg	0.9 to 1.1 hours	Sleepiness
Benzodiazepines			
Estazolam (ProSom®)*	0.5–1 mg daily	8 to 24 hours	Daytime sedation
Flurazepam (Dalmane®)	15 mg daily	Long	Psychomotor impairment
Quazepam (Doral®)	7.5–15 mg daily	25 to 41 hours	Delirium
Temazepam (Restoril®)	7.5–15 mg daily	10 to 20 hours	
Triazolam (Halcion®)*	0.0625–0.125 mg daily	1.6 to 5.4 hours	
Antidepressants			
Amitriptyline (Elavil®)	10–25 mg	10–50 hours	Anticholinergic effects Orthostatic hypotension/
Doxepin (Sinequan®)	10–25, up to 75 mg	6 to 8 hours	dizziness
Trazodone (Desyrel®)	25–50, up to 150 mg	5 to 9 hours	Daytime sleepiness
Remeron (Mirtazapine®)	7.5–15, up to 45 mg daily	20 to 40 hours	
Antihistamines			
Diphenhydramine	25 mg	30 to 60 minutes	Tolerance develops in 1–2 weeks Daytime somnolence Anticholinergic Effects

*Examples of triazolobenzodiazepines

Note. Adapted from "Lexi-Comp's Geriatric Dosage Handbook: Monitoring, Clinical Recommendations, and OBRA Guidelines," (9th ed.), by T. P. Semla, M. D. Higbee, and J. L. Beizer, 2003, Hudson, OH: Lexicom, and from "Pharmacotherapy: A pathophysiologic approach" by R. T. DiPiro, R. L. Talbert, G. C. Yee, G. R. Matzke, B. G. Wells, & L. M. Posey, 2002, NJ: McGraw Hill, and from PDR 2004 (58th ed.). Montvale, NJ: Thomson PDR, 2003.

▪ GENERAL RECOMMENDATIONS FOR MEDICATION USE FOR INSOMNIA

As with all principles of prescribing medication among older adults, treatment should "start low and go slow." Preferred agents include temazepam, zaleplon, and zolpidem (Geriatric Pharmaceutical Care Guidelines, 2003). The effect of age-related physiological changes on the pharmacokinetic characteristics of temazepam are minimal, and this drug is not associated with as severe or frequent adverse side effects as the long-acting benzodiazepines and triazolobenzodiazepines. Of all treatment options zaleplon and zolpidem are preferred agents for the short-term treatment of insomnia. They have a more favorable side-effect profile and induce the most natural sleep. At recommended doses, zolpidem and zaleplon rarely cause withdrawal effects or rebound insomnia when discontinued, and there is less likely to be tolerance to these drugs over time.

In light of the significant side effects and risks associated with usage of benzodiazepines, chloral hydrate, and diphenhydramine, these drugs and drug groups are not recommended sleep agents for older adults. The associated risks include anticholinergic side effects, residual sedation, tolerance over time, and risk of falling and subsequent fracture. These drugs should *not* be recommended for older adults in any setting unless other agents and/or behavioral interventions have been attempted without success.

▪ PHARMACOTHERAPY FOR INSOMNIA

Nonbenzodiazepine and Nonbarbiturate Hypnotics

Nonbenzodiazepine and nonbarbiturate hypnotic medications are the most common treatment choices for individuals with insomnia. These drugs are very effective in inducing and maintaining sleep. They decrease the frequency and duration of REM sleep, however, and can cause daytime sedation and memory impairment. The two newer and very popular hypnotics in this group that are commonly prescribed for older adults are zolpidem (Ambien) and zaleplon (Sonata). These drugs are chemically unrelated to benzodiazepines and have a shorter half-life, fewer side effects (specifically less morning sedation and less likelihood of incurring cognitive changes), and preserve normal sleep stages (Geriatric Pharmaceutical Care Guidelines, 2003). The maximal concentration and elimination half-life of zolpidem is increased in older adults compared to that of zaleplon so the drug effects may last longer (Product information: GD Searle, 2004).

Chloral hydrate is another nonbenzodiazepine/nonbarbiturate sedative. The mechanism of action of chloral hydrate is unknown. This drug does decrease sleep latency and nighttime awakening with minimal effects on rapid eye movement. Chloral hydrate is absorbed readily and metabolized in the liver and kidney to active and inactive metabolites. The drug and the metabolites are excreted primarily in the urine, so it should be avoided in patients with a creatinine clearance of less than 50 ml/minute. This drug can result in significant sedation in older individuals, may be habit forming and should be used cautiously in individuals prone to such addictions. Older individuals may become disoriented, sedated, ataxic, dizzy, have nightmares, and complain of residual sleepiness with normal doses of chloral hydrate. As previously indicated, use of chloral hydrate is not recommended for older adults and when used should be done with caution and only after trying other interventions to promote sleep.

Benzodiazepines

Benzodiazepines act at the limbic, thalamic, and hypothalamic levels of the central nervous system (CNS), causing CNS depression and producing anxiolytic, sedative, hypnotic, skeletal muscle relaxant, and anticonvulsant effects. Benzodiazepines are metabolized in the liver and the elimination half-life of these drugs may be longer in older adults and in individuals with liver impairment. Consequently these agents can accumulate in the body with continued use. Flurazepam and quazepam have active metabolites that can also have long half-lives. Benzodiazepines are potentially addictive and have a negative side-effect profile so should certainly be avoided if at all possible, particularly with older adults. Benzodiazepines with a relatively long elimination half-life, for example, are more likely to be associated with residual daytime sedative effects, impaired psychomotor and mental performance, and subsequent ataxia, falls, and fractures (Beers, 1997; Gurvich & Cunningham, 2000; Mort & Aparasu, 2000; Ray, 1992). Although long-term treatment is not recommended, one effective option to avoid continuous use is to use cycled treatment of 5 days taking the medication and 2 days off (Cluydt, Peeters, DeBouyalsky, & Lavoisy, 1998).

Barbiturates

Barbiturates can be classified into three groups: short acting (pentobarbital and secobarbital), intermediate-acting (amobarbital, aprobarbital, and butabarbital), and long-acting (phenobarbital and mephobarbital). The onset of action can range from 10 to 60 minutes and the half-life of barbiturates ranges from 11 to 140 hours. All barbiturates have been shown to be relatively equivalent in efficacy (Geriatric Pharmaceutical Care Guidelines, 2003). Barbiturates are indicated for the short-term treatment of insomnia because their efficacy does appear to diminish after 2 weeks and they have significant adverse drug side effects. Adverse effects associated with barbiturates include somnolence, confusion, and CNS depression. Residual sedation is not uncommon, particularly when used with older adults, and there may be acute changes in mood, impaired judgment, and impaired motor skills that can persist for hours (Geriatric Pharmaceutical Care Guidelines, 2003). Due to this side-effect profile these drugs are not recommended as first-line treatment for insomnia in older adults.

Antidepressants

Sedating antidepressants have been used to facilitate sleep among older adults, particularly those who also have concomitant depression. The drugs most commonly used to induce sleep include trazodone (Desyrel), or mirtazapine (Remeron). Mirtazapine, for example, when used in a small group of patients with known Alzheimer's disease, improved sleep patterns, decreased anxiety, and improved appetite (Raji & Brady, 2001). In a study by Saletu-Zyhlarz et al. (2002), trazodone, a serotonin reuptake inhibitor, was found to increase sleep efficiency and decrease wakefulness during the night and early morning awakening. There was no change in rapid eye movement (REM) sleep with the exception of an increase in the REM duration in minutes. Trazodone also improved subjective sleep quality, affectivity, numerical memory, and somatic complaints (Saletu-Zyhlarz et al., 2002). Sedating antidepressants, however, should be used cautiously as they have significant anticholinergic side effects, including hypotension, dry mouth, constipation, and urinary retention, and they can exacerbate restless legs syndrome and periodic limb movement disorders in some individuals.

Antihistamines

The histamine-1 receptor antagonist diphenhydramine (e.g., Benadryl) has been approved by the U.S. Food and Drug Administration for the treatment of insomnia. Many over-the-counter sleep aids contain diphenhydramine, alone or in combination with acetaminophen. Diphenhydramine antagonizes histamine at the H1 receptor site and has a sedative effect, is well absorbed following oral administration, and has an onset of action of approximately 15 to 30 minutes. It is metabolized extensively in the liver and has a half-life of approximately 12 to 14 hours.

Although diphenhydramine is often assumed to be safe by many older individuals because it is sold over the counter, older adults should be informed about the potential side effects of sleep aids containing these drugs. Diphenhydramine is not only highly sedating, it has significant anticholinergic properties and causes dry mouth, dizziness, syncope, hypotension, constipation, and urinary retention. These side effects must be anticipated in individuals and treatment options provided. For example, older adults who have a history of urinary retention may note exacerbation of this problem when using diphenhydramine for sleep.

CONSIDERATION FOR USE OF SEDATIVE–HYPNOTICS AMONG INSTITUTIONALIZED OLDER ADULTS

The Center for Medicare and Medicaid Services (CMS) has published guidelines for the use of sedative–hypnotics in institutionalized older adults (i.e. in nursing facilities). These guidelines recommend that the drugs be used for 10 days and then attempts should be made to decrease and/or eliminate use. Specific recommended doses of agents for use with older adults have been recommended and use should not exceed these dosages (Table 16-6). It is strongly recommended that alternatives to sleeping agents be incorporated into care. Prior research has shown that using behavioral alternatives such as a back rub, warm beverage, or relaxing music resulted in a 23% reduction in the administration of sedative–hypnotics to older individuals in institutional settings (McDowell, Mion, Lydon, & Inouye, 1998).

DISCONTINUATION OF SEDATIVE–HYPNOTICS

As soon as possible after initiating a sleep agent into use, attempts should be made to incorporate behavioral interventions to regain natural sleep patterns. Benzodiazepines that have shorter half-lives (estazolam, temazepam, and triazolam) are more likely to be associated with rebound anxiety and insomnia after discontinuation (Vogel & Morris, 1992; Wang, Bohn, Glynn, Mogun, & Avorn, 2001). Discontinuation of triazolobenzodiazepines such as triazolam and estazolam are more likely to be associated with delirium in older adults than other benzodiazepines (Wang et al.). This is particularly true when the drug is used in greater-than-recommended doses and over a longer period of time. For patients on chloral hydrate, attempts to discontinue use should be done by tapering the dose initially and weaning the individual off this agent. Withdrawal symptoms (convulsions, tremor, vomiting, and sweating) can occur following abrupt discontinuation of any benzodiazepine. The more severe withdrawal symptoms usually have been seen in patients who received excessive doses over an extended period of time.

REVIEW ALL PHARMACEUTICAL AGENTS USED TO AVOID EXACERBATIONS OF INSOMNIA

While drug treatment is appropriate for the management of insomnia in some cases, the discontinuation of some medications is also a possible treatment option. Table 16-7 lists those medications that can aggravate sleep disorders in older adults. While individuals are often willing to work with providers to eliminate or alter prescribed medications, the use of alcohol, caffeine, and nicotine are generally less likely to be discontinued altogether by these individuals. Changing beliefs and

TABLE 16-7 Drugs that Decrease Sleep	
Prescribed	**Over the Counter**
Antidepressants	Histamine-2 receptor blockers
Antihypertensives	Smoking-cessation aids
Antineoplastics	Nicotine
Bronchodilators	Some herbs and supplements
Central nervous system stimulants	Non steroidal anti-inflammatory drugs
Corticosteroids	Alcohol
Diuretics	Caffeine
	Anticholinergics
	Decongestants

attitudes about sleep and poor sleep habits can be a slow and often difficult process. Using a step approach and establishing patient-centered short-term and long-term goals can facilitate behavior change. For example, a history and physical may reveal that an individual is currently a smoker, drinks two to four alcoholic beverages in the evening to relax, and does not engage in regular exercise. While changing all three of these behaviors may be an appropriate long-term goal, breaking this long-term goal into smaller short-term goals is less challenging and will result in greater outcomes over time.

PATIENT EDUCATION AND COUNSELING

Patients with sleep disorders need encouragement and education on how to incorporate the use of a variety of techniques to facilitate sleep: complementary treatments, environmental interventions, and short-term use of medications if necessary. Specific information regarding medication management is particularly important. Patients should be informed that the long-acting benzodiazepines are likely to result in drug–drug interactions due to their biotransformation by the cytochrome P450 oxidase system. A table of such drug interactions could be reviewed

with the patient as appropriate. The bioavailability of zolpidem and zoleplon are significantly reduced when given with food and therefore they should not be taken within two hours of an evening snack. Dosage adjustments may be needed in these situations. Patients should be informed that barbiturates, available in liquid, tablet, and intravenous preparations, are well known to interact with other CNS depressants. Moreover, these drugs can interact with anticoagulants, antihistamines, narcotics, alcohol, and tranquilizers. Dosage adjustments should be considered when used with these other agents, and for any patient who has liver or renal impairment.

REFERRAL AND CONSULTATION

Identification of problems such as depression, alcohol abuse, or chronic pain that impact sleep may be best managed through referrals to appropriate counselors for individual and/or group therapy. In addition, support groups for specific problems such as restless legs syndrome as well as insomnia may be useful in helping these individuals and/or their caregivers best manage and cope with both the underlying disorder and the associated problem with sleep.

■ EVALUATION OF TREATMENT EFFECTIVENESS WITH FOLLOW-UP

Follow-up is particularly important for older adults with sleep disorders due to the long-term impact of medication management and the tendency for the effectiveness of these drugs to decrease over time. Patients should be helped to decrease medication use as soon as there is evidence that the underlying cause of the insomnia is resolving. At the same time, patients will need to be encouraged to continue with appropriate sleep hygiene techniques, promote positive health behaviors such as exercise and limited use of alcohol, and utilize complementary treatments. In so doing, older adults will enjoy optimal sleep, which should improve their overall health and quality of life.

REFERENCES

American Massage Therapy Association (1999). Massage therapy: Enhancing your health with therapeutic massage. Retrieved February, 2004, from http://www.amtamassage.org/publications/enhancing-health.htm

Ancoli-Israel, S., & Roth, T. (1999). Characteristics of insomnia in the United States: Results of the 1991 National Sleep Foundation Survey I. *Sleep, 22*(Suppl. 2), S347–S353.

Barthlen, G. M. (2002). Sleep disorders: Obstructive sleep apnea syndrome, restless legs syndrome and insomnia in geriatric patients. *Geriatrics, 57*(11), 34–40.

Beers, M. (1997). Explicit criteria for determining potentially inappropriate medication use by the elderly. *Archives of Internal Medicine, 51*, 1531–1536.

Cluydt, R., Peeters, K., DeBouyalsky, I., & Lavoisy, J. (1998). Comparison of continuous versus intermittent administration of zolpidem in chronic insomniacs: A double blind randomized pilot study. *Journal of Internal Medicine Research, 26*, 13–24.

Cochran, H. (2003). Diagnose and treat primary insomnia. *The Nurse Practitioner, 28*(9), 15–27.

Dattilo D. J., & Drooger, S. A. (2004). Outcome assessment of patients undergoing maxillofacial procedures for the treatment of sleep apnea: Comparison of subjective and objective results. *Journal of Oral Maxillofacial Surgery, 62*(2), 164–168.

DiPiro, R. T., Talbert, R. L., Yee, G. C., Matzke, G. R., Wells, B. G., & Posey, L. M. (2002). *Pharmacotherapy: A pathophysiologic approach.* NY: McGraw Hill.

Edinger, J., Wohlgemuth, W., Radtke, R., Mahr, G., & Quillian, R. (2001). Cognitive behavioral therapy for treatment of chronic primary insomnia: A randomized controlled trial. *Journal of the American Medical Association, 285*(14), 1856–1864.

Ernst, E. (2002). The risk-benefit profile of commonly used herbal therapies: Ginkgo, St. John's wort, ginseng, echinacea, saw palmetto, and kava. *Annals of Internal Medicine, 136*(1), 42–53.

Floyd, J. A. (2002). Sleep and aging. *Nursing Clinics of North America, 37*(4), 719–731.

GD Searle. Ambien product information. Retrieved July 31, 2004, from http://www.rxlist.com/generic/zolpid.htm

Garcia-Borreguero D., Larrosa, O., de la Llave, Y., Verger, K., Masramon, X., Hernandez, G. (2002). Treatment of restless legs syndrome with gabapentin: A double-blind, cross-over study. *Neurology, 59*(10), 1573–1579.

Geriatric Pharmaceutical Care Guidelines (2003). *The Omnicare formulary.* Covington, KY: Omnicare.

Gurvich, T., & Cunningham, J. A. (2000). Appropriate use of psychotropic drugs in nursing homes. *American Family Physician, 61*(5), 1437–1446.

Hoffman, S. (2003). Sleep in the older adult: Implications for nurses. *Geriatric Nursing, 24*, 210–214.

King, A., Oman, R., Brassington, G., Bliwise, D., & Haskell, W. (1997). Moderate-intensity exercise and self-rated quality of sleep in older adults: A randomized controlled trial. *Journal of the American Medical Association, 277*(1), 32–37.

Lattimore, J. D., Celermajer, D. S., & Wilcox, I. (2003). Obstructive sleep apnea and cardiovascular disease. *Journal of the American College of Cardiology, 41,* 1429–1437.

Lund, I., Yu, L. C., Uvnas-Moberg, K., Wang, J., Yu, C., Kurosawa, M., et al. (2002). Repeated massage-like stimulation induces long-term effects on nociception: Contribution of oxytocinergic mechanisms. *European Journal of Neuroscience, 16,* 330–338.

Matthews, E., Farrell, G., & Blackmore, A. (1996). Effects of an environmental manipulation emphasizing client-centered care on agitation and sleep in dementia sufferers in a nursing home. *Journal of Advanced Nursing, 24*(3), 439–447.

McDowell, J., Mion, L., Lydon, T., & Inouye, S. (1998). A nonpharmacologic sleep protocol for hospitalized older patients. *Journal of the American Geriatric Society, 46,* 700–705.

Minnick, M. E. (2003). Restless legs syndrome: Recognition and management in primary care. *Advance for Nurse Practitioners, 11*(3), 71–75.

Montgomery, P., & Dennis, J. (2003a). Physical exercise for sleep problems in adults aged 60+ (Cochrane Review). *The Cochrane Library, 3.* Retrieved February, 2004, from http://www. update-software.com/abstract/ab003404.htm

Montgomery, P., & Dennis, J. (2003b). Bright light therapy for sleep problems in adults aged 60+ (Cochrane Review). *The Cochrane Library, 3.* Retrieved February, 2004, from http://www. update-software.com/abstract/ab003404.htm

Morgan, K. (2003). Daytime activity and risk factors for late-life insomnia. *Journal of Sleep Research, 12,* 231–238.

Morin, C., Rodrigue, S., & Ivers, H. (2003). Role of stress, arousal, and coping skills in primary insomnia. *Psychosomatic Medicine, 65,* 259–267.

Mort, J., & Aparasu, R. (2000). Prescribing potentially inappropriate psychotropic medications to the ambulatory elderly. *Archives of Internal Medicine, 160,* 2825–2831.

National Institute of Aging. Exercise: A guide from the National Institute of Aging (2001). Retrieved February, 2004, from http://www.nia.nih.gov/exercisebook

O'Rourke, D., Klaasen, K., & Sloan, J. (2001). Redesigning nighttime care for personal care residents. *Journal of Gerontolgical Nursing, 27*(7), 30–37.

PDR 2004 (58th ed.) (2003). Montvale, NJ: Thomson PDR.

Penninx, B. W., Rejeski, W. J., Pandya, J., Miller, M. E, Di Bari, M., Applegate, W. B., et al. (2002). Exercise and depressive symptoms: A comparison of aerobic and resistance exercise effects on emotional and physical function in older persons with high and low depressive symptomatology. *Journal of Gerontology: Psychological Sciences and Social Sciences, 57B,* 124–132.

Raji, M. A., & Brady, S. R. (2001). Mirtazapine for treatment of depression and comorbidities in Alzheimer's disease. *Annals of Pharmacotherapy, 35*(9), 1024–1027.

Ray, W. (1992). Psychotropic drugs and injuries among the elderly: A review. *Journal of Clinical Psychopharmacology, 12,* 386–396.

Richardson, S. (2003). Effects of relaxation and imagery on the sleep of critically ill adults. *Dimensions of Critical Care Nursing, 22*(4), 182–190.

Rothdach, A. J., Trenkwalder, C., Haberstock, J., Keil, U., & Gerger, K. (2000). Prevalence and risk factors of RLS in an elderly population: The MEMO study. *Neurology, 54*(5), 1064–1068.

Saletu-Zyhlarz, G. M., Abu-Bakr, M. H., Anderer, P., Gruber, G., Mandl, M., Strobl, R., et al. (2002). Insomnia in depression: Differences in objective and subjective sleep and awakening quality to normal controls and acute effects of trazodone. *Progress in Neuropsychopharmacology Biology Psychiatry, 26*(2), 249–260.

Schneider, D. L. (2002). Insomnia: Safe and effective therapy for sleep problems in the older patient. *Geriatrics, 57*(5), 24–35.

Scott, G. N., & Elmer, G. W. (2002). Update on natural product—drug interactions. *American Journal of Health Systems Pharmcology, 59*(4), 339–347.

Semla, T. P., Higbee, M. D., & Beizer, J. L. (2003). Lexi-Comp's geriatric dosage handbook: Monitoring, clinical recommendations, and OBRA guidelines (9th ed.). Hudson, OH: Lexi-Comp.

Sleep in America (1995). Princeton, NJ: Gallup Organization.

Van Cauter, E. (2000). Slow wave sleep and release of growth hormone. *Journal of the American Medical Association, 284*(21), 2717–2718.

Van Tulder, M., Malmivaara, A., Esmall, R., & Koes, B. (2003). Exercise therapy for low back pain (Cochrane Review). *The Cochrane Library, 3.* Retrieved February, 2004, from http://www.update-software.com/abstract/ab000335.htm

Vgontzas, A. N., & Kales, A. (1999). Sleep and its disorders. *Annual Review of Medicine, 50,* 387–400.

Vogel, G., & Morris, D. (1992). The effects of estazolam on sleep performance and memory: A long term sleep laboratory study of elderly insomniacs. *Journal of Clinical Pharmacology, 32,* 647–651.

Wang, P., Bohn, R., Glynn, R., Mogun, H., & Avorn, J. (2001). Hazardous benzodiazepine regimens in the elderly: Effects of half life dosage and duration on risk of hip fracture. *American Journal of Psychiatry, 158,* 892–898.

Williamson, A., Fletcher, P., & Dawson, E. (2003). Complementary and alternative medicine. Use in an older population. *Journal of Gerontological Nursing, 29*(2), 20–28.

Wolsko, P., Eisenberg, D., Davis, R., Kessler, R., & Phillips, R. (2003). Patterns and perceptions of care for treatment of back and neck pain: Results of a national survey. *Spine, 28,* 292–297.

Wong, A., Smith, M., & Boon, H. (1998). Herbal remedies in psychiatric practice. *Archives of General Psychiatry, 55*(11), 1033–1044.

CHAPTER 17

Problem and Pathological Gambling Among Older Adults

Cindy Sullivan Kerber, PhD, APN, CS

▰▰ INTRODUCTION

A Brief History of Gambling in the United States

The United States has seen three eras of legalized gambling. Gambling first began in precolonial times with lotteries used to subsidize explorations to and settlements within the New World. The second era was after the Civil War, when money from gambling proceeds was used for reconstruction. In each of the above episodes, gambling-related scandals ended legalized gambling. The third era began in 1931 when Nevada relegalized casinos (National Opinion Research Council [NORC], 1999).

Initially, legalized gambling was limited to Nevada casinos, church bingo, and pari-mutuel betting (horse and dog track racing). Then in 1964, New Hampshire opened the first state lottery. By century's end, 37 states had lotteries and 21 had casinos (NORC, 1999). Gambling is now legal in 48 states, excluding Utah and Hawaii.

Gambling Accessibility

The expansion of legalized gambling in the United States has increased the availability of gambling sites. The games that were available only in a few states have become accessible from home computers, at grocery stores and gas stations, in churches, and aboard gambling boats close to home. Citizens are made aware of gambling opportunities through state highway signs and announcements of lotto numbers in the newspapers and on the evening news. Because there are more opportunities to gamble, more people gamble today than they did in the past (NORC, 1999).

Gambling Accessibility and Older Adults

In 1975, only 35% of people 65 years and older had gambled in their lifetime. By 1998, 80% had gambled, tying the percentage of 18–24 year olds and more than doubling the percentage of lifetime gambling among older adults in 1975 (NORC, 1999). The increase in access to gambling venues has had a greater impact on the prevalence of gambling throughout the older adult's lifetime than other age groups (Table 17-1).

In addition to lifetime gambling, the National Research Council surveyed individuals to determine if they had gambled in the past year. The percentage of older adults who

TABLE 17-1   Lifetime Gambling in 1975 and 1998 by Age Category

Age	Lifetime gambling in 1975	Lifetime gambling in 1998
>65	35%	80%
45–64	67%	88%
25–44	74%	88%
18–24	75%	80%

Note. From *"Pathological Gambling: A Critical Review,"* by the National Opinion Research Council, 1999, Washington, DC: National Academy Press.

gambled in the past year more than doubled between 1975 and 1998, with 23% reporting positively in 1975 and 50% in 1998. Legalization and access to gambling activities in the United States is paralleled by the increased prevalence of gambling activities by citizens.

Gambling can be an innocent recreational activity for many individuals. However, for some, gambling becomes a compulsive, pathological behavior. As the availability of gambling opportunities has increased, so too have the problems associated with excessive or compulsive gambling. These problems affect all aspects of a person's life. Increased stress, financial strains, disagreements with family, problems at work, and legal difficulties are problems experienced when gambling becomes more than an occasional entertainment option (NORC, 1999).

■ PREVALENCE OF PATHOLOGICAL GAMBLING IN THE GENERAL POPULATION

Prevalence studies for pathological gambling began in the 1970s as an increasing number of states legalized gambling activities. In 1988, a project funded by the National Institute of Mental Health used the South Oaks Gambling Screen (SOGS) (Table 17-2) to study the prevalence of pathological gambling in five states (Volberg, 1994). The SOGS uses a scale with

scores ranging from 0 to 20; scores of 3 or 4 are indicative of potential "problem" gambling, while scores of 5 or more are indicative of probable "pathological" gambling. The study found that prevalence rates of problem gamblers varied from 2.9% in California to 1.6% in Iowa. Rates for pathological gamblers ranged from 2.3% in Massachusetts to 0.1% in Iowa (Volberg, 1994).

Lesieur (1994) critiqued epidemiological studies, making the case that previous research underestimates the incidence of problem and pathological gambling. He raised the concern that these studies have not been comprehensive, suggesting the need for supplemental surveys to obtain data from inpatient and intensive outpatient treatment programs as well as from prison and jail populations. Lesieur (1994) also pointed out that military personnel and the homeless had been excluded from epidemiological studies. The exclusion of these high-risk populations, he argued, has led to an underestimation of the proportion of the population that may be problem or pathological gamblers.

■ PREVALENCE OF PATHOLOGICAL GAMBLING AMONG OLDER ADULTS

No age group is immune to problem gambling but older adults appear to be among the

TABLE 17-2   South Oaks Gambling Screen

This is a questionnaire about types of gambling, the incidence of gambling and related behaviors. Please answer each item as it relates to you. Thank you.

1. Please indicate which of the following types of gambling you have done in your lifetime. For each type, mark one answer: "not at all," "less than once a week," or "once a week or more."

	Not at all	Less than once a week	Once a week or more	
a.	____	____	____	play cards for money
b.	____	____	____	bet on horses, dogs, or other animals (at OTB, at the track, or with a bookie)
c.	____	____	____	bet on sports (parlay cards, with a bookie, or at jai alai)
d.	____	____	____	played dice games (including craps, over and under, or other dice games) for money
e.	____	____	____	gambled in a casino (legal or otherwise)
f.	____	____	____	played the numbers or bet on lotteries
g.	____	____	____	played bingo for money
h.	____	____	____	played the stock, options and/or commodities market
i.	____	____	____	played slot machines, poker machines, or other gambling machines
j.	____	____	____	bowled, shot pool, played golf, or played some other game of skill for money
k.	____	____	____	pull tabs or "paper" games other than lotteries
l.	____	____	____	gambled on internet
m.	____	____	____	some form of gambling not listed above (please specify) _____

2. What is the largest amount of money you have ever gambled with on any one day?
   ____ never have gambled
   ____ $1 or less
   ____ more than $1 up to $10
   ____ more than $10 up to $100
   ____ more than $100 up to $1000
   ____ more than $1000 up to $10,000
   ____ more than $10,000

3. Check which of the following people in your life has (or had) a gambling problem.
   ____ father   ____ mother   ____ brother or sister   ____ grandparent
   ____ my spouse/partner   ____ my children   ____ another relative
   ____ a friend or someone else important in my life   ____ does not apply

4. When you gamble, how often do you go back another day to win back money you lost?
   ____ never
   ____ some of the time (less than half the time) I lost
   ____ most of the time I lost
   ____ every time I lost

continues

TABLE 17-2   South Oaks Gambling Screen (*continued*)

5. Have you ever claimed to be winning money gambling but weren't really? In fact, you lost?
   ____ never (or never gamble)
   ____ yes, less than half the time I lost
   ____ yes, most of the time

6. Do you feel you have ever had a problem with betting money or gambling?
   ____ no
   ____ yes, in the past, but not now
   ____ yes

CIRCLE YES OR NO FOR EACH OF THE FOLLOWING:

7. Did you ever gamble more than you intended to?   yes   no

8. Have people criticized your betting or told you that you had a gambling problem, regardless of whether or not you thought it was true?   yes   no

9. Have you ever felt guilty about the way you gamble or what happens when you gamble?
                                   yes   no

10. Have you ever felt like you would like to stop betting money or gambling but didn't think you could?
                                   yes   no

11. Have you ever hidden betting slips, lottery tickets, gambling money, I.O.U.s or other signs of betting or gambling from your spouse, children, or other important people in your life?   yes   no

12. Have you ever argued with people you live with over how you handle money?   yes   no

13. (If you answered yes to question 12): Have money arguments ever centered on your gambling?
                                   yes   no

14. Have you ever borrowed from someone and not paid them back as a result of your gambling?
                                   yes   no

15. Have you ever lost time from work (or school) due to betting money or gambling?
                                   yes   no

16. If you borrowed money to gamble or to pay gambling debts, who or where did you borrow from? (check "yes" or "no" for each)

	No	Yes
a. from household money	( )	( )
b. from your spouse	( )	( )
c. from other relatives or in-laws	( )	( )
d. from banks, loan companies, or credit unions	( )	( )
e. from credit cards	( )	( )
f. from loan sharks	( )	( )
g. you cashed in stocks, bonds, or other securities	( )	( )
h. you sold personal or family property	( )	( )
i. you borrowed on your checking account (passed bad checks)	( )	( )
j. you have (had) a credit line with a bookie	( )	( )
k. you have (had) a credit line with a casino	( )	( )

17. About how much money do you owe which is possibly a result of gambling? $_____

18. At what age did you first gamble?   _____

South Oaks Gambling Screen Score Sheet

Scores on the SOGS itself are determined by adding up the number of questions which show an "at risk" response:

Questions 1, 2, & 3 not counted:

_____ Question 4 – most of the time I lose or every time I lose

_____ Question 5 – yes, less than half the time I lose or yes, most of the time

_____ Question 6 – yes, in the past but not now or yes

_____ Question 7 – yes

_____ Question 8 — yes

_____ Question 9 — yes

_____ Question 10 — yes

_____ Question 11 — yes

Question 12 not counted

_____ Question 13 — yes

_____ Question 14 — yes

_____ Question 15 — yes

_____ Question 16a — yes

_____ Question b — yes

_____ Question c — yes

_____ Question d — yes

_____ Question e — yes

_____ Question f — yes

_____ Question g — yes

_____ Question h — yes

_____ Question i — yes

Question 16j & k not counted

_____ Total (there are 20 questions which are counted)

0 = no problem

3-4 = some problem

5 or more = probable pathological gambler

Note. From "Revising the South Oaks Gambling Screen in a different setting," by H. R. Lesieur and S. B. Bloom, 1993, *Journal of Gambling Studies, 9,* pp. 213–223. Reprinted with permission.

most vulnerable. Few studies address older adult gambling. Research about gambling problems among the older adult population is rare in literature. Researchers from the University of Nebraska (McNeilly & Burke, 2001) studied 315 older adults from gambling venues and within the community. Older adults at casinos were more likely to have gambling problems (17%) than those surveyed in the community (4%). Older adults cited relaxation, boredom, passing time, and getting away for the day as motivations for gambling. Bazargan, Bazargan, & Akanda (2000) studied 80 independently living African-American older adults from two senior citizen centers that provide inexpensive or free trips to gambling sites. They found 17% of their older adult population to be heavy to pathological gamblers, 19% to be light to moderate gamblers, and 64% to be non- or occasional gamblers. Onset of gambling as an older adult has been found to be a predictor of developing pathological gambling within one year (Grant & Kim, 2001).

As the prevalence of older adult gambling increases, the problems associated with excessive gambling increase as well. According to the NORC (1999), gamblers' bets increase with age. Older adults with retirement moneys, some with lump-sum amounts, are vulnerable to gambling. Casinos offer affordable trips and entice with free drinks, meals tokens, and medication discounts. This makes for a popular day trip for senior centers. Casinos market to senior centers near the third of the month, when seniors receive their Social Security checks (Gosker, 1999). Stewart and Oslin (2001) found that 65% of losses in Atlantic City casinos were incurred by older adults.

A study by Sullivan et al. (1994) focused on elevated suicide and attempted suicide rates among pathological gamblers. Older adults who are already at higher risk for depression and suicide may be at increased rates if they develop problem gambling behavior. Assessment of older adults for potential gambling-related problems is therefore vital.

■■■■ ASSESSMENT OF
PATHOLOGICAL GAMBLING

There is an urgent need to increase clinicians' awareness of the prevalence, diagnosis, and treatment for patients with pathological gambling (Petry & Armentano, 1999). For comprehensive assessment of problem gambling behaviors, the South Oaks Gambling Screen (SOGS) is most often used (Table 17-2). The SOGS developed in the 1980s and revised in 1993 is based on DSM-III criteria (Lesieur & Blume, 1993). It has been the primary tool for screening for problem and pathological gambling. It is a valid and reliable 20-item screen that has been used in various studies including epidemiological studies in the United States and Canada. The NORC/DSM-IV Screen (NODS) is also a comprehensive assessment (Gerstein et al., 1999; Toce-Gerstein, Gerstein, & Volberg, 2003) (Table 17-3). It is a newer instrument and was developed to closely reflect the DSM-IV criteria. There are no tools specifically designed for older adults.

According to the Diagnostic and Statistical Manual-IV-TR (American Psychiatric Association [APA], 2000), the diagnosis of pathological gambling is an illness within the category of impulse-control disorders and is based upon the following 10 criteria.

A pathological gambler has persistent and recurrent maladaptive gambling behavior as indicated by five or more of the following criteria:

- Is preoccupied with gambling (e.g., preoccupied with reliving past gambling experiences, handicapping or planning the next venture, or thinking of ways to get money with which to gamble)

- Needs to gamble with increasing amounts of money in order to achieve the desired excitement

- Has repeated unsuccessful efforts to control, cut down, or stop gambling

- Is restless or irritable when attempting to cut down or stop gambling

- Gambles as a way of escaping from problems or of relieving a dysphoric mood (e.g., feelings of helplessness, guilt, anxiety, depression)

- After losing money gambling, often returns another day to get even ("chasing" one's losses)

- Lies to family members, therapists, or others to conceal the extent of involvement with gambling

TABLE 17-3   The NORC Diagnostic Screen for Gambling Problems

INSTRUCTIONS: For each question asked, circle YES or NO. When interview is complete, for questions for which R said YES, mark the corresponding box in the right-hand margin, ignoring items that do not have a corresponding box. Add up the number of marked boxes to determine R's score. A score of 0 indicates that results are not consistent with problematic levels of gambling. A score of 1 or 2 means that results are consistent with mild but subclinical risk for gambling problems. A score of 3 or 4 indicates results are consistent with moderate but subclinical gambling problems. A score of 5 or higher means that results are consistent with a likely diagnosis of pathological gambling, consistent with the diagnostic criteria of the DSM-IV. The highest score possible is 10.

1. Have there ever been periods lasting 2 weeks or longer when you spent a lot of time thinking about your gambling experiences, or planning out future gambling ventures or bets?
   YES   SKIP TO 3   1 ❑
   NO   GO TO 2

2. Have there ever been periods lasting 2 weeks or longer when you spent a lot of time thinking about ways of getting money to gamble with?
   YES   2 ❑
   NO

3. Have there ever been periods when you needed to gamble with increasing amounts of money or with larger bets than before in order to get the same feeling of excitement?
   YES   3 ❑
   NO

4. Have you ever tried to stop, cut down, or control your gambling?
   YES   GO TO 5
   NO   SKIP TO 8

5. On one or more of the times when you tried to stop, cut down, or control your gambling, were you restless or irritable?
   YES   5 ❑
   NO

6. Have you ever tried *but not succeeded* in stopping, cutting down, or controlling your gambling?
   YES   GO TO 7
   NO   SKIP TO 8

7. Has this happened three or more times?
   YES   7 ❑
   NO

8. Have you ever gambled to relieve uncomfortable feelings such as guilt, anxiety, helplessness, or depression?
   YES   SKIP TO 10   8 ❑
   NO   GO TO 9

continues

TABLE 17-3   The NORC Diagnostic Screen for Gambling Problems (*continued*)

9. Have you ever gambled as a way to escape from personal problems?
   YES   9 ❑
   NO

10. Has there ever been a period when, if you lost money gambling one day, you would often return
   another day to get even?
   YES   10 ❑
   NO

11. Have you ever lied to family members, friends, or others about how much you gamble or how much
   money you lost on gambling?
   YES   GO TO 12
   NO   SKIP TO 13

12. Has this happened three or more times?
   YES   12 ❑
   NO

13. Have you ever written a bad check or taken money that didn't belong to you from family members or
   anyone else in order to pay for your gambling?
   YES   13 ❑
   NO

14. Has your gambling ever caused serious or repeated problems in your relationships with any of your
   family members or friends?
   YES   SKIP TO 17   14 ❑
   NO   GO TO 15

15. Has your gambling ever caused you any problems in school, such as missing classes or days of school
   or your grades dropping?
   YES   SKIP TO 17   15 ❑
   NO   GO TO 16

16. Has your gambling ever caused you to lose a job, have trouble with your job, or miss out on an impor-
   tant job or career opportunity?
   YES   16 ❑
   NO

17. Have you ever needed to ask family members or anyone else to loan you money or otherwise bail you
   out of a desperate money situation that was largely caused by your gambling?
   YES   ❑
   NO

Note. From "*Gambling Impact and Behavior Study: Report to the National Gambling Impact Study Commission,*" by
D. Gerstein, R. Volberg, M. Toce, H. Harwood, R. Johnson, T. Buie, et al., 1999, Chicago: National Opinion Research
Center. The NORC NODS instrument is in the public domain.

- Has committed illegal acts such as forgery, fraud, theft, or embezzlement to finance gambling
- Has jeopardized or lost a significant relationship, job, or educational or career opportunity because of gambling
- Relies on others to provide money to relieve a desperate financial situation caused by gambling (APA, 2000, p. 674).

◼ ASSESSMENT OF THIS DISORDER AS IT RELATES TO OLDER ADULTS

Older adults tend not to seek help for addictions in behavioral-health settings (Stewart & Oslin, 2001). Unwin, Davis, and De Leeuw (2000) recommend screening patients for pathological gambling if financial problems, alcoholism, or depression are present. Instead of asking clients if they gamble, Stewart and Oslin (2001) suggest asking clients: "What type of gambling do you do?" If the patient offers information about gambling behaviors, follow with the Lie/Bet questionnaire (Johnson, Hamer, Nora, & Tan, 1997). It comprises two questions:

1. Have you ever had to lie to people important to you about how much you gamble?
2. Have you ever felt the need to bet more and more money?

This two-question screen has shown both sensitivity and specificity in identifying pathological gamblers. If your client answers yes to either of the Lie/Bet questions, follow with a review of the DSM-IV criteria for verification of the diagnosis. The pathological gambling diagnostic screens (SOGS, NODS, and Lie/Bet), while not designed specifically for older adults, are considered tools of choice for the adult population in general.

A recent study by Volberg (2003) of gambling and problem gambling among seniors in Florida sought to improve methods to identify older adults with problem gambling behaviors. They found two topics to assess that were endorsed by 95% of older adults who identified any gambling problem: (1) borrowing from or using credit cards to gamble, and (2) experiencing feelings of shame related to gambling.

A New Zealand study (Sullivan, Abbott, McAvor, & Arroll, 1994) found that few pathologic gamblers reveal their problem to a primary care provider. Therefore, it is essential to look for physical and emotional signs associated with problem and pathological gambling behavior. People with pathological gambling usually present with comorbid illnesses. Therefore, pathological gambling may present as signs of deteriorating health common in advanced age (Fessler, 1996). Physical symptoms such as insomnia, gastrointestinal disorders, cardiac problems, high blood pressure, and headaches are frequently found in patients with pathological gambling (Cunningham-Williams, Cottler, Compton, & Spittnagel, 1998; Lorenz & Yaffee, 1986).

Mental health concerns such as anxiety, distractibility, increased isolation, and depressed mood are common psychological signs of pathological gambling. Problem and pathological gambling is often comorbid with other mental illnesses. Lesieur (1989) found a significant correlation between depression and gambling in most studies reviewed. Fifty percent of gamblers have also been found to have substance abuse disorders (Cunningham-Williams et al., 1998; Lesieur, Blume, & Zoppa, 1986; Ramirez, McCormick, & Russo, 1984).

Black and Moyer (1998) in their study of 30 individuals with pathological gambling found a 60% lifetime prevalence of mood disorders, a 64% lifetime prevalence of substance abuse disorders, and a 40% lifetime prevalence of anxiety disorders. They found 87% of their population had a personality disorder. The most common personality disorders were obsessive–compulsive, avoidant, schizotypal, and paranoid. In addition, other impulse-control disorders such as compulsive shopping and sexual behavior were commonly found. Volberg and Abbott (1997) found socioeconomic status factors in a group of variables that are predictive of probable pathological gambling.

Lesieur (1989) found almost a significant correlation between depression and gambling in most studies reviewed. This becomes an issue of extreme importance because older adults are at higher risk for suicide, as are pathological gamblers. McCormick, Russo, Ramirez, and Taber (1984) found that 76% of gamblers in treatment met the criteria for a major affective disorder. In 86% of those with major affective disorder, the onset of pathological gambling preceded depression.

▰▰▰ THERAPEUTIC NURSING INTERVENTIONS FOR PROBLEM AND PATHOLOGICAL GAMBLING

Little research has been done to identify specific treatments for problem and pathological gambling. However, as the number of pathological gamblers has increased, so has interest in how best to treat this illness. Inpatient treatment is available in only a few states. Outpatient treatment through counseling and Gamblers Anonymous is the most common treatment (NORC, 1999). There are only 12 inpatient and 100 outpatient treatment facilities in the United States dedicated to gambling addiction, compared with 13,000 programs dedicated to drug and alcohol addictions (Burke, 1996). There are, however, other approaches, including individual and group therapy, support groups, and pharmacotherapy that have been used to treat problem and pathological gambling. Only a few studies have evaluated the effectiveness of treatments and none has focused specifically on older adults.

Support Groups

The support group for people with gambling pathology is Gamblers Anonymous (GA, 1998). GA meetings are available in larger cities as well as Gam-Anon and Gam-A-Teen meetings for families. The first GA meeting was held in 1957 (GA, 1998). Nationwide in 1995 there were 963 such meetings. By 1998 that number had increased to 1307 (NORC, 1999). Although there has been an increase in number and popularity of GA meetings, there is still a significant population that is unaware of this treatment option for people with gambling problems. Therefore, advanced practice nurses should provide information about GA support groups and availability of meetings for the patient. The Gamblers Anonymous International Service Office can be reached at P.O. Box 17173, Los Angeles, CA 90017; by telephone at (213) 386-8789, or by fax at (213) 386-0030. The Official Gamblers Anonymous Home Page is http://www.gamblersanonymous.org. It includes a meeting directory icon listing meetings by state. GA, like Alcoholics Anonymous (AA) uses a 12-step program and supports abstinence as a means to recovery. Nurses can refer patients to GA and their family members to Gam-Anon and Gam-A-Teen.

Indications for Pharmacological Therapies

There are only a few pharmacological studies of pathological gambling, with no studies focused specifically on older adults. Zimmerman (2002) found that gamblers both with and without major depressive disorder responded to citalopram (Celexa). Fluvoxamine (Luvox) was found effective in reducing gambling urges in 7 of 10 patients (Hollander et al., 1998). Black (2004) gave bupropion to 10 persons with pathological gambling. Seven were judged to have had much or very much improvement, indicating that their gambling behavior was significantly better controlled. Naltrexone (Narcan) has been found to be effective in reducing the euphoria associated with pathological gambling (Kim, 1998).

Counseling

Individual or group counseling can be of help to those with gambling problems. The majority of counselors recommend combining counseling with GA. Interventions for pathological gambling such as relapse prevention, problem solving, and social skill training are common to both pathological gambling and to other addictions (Tavares, Zilberman, & el-Guebaly, 2003).

Psychotherapy techniques specific to pathological gambling should address cognitive distortions. Gamblers believe that their actions, betting choices, or personal attributes are likely to influence outcomes. The goal is to help the client to identify false beliefs about gambling and replace those thoughts with a realistic understanding of the randomness, unpredictability, and independence of events.

Cue exposure, whether in vivo or imagined, may help clients deal with gambling triggers (Tavares et al., 2003). Individual counseling aims to change the lifestyle of the gambler and provide insight into irrational, fantasy-based ways of thinking (Ladouceur, Sylvain, Boutin, & Doucet, 2002). Aversion therapy, cognitive, behavioral, and cognitive–behavioral therapies are all used to treat problem gambling behavior, though no one method has been found to be superior in treating problem gambling (Lesieur, 1998). In the elderly population it is important to differentiate the altered cognitions seen in pathological gambling from other mental conditions such as depression and dementia.

Ideally, a pathological gambler should be treated by an advanced practice nurse or counselor who is certified to treat gambling problems. The National Council on Problem Gambling (NCPG) offers certification for training and 2000 hours of supervised clinical practice (NORC, 1999). The National Council on Problem Gambling (NCPG) Web site (http://www.ncpgambling.org) offers information about how to identify and treat gambling problems. They also offer a certification program for counselors wishing to specialize in the treatment of pathological gambling. Certified counselors can be found at the NCPG Web site by city and state.

Alternative Therapies

Natural recovery from addictive disorders is becoming increasingly recognized as a common occurrence (McCartney, 1996). Hodgins and el-Guebaly (2000) compared natural and treatment-assisted recovery from gambling problems among resolved and active gamblers. They speculated that since natural recovery can occur from alcohol problems and most smokers quit on their own, a natural recovery phenomenon may occur with gambling as well. They cited two major reasons for quitting: negative emotions (such as anxiety, depression, and guilt) and financial constraints. The two actions taken by the natural recovery group were stimulus control (avoiding gambling activities and advertisements) and new activities to replace gambling.

Education

Education about the risks of gambling is highly recommended for older adults given the reported risk of addiction (Gosker, 1999; Higgins, 2001). The first step in treatment may be education about the problems or consequences of pathological gambling. Higgins recommends a gambling education program for seniors, especially those living in residential communities. She also recommends peers to serve as mentors in senior center-sponsored gambling trips.

EVALUATION OF TREATMENT EFFECTIVENESS WITH FOLLOW-UP

Treatment effectiveness can be measured by the following outcomes. If treatment is effective, the client:

- Avoids exposure to gambling cues, situations, and other gamblers.
- Participates in stress management or relaxation training if coping with stress by gambling.
- If dysphoric or depressed, seeks treatment through counseling and/or antidepressants.
- Challenges false beliefs, attitudes, and expectations regarding gambling.
- Participates in marriage or family counseling to reestablish trust between partners.
- Accepts financial responsibility to meet financial obligations without gambling.
- Develops nongambling leisure activities.
- Addresses addiction to alcohol or other drugs if present.
- Attends Gamblers Anonymous meetings and spouse or significant other attends GamAnon meetings (Blaszczynski & Silove, 1995).

RESEARCH ISSUES PERTAINING TO PROBLEM AND PATHOLOGICAL GAMBLING IN OLDER ADULTS

A newer type of gambling is gambling on the Internet. Internet gambling is available to those who want to place a bet without leaving home. Online gambling offers unprecedented access and individuals are lured to "just play for fun" initially. Pop-up advertisements then encourage "playing for real," which only requires a credit card number. The companies running gambling Web sites are based outside the country therefore avoiding the illegalities of their operation in the United States (Tresniowski et al., 2003). It is unknown to what degree older adults are involved in gambling online.

An ethical issue about gambling relates to senior center gambling trips. Should a gambling outing be sponsored by a senior center? Trips to casinos seem to be affordable and especially enticing to those on a fixed income, but this form of recreation is not without risk. These outings are popular off-site activities (McNeilly & Burke, 2001). They provide a day out, socialization, reasonably priced meals, and chances to win money. Older adults cited motivations for gambling as relaxation, escaping boredom, passing time, and getting away for the day (McNeilly & Burke). Activity directors at senior centers may encourage residents to attend for the social benefit and to obtain a reasonably priced meal. In addition, some casinos provide bus service if there are enough individuals to fill the bus, so an added benefit is that there may be no financial obligation from the senior center. However, the risks may easily outweigh the benefits at several levels. Individuals at senior centers most likely do not know where to go for help, how to identify problems, or what treatments are available to treat gambling problems. Senior centers may be at risk for sending residents into an environment to participate in a potentially addictive activity. If a resident loses large sums of money on center-sponsored trips, family members may consider the center that is responsible for caring for the older adult responsible for losses. These centers are not likely to have an outing to the local tavern and would not take a known alcoholic to a bar, however they might not know if they were taking a problem or pathological gambler to the casino.

▰ SUMMARY

In conclusion, nurses need to assess older adults for possible gambling problems and provide treatment for pathological gambling and comorbid illnesses. Treatment for patho-logical gambling is available from certified counselors and by attending GA meetings. Careful assessment for depression and possible suicidal thoughts or plans are vital for every older adult with gambling pathology.

REFERENCES

American Psychiatric Association. (2000). *Diagnostic and statistical manual of mental disorders.* (4th ed., Rev. ed.). Washington, DC: Author.

Bazargan, M., Bazargan, S., & Akanda, M. (2000). Gambling habits among aged African Americans. *Clinical Gerontologist, 22*(3/4), 51–62.

Black, D. W. (2004). An open-label trial of bupropion in the treatment of pathological gambling. *Journal of Clinical Psychopharmacology, 24*, 108–109.

Black, D. W., & Moyer, B. A. (1998). Clinical features and psychiatric comorbidity of subjects with pathological gambling behavior. *Psychiatric Services, 49*(11), 1434–1439.

Blaszczynski, A., & Silove, D. (1995), Cognitive and behavioral therapies for pathological gambling. *Journal of Gambling Studies, 11*, 195–220.

Burke, J. D. (1996). Problem gambling hits home. *Wisconsin Medical Journal,* (Sept.), 611–614.

Cunningham-Williams, R. M., Cottler, L. B., Compton, W. M., III, & Spittnagel, E. L. (1998). Taking chances: Problem gamblers and mental health disorders—Results from the St. Louis Epidemiologic Catchments Area Study. *American Journal of Public Health, 88*(7), 1093–1096.

Fessler, J. L. (1996). Gambling away the golden years. *Wisconsin Medical Journal* (Sept.), 618–619.

GA (1998). *Gamblers Anonymous: A new beginning.* Los Angeles: Gamblers Anonymous.

Gerstein, D., Volberg, R., Toce, M., Harwood, H., Johnson, R., Buie, T., et al. (1999). *Gambling impact and behavior study: Report to the National Gambling Impact Study Commission.* Chicago: National Opinion Research Center and partners. Retrieved July 12, 2004 from http://www.purl.oclc.org/norc/dlib/ngis.htm.

Gosker, E. (1999). The marketing of gambling to the elderly. *The Elder Law Journal, 7*, 185–216.

Grant, J. E., & Kim, S. W. (2001). Demographic and clinical features of 131 adult pathological gamblers. *Journal of Clinical Psychiatry, 62*(12), 957–962.

Higgins, J. (2001). A comprehensive policy analysis of and recommendations for senior center gambling trips. *Journal of Aging & Social Policy, 12*(2), 73–91.

Hodgins, D. C., & el-Guebaly, N. (2000). Natural and treatment-assisted recovery from gambling problems: A comparison of resolved and active gamblers. *Addiction, 95*(5), 777–789.

Hollander, E., DeCaria, C. M., Mari, E., Wong, C. M., Mosovich, S., Grossman, R., & Begaz, T. (1998). Short-term single-blind fluvoxamine treatment of pathological gambling. *American Journal of Psychiatry, 155*, 1781–1783.

Johnson, E. E., Hamer, R., Nora, R. M., & Tan, B. (1997). The lie/bet questionnaire for screening pathological gamblers. *Psychological Reports, 80*, 83–88.

Kim, S. (1998). Opioid antagonists in the treatment of impulse-control disorders. *Journal of Clinical Psychiatry, 59*, 159–164.

Ladouceur, R., Sylvain, C., Boutin, C., & Doucet, C. (2002). *Understanding and treating the pathological gambler.* Quebec, Canada: John Wiley & Sons.

Lesieur, H. R., & Blume, S. B. (1993). Revising the South Oaks Gambling Screen in a different setting. *Journal of Gambling Studies, 9*, 213–223.

Lesieur, H. R. (1994). Epidemiological surveys on pathological gambling: Critique and suggestions for modification. *Journal of Gambling Studies, 10*, 385–398.

Lesieur, H. R. (1998). Cost and treatment of pathological gambling. *The Annals, 556*, 153–169.

Lesieur, H. R. (1989). Current research into pathological gambling and gaps in the literature. In H.

Shaffer, S. Stein, B. Gambino, & T. Cummings, (Eds.), *Compulsive Gambling* (pp. 225–258). Lexington, MA: Health.

Lesieur, H. R., Blume, S. B., & Zoppa, R. M. (1986). Alcoholism, drug abuse, and gambling. *Alcoholism: Clinical and Experimental Research, 10,* 33–38.

Lorenz, V. C., & Yaffee, R. A. (1986). Pathological gambling: Psychosomatic, emotional, and marital difficulties as reported by the gambler. *Journal of Gambling Behavior, 2,* 40–49.

McCartney, J. (1996). A community study of natural change across the addictions. *Addiction Research, 4,* 65–83.

McCormick, R. A., Russo, A. M., Ramirez, L. R., & Taber, J. I. (1984). Affective disorders among pathological gamblers seeking treatment. *American Journal of Psychiatry, 141,* 215–218.

McNeilly, D. P., & Burke, W. J. (2001). Gambling as a social activity of older adults. *International Journal of Aging and Human Development, 52*(1), 19–28.

National Opinion Research Council (1999). *Pathological gambling: A critical review.* Washington, DC: National Academy Press.

Petry, N., & Armentano, C. (1999). Prevalence, assessment and treatment of pathological gambling: A review. *Psychiatric Services, 50,* 1021–1027.

Ramirez, L. F., McCormick, R. A., & Russo, A. M. (1984). Patterns of substance abuse in pathological gamblers undergoing treatment. *Addictive Behavior, 8,* 425–428.

Stewart, D., & Oslin, D. (2001). Recognition and treatment of late-life addictions in medical settings. *Journal of Clinical Geropsychology, 7*(2), 145–158.

Sullivan, S., Abbott, M., McAvor, B., & Arroll, B. (1994). Pathological gamblers—Will they use a new telephone hotline? *New Zealand Medical Journal, 107,* 313–315.

Tavares, H., Zilberman, M. L., & el-Guebaly, N. (2003). Are there cognitive and behavioural approaches specific to the treatment of pathological gambling? *Canadian Journal of Psychiatry, 48*(1), 22–28.

Toce-Gerstein, M., Gerstein, D., & Volberg, R. (2003). A hierarchy of gambling disorders in the community. *Addiction, 98*(12), 1661–1672.

Tresniowski, A., Arias, R., Morrison, M., Billups, A., Bass, S., Howard, C., et al. (2003). Gambling online: How to go deep into debt without ever leaving your living room. *People,* (Oct. 13), 119–122.

Unwin, B. K., Davis, M. K., & De Leeuw, J. B. (2000). Pathologic gambling. *American Family Physician, 61*(3), 741–749.

Volberg, R. A. (1994). The prevalence and demographics of pathological gamblers: Implications for public health. *American Journal of Public Health, 84*(2), 237–241.

Volberg, R. A., & Abbott, M. W. (1997). Gambling and problem gambling among indigenous peoples. *Substance Use & Misuse, 32*(11), 1525–1538.

Volberg, R. A. (2003). *Gambling and problem gambling among seniors in Florida.* Maitland, FL: Florida Council on Compulsive Gambling.

Zimmerman, (2002). An open-label study of citalopram in the treatment of pathological gambling. *Journal of Clinical Psychiatry, 63*(1), 44–48.

CHAPTER 18

Elder Mistreatment

Terry Fulmer, PhD, RN, FAAN
Lisa Guadagno, MPA
Marguarette M. Bolton, BA

INTRODUCTION

Elder mistreatment (EM) is a major health care problem that can lead to severe physical disability, psychological problems, and even death in the older adult. Surgeon General Louis Sullivan played a major role in "medicalizing" the issue, which has helped sensitize American health care professionals about the important role they have in assessing and managing cases of EM (Sullivan, 1992). Although legal definitions of EM vary from state to state, EM is generally considered to include:

a. Intentional actions that cause harm or create serious risk of harm (whether or not harm is intended) to a vulnerable elder by a caregiver or other person who is in a trust relationship to the elder, or

b. Failure by a caregiver to satisfy the elder's basic needs or to protect himself or herself from harm (National Research Council, 2003).

EM is the outcome of the actions of abuse, neglect, exploitation, or abandonment of older adults by a known caregiver, as distinct from "stranger violence." The existence of a caregiving relationship is inherent in the definition. Spouse abuse in older adults may be a longstanding issue and is generally not considered in the EM literature. There is a lack of consensus about whether self-neglect, the failure of a mentally competent elder to protect himself or herself from harm, is a subcategory of EM. The National Center on Elder Abuse and various states include it in the definition of EM since outcomes may be similar to mistreatment by caregivers (The National Center on Elder Abuse, 2001). However, the Panel to Review Risk and Prevalence of Elder Abuse and Neglect (National Research Council, 2003) considers self-neglect as a separate domain from EM, albeit one that also often warrants intervention.

TYPES OF EM

EM occurs in both domestic and institutional settings, though much of the research on the causes and outcomes has focused on the domestic setting. Table 18-1 lists several different subtypes of elder mistreatment of which clinicians should be aware.

TABLE 18-1 Subtypes of EM		
Type of Mistreatment	Definition	Examples
Physical Abuse	Acts of violence that may result in pain, injury, impairment, or disease	Pushing, slapping, striking, improper use of restraints, force-feeding
Sexual Abuse	Sexual contact or exposure without the older person's consent or when the person is incapable of giving consent	Unwanted touching, sexual assault or battery, rape, coerced nudity
Physical Neglect	Failure to provide for the needs of an older person that may result in harm	Failure to provide clothing, food, shelter, hygiene; withholding of health maintenance care, social interaction
Psychological Abuse	Infliction of mental anguish, pain, or distress on an older person	Harassment, intimidation, threats, isolating the person, treating the person like a child
Psychological Neglect	Failure to provide the older person with sufficient social stimulation	Leaving the person alone, ignoring the person, giving the "silent treatment," failure to provide news or companionship
Financial/Material Abuse or Exploitation	Misuse of the older person's funds, income, or assets	Stealing money, cashing the person's checks for personal gain, forging the person's signature on documents, improper use of guardianship or power of attorney

Note. From *Diagnostic and Treatment Guidelines on Elder Abuse and Neglect* (p. 9), by the American Medical Association, 1992, Chicago: Author. Adapted with permission.

INCIDENCE AND PREVALENCE

Precise estimates on the number of cases of EM are difficult to obtain for a variety of reasons, including the social stigma and fear of retribution from the abuser. The incidence of EM has been estimated at over 500,000 per year, with a prevalence of 32 per 1000 (Jogerst et al., 2003; Pillemer & Finkelhor, 1988; Tatara, 1993; The National Center on Elder Abuse [at The American Public Human Services Association in Collaboration with Westat, Inc.], 1998). Others have estimated the number of cases of EM to be between 1.5 and 2 million annually (American Medical Association, 1992). A major barrier in determining the true number of cases of EM is the fact that many cases are never reported. Many states do not record separate data on elders nor are their reports uniform across states for accurate data collection (Jogerst et al., 2003; Wolf & Li, 1999). In one study, only 21% of EM cases were reported and substantiated by Adult Protective Service (APS) agencies (The National Center on Elder Abuse, 1998). Others estimate that only 1 in 14 cases of domestic EM come to the attention of authorities (Pillemer & Finkelhor, 1988). Most of these prevalence and incidence estimates are extrapolated from literature on domestic violence.

POPULATION AT RISK

Risk factors for EM include low socioeconomic status, low educational level, impaired functional or cognitive status, and a history of domestic violence, stressful events and depression in the older adult or the caregiver (Dyer, Pavlik, Murphy, & Hyman, 2000; Pillemer & Finkelhor, 1989). EM victims are more likely to be female (Dunlop, Rothman, Condon, Hebert, & Martinez, 2000), over 80 years old (The National Center on Elder Abuse, 1998; Teaster, Roberto, Duke, & Myeonghwan, 2000), and to live with the caregiver who mistreats them (Lachs, Williams, O'Brien, Hurst, & Horwitz, 1997; Pillemer & Finkelhor, 1988; Vladescu, Eveleigh, Ploeg, & Patterson, 1999). Furthermore, chronic, disabling illnesses that impair function have been shown to be a risk factor for being mistreated (Fulmer & O'Malley, 1987).

There are several characteristics that have been shown to be more common among perpetrators of EM. These individuals are more likely to have impairment such as mental illness, depression, or substance abuse (Brownell, 1999; Cohen, Llorente, & Eisdorfer, 1998; Pillemer & Finkelhor, 1989; Reis & Nahmiash, 1998). They are also more likely to be financially dependent on the older adult (Brownell, 1999; Pillemer & Finkelhor, 1989; Seaver, 1996; Wolf & Pillemer, 1997). Many studies have reported that the majority of perpetrators are male, particularly in the case of sexual abusers (Brownell, 1999; Ramsey-Klawsnik, 1991; Teaster et al., 2000; The National Center on Elder Abuse, 1998).

THEORIES OF EM

The etiology of EM can be examined through a number of different theories. "Transgenerational" violence, a phenomenon whereby children who were abused grow up and mistreat their abusing parents, has been postulated as a possible theory (O'Malley, O'Malley, Everitt, & Sarson, 1984). Others theorize that psychopathology in the abuser may be the contributing factor. Perpetrators have been shown to be more likely to have substance

abuse issues and psychopathology (Lachs & Fulmer, 1993). Caregiver stress may also account for cases of EM. Caregivers may become overburdened or overwhelmed by their caregiving responsibilities, which may cause them to become violent. The phenomenon of "generational inversion," where children must suddenly reverse their roles and become the caregiver instead of being cared for by the parent, may be a contributing factor to caregiver stress and may lead to a higher risk of EM occurrence (Steinmetz, 1990). Another theory of etiology for EM includes dependency as a central issue. Older adults who are dependent on their caregivers for ADLs and IADLs are more vulnerable to being mistreated. Caregivers who are emotionally and/or financially dependent on the older adult they care for are more likely to become perpetrators of EM. This is sometimes described as a "web of dependency," where victim and perpetrator are equally dependent upon one another, which creates a situation that might give rise to EM (O'Malley, Everitt, O'Malley, & Campion, 1983). Lastly, it has been noted that isolation plays a key role in EM. Older adults who are isolated may be at risk since there are no outsiders monitoring their quality of life; therefore, they may not be identified by the health care system or reporting agencies (The National Center on Elder Abuse, 1998).

INSTITUTIONAL MISTREATMENT

Research on the extent of EM in nursing homes and other long-term care facilities is scarce. However, the studies that have been conducted include implications that EM may be a widespread phenomenon in institutional settings. In a survey of nursing home staff, 10% of the staff members reported committing an act of physical abuse against a resident in the previous year, and 40% admitted to having committed an act of psychological abuse. Moreover, 81% had witnessed at least one incident of psychological abuse by another staff member and 36% had witnessed at least one incident of physical abuse (Pillemer & Moore, 1989). In this study, older adult aggressiveness was a predictor of physical and psychological abuse by staff members, and abusers were more likely to be younger than nonabusers.

Reporting of EM in nursing homes is a problem and long delays in the reporting of incidents are common (United States General Accounting Office Report to Congressional Requesters, 2002). In addition, great delays were reported in the length of time it takes for nursing homes to report incidents of EM to law enforcement and state agencies and the time it takes for state survey agencies to follow up and make determinations about reports of mistreatment (United States General Accounting Office Report to Congressional Requesters, 2002). These delays in reporting hamper efforts of state survey agencies to collect evidence and may put other nursing home residents at risk of being mistreated. No federal law requiring criminal background checks of nursing home employees exists, though several states require them and a proposed federal Patient Abuse Prevention Act would mandate these background checks (Library of Congress, n.d.).

The Minimum Data Set (MDS) requirements for long-term care facilities, which include a section on resident abuse, have done much to help in the assessment of EM (Centers for Medicare and Medicaid Services, 2000). Every institution is required to complete in-service training on resident abuse with every new employee and annually thereafter. All staff members are instructed on the institutional guidelines for reporting suspected EM. In some instances there may be delays in reporting EM in nursing homes. Staff members may fear losing their jobs or facing reprisal by other staff members and management if they report EM. Residents may be afraid of retribution and family members may fear having to find a new nursing home for the resident. Finally, managers of nursing homes may want to avoid adverse publicity (Burgess, Dowdell, & Prentky, 2000). None of these are acceptable reasons for nonreporting and could result in state agencies penalizing the institution for noncompliance or even obstruction of justice. Reporting should be presented as a positive feature in any nursing home that strives to create a safe and supportive environment.

CLINICAL PRESENTATIONS

History

Successful assessment for EM begins with a thorough history. It seems obvious that unless older adults are asked about any elder mistreatment, they are unlikely to discuss it. There are a number of appropriate times during the history to ask older adults about EM and the nurse should use his or her judgment with regard to the timing given the rapport he or she has with the older adult. In a busy emergency department setting, elder mistreatment should be explored during the history taking. After review of the chief complaint, it is appropriate to ask about physical violence in the same context as one would ask about guns in the home, drugs and alcohol history, and other high risk or dangerous aspects of a person's life. The nurse should be direct and help the older adult by using phrases such as:

- "Is there any family violence you would like to talk about?"

- "Have you ever been abused by any of your family members or friends? If so, has it been physical or emotional?"

The discussion should be continued in that manner. As with any good history, when there is a positive response to a screening question, the nurse should proceed to get a sense of the onset of the problem, the circumstances, how long it has been going on, the characteristics of the problem, the associated or aggravating issues that bring on the EM, things that relieve the situation, and what the appropriate types of interventions would be based on that individual's life circumstances.

The Institute of Medicine discusses screening assessments in Appendix A of its 2002 report (Institute of Medicine, 2002), and a review article presenting current providers with a succinct analysis of available instruments was recently published in *The Journal of American Geriatrics Society* (Fulmer, Guadagno, Bitondo Dyer, & Connolly, 2004). The American Medical Association has published diagnostic and treatment guidelines on elder abuse and neglect (American Medical Association, 1992) that are extremely useful in developing an approach to screening for EM.

The clinician is urged to incorporate routine questions related to EM into his or her daily practice and to be sure to pay special note to older adults who have cognitive impairment, which itself is a risk factor for EM. In the case where older adults do not hear well or have diseases that might impair their ability to communicate, such as Parkinson's or a cerebral vascular accident, it is even more important to get accurate information in the history. In the event the information is not obtained in the first interview, the nurse needs to create a follow-up plan as to how he or she will obtain the information as soon as possible. This may require an interdisciplinary approach. For example, if the emergency department nurse does not get the answer to a screening question about EM, he or she should contact the social worker who would be in touch with the older adult on the unit, or who will communicate with the older adult after returning home, so that information can be obtained and a follow-up plan can be developed as needed. (See Table 18-2.)

In an older adult with severe dementia, the nurse needs to seek out a proxy who can comment on the possibility of EM. It is very important that the nurse be sensitive to the fact that proxies could potentially be the abusers and that caution should be exercised in order to avoid creating a dangerous situation for the older adult. It is extremely important that the nurse determine how serious and dangerous the current situation is for the older adult. For example, in the clinic or emergency department, when the older adult is being treated and released, an alternative plan needs to be developed if the older adult is at risk for injury and harm from EM. Such a plan needs to be created rapidly in order to avoid having the older adult return to an unsafe situation. In some circumstances, shelters may be

TABLE 18-2   Screening Questions
• Has anyone at home ever hurt you?
• Has anyone ever touched you without your consent?
• Has anyone ever made you do things you didn't want to do?
• Has anyone taken anything that was yours without asking?
• Has anyone ever scolded or threatened you?
• Have you ever signed any documents that you didn't understand?
• Are you afraid of anyone at home?
• Are you alone a lot?
• Has anyone ever failed to help you take care of yourself when you needed help?

Note. From *Diagnostic and Treatment Guidelines on Elder Abuse and Neglect* (p. 9), by the American Medical Association, 1992, Chicago: Author. Adapted with permission.

needed or it may be necessary to arrange a protective service admission into the hospital. All this needs to be done in the context of state reporting laws as well as in the context of the older adult's rights and wishes. There are mandatory EM reporting laws in 46 states (Capezuti, Brush, & Lawson, 1997; Jogerst et al., 2003; Roby & Sullivan, 2000). Protocols need to be followed not only for the state requirements, but also within the context of any institutional guidelines at the hospital, clinic, or practice setting.

The nurse needs to safeguard the older adult against care plans that are not in their best interest or contrary to the older adult's wishes. For example, older adults who have cognitive impairment and live in a home with an abusive relative may be reviewed for nursing home placement (Centers for Medicare and Medicaid Services, 2000). While there are times when this may be appropriate, it should not be considered the only plan of care. Older adults should not be forced out of their homes because of other people's detrimental behavior. Depending on the situation, it may be possible to alleviate the situation through adult day health services or home care services, while still allowing the older adult to maintain independence and live at home. In some cases, adult children are misusing the resources and the living space of older adults in a negative way that disrupts the older adult's life. Steps can be taken to obtain restraining orders against adult children or other individuals who are harming the older adult. Older adults may feel guilty about doing this to a relative, even when they are at increased risk. EM cases are complicated and require a team approach that may involve a multidisciplinary assessment and regular team follow-up to ensure the older adult's well-being. Legal services or police protection may be needed and will require expertise from the team to be alert for any signs of depression, suicidal tendencies, or self-neglect in these potentially devastating circumstances.

Physical Examination

Once the history has been completed, the physical examination should be conducted in a comprehensive manner in order to determine if there are any signs of EM. Table 18-3 provides an overview of high-risk signs for physical abuse, neglect, financial and material abuse, or neglect and violation of rights.

There are signs that can be misconstrued as EM in older adults given comorbidities and multiple medications. For example, a bruise may be misinterpreted as a sign of abuse but in fact, the older adult may be on Coumadin or have a history of falls. The nurse should question the older adult about the causes of any suspicious bruises or skin lesions. Older adults who are incontinent may have urine burns or excoriations on their skin as a result of neglect. The causes of these findings should be explored thoroughly to determine if neglect exists. In the past, clinical assessment of older adults has been extraordinarily "forgiving" of symptoms such as dehydration, skin tears, poor hygiene, and other presentations that would never be overlooked in a younger person. A physical assessment of an older adult requires precise documentation of findings that may indicate that the older adult is a victim of abuse or neglect.

Psychological Assessment

A psychological assessment for EM is extremely important and needs to be done with precision and specificity. Older adults may present with signs such as sucking, rocking, or other redundant behaviors that are unexplained by mental illness. In cases such as these, it is useful to call a psychiatric liaison nurse, a social worker, a psychiatrist, or other mental health professional to conduct an assessment of the symptoms in the context of the older adult's mental health. In some cases, the behavior may be longstanding and result from childhood trauma or child abuse. The Childhood Trauma Questionnaire (Bernstein

TABLE 18-3	Examples of High-Risk Signs and Symptoms
Abuse	Unexplained bruises, repeated falls, lab values inconsistent with history, fractures or bruises in various stages of healing (any report by patient of being physically abused should be followed up immediately)
Neglect	Listlessness, poor hygiene, evidence of malnourishment, inappropriate dress, decubiti, urine burns, reports of being left in an unsafe situation, reports of inability to get needed medications
Exploitation	Unexplained loss of Social Security or pension checks, any evidence that material goods are being taken in exchange for care, any evidence that personal belongings of elder (house, jewelry, car) are being taken over without consent or approval of elder

Other High Risk Situations

- Drug or alcohol addiction in the family
- Isolation of the elder
- History of untreated psychiatric problems
- Evidence of unusual family stress
- Excessive dependence of elder on caretaker

Note. From *Inadequate Care of the Elderly: A Health Care Perspective on Abuse and Neglect* (pp. 18–19), by T. Fulmer and T. O'Malley, 1987, New York: Springer. Adapted with permission.

& Fink, 1998) is a useful screen to determine whether an older adult has suffered from traumatic life circumstances in childhood and may have issues that are still unresolved. This instrument has been used and validated with older adult samples including HMO members, female pain patients, adult psychiatric outpatients, and adult substance abusers. The instrument can be used in adult populations to assess for traumatic histories and formulate a treatment plan (Bernstein & Fink, 1998).

Laboratory and Diagnostic Testing

Laboratory tests for older adults should be selected and conducted based on the history and the presentation in the clinical setting. Routine blood work should be ordered as appropriate for annual physical examinations. When signs of EM are evident, as in severe dehydration or multiple bruises, X-rays or blood chemistries should be obtained to explore the presentation more thoroughly. If an older adult presents with an open wound that

appears to be untreated, a culture of that wound may be required.

■ EVALUATION AND REFERRAL

Whenever an older adult screens positive for elder mistreatment, the nurse needs to be knowledgeable about the state reporting laws, the institutional guidelines in the workplace, and the follow-up required to ensure the well-being of the adult. The APS network in the United States is extremely effective in follow-up of suspected cases of EM, and in some cases, can provide support services that can create a safer home environment for the adult. Community-based services such as respite care, hospice care, adult day health care centers, and less formal organizations such as church groups can all offer useful interventions in cases of EM. The Alzheimer's Association, with its extensive network of chapters throughout the United States, is an excellent resource for older adults and their families or caregivers who need support and guidance in understanding community services. This as-sociation should not be overlooked as a major resource for these issues.

LEGAL CONSIDERATIONS

When a nurse obtains a positive history for EM, he or she will need to work with the administration of his or her organization to determine the best way to engage law enforce-ment and legal assistance. Assault and battery is against the law, and the procedures for working with the police should be known in advance. Rape is a felony and should never be labeled as a type of elder mistreatment without following the appropriate rape proce-dures already in place for any other age group. Careful documentation of the history, physical, and laboratory findings in such cases cannot be underscored enough.

PREVENTION

Every time an older adult presents in any nursing care setting, there is opportunity to screen for EM and to remind older adults that they have the right to live a life free from fear of mistreatment. It is helpful to have teaching materials that can be distributed to the older adult with contact information that can be used in the event that they are victims of EM or have concerns regarding EM. In some cir-cumstances, the older adult may give a his-tory of EM and yet demand that "no one be told," or refuse services. This presents an ethi-cal dilemma for any nurse who is concerned about the older adult. The fear of discharging an older adult to an unsafe setting or leaving a person in his or her residence when there is known abuse is antithetical to nursing prac-tice. However, in the absence of dementia or other serious cognitive impairments, the older adult has the right to self-determination no matter how distasteful it is to the nurse. In such situations teaching materials with con-tact telephone numbers that can be used on a

24-hour emergency basis are essential in the clinical interaction. It is tempting for any clini-cian to assume cognitive impairment when the older adult chooses an EM situation over a protected environment, but it is a possibility. In these circumstances, counseling services should be obtained to address the nature of the EM situation and to suggest alternatives to the older adult.

In cases of EM where the older adult does have documented dementia or cognitive im-pairment, a geropsychiatric consultation will be needed. Geropsychiatric nurses are in a unique position to complete a detailed assess-ment and diagnose impairments that preclude self-determination at a given moment. Regu-lar re-evaluation of cognitive status is manda-tory given the fluctuating cycles that take place over time. The plan of care will be highly dependent on the context including the site of care, the residence of the older adult, his or her living circumstances, and any guardianship or conservatorship proxies in place. When an older adult is screened and diagnosed in the emergency department, the concern regarding a treat-and-release situation will be especially high. Plans for fol-low-up should be carefully coordinated with home care nursing and social services. Older adults need to be informed that nurses are mandatory reporters for suspected EM and that appropriate reports will be made. They should be informed that if Adult Protective Services makes contact, they could refuse ser-vices. If there is suspected criminal activity such as assault or theft, police will be con-tacted. This may be distressing for the older adult, just as it is to parents when child abuse reports are made. Nurses can alleviate some of the tension by explaining that their actions are being made in good faith.

In summary, elder mistreatment presents major challenges for both the older adult and the nurse. Comprehensive assessment, sensi-tivity, care planning, and follow-up can make the difference in health outcomes for the older adult.

REFERENCES

American Medical Association. (1992). *Diagnostic and treatment guidelines on elder abuse and neglect.* Chicago, IL: Author.

Bernstein, D., & Fink, L. (1998). *Childhood Trauma Questionnaire: A retrospective of self-report.* San Antonio, TX: Psychological Corporation.

Brownell, P. (1999). Mental health and criminal justice issues among perpetrators of elder abuse. *Journal of Elder Abuse & Neglect, 11*(4), 81–94.

Burgess, A. W., Dowdell, E. B., & Prentky, R. A. (2000). Sexual abuse of nursing home residents. *Journal of Psychosocial Nursing and Mental Health Services, 38*(6), 10–18, 48–49.

Capezuti, E., Brush, B. L., & Lawson, W. T. (1997). Reporting elder mistreatment. *Journal of Gerontological Nursing, 23*(7), 24–32.

Centers for Medicare and Medicaid Services. (2000). *Minimum Data Set (MDS) Long-Term Care User's Facility Manual.* Baltimore, MD: DHHS.

Cohen, D., Llorente, M., & Eisdorfer, C. (1998). Homicide-suicide in older persons. *The American Journal of Psychiatry, 155*(3), 390–396.

Dunlop, B., Rothman, M. B., Condon, K. M., Hebert, K. S., & Martinez, I. L. (2000). Elder abuse: Risk factors and use of case data to improve policy and practice. *Journal of Elder Abuse & Neglect, 12*(3/4), 95–122.

Dyer, C. B., Pavlik, V. N., Murphy, K. P., & Hyman, D. J. (2000). The high prevalence of depression and dementia in elder abuse or neglect. *Journal of the American Geriatrics Society, 48*(2), 205–208.

Fulmer, T., Guadagno, L., Bitondo Dyer, C., & Connolly, M. T. (2004). Progress in elder abuse screening and assessment instruments. *Journal of American Geriatrics Society , 52*(2), 297–304.

Fulmer, T., & O'Malley, T. (1987). *Inadequate care of the elderly: A health care perspective on abuse and neglect.* New York: Springer.

Institute of Medicine. (2002). *Confronting chronic neglect: The education and training of health professionals on family violence.* Washington, DC: National Academy Press.

Jogerst, G. J., Daly, J. M., Brinig, M. F., Dawson, J. D., Schmuch, G. A., & Ingram, J. G. (2003). Domestic elder abuse and the law. *American Journal of Public Health, 93*(12), 2131–2136.

Lachs, M. S., & Fulmer, T. (1993). Recognizing elder abuse and neglect. *Clinical Geriatric Medicine, 9*(3), 665–681.

Lachs, M. S., Williams, C., O'Brien, S., Hurst, L., & Horwitz, R. I. (1997). Risk factors for reported elder abuse and neglect: A nine-year observational cohort study. *Gerontologist, 37*(4), 469–474.

Library of Congress (n.d.) Bill summary and status for the 108th Congress. Retrieved September 7, 2004, from http://thomas.loc.gov/cgi-bin/bdquery

The National Center on Elder Abuse. (2001). *Creating and promoting an elder abuse action agenda.* Washington, DC: National Policy Summit on Elder Abuse.

The National Center on Elder Abuse at The American Public Human Services Association in Collaboration with Westat, Inc. (1998). *The National Elder Abuse Incidence Study; Final report: September 1998.* Washington, DC: National Aging Information Center.

National Research Council. (2003). *Elder mistreatment: Abuse, neglect, and exploitation in an Aging America.* Panel to Review Risk and Prevalence of Elder Abuse and Neglect. Bonnie, R. J., & Wallace, R. B. (Eds.). Committee on National Statistics and Committee on Law and Justice, Division of Behavioral and Social Sciences and Education. Washington, DC: The National Academies Press.

O'Malley, T. A., Everitt, D. E., O'Malley, H. C., & Campion, E. W. (1983). Identifying and preventing family-mediated abuse and neglect of elderly persons. *Annals of Internal Medicine, 98*(6), 998–1005.

O'Malley, T. A., O'Malley, H. C., Everitt, D. E., & Sarson, D. (1984). Categories of family-mediated abuse and neglect of elderly persons. *Journal of the American Geriatrics Society, 32*(5), 362–369.

Pillemer, K. A., & Finkelhor, D. (1988). The prevalence of elder abuse: A random sample survey. *Gerontologist, 28*(1), 51–57.

Pillemer, K. A., & Finkelhor, D. (1989). Causes of elder abuse: Caregiver stress versus problem relatives. *American Journal of Orthopsychiatry, 59*(2), 179–187.

Pillemer, K. A., & Moore, D. W. (1989). Abuse of patients in nursing homes: Findings from a survey of staff. *Gerontologist, 29*(3), 314–320.

Ramsey-Klawsnik, H. (1991). Elder sexual abuse: Preliminary findings. *Journal of Elder Abuse & Neglect, 3*(3), 73–90.

Reis, M., & Nahmiash, D. (1998). Validation of the Indicators of Abuse (IOA) screen. *Gerontologist, 38*(4), 471–480.

Roby, J. L., & Sullivan, R. (2000). Adult protection service laws: A comparison of state statutes from definition to case closure. *Journal of Elder Abuse & Neglect, 12*(3/4), 17–51.

Seaver, C. (1996). Muted lives: Older battered women. *Journal of Elder Abuse & Neglect, 8*(2), 3–21.

Steinmetz, S. K. (1990). Elder abuse by adult offspring: The relationship of actual vs. perceived dependency. *Journal of Health & Human Resources Administration, 12*(4), 434–463.

Sullivan, L. (1992) *Nursing Home Resident Protection.* Retrieved April 22, 1999, from http://www.hhs.gov/news.../pre1995pres/92025.txt

Tatara, T. (1993). Understanding the nature and scope of domestic elder abuse with the use of state aggregate data: Summaries of key findings of a national survey of state APS and aging agencies. *Journal of Elder Abuse and Neglect, 5,* 35–57.

Teaster, P., Roberto, K., Duke, J., & Myeonghwan, K. (2000). Sexual abuse of older adults: Preliminary findings of cases in Virginia. *Journal of Elder Abuse & Neglect, 12*(3/4), 1–16.

United States General Accounting Office Report to Congressional Requesters. (2002). *Nursing homes: More can be done to protect residents from abuse.* Washington, DC: GAO-02-312.

Vladescu, D., Eveleigh, K., Ploeg, J., & Patterson, C. (1999). An evaluation of a client-centered case management program for elder abuse. *Journal of Elder Abuse & Neglect, 11*(4), 5–22.

Wolf, R. S., & Li, D. (1999). Factors affecting the rate of elder abuse reporting to a state protective services program. *Gerontologist, 39*(2), 222–228.

Wolf, R. S., & Pillemer, K. A. (1997). The older battered woman: Wives and mothers compared. *Journal of Mental Health & Aging, 3*(3), 325–336.

CHAPTER 19

End of Life

Michelle Doran, MS, APRN, BC, ANP, GNP, PCM
Karyn Geary, MS, APRN, BC, ANP, GNP, PCM

▰ INTRODUCTION

Over the past century, how people die and where they die has changed dramatically. Before World War II, people usually died in the comfort of their own home, cared for by family members. Deaths often occurred rapidly as a result of communicable illnesses or acute events. In 1900, the average life expectancy for both men and women was less than 50 years of age (Berry & Matzo, 2004; Bookbinder & Kiss, 2001). In the earlier half of the 1900s infant and childhood death was not an uncommon experience for a family to endure, with 53% of all deaths occurring in children under the age of 15 (Krisman-Scott, 2003). In the absence of advanced medical technology, symptom management was a major focus of care. Families were skilled at providing the care and attention necessary for achieving comfortable, peaceful, and digni-fied death experiences for their loved ones. Death was often accepted to be as much a part of life as birth. Families embraced the oppor-tunity to provide meaningful end-of-life care (Sherman & Laporte, 2001).

By the mid-1900s, several developments had taken place that would contribute to changing the death experience in the United States.

Growth in science and industry resulted in improved living and working conditions. Dis-ease prevention, treatment, and life-saving or prolonging treatments evolved with the development of vaccinations, antibiotics, cardiopulmonary resuscitation, advances in surgery, and anesthesia. As a result, the focus of care shifted from symptom management to curative interventions. With these changes, patients, families, and health care profession-als not only began to have higher expectations for curable illnesses, but also for those that were incurable. Death became equated with medical failure. Medical treatments were sought that resulted in a shift for the dying from care at home to hospitalization. End-of-life care became the responsibility of health care providers who often were not educated in care of the dying and hospitals that were ill equipped to meet the complex physical, emo-tional, and spiritual needs of the terminally ill (Bookbinder & Kiss, 2001; Ferrell, Virani, & Grant, 1999; Krisman-Scott, 2003; Rabow, Hardie, Fair, & McPhee, 2000; Super, 2001).

With the advances in medical technology and treatments, many other aspects of dying were impacted. Infant and childhood mortal-ity rates decreased markedly and causes of death changed dramatically. In the first half of the 1900s, most deaths were the result of influenza and pneumonia. Death from communicable disease became far less common with developments in sanitation, antibiotics, and immunizations (Berry & Matzo, 2004; Bookbinder & Kiss, 2001; Krisman-Scott, 2003). As a result, people began to live longer, with chronic, degenerative, and progressive illnesses. By 2001, the 10 leading causes of death in the United States (in rank order) were identified as: heart disease, malignant neoplasms, cerebrovascular diseases, chronic lower respiratory diseases, accidents or unintentional injuries, diabetes mellitus, influenza/pneumonia, Alzheimer's disease, kidney disease, and sepsis. These diseases accounted for close to 80% of all deaths. This, coupled with increased life expectancies and a growing, aging population, resulted in larger numbers of older Americans experiencing a longer, slower dying process (Amella, 2003; Anderson & Smith, 2003).

Changes, such as the decline in infant and childhood mortality, mobility of our society, distancing of extended families, late experiences with death, and hospitalization of the dying, resulted in Americans becoming estranged from death. These factors, as well as medical advances, made it easier for patients, families, and health care providers to deny the inevitability of death. It became common practice to use aggressive technology and curative therapies in patients with incurable illness. It was not unusual for patients to be kept alive with technology with the expectation that developments for a cure could be in progress. In the 1960s, families as well as professionals began to question the medicalization of the dying and the technical, depersonalized deaths occurring in hospitals. In 1969, Dr. Elizabeth Kubler-Ross published her best-selling work on dying patients, *On Death and Dying*, which revealed the tragedy of the hospitalized dying experience and the inability of the American health care system to focus on appropriate care when cure was no longer possible.

It is overwhelmingly clear that care for the dying in this country remains inadequate and much work remains to be done. Nurses in general, and advanced practice nurses (APNs), particularly those with expertise in palliative care, have been recognized as an essential resource for meeting the complex needs of dying patients and their families. One key component of nurses' willingness to actively take part in end-of-life care comes with the acceptance of death as a natural part of the life cycle. With this acceptance, a journey of growth can begin with the recognition of death as an opportunity and achievement, rather than a medical failure. Nursing professionals are crucial in ensuring that patients and families are not deprived of such opportunities for growth at the end of life (Byock, 1997).

GOLD STANDARD FOR END-OF-LIFE CARE: HOSPICE AND PALLIATIVE CARE

Hospice

Hospice began in the United States as a grassroots movement to improve the quality of care being provided to dying patients and surviving families. The contemporary hospice movement, founded by Dame Cicely Saunders in London in the 1950s and '60s, continues to be the gold standard for end-of-life care. Dame Saunders was instrumental in the development of the first organized hospice program in the United States, which opened in Connecticut in 1975 (Egan & Labyak, 2001; Krisman-Scott, 2003). At the center of hospice care is the belief that dying is a normal part of the life cycle. When cure is no longer possible or realistic, focusing on curative care becomes inappropriate. Instead, patients elect to focus on quality of remaining life, relief of suffering, and symptom control. An interdisciplinary hospice team helps not only with physical care, but also psychosocial and spiritual support, as well as grief and bereavement for surviving family members. Hospice teams include physicians, nurses, chaplains, social workers, nursing assistants, bereavement counselors, and volunteers. The plan of care is based on knowledge of patient and family preferences and goals of end-of-life care.

The delivery of hospice care can occur in a variety of settings. The majority of hospice care continues to be provided in the home setting by family and friends. However, as the population ages, hospices are serving an older-adult population who can no longer live alone or with frail caregivers. In such cases, the definition of *home* may commonly be a rest home, assisted living facility, or nursing home. In addition, inpatient hospital hospice units and hospice residences are emerging as other options for patients who are no longer able to stay in their own homes at end of life. Hospice services are available to patients of any age, religion, race, illness, and financial situation. Many hospice programs provide free care to specific patients without insurance or financial resources.

The Medicare Hospice Benefit provides hospice care to patients who elect it and are certified to be terminally ill with a prognosis of six months or less if the disease runs its usual course. Under the Medicare Hospice Benefit, beneficiaries elect to receive noncurative treatment and services for a variety of life-limiting illnesses ranging from cancer to dementia. The Medicare Hospice Benefit includes home visits by the interdisciplinary team, medical equipment, medical supplies, medications that relate to the hospice diagnosis, volunteer and bereavement support, and therapy services, when appropriate. The benefit reimburses for inpatient care in a variety of settings when patients are very close to end of life or have acute symptoms that require intensive management for a limited time, usually a few weeks. Additionally, the routine hospice benefit covers services delivered in a variety of settings including home, nursing home, assisted living, and residences, but does not cover room and board. Patients and families are also eligible for respite care in a Medicare-approved facility for up to five days at a time. Patients continue to receive hospice care for their illnesses as long as these services remain appropriate, which can range from days to months to years. Patients may revoke their hospice benefit at any time. Various insurance companies are realizing the importance of hospice and include a hospice benefit similar to the Medicare benefit.

Palliative Care

Palliative care is specialized, interdisciplinary care for patients with serious, life-limiting or chronic debilitating illnesses. It involves the comprehensive management of the patient's physical, psychological, social, and spiritual needs. The goal of palliative care is to maximize quality of life through expert control of pain and other distressing physical symptoms, management of psychosocial stressors, and attention to spiritual needs. The original model of palliative care is hospice care. However, unlike hospice care, palliative care can occur any time during a patient's illness, even if life expectancy extends to years and aggressive or curative treatment is being pursued. Typically, the intensity and range of palliative interventions will change as the illness progresses and the complexity of care increases.

Palliative medicine and nursing are well-established specialties in Great Britain and Australia. In more recent years, palliative care has been emerging as a distinct medical and nursing specialty in the United States. The number of palliative-care programs in this country continues to grow. Palliative care is being offered in specialized inpatient units, in the form of consultative services in acute, long-term-care, and home settings, and in outpatient clinics. Physicians and nurses with specialized training and experience are eligible to sit for board certification in palliative care. Palliative care should be provided by a specially trained, interdisciplinary team that includes physicians, nurses, social workers, and chaplains.

There is overwhelming evidence that the majority of health care providers in general receive little or no training in pain and symptom management and other complex issues related to end-of-life care. As a result, there is often unfamiliarity with concepts of advanced pain and symptom control and discomfort with complex topics such as prognostication, communicating bad news, resuscitation wishes, artificial hydration and nutrition, placement of feeding tubes, implications of initiating and withdrawing treatments, medical futility, resolving communication conflicts, and discussions surrounding burdens versus benefits of treatments. In addition, due to the complexity and time intensity of these discussions, primary care providers are often left without the proper time to facilitate these lengthy, emotional discussions. With advanced training and certification, palliative-care providers are the ideal specialists to be consulted to provide this level of care in conjunction with the primary heath care team. Geropsychiatic nurses may be important members of the palliative-care team providing mental health services to older adults with psychiatric or mental health problems and their families.

Barriers to Quality Care at End of Life

Despite the fact that hospice care is the gold standard for end of life and that it is widely available in the United States, many barriers prevent uniform access. Perhaps the most eye-opening recognition of these barriers came with the results of the Study to Understand Prognoses and Preferences for Outcomes and Risks of Treatments (SUPPORT, 1995). SUPPORT was a 5-year study of more than 9000 hospitalized adults with one or more of nine life-threatening cancer and noncancer diagnoses. All of the patients involved were terminally ill and had predictable courses of illness. The objective of the study was to improve end-of-life decision making and reduce the frequency of a mechanically supported, painful, and prolonged process of dying. The goal was to develop a model intervention that would improve the frequency and effectiveness of communication between physicians and patients about medical decisions. This landmark study provided overwhelming empirical evidence that detailed many problems with end-of-life care of seriously ill, hospitalized patients.

SUPPORT data suggested that most of the patients who participated in the study died in the hospital under unfavorable conditions. Almost half of all Do Not Resuscitate (DNR) orders were written within the last two days of life, and for patients preferring DNR status, less than 50% of their physicians were aware of this preference. Almost half of patients spent more than eight days at the end of life in an intensive care unit (ICU) receiving mechanical ventilation, and/or in a comatose state. For 50% of patients who had been conscious at the end of life, families reported at least half their final days were spent in moderate to severe pain. The study demonstrated that well-planned interventions did not improve outcomes, as patients in the intervention group did not have better experiences than the control group. The findings from this study have contributed to the development of many initiatives to improve the care of the dying.

The inadequacy of care of the dying in the United States was further documented in 1997 when the Institute of Medicine published a report that summarized the priorities necessary for improving end-of-life care. Four major barriers to quality end-of-life care were identified: (1) many people suffer at end of life because they do not receive appropriate palliative care or they receive inappropriate or ineffective care; (2) legal, organizational, and financial barriers prevent excellent end-of-life care; (3) physicians, nurses, and other health care professionals do not receive proper education and training to care for dying patients and their families; and (4) there is insufficient knowledge to guide consistent practice of evidence-based care at end of life (Field & Cassel, 1997).

Misperceptions by health care providers and the public in general about hospice and palliative-care services remain a tremendous barrier to adequate end-of-life care. Many providers believe that hospice is for patients with a cancer diagnosis only or those very close to death. Hospice and palliative-care experts are often called in very late, when patients are expected to live days to weeks rather than months. At this point, services become focused on crisis work because of limited time with dying patients and surviving family members. The challenge is to educate health care providers to refer patients early, so they can benefit from the full range of services for months rather than days. The majority of providers are unfamiliar with the National Hospice Organization's (NHO) specific guidelines for noncancer diagnoses. This includes eligibility for patients with heart failure, dementia, terminal debility, and all advanced diseases. Improving the awareness among providers and the general public can improve use of the hospice benefit.

ADVANCED-CARE PLANNING

Advanced-care planning enables patients to consider and communicate preferences regarding medical interventions that relate to illnesses and end-of-life care. Typically, patients make decisions with regard to specific life-sustaining therapies, such as cardiopulmonary resuscitation (CPR) and mechanical ventilation, or about the general level of care they wish to receive, such as life prolonging or palliative (Lamont & Siegler, 2000). Additionally, discussions about advanced-care planning involve appointing a person as decision-maker in the event the patient becomes unable to communicate.

The Patient Self-Determination Act of 1990 guarantees the right of patients to determine the kinds of medical care they will and will not want if they lose the capacity to participate in decision making by virtue of disease progression or other causes (Grant, 1992). Health care providers are required to discuss and document such advanced directives. Despite the Patient Self-Determination Act, and the widely held notion that completing advanced directives is important to providing good medical care, few people have done so. According to the U.S. Living Will Registry (2000) only 20% of the general population had an advanced directive. Another survey demonstrated that 16% of the public have engaged in these discussions with their health care providers and 11% have completed an advanced directive (Schlegel & Shannon, 2000).

The two types of advanced directives are the durable power of attorney (DPA) for health care and the living will. The DPA for health care, also commonly known as the health care proxy, is a simple legal document naming an agent to make decisions relating to medical care in the event that the patient becomes unable to communicate preferences. Any competent adult 18 years of age or older can fill out a health care proxy. The document becomes legal when completed by the person and does not require an attorney. It is essential that the patient discuss their wishes for specific medical care with the designated agent. The agent's role is to make decisions with regard to particular medical treatments, based on the patient's previous stated preferences and wishes. If the patient did not specify specific treatment preferences, the proxy should use substituted judgment to make decisions.

The living will is a legal statement that lists specific treatments and preferences by the individual patient. Patients are given the opportunity to think about specific medical interventions in the event of terminal illness, imminent death, vegetative state, and other specific states of health. The legalities of living wills may vary from state to state. Although this specific advanced directive may not be legally binding in many states, it can be helpful in guiding care. Providers should familiarize themselves with their individual state laws in relation to such advanced directives.

There are numerous barriers to providers and patients participating in advanced care planning. These discussions can be time consuming and are often not reimbursed (Buttersworth, 2003). Patient's preferences for end-of-life care are often misunderstood or misinterpreted, as demonstrated by the SUPPORT study. Discussing end-of-life issues forces providers to face their own mortality, which can be a deterrent to engaging in such discussions (Buttersworth, 2003). The general public often shares unrealistic expectations of medical interventions in relation to terminal illness. Lack of education for providers is a common barrier to advanced-care planning. According to one study, only 26% of providers have received any end-of-life training in their educational programs (Schlegel & Shannon, 2000). Additionally, the cultures of health care systems, as well as patient's individual cultural beliefs, are a common obstacle to engaging in planning.

A prevalent impediment to advanced-care planning is the public's misconception of the success rate for cardiopulmonary resuscitation (CPR), mechanical ventilation, and other aggressive interventions. In contrast to the popular belief, resuscitation is not an easy procedure with a high success rate. It is known that CPR under the best circumstances has a survival rate of about 15% (Cranston, 2001). Furthermore, CPR is fraught with a variety of complications including rib fractures, major heart or lung injuries, and patients who end up in a persistent vegetative state (Cranston). Patients at end of life, with advanced illnesses, have little to no chance of survival by having CPR performed, and in

such cases CPR may violate a patient's right to die with dignity. The literature supports the notion that for CPR to have any remote possibility of success, the event must be witnessed and unexpected, meaning that terminally ill patients without vital signs do not have any possible life-saving benefit from CPR (Gordon, 2003). If it is clear that death is approaching and the goals of care have been identified as comfort focused, then CPR is not an appropriate medical intervention and health care providers should recommend against such an intervention. Artificial ventilation is also not considered appropriate treatment for terminally ill patients who are nearing the end of life. If artificial ventilation fails to benefit the patient, and the process of death is proceeding, such interventions should be discontinued or withheld and the focus of care should be on aggressive comfort interventions. Discussions should take place in advance with patients and families based on preferences, values, and goals of care.

Artificial nutrition and hydration (ANH) at end of life are 20th-century technologies. ANH have been considered necessary components to good medical care, with the primary intention of benefiting patients. Withholding or withdrawing hydration is a difficult issue for many providers, perhaps because offering food and fluids is linked to sustaining life and providing patient care (Bennett, 2000). It is almost reflexive for health care providers and families to request such interventions for patients who lose the ability to swallow, though the evidence base for utilizing such techniques is weak at best. When a person is approaching death, ANH can be potentially harmful and may provide little to no benefit to patients and at times may make dying more uncomfortable (AAHPM, 2001).

There are numerous benefits of terminal dehydration found in the literature. Many of the potential benefits of dehydration include decreased pain or no pain due to the anesthetic effect that electrolyte imbalances may provide. At the end of life, the brain converts the derivative of metabolic fat to gamma-hydroxybutyrate, a substance with anesthetic properties (Fox, 1996). Electrolyte imbalances may serve as a natural anesthetic, facilitating a reduction in pain medication (Sutcliffe, 1994). Decreased urine output is a beneficial side effect of becoming fluid deficient at the end of life. Reduced urine output lessens incontinence, decreases the need for catheterization, and preserves skin integrity. Dehydration at the end of life decreases pharyngeal, pulmonary, and gastrointestinal secretions, leading to reduction in nausea, emesis, and pulmonary congestion (Meares, 1994; Zerwekh, 1983). Parenteral fluid and nutrition can cause discomfort with repeated venipunctures and iatrogenic infections (HPNA, 2003). Having an intravenous line is invasive and terminally ill patients may need to be restrained because of the risk of injury from pulling at the line. It is also argued that the dying patient experiences multisystem failure, so electrolyte balance may be impossible to maintain even in the presence of artificial hydration (Sutcliffe, 1994).

There is limited support in the literature for using ANH at the end of life. Two common reasons for utilizing it are concerns for discomfort related to thirst and dry mouth. Some authors propose thirst is attributable to a feeling of dry mouth, rather than to actual dehydration (Sutcliffe, 1994). Most experts agree that such oral discomfort can be eased with saliva substitutes, moisturizers, mouth care, ice chips, and petroleum jelly. Some medical consequences of dehydration at end of life include confusion, restlessness, and neuromuscular irritability (Huffman & Dunn, 2002). Occasionally, patients may benefit from a trial of intravenous fluids at end of life, to improve renal clearance when opioid metabolite accumulation is the suspected cause of confusion, or when patients have rapid fluid loss resulting in syncope and confusion (Huffman & Dunn).

In providing care to terminally ill patients close to the end of life, only essential medications should be administered (Cherny, Coyle, & Foley, 1996). These include medications for treatment of pain and other common symptoms. Medications that are offering no benefit to the patient should be discontinued. Antibiotic use at the end of life is often an issue met with controversy. In some cases, oral antibiotics may be a useful adjunct when the goal is palliation of the symptoms of infection, versus eradication of the infection. Oral antibiotics may be useful to reduce tachypnea, cough, sputum, fever, and shaking chills associated with infections. However, if antibiotics cause increased burden and physical distress due to nausea, diarrhea, or pruritis, for example, they should be discontinued. Parenteral antibiotic use is often not indicated unless there is an identified organism, there are clear goals to be met, the likelihood of success is high, and the patient is expected to live long enough to achieve the benefits of treatment.

DETERMINING PROGNOSIS

Prognostication, or estimating life expectancy, is crucial in clinical practice, particularly in regards to end-of-life care. Accurate prediction of life expectancy is important for both providers and patients to make good clinical decisions when dealing with terminal illness (Christakis, 1999; SUPPORT, 1995). Prognostication involves exploring the natural history or clinical course of a particular disease, determining its average prognosis in most patients, and then applying it to a specific patient and his or her treatment decisions. However, true prognosis can never be absolutely established. Diagnosis, treatment, and prognosis are interrelated, though diagnosis and treatment receive much more attention in patient care, medical education, and research.

Prognosis is often linked to ethical decisions in clinical practice. It may affect decisions to initiate, withhold, or withdraw life-sustaining treatments in the terminally ill. Patients want information regarding prognosis to evaluate treatment decisions and determine when they should be referred for hospice care. With the lack of or an inaccurate prognosis, patients may receive unnecessary or burdensome treatments and may not receive beneficial ones. Unfortunately, no established method exists to definitively determine prognosis. Aside from disease-specific criteria, functional status and nutritional status can be good predictors of prognosis. Patients and families should understand that prognostication is not an exact science and can vary widely from one patient to another, particularly with chronic, progressive illness. Patients and families may need prognostic information to make and complete important plans such as saying goodbye, completing relationships, writing wills, arranging finances, and making funeral plans (AAHPM, 2003).

Despite the complexity inherent in the issue of prognostication, a more simplistic

---

ANA Position Statements on Nurses' Role in End-of-Life Decisions

The American Nurses Association (ANA) (1996) has developed position statements on the nurses' role in end-of-life decisions, including:

Nursing and the Patient Self-Determination Acts: The ANA believes that nurses should play a primary role in implementation of the Patient Self-Determination Act, passed as part of the Omnibus Budget Reconciliation Act of 1990. It is the responsibility of nurses to facilitate informed decision making for patients making choices about end-of-life care. The nurse's role in education, research, patient care and advocacy is critical to implementation of the Patient Self-Determination Act within all health care settings.

Promotion of Comfort and Relief of Pain in Dying Patients: Nurses should not hesitate to use full and effective doses of pain medication for the proper management of pain in the dying patient. The increasing titration of medication to achieve adequate symptom control, even at the expense of life, thus hastening death secondarily, is ethically justified.

Foregoing Nutrition and Hydration: The ANA believes that the decision to withhold artificial nutrition and hydration should be made by the patient or surrogate with the health care team. The nurse continues to provide expert care to patients who are no longer receiving artificial nutrition and hydration.

Nursing Care and Do-Not-Resuscitate Decisions: Nurses bear a large responsibility at the time a patient experiences cardiac arrest for either initiating resuscitation or ensuring that unwanted attempts to resuscitate do not occur. Nurses face ethical dilemmas concerning confusing or conflicting DNR orders and this statement includes specific recommendations for the resolution of some of these dilemmas.

Assisted Suicide: The ANA believes that the nurse should not participate in assisted suicide. Such an act is in violation of the *Code for Nurses with Interpretive Statements (Code for Nurses)* (ANA, 1985) and the ethical traditions of the profession. Nurses, individually and collectively, have an obligation to provide comprehensive and compassionate end-of-life care that includes the promotion of comfort and the relief of pain, and at times, foregoing life-sustaining treatments.

Active Euthanasia: The ANA believes that the nurse should not participate in active euthanasia because such an act is in direct violation of the *Code for Nurses with Interpretive Statements (Code for Nurses)*, the ethical traditions and goals of the profession, and its covenant with society. Nurses have an obligation to provide timely, humane, comprehensive and compassionate end-of-life care.

Note. From American Nurses Association. *Position Statements on the Nurse's Role in End-of-Life Decisions*, 1996, Washington, DC: Author. Retrieved August 3, 2004, from http://www.nursingworld.org. Reproduced with permission.

approach can serve as a beginning step toward improving end-of-life care and opportunities. With each patient encounter, consider the question "Would I be surprised if this patient died in the next few months?" Those who may be sick enough to die should be informed and counseled about possibilities to eliminate misconceptions and anxiety. Efforts should focus on prioritizing the patient's concerns, which may include symptom control, family support, and advanced-care planning or spiritual issues. To clearly understand the patient, the nurse should ask "What do you hope for as you live with this condition? What do you fear?" Patients should understand that it is often difficult to know when death is close and should be asked to contemplate "If you were to die soon, what would be left undone?" Prognostication can help providers and patients to focus on life yet to be lived and what can be done to make it better (Lynn, Schuster, & Kabcenell, 2000).

PATIENT–FAMILY ASSESSMENT

The number one priority in patient assessment in end-of-life care is to identify areas of suffering so that appropriate plans for symptom relief can be formulated and necessary interdisciplinary team members can be consulted, such as palliative-care specialists, psychiatric specialists, chaplains, or social workers. To ensure a holistic assessment, the American Medical Association's Education for Physicians on End of Life Care Curriculum (EPEC, 1999) has developed an assessment tool made up of nine dimensions. The assessment dimensions include illness/treatment summary, physical, psychological, decision making, communication, social, spiritual, practical, and anticipatory planning for death. A few of these dimensions will be addressed in detail.

Physical assessment in end-of-life care is primarily concerned with physical symptoms and how they impact on an individual's daily life and ability to function. There is less focus on physical assessment from an anatomic or organ system approach, because the major relevance in palliative care is the control of symptoms. Symptoms, such as pain, that are poorly managed will prevent patients from achieving quality of remaining life and participating in meaningful activities as end of life approaches. Some commonly encountered symptoms in advanced terminal illness are pain, fatigue, dyspnea, insomnia, anorexia, nausea, constipation, anxiety, depression, and delirium. Inquiry about each symptom is crucial. The patient's self-report and self-measurement of the intensity or severity of the symptom should be accepted, as these are subjective phenomena.

Performing a psychological assessment is essential to providing good care at end of life. Nurses may begin to make some notes at the beginning of the interview. Observations should be made about cognitive status, mood, and presence of any confusion or delirium and these should be addressed if noted. History should be gathered about past or present mood disorders. Screening questions about suicidal ideation may be appropriate. Assessing for anxiety, depression, and delirium is essential, with more in-depth assessments using validated tools. It is essential for the nurse to address common fears, such as loss of control, loss of dignity, loss of independence, loss of relationships, becoming a burden, and physical suffering. Individuals also commonly face unresolved issues in personal matters and relationships as end of life approaches. Sometimes these issues may prevent patients from achieving a peaceful frame of mind. Identification of these issues will allow for development of an individualized care plan. Referral should be considered in any situation in need of higher levels of psychiatric expertise, preferably to providers also skilled in end-of-life care.

Spiritual assessment is essential to understanding the role of religion in a patient's life and the resources that affiliation may bring.

Past spiritual involvement, as well as current desires, should be explored. Questioning should explore whether the patient would like a chaplain to visit, and whether there are any important religious rituals to honor. It should be recognized that some patients might experience significant spiritual growth at end of life, while others may struggle with spiritual distress. Spiritual crises may arise as people face death and begin to question the meaning and purpose in life. Patients may also question their faith, or express guilt and a desire for forgiveness. Others may feel abandoned by God. Spiritual needs may be assessed through questions such as "Are you a spiritual person?" "What role does religion play in your life?" "Have you thought about what will happen after you die?" or "Have you tried to make sense of what's happening to you?" The identification of spiritual suffering is crucial and enables obtaining appropriate religious support and resources for comprehensive spiritual care.

Assessment of decision-making capacity follows naturally from the psychological assessment. Even patients with some degree of mental compromise may show clear insight into information and may be able to give meaningful consent. To assess a patient's decision-making capacity, it must be determined whether the patient can understand that he is authorizing the decision, can demonstrate rational use of the information including risks, can demonstrate insight into the possible consequences of the decision, and that the decision is made without the influence of coercion. In the absence of capacity, an authorized proxy must decide on the patient's behalf using the patient's prior stated preferences or substituted judgment. Goals of care should be discussed with the patient and family so they may be tailored to matters of personal meaning. Patients may be asked, "What are the most important things to be accomplished?" Common responses may include aggressive symptom management or the desire to prolong life until an important event such as a family wedding or anniversary. Advanced-care planning for future medical care should also be addressed. Preferences should be discussed, preferably in the presence of the future proxy decision maker, in the event that there may be a time when the patient may not be able to make decisions for himself. Having already identified goals of care will make it easier for the patient to make decisions about future medical care that may or may not help him to achieve his goals.

▮ PAIN

Pain can be defined in many ways, though most succinctly it is "whatever the person says it is, experienced whenever they say they are experiencing it" (McCaffery & Pasero, 1999). It is a completely subjective experience and patient self-reports remain the only valid measure of pain. Some patients may not be able to report their pain, and in such cases it is acceptable to ask family and caregivers if they believe the person is in pain. Adequate relief of pain begins with comprehensive assessment. Assessment parameters should include pain history, onset, location, intensity, quality, pattern, aggravating or alleviating factors, medication history, and meaning of the pain to the patient. Whenever possible, it is best to ask patients to quantify pain severity with a validated tool such as a 0–10 intensity rating scale. A thorough medication history should be taken to determine what medications have already been tried, at what doses and timing intervals. Any report of allergic reaction to analgesics should be explored as true allergies are rare and the experience may have been a manageable side effect such as nausea. Physical examination should focus on nonverbal pain cues, inspection of site or sites of pain, palpation, auscultation, percussion, and focused neurological exam as needed, if there is suspicion for neuropathic pain and/or neurological compromise. Pharmacological principles and therapies are numerous and beyond the scope of this chapter.

THE DYING PROCESS

The art of nursing care includes the opportunity to be present when a patient is actively dying. This can be both a time of grief and sorrow, and a time of love and personal growth for all involved. As a patient's illness progresses and death nears, the focus of care changes. The philosophy of care shifts from living well and quality of life to the process of dying well. Physical, social, and spiritual needs will change, as the end of life grows closer. Pain and symptom management issues become more complex and involving hospice and palliative-care experts becomes essential to good end-of-life care.

It is often difficult for health care providers to recognize and acknowledge imminently approaching death. This may be a self-protective mechanism used by providers, patients, and families. However, in an era of technically disguised dying, the dying process may be surprisingly difficult to recognize (Dunn & Milch, 2002). One of the most reliable signs that a patient is dying is their own report. It is important for health care providers to pay close attention, as patients often allude to when they anticipate dying. Often patients who are very near death share having visions of people who have passed on waiting in the room. They may have conversations with people who are not visible. These experiences may be comforting to both patients and families at the end of life.

Although prognosticating when death will occur is often inaccurate, there are some predictable signs that death is nearing. Commonly, physical changes can assist patients and families in the preparation for death. Months before death may occur, patients may become more withdrawn. Patients may begin to decrease their food and fluid intake and require more sleep. When death draws closer, within days to weeks, patients commonly are profoundly weak, often becoming bedbound. At this point, patients become dependent with all care, including feeding and continence.

Additionally, patients may experience reduction in awareness, disinterest in food and fluids, and dysphagia. Patients' skin often becomes clammy and appearance changes from pale to mottled (Pitorak, 2003). Mottling, a sign that death is imminent, is secondary to decreases in the peripheral circulation. It is commonly seen first on the heels of the patient and over bony prominence. Agitation and restlessness in the final hours of life are common symptoms. This may be due to medications, electrolyte imbalances, organ failure, infections, or various other reasons (Pitorak, 2003). (See Table 19-1.)

TABLE 19-1 Changes Consistent with Death Approaching Within Weeks to Days
Progressive, profound weakness
Bedbound
Increased sleeping
Disinterest in food and fluids
Dysphagia
Weakening voice
Inability to close eyes
Incontinence
Oliguria
Diminished attention span
Vivid dreams
Reports of seeing previously deceased people
Speech content containing references to home or travel to a final destination

Changes Consistent with Death Approaching Within Hours

Cheyne-Stokes respirations
Apnea
Mottling
Cool skin
Restlessness, agitation
Death rattle
Hypotension
Tachycardia
No radial pulse

Note. Summarized from "Is This a Bad Day, or One of the Last Days? How to Respond to Approaching Demise," by G. Dunn and R. Milch, 2002. *Journal of American College of Surgeons, 196*(6), pp. 879–887.

Death vigils are an important opportunity for friends and families to begin the grieving process. Sitting at the bedside and being present can be the greatest gift to patients. Often time is spent sharing memories, telling stories, and touching the dying individual. Nurses should encourage and take part in death vigils when appropriate. It is believed that hearing is the last remaining sense, so continual communication with the dying patient should be encouraged, even when comatose. It is essential that discussions are held with patients and families prior to the dying process regarding where they wish to die, whom they would like present, and whether they would like to listen to music and, if so, what type. Immediately after the patient dies, it is important that the health care team allow time for family members and friends to spend with the patient's body.

▮▮▮ GRIEF AND BEREAVEMENT

Two very important aspects of end-of-life care are often overlooked. First, nursing care and responsibilities to the patient and family do not come to an end upon the death of the patient. Second, a bereavement needs assessment of the family and friends of the dying patient should ideally begin at the time of diagnosis, and continue throughout the course of the illness. Bereavement is the range of emotions and behavior a person experiences when he or she suffers a loss, particularly the death of another person. It consists of the grief a person feels and the outward expression of mourning exhibited. It occurs over the period of time that it takes to experience grief of the loss, and to adjust to life without the deceased. Grief is the emotional response or reaction that occurs as a result of the loss (Corliss, 2001; Egan & Arnold, 2003; Potter, 2001). All dying patients may feel loss due to many factors such as loss of physical control or function, loss of independence, loss of employment and finances, and eventually loss of life. Grief is often felt by patients and families in response to these losses and in response to approaching death. Grief and bereavement are normal, individualized experiences and processes. Resolution of grief is often dependent upon support and resources available to aid in dealing with grief. Bereavement care should be offered to friends and family before death to increase support and information in order to try to prevent complicated grief and bereavement (Egan & Arnold, 2003).

There are various types of grief and nurses should be able to assess for and determine the type, in order to implement appropriate interventions. Anticipatory grief usually occurs before a loss, such as at the time of diagnosis. It may occur in response to anticipated or actual loss of health, function, or independence. Anticipatory grief may provide some benefits such as providing time for acknowledgment of death, preparation for death, adaptation to change that will occur over the course of an illness, and resolution of conflicts.

Normal or uncomplicated grief is characterized by expected emotional and behavioral responses to a loss. Responses to loss may be physical, psychological, cognitive, or spiritual. The responses will vary widely among individuals in terms of coping strategies, expressions, and behaviors. They are influenced by past experience with loss and death, and cultural and social factors (Clements et al., 2003; Corliss, 2001).

Complicated grief may occur if reactions persist over long periods of time, are overwhelming or interfere with physical or emotional well-being. Some manifestations of complicated grief include severe or prolonged depression, suicidal ideation, extreme isolation, or avoidance of any reminder of the deceased. Some risk factors for complicated grief include sudden or traumatic death, multiple losses, unresolved grief from earlier losses, suffering at end of life by the loved one, lack of supports, and lack of faith beliefs.

Complicated grief may be further subdivided into chronic, delayed, exaggerated, masked, and disenfranchised grief. Chronic grief may begin as normal grief, but persists over an excessively long period of time. Delayed grief occurs when normal grief reactions are suppressed or postponed, either consciously or subconsciously, to avoid the pain of the loss. Exaggerated grief is characterized by the use of potentially harmful coping strategies or self-destructive behavior in attempt to alleviate pain. It may manifest as substance abuse, suicidal ideation or attempts, or unsafe sex practices. Masked grief results when a person is unaware that his ability to function normally is being affected by his response to loss. Manifestations may include maintaining physical distance, avoiding relationships, and rejecting help (Arnold & Egan, 2004; Ferris, Von Gunten, & Emanuel, 2003). Disenfranchised grief occurs when a loss has been experienced and cannot be openly acknowledged or shared because the relationship has not been accepted by or revealed to family or friends. People who may be at risk for this type of grief include gay and lesbian partners. It is often manifested as anger, sadness, and isolation (Egan & Arnold, 2003).

Nursing assessment of grief should include the patient, family, significant others, friends, and professional caregivers, such as nursing home or home care staff. Ideally, it should start at the time of diagnosis of serious illness and should continue throughout the course of the illness. Following the death of the patient, it should extend into the bereavement period for the survivors. Following assessment, bereavement interventions should be implemented to facilitate the grieving process. This should start with helping survivors to recognize that grief is a normal response and that there is no standard or "right" way to grieve. It is helpful for survivors to understand that symptoms of grief that they may be experiencing are expected, such as trouble sleeping or concentrating or sudden waves of sadness or emotion. Education should include information such as the fact that grieving may go on for months to years and may become more intense or resurface on significant dates such as holidays, birthdays, or the anniversary of the death (Egan & Arnold, 2003). Nursing interventions should include facilitation of identification and expression of feelings, which may help survivors manage stress and deal with the emotional pain that is a necessary component of grief. Facilitation of and participation in funerals, memorial services, or other rituals are important bereavement interventions to help survivors acknowledge the death and memorialize their loved one (Arnold & Egan, 2004).

There are generally four tasks that the bereaved must complete in order to deal with their loss in an effective manner. The first task involves realizing and accepting that the loss or death has actually occurred. Second, it is important that they are able to experience the pain that the loss has caused. Third, they need to acknowledge how the loss is significant to them and how it is going to impact their lives. Finally, as grief evolves, they need to be able to concentrate their energy into new relationships and activities. Although these tasks may seem simple to approach, they can be extremely difficult for emotionally overwhelmed, grieving individuals without appropriate support from caregivers, friends and family (Ferris, Von Gunten, & Emanuel, 2003).

FUTURE END-OF-LIFE CARE

The future of end-of-life care remains ever-changing. End-of-life care will become more significant as our population ages. The trend will continue to change from dying in hospital settings to dying in homes, nursing homes, and various other settings. Curative interventions will be developed and terminal illnesses may transition to chronic illnesses. While the medical community searches for a quick fix to our inevitable mortality through the discovery of miracle cures for terminal illness, little discussion takes place about the alternatives for care of persons who will not survive their disease, known as palliative care (Walsh & Gordon, 2001). Palliative care must become a health care priority, and public policy and health care funding must be redirected to respond (Walsh & Gordon, 2001). This includes more research to guide pain and symptom management, and quality end-of-life care.

As we begin the 21st century, health care providers are all faced with many challenges within the health care system. A major challenge ahead is the rapidly growing population of aging, chronically, and terminally ill people in the United States. Americans are living longer in general and living longer with complex, debilitating illness. As a result, there is an increased need for specialized pain and symptom control and complex care discussions and planning. A challenge in meeting this need is the scarcity of health care providers with the expertise required providing this level of care. The "Promoting Excellence in End-of-Life Care" national program of the Robert Wood Johnson Foundation (2002), "dedicated to long-term changes in health care to improve care of the dying and their families" (para. 11), has examined this issue and recognizes that nurses, and especially advanced practice nurses with expertise in palliative care, represent a crucial resource for meeting the needs of chronically and terminally ill Americans and their families.

REFERENCES

Amella, E. (2003). Geriatrics and palliative care: Collaboration for quality of life until death. *Journal of Hospice and Palliative Nursing, 5*(1), 40–48.

American Academy of Hospice and Palliative Medicine (AAHPM). (2003). *Pocket guide to hospice/palliative medicine.* Glenview, IL: Author.

American Academy of Hospice and Palliative Medicine (2001). Position statement: Statement on the use of nutrition and hydration. Retrieved December 24, 2004, from http://www.aahpm.org/positions/nutrition.html

American Nurses Association. (1985). *Code for nurses with interpretive statements.* Kansas City, MO: Author.

American Nurses Association. (1996). *Position statements on the nurse's role in end-of-life decisions.* Washington, DC: Author.

Anderson, R., & Smith, B. (2003). Deaths: Leading causes for 2001. *U.S. Department of Health and Human Services; National Vital Statistics Report, 52*(9), 1–10.

Arnold, R. & Egan, K. (2004). Suffering, loss, grief, and bereavement. In M. Matzo & D. Sherman (Eds.), *Gerontologic pallative care nursing* (pp. 148–164). St. Louis, MO: C.V. Mosby.

Bennett, J. A. (2000). Dehydration: Hazards and benefits. *Geriatric Nursing, 21*(2), 84–88.

Berry, P., & Matzo, M. (2004). Death and an aging society. In M. Matzo & D. Sherman (Eds.), *Gerontologic palliative care nursing* (pp. 31–51). St. Louis, MO: C.V. Mosby.

Bookbinder, M., & Kiss, M. (2001). Death and society. In M. Matzo & D. Sherman (Eds.), *Palliative care nursing: Quality care to the end of life* (pp. 89–117). New York: Springer.

Buttersworth, A. M. (2003). Reality check: Ten barriers to advanced care planning. *The Nurse Practitioner, 28*(5), 42–43.

Byock, I. (1997). *Dying well: Peace and possibilities at the end of life.* New York: Berkley.

Cherny, N. I., Coyle, N., & Foley, K. M. (1996). Guidelines in the care of the dying cancer patient. *Hematology/Oncology Clinics of North America, 10*(1), 261–287.

Christakis, N. (1999). *Death foretold: Prophecy and prognosis in medical care.* Chicago: University of Chicago Press.

Clements, P., Vigil, G., Manno, M., Henry, G., Wilks, J., Das, S., et al. (2003). Cultural perspectives of death, grief, and bereavement. *Journal of

Psychosocial Nursing and Mental Health Services, 41(7), 18–26.

Corliss, I. (2001). Bereavement. In B. Ferrell & N. Coyle (Eds.), *Textbook of palliative nursing* (pp. 352–362). New York: Oxford University Press.

Cranston, R. E. (2001). Advanced directives and do not resuscitate orders. Retrieved December 22, 2003, from http://www.cbhd.org/resources/endoflife/cranston_2001-12-14.htm

Dunn, G., & Milch, R. (2002). Is this a bad day, or one of the last days? How to recognize and respond to approaching demise. *Journal of American College of Surgeons, 195*(6), 879–887.

Education for Physicians on End-of-Life Care Curriculum (EPEC). (1999). *Whole patient assessment. Trainer's guide.* Chicago: American Medical Association.

Egan, K., & Arnold, R. (2003). Grief and bereavement care: With sufficient support, grief and bereavement can be transformative. *American Journal of Nursing, 103*(9), 42–52.

Egan, K., & Labyak, M. (2001). Hospice care: A model for quality end-of-life care. In B. Ferrell & N. Coyle (Eds.), *Textbook of palliative nursing* (pp. 7–26). New York: Oxford University Press.

Ferrell, B., Virani, R., & Grant, M. (1999). Analysis of end-of-life content in nursing textbooks. *Oncology Nursing Forum, 26,* 869–876.

Ferris, F., Von Gunten, C., & Emanuel, L. (2003). Competency in end-of-life care. *Journal of Palliative Medicine, 6*(4), 605–613.

Field, M., & Cassel, C. (Eds.). (1997). *Approaching death: Improving care at the end of life.* Committee on Care at the End of Life, Division of Health Care Services, Institute of Medicine. Washington, DC: National Academy Press.

Fox, E. T. (1996). IV hydration in the terminally ill: Ritual or therapy. *British Journal of Nursing, 5*(1), 41–45.

Gordon, M. (2003). CPR in long-term care: Mythical benefits or necessary ritual? *Annals of Long-Term Care, 11*(4), 41–49.

Grant, K. D. (1992). The Patient Self-Determination Act: Implications for physicians. *Hospital Practice, 27*(44), 44–48.

Hospice and Palliative Nurses Association. (2003). *Position statement on artificial nutrition and hydration.* Retrieved June 23, 2003, from http://www.hpna.org/position_artificialnutrition

Huffman, J. L., & Dunn, G. P. (2002). The paradox of hydration in advanced terminal illness. *Journal of American College of Surgeons, 194*(6), 835–839.

Krisman-Scott, M. (2003). Origins of hospice in the United States. *Journal of Hospice and Palliative Nursing, 5*(4), 205–210.

Kubler-Ross, E. (1969). *On death and dying.* New York: Macmillan.

Lamont, E., & Siegler, M. (2000). Paradoxes in cancer patients' advanced care planning. *Journal of Palliative Medicine, 3*(1), 27–35.

Lynn, J., Schuster, J., & Kabcenell, A. (2000). *Improving care for the end of life: A sourcebook for health care managers and clinicians.* New York: Oxford University Press.

McCaffery, M., & Pasero, C., (1999). *Pain clinical manual.* (2nd ed.). St. Louis, MO: C.V. Mosby.

Meares, C. J. (1994). Terminal dehydration: A review. *American Journal of Hospice and Palliative Care, 11*(3), 10–14.

Omnibus Reconciliation Act of 1990. (Publication No. 101-508, Sect. 4206, 4751)

Pitorak, E. F. (2003). Care at the time of death. *American Journal of Nursing, 103*(7), 42–52.

Potter, M. (2001). Loss, suffering, bereavement, and grief. In M. Matzo & D. Sherman (Eds.), *Palliative care nursing: Quality care to the end of life* (pp. 275–321). New York: Springer.

Promoting Excellence in End of Life Care (2002). *A position statement from American nursing leaders: Recommendations.* Retrieved August 3, 2004, from http://www.PromotingExcellence.org

Rabow, M., Hardie, G., Fair, J., & McPhee, S. (2000). End-of-life care content in 50 textbooks from multiple specialties. *Journal of the American Medical Association, 283,* 771–778.

Schlegel, K. L., & Shannon, S. E. (2000). Legal guidelines related to end-of-life decisions: Are nurse practitioners knowledgeable? *Journal of Gerontological Nursing, 26*(9), 14–24.

Sherman, D., & Laporte, M. (2001). Palliative care nursing: Changing the experience of dying in

America. In M. Matzo & D. Sherman (Eds.), *Palliative care nursing: Quality care to the end of life* (pp. xvii–xxiv). New York: Springer.

Super, A. (2001). The context of palliative care in progressive illness. In B. Ferrell & N. Coyle (Eds.), *Textbook of palliative nursing* (pp. 27–36). New York: Oxford University Press.

SUPPORT Principal Investigators. (1995). A controlled trial to improve care for seriously ill hospitalized patients: The Study to Understand Prognoses and Preferences for Outcomes and Risks of Treatments (SUPPORT). *Journal of the American Medical Association*, 274(20), 1591–1598.

Sutcliffe, J. (1994). Terminal dehydration. *Nursing Times*, 90(6), 60–63.

U.S. Living Will Registry (2000). U.S. Living Will Registry helps hospitals educate public about advance directives. Retrieved December 27, 2004, from www.livingwillregistry.com/pr_hospital.shtm

Walsh, D., & Gordon, S. (2001). The terminally ill: Dying for palliative medicine? *American Journal of Hospice and Palliative Care*, 18(3), 203–205.

Zerwekh, J. V. (1983). The dehydration question. *Nursing*, 13(1), 46–51.

CHAPTER 20

Social, Health, and Long-Term Care Programs and Policies Affecting Mental Health in Older Adults

Kathy J. Fabiszewski, PhD, APRN, BC

INTRODUCTION

Mental health is the successful performance of mental function, resulting in productive activities, fulfilling relationships with other people, and the ability to adapt to change and to cope with adversity; from early childhood until late life, mental health is the springboard of thinking and communication skills, learning, emotional growth, resilience, and self-esteem (Satcher, 2000, p. 89).

Mental health is an essential part of overall health. Older adults suffer from many of the same mental disorders as their younger counterparts. However, the prevalence, nature, and course of each disorder might be very different in older adults and assessment and management strategies are complicated by medical comorbidities, inadequate social support systems, and controversial health policy issues. Millions of older Americans—the frail elderly, disabled and chronically ill persons, and mentally ill individuals—have difficulty living fully independent lives. Studies have shown that older individuals with chronic health conditions, such as heart disease, cancer, and arthritis, have better outcomes and treatment compliance if co-occurring mental health disorders are identified and treated

effectively (Lantz, 2002; Lin et al., 2003). This chapter discusses social, health, and long-term care programs and policies affecting mental health in older adults.

ROLE OF THE PROFESSIONAL NURSE

Nurses have become increasingly involved not only in the clinical assessment and management of mental health issues of older adults but also in affecting health policy change. As the demographics of aging populations evolve, professional nursing remains responsive to the needs and demands for health care in the fastest growing segment of our population, the oldest-old. The number of Americans that are expected to be age 65 and older in the year 2020 is estimated to be about 50 million—one in five Americans, or 20% of the population. The number of Americans age 85 and over was 2.7 million in 1985 and is projected to increase to over 7 million by 2020 (NIA, 1993). As many as 58% of Americans between the ages of 75 and 89 may be affected by Alzheimer's disease (Hebert, Scherr, Bienias, Bennett, & Evans, 2003); 20% of older adults suffer from some sort of anxiety; and approximately 1% are diagnosed with schizophrenia (NIA, 1993). In upholding the *Standards of Gerontological Nursing Practice* (ANA, 2001) and the *Standards of Advanced Practice Registered Nursing* (ANA, 1996), professional nurses engaged in gerontological practice are expected to "identify the settings in which services may be safely and appropriately delivered" to the older adult and "propose alternatives for continuity of care for long-term needs" (ANA, 2001, p. 15).

The need for effective and humane policy that will guide the design and delivery of mental health care for all age groups and generations at the local, state, and national levels has long been recognized in the profession of nursing. There is a desire and a need for many changes but the financing, delivery, regulation, and evaluation of implemented social and mental health programs and services create another dimension of health care for nursing scrutiny. From this scrutiny many policy questions arise including:

- Does the current reimbursement system adequately provide for older citizens with mental illness? In the community? In institutions?

- To what extent do mental health care programs and private third-party payers cover the services of nurses?

- To what extent is the quality and cost of primary and mental health care delivered by nurses comparable to that of other providers?

- What lessons can be learned about the impact of state variations in Medicaid reimbursement rates and mental health outcomes in older adults?

Policy making for persons with mental illness is a very challenging process because sociocultural, environmental, and even geographic factors weigh so heavily on how the illness is experienced and how life experiences shape what is believed to be the best approach to care and treatment. Policies that address this parity are needed but are only one piece of a very complex and convoluted puzzle (Smoyak, 2000). Nurses interested in client advocacy should be aware of the emerging issues that challenge their best efforts and must continue finding ways to meet client's needs even when policies seem to make this impossible (Edmunds, 2003). Cognizance of the strengths and weaknesses in the mental health system and savvy in educating and advocating for clients attempting to access care and services enhances nursing's posture. The politically dynamic nurse no longer uncritically accepts mediocrity, the status quo, simply because of knowledge about skyrocketing health care costs. Nurses know that reform is badly needed. Unfortunately reforms are often driven and shaped by economic and political considerations and not by coherent, internally consistent health care policy.

▬ FEDERAL PROGRAMS SUPPORTING AND FINANCING MENTAL HEALTH CARE

The federal government provides an extensive range of programs that support and finance mental health care to meet the complex needs of adults with serious mental illnesses. Unfortunately, the responsibility for these programs is scattered across many departments and agencies, resulting in the "layering on" of multiple, well-intentioned programs without overall direction, coordination, or consistency (President's New Freedom Commission on Mental Health, 2003). An integrated system that effectively addresses the needs of people with mental illnesses, especially older adults who may coexperience physical frailty, functional impairment, and financial limitation, must include a comprehensive range of mental health services including ancillary supports such as housing, education, substance abuse treatment, income support, and other basic services. Mental health care utilization and Medicare expenditures have changed over recent years including a 136% increase in Medicare Part B payments between 1987 and 1992 (Rosenbach & Ammering, 1997). Yet, the lack of federal program focus on adults, and in particular older adults, with serious mental illnesses has resulted in a mental health system that is severely fragmented and uncoordinated because of the underlying structural, financial, and organizational inconsistencies or conflicts that exist in the programs that support it (President's New Freedom Commission on Mental Health, 2003).

Furthermore, there is a paucity of programs targeted specifically to meeting the needs of older adults with mental health problems. "The tragic consequences of system fragmentation and service gaps have produced unnecessary human suffering, disability, homelessness, criminalization of mental illnesses, and other severe consequences" (President's New Freedom Commission on Mental Health, 2003, p. i). Some have portrayed federal programs as isolated funding streams that are difficult or impossible to coordinate, generating a large administrative burden for state and local agency and provider staff, and denying consumers and family members access to integrated and essential services (President's New Freedom Commission on Mental Health).

The financing of mental health care amounts to at least $80 billion annually in the United States (U.S. Surgeon General, 1999). Sources of funding include Medicaid, Medicare, the Department of Veterans Affairs (DVA), state agencies, local agencies, foundations, and private insurance. Unfortunately, each source of funding of mental health care has its own complex, sometimes contradictory, set of rules. Taken as a whole, the system is supposed to function in a coordinated manner; it is supposed to deliver optimal treatments, services, and supports—but it

often falls short (President's New Freedom Commission on Mental Health, 2003).

Over 40 programs exist in the federal program armamentarium to support and finance mental health care in general. Those programs specifically targeting mental health and older adults are displayed in Table 20-1. Each program varies in terms of who or what entity is eligible to receive funds, the allowable uses of funds, the application process, the payment methodology, and funding requirements or limitations. Some programs provide grants to states, localities, private providers, and/or public providers; others offer direct services or funds/income directly to individuals; and others are flexible so that funds can be distributed to either entities or individuals. "Despite the existence of many federal programs, all too often federal funds are unavailable to meet even the most basic needs of consumers and families" (President's New Freedom Commission on Mental Health, 2003, p. ii). There is a consensus among providers, advocates, and policymakers that the system could improve. The following are descriptions of the few social, health, and long-term care programs among the 40 that have direct applicability to older adults with mental illness (President's New Freedom Commission on Mental Health).

Administration on Aging: State and Community Programs

The Older Americans Act authorizes a range of programs that offer services and opportunities for older Americans, especially those at risk of losing their independence. Under Title III, State and Community Programs, the Administration on Aging (AoA) works closely with its nationwide network on aging composed of Regional Offices, State Agencies on Aging, and Area Agencies on Aging, to plan, coordinate, and develop community-level systems of services designed to assist older persons at risk of losing their independence.

TABLE 20-1   Sample of Major Federal Programs Supporting and Financing Mental Health Care for Older Adults

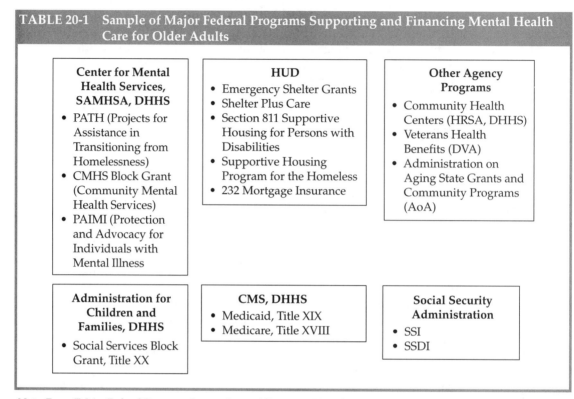

Center for Mental Health Services, SAMHSA, DHHS	HUD	Other Agency Programs
• PATH (Projects for Assistance in Transitioning from Homelessness) • CMHS Block Grant (Community Mental Health Services) • PAIMI (Protection and Advocacy for Individuals with Mental Illness	• Emergency Shelter Grants • Shelter Plus Care • Section 811 Supportive Housing for Persons with Disabilities • Supportive Housing Program for the Homeless • 232 Mortgage Insurance	• Community Health Centers (HRSA, DHHS) • Veterans Health Benefits (DVA) • Administration on Aging State Grants and Community Programs (AoA)
Administration for Children and Families, DHHS	**CMS, DHHS**	**Social Security Administration**
• Social Services Block Grant, Title XX	• Medicaid, Title XIX • Medicare, Title XVIII	• SSI • SSDI

Note. From "Major Federal Programs Supporting and Financing Mental Health Care," adapted from the President's New Freedom Commission on Mental Health, 2003. Retrieved December 1, 2003, from http://www.mentalhealthcommission.gov/reports/reports/htm

The AoA awards Title III funds to 57 state Agencies on Aging, based on the number of older persons residing in the state, to plan, develop, and coordinate systems of supportive in-home and community-based services for older persons. States receive funds on a formula grant basis. All individuals age 60 and over are eligible for services, although priority is given to those with the greatest economic and social need with particular attention to low-income minority older persons. There are no mandatory fees for services. Older persons are, however, encouraged to contribute to help defray the costs of services. Core service activities include:

1. Supportive services
   - Access services (transportation, outreach, information and assistance, and case management)
   - In-home services (homemaker and home health aides, chore maintenance, and supportive services for families of older individuals with Alzheimer's disease)
   - Community services (adult day care, legal assistance, and recreation)
2. Congregate and home-delivered meals
3. In-home services for frail elderly
4. Disease prevention and health promotion services

- Support public health and educational organizations, community-based agencies, hospitals and medical institutions, and senior centers

Area Agencies on Aging may be contacted for information and referral to services for older adults in the community. In addition, a nationwide toll-free hotline may be found at www.aoa.gov that provides information about assistance for older individuals anywhere in the nation (Administration on Aging, 2003).

Community Health Centers

CHCs provide primary and preventive health care services to people living in rural and urban medically underserved communities where economic, geographic, or cultural barriers limit access to primary health care for a substantial portion of the population. Major CHC activities include provision of:

- Primary and preventive health care
- Outreach
- Pharmacy services
- Linkage to other services such as welfare income assistance, Medicaid, mental health, substance abuse treatment, and nutrition programs
- Specialty care services, including mental health services

CHCs deliver care regardless of clients' ability to pay. Charges for health care services are income-based, with services to the poorest clients provided at no cost.

The Health Resources and Services Administration (HRSA) assists in the preparation of program applications, providing consultation about grants administration and managing the grant process. The method of payment is direct grants from HRSA to CHC grantees.

Community Mental Health Block Grants

The Community Mental Health Services Block Grant is the single largest federal contribution dedicated toward improving mental health service systems in the United States. It is a formula grant to states to support delivery of a broad range of community mental health services determined by the individual states. While there are no provisions requiring tailored outreach to the older adult, this program supports comprehensive, community-based systems of care for adults with serious mental illnesses and represents the major federal effort to work in partnership with the states to plan and deliver state-of-the-art systems of community-based mental health services for adults.

HUD Section 232: Mortgage Insurance for Board and Care, Assisted-Living, and Other Facilities

HUD Section 232 provides government-backed mortgage loan insurance to facilitate both the construction and rehabilitation, acquisition, or refinancing of nursing homes, intermediate care facilities, board and care homes, assisted-living, and other facilities. "Eligible mortgage borrowers include investors, builders, developers, public entities, and private nonprofit corporations and associations" (President's New Freedom Commission on Mental Health, 2003, p. 8). Eligible residents under HUD Section 232 must require skilled nursing, custodial care, assistance with activities of daily living, or be eligible to live in facilities insured under this program.

Medicaid (Title XIX)

Medicaid (Title XIX of the Social Security Act) is 56 jointly administered state–federal welfare entitlement programs that provide medical care and medically related services to the most vulnerable populations. Although the

Centers for Medicare and Medicaid Services (CMS) officially preside over Medicaid, each state has a different Medicaid formula for benefits and for the rates of federal reimbursement. Since each state administers its Medicaid program under federal guidelines, and since latitude is provided to the states in the design of their Medicaid programs, each program has different eligibility standards, benefit packages, and reimbursement rates. Medicaid programs provide: (1) health insurance for low-income families and for disabled individuals (those eligible for Supplemental Security Income [SSI]); (2) long-term care (community-based or institutional) for older adults and disabled individuals; and (3) supplemental copayment coverage for low-income Medicare beneficiaries (dual eligibility). Payment methodologies may vary and are state determined based on broad federal limits. Beneficiaries may make nominal copayments.

Medicaid provides a comprehensive package of health insurance benefits for eligible persons. In general, each state must cover 10 categories of "mandatory services" identified in statute, such as inpatient and outpatient hospital services, physician or advanced practice nurse (APN) services, laboratory and radiology services, and nursing facility services. In addition, states have the discretion to cover one or more of up to 33 "optional services" under Medicaid including case management services, personal care services, transportation services, prescription drugs, and a variety of professional services (including psychologist services) (President's New Freedom Commission on Mental Health, 2003).

While some mental health services are included among the "mandatory services" (e.g., limited outpatient mental health services and inpatient psychiatric care) required by federal law, most community-based mental health services are among the various "optional services" that states may choose to include in their Medicaid programs. Optional mental

health services that states may provide include care by a psychologist, clinic services, and inpatient hospital and nursing facility services for individuals 65 years of age and over in an institution for mental diseases, case management services, and community-supported living arrangements. In practice, since states have primary responsibility for the care and financing of persons with severe mental illness, most states have made extensive use of optional Medicaid benefits to provide services for the mentally ill population. In addition, some state Medicaid programs provide mental health services through contracts with managed care organizations (MCOs) (Centers for Medicare and Medicaid Services, 2004).

Medicaid is the third largest source of health insurance in the United States behind Medicare and employer-sponsored coverage. It is the largest source of funding for medical and health-related services for people with limited income (Center for Medicare and Medicaid Services, 2004). Combined federal and state Medicaid expenditures accounted for 20% of all mental health spending in 1997. Currently, 35 million Americans are eligible for Medicaid benefits. In 1998, persons who were aged, blind, or disabled accounted for 26% of all Medicaid beneficiaries, but 71% of all program expenditures. Most of the Medicaid payments for older adults are for the small portion of the population that requires long-term institutional care (President's New Freedom Commission on Mental Health, 2003).

Medicare (Title XVIII)

As part of the Social Security Amendments of 1965, Medicare legislation established a national health insurance program for older adults to complement the retirement, survivors, and disability insurance benefits provided under other titles of the Social Security Act (Melillo, 1996). Medicare is administered nationally by the Centers for Medicare and

Medicaid Services (CMS). Medicare is a broad but limited package of health insurance benefits for: (1) persons aged 65 and older, (2) severely disabled persons under age 65 (Social Security Disability Insurance [SSDI] definition), and (3) people of any age with end-stage renal disease (ESRD). It provides acute care to older adults and the disabled regardless of income. Unlike Medicaid, Medicare has national eligibility, coverage, and reimbursement standards. The program offers two basic choices to enrollees: (1) Standard Medicare, also known as the Original Medicare Plan (traditional or fee-for-service Medicare); and (2) Medicare + Choice (which includes Managed Medicare Care Plan and Medicare Private Fee-for-Service Options). Standard Medicare is offered nationwide and comprises two parts:

- Part A (Hospital Insurance) provides hospital insurance that helps pay for most inpatient care as well as care in skilled nursing facilities (SNFs), hospice care, and some home health care. Most people with any work history do not have to pay for Part A benefits.

- Part B (Supplementary Medical Insurance) is optional and provides medical insurance that helps pay for physician/APN services, outpatient hospital care, and some medical services not covered by Part A. Most enrollees pay a monthly premium of $66.60 (in 2004) for coverage (Medicare, n.d.)

Many beneficiaries with Standard Medicare electively purchase Medigap insurance. Medigap insurance covers expenses not reimbursed by Part A or B. Persons eligible for Medicare with low incomes or assets may also qualify for Medicaid coverage. Such beneficiaries are categorized as being *dual-eligible*.

Medicare + Choice plans are offered in many but not all areas of the country. Within Medicare + Choice plans, each participating health care organization receives a capitated payment or predetermined lump sum from Medicare for the health care services for each enrolled beneficiary (usually paid per member per month), regardless of the number of health care encounters the client requires. Providers establish their own payment agreements with the health plans. Beneficiaries pay monthly premiums as well as nominal copayments for services. The capitation method of payment introduces flexibility in the financing and delivery of care that is not present under the fee-for-services method. In Medicare + Choice plans, the Medicare benefit becomes a floor rather than a ceiling of coverage (HMO Workgroup on Care Management, 1998). That is, the same benefits and coverage rules that apply to fee-for-service enrollees apply, but additional benefits, over and above what Standard Medicare covers, such as outpatient prescription drugs, hearing aids, and other services may also be provided. Capitated payments provide an incentive to avoid expensive services, particularly inpatient admissions, by encouraging early identification of health problems among patients. For example: the resources devoted to screening and self-care may reduce the use of a hospital, and transportation to obtain outpatient mental health care costs less in a taxi or van than in an ambulance, particularly when the destination is a health care provider's office rather than an emergency room (HMO Workgroup on Care Management, 1998).

Standard Medicare covers outpatient, inpatient, and partial hospitalization benefits for mental health care. Medicare pays for mental health services provided by certain specialty providers such as psychiatrists, psychiatric advanced practice nurses (both clinical nurse specialists and nurse practitioners), clinical psychologists, and clinical social workers (Centers for Medicare and Medicaid Services, 2003). Unfortunately, "most outpatient mental health services are subject to higher beneficiary copayments than other outpatient care (50/50 copayments for mental health versus 80/20 for other covered benefits). Inpatient mental health care is limited to a lifetime maximum of 190 days of care in a specialty psychiatric hospital" (President's New Freedom Commission on Mental Health, 2003, p. 52). Under certain circumstances, partial hospitalization is covered as an outpatient service for seriously ill beneficiaries who would otherwise require hospitalization (Centers for Medicare and Medicaid Services, 2004).

The Chronic Care Improvement (CCI) Program is a component of the Medicare Modernization Act of 2003 that represents the first large-scale chronic care initiative aimed at improving and strengthening Standard Medicare. In this program the CMS will select organizations to offer coordinated care to hundreds of thousands of chronically ill Medicare beneficiaries. The objectives of the program include not only collaboration with participants' providers to enhance communication of relevant clinical information but also to increase adherence to evidenced-based care, reduce unnecessary hospital stays and emergency room visits, and help enrollees avoid costly and debilitating comorbidities and complications. While initially the program will focus on those older and disabled adults with medical conditions such as congestive heart failure, diabetes, and chronic obstructive pulmonary disease, other prevalent entities that pose a high risk of experiencing poor clinical and financial outcomes such as depression, substance abuse, dementia, and other age-related psychiatric conditions will ultimately be targeted for inclusion in the initiative (Centers for Medicare and Medicaid Services, 2004).

Medicare is a major payer in the United States health care system. In 2000, approximately 39.6 million persons were enrolled in Medicare. Of all Medicare beneficiaries in 2000, only 5.4 million (13.6%) were disabled persons under age 65; 6.2 million (15.7%) were enrolled in Medicare + Choice plans; and approximately 6 million were dually eligible for Medicare and Medicaid (Medicare, n.d.).

Medicare accounts for approximately 28% of all hospital and 20% of all health care provider payments. It also covers 45% of health care spending for older adults overall, but less for the oldest-old, who require more nursing home care (U.S. Surgeon General, DHHS, 1999). Unlike Medicaid, Medicare does not pay for long-term care—either in the community or in an institutional-based setting when care is primarily used for assisting patients with activities of daily living that could be provided by informal or nonprofessional caregivers.

"In FY 1997, total mental health expenditures for Medicare beneficiaries were $9.0 billion. According to an American Association of Retired Persons (AARP) funded report, 45% of total Medicare mental health expenditures are for disabled beneficiaries under age 65, who comprise 12% of all beneficiaries. While women represent 60% of all beneficiaries age 65 and older, they receive 68–73% of outpatient mental health services, depending upon the specific service delivery site" (President's New Freedom Commission on Mental Health, 2003, p. 53).

As part of the Medicare Prescription Drug, Improvement, and Modernization Act of 2003, beginning in mid-2004, Medicare beneficiaries can enroll in the Medicare-approved Prescription Drug Discount Program (PDDP). In this program, designed to offer interim relief to older adults until the full Medicare prescription drug benefit goes into effect in 2006, private pharmaceutical and insurance companies offer discount cards to Medicare enrollees. The private companies decide which drugs will be discounted and the amount of the discount. As of May 1, 2004 there were 36 national discount cards and 35 cards only to be used in certain states, available for a $30 program enrollment fee (for those not meeting low-income qualifications). Single older adults with an annual income of less than $12,569 or married individuals with an income of less than $16,862 may qualify to enroll in the program at no charge. In addition, some low-income seniors may qualify to receive a $600 prescription drug credit from Medicare. Some cards offer a substantial discount on one drug, but no discount on another; other cards offer substantial discounts, but may not utilize pharmacies near the beneficiaries' home. Each Medicare enrollee can only sign up for one card, and may not switch from one card to another, so it is important that the one card that best meets an older adult's needs be selected. While high out-of-pocket prescription drug spending by Medicare beneficiaries with medical and psychiatric illness without drug coverage has been a long-standing health policy concern, the complexity of the PDDP may pose an overwhelming obstacle for some older adults, especially those with cognitive impairment or mental illness. Only modest savings for beneficiaries without drug coverage, such as an average savings of 17.4% over current retail prices, is predicted (Cubanski, Frank, & Epstein, 2004).

PATH (Projects for Assistance in Transition from Homelessness)

Of the 600,000 Americans who are homeless on any given night, an estimated 33% have serious mental illnesses and more than half have alcohol- or drug-related problems (President's New Freedom Commission on Mental Health, 2003). PATH was established in 1990 to address the multiple needs of people who are homeless and mentally ill. It provides formula grants to states and territories, which are required to match funds with $1 for every $3 received in federal funds. PATH develops innovative programs for persons with mental illness who are homeless. Services such as outreach, screening and diagnosis, rehabilitation, community mental health treatment, case management, and limited housing assistance are available to individuals with severe mental illness including those with co-occurring substance abuse disorders who are homeless or at risk of becoming homeless. Individual states and territories determine the payment methodology.

PAIMI (Protection and Advocacy for Individuals with Mental Illness)

PAIMI state formula grants support Protection and Advocacy (P&A) systems designated by the governor of each state to protect and to advocate for the rights of persons diagnosed with a significant mental illness or emotional impairment. Grants support P&A systems to pursue administrative, legal, and legislative activities or other remedies to redress complaints of abuse, neglect, and civil rights violations.

Service beneficiaries include those who are:

- Diagnosed with a significant mental illness or emotional impairment by a mental health professional

- Inpatients or residents in public or private residential facilities that provide care or treatment to individuals with mental illness

- Residents in a community-based setting, including their home

- Abused, neglected, or had their rights violated or were in danger of abuse, neglect, or rights violations while receiving care or treatment in a public or private residential facility (President's New Freedom Commission on Mental Health, 2003).

Social Services Block Grant (Title XX)

"The Social Services Block Grant (SSBG) program provides formula grants to states for the provision of social services directed at achieving economic self-support or self-sufficiency, preventing or remedying neglect, abuse, or the exploitation of adults, preventing or reducing inappropriate institutionalization, and securing referral for institutional care, where appropriate" (President's New Freedom Commission on Mental Health, 2003, p. 60). SSBG allocations are determined by a statutory formula based on each state's population. States are fully responsible for determining the use of their funds. In FY 2001, Congress appropriated $1.8 billion for this program (President's New Freedom Commission on Mental Health).

Supplemental Security Income (Title XVI)

This program is a federal income supplement program that provides monthly financial assistance payments to individuals who are aged, blind, or disabled and have little or no income to meet basic needs (i.e., food, clothing, and shelter). In 2004 SSI provided payments of $564 per individual or $846 per couple per month plus Medicaid and Food Stamp Program eligibility (Medicare, n.d.). Income limits are state determined. Payments are sent to eligible individuals monthly from the Social Security Administration (SSA).

Approximately 6.7 million individuals received SSI in December 2001; 30% of beneficiaries were over the age of 65. More than one-third (36%) of all adult beneficiaries were eligible because of mental disorders. Overall, approximately 1.2 million adult beneficiaries were disabled for reasons of mental disorders. Total federal expenditures for SSI in 2001 were approximately $32 billion, which included about $3 billion in state supplementation (President's New Freedom Commission on Mental Health, 2003).

Veterans' Benefits

The Department of Veterans Affairs (DVA) was established in 1989, succeeding the Veterans Administration (VA). It is the second largest of the 15 Cabinet departments and operates nationwide programs for health care, financial assistance, and burial benefits at its 1300 inpatient and outpatient health care facilities. In 2003, projected spending in the DVA was $59.6 billion with $25.9 billion earmarked for health care and $32.8 billion for disability benefits (Department of Veterans Affairs, 2003). There are an estimated 26 million veterans alive, with more than 6.8 million enrolled to receive DVA health care benefits. The aging of the veteran population is a major issue confronting the DVA. About 9.2 million veterans are age 65 or older, representing 35% of the total veteran population. By 2020 the proportion of older veterans will increase dramatically, to 51% of the total veteran population. More than 100,000 homeless veterans receive DVA health care and benefits. About 45% of homeless veterans suffer from mental illness and over 68% suffer from alcohol or drug abuse problems; 33% have both psychiatric and substance-abuse disorders. The DVA offers a spectrum of geriatric and extended-care services to veterans with nearly 65,000 veterans receiving long-term care annually through inpatient programs of the DVA or state veterans' homes (DVA, 2003).

The Veterans Health Care Eligibility Reform Act of 1996 created a standard enhanced health benefits plan available to enrolled veterans that provides health services that promote, preserve, and restore health with no prescribed day or visit limits. Those eligible include veterans discharged from active military service under honorable conditions. If discharged after September 7, 1980, a minimum service of two years is required. Once enrolled, veterans can receive care anywhere in the DVA system. In general, mental health benefits provided within the Medical Benefits Package are quite comprehensive. A substantial percentage of DVA health care service and funds are utilized for psychiatric care.

Most services are provided through DVA operated facilities. Recipient cost-sharing varies based upon the service received and eligibility status of the individual. In FY 2001, approximately 4.2 million veterans received health care through the DVA health care system, which comprised 172 hospitals, 859 outpatient clinics, 137 nursing homes, and several dozen other types of health care facilities. Twenty-one percent (886,019) received mental health care, 712,045 (80.4%) of whom were treated in specialized mental health programs and the remaining 173,974 (19.6%) of whom received care in general medical settings. Of the overall total of veterans receiving mental health care in 2001, 285,161 (32.2%) met the DVAs utilization criteria for serious mental illness and 72,252 (8.2%) received inpatient care, including 8627 (1.0%) in substance-abuse units (President's New Freedom Commission on Mental Health, 2003, p. 69).

Managed Care Organizations (MCOs)

Managed care refers to health care systems that integrate the financing and delivery of appropriate health care services to covered individuals by arrangement with selected providers to furnish a comprehensive set of health care services. Federal initiatives are promoting the growth of Medicare managed care even though little is known about the ability of these plans to deliver quality mental health services (Colenda, Banazak, & Mickus, 1998). The rapid growth in the number of older adults enrolling in managed health care plans presents a number of opportunities and challenges (HMO Workgroup on Care Management, 1998). It has long been recognized that older HMO enrollees have needs that differ from those of younger members. Not only do older adults experience more chronic health conditions but they also have an increased likelihood of functional impairment, and experience differences in their living arrangements. The health needs of older adults often extend beyond medical care and may include other domains shown to influence health and functional status, including relationships with families, formal and informal caregivers, community agencies, and

long-term care institutions (HMO Workgroup on Care Management, 1998). The HMO Workgroup on Care Management (1998) has described the types of services that should realistically be available to older adults who are enrolled in Medicare + Choice programs in order to meet the goals of gerontological health care. The essential components of a health care system for an older adult population that have particular applicability to mental health care are identified as:

- A systematic program for identifying enrollees at high risk for adverse health outcomes
- Available geriatric case management to proactively serve high-risk enrollees in all settings to ensure seamless use of health services
- Mechanisms to identify and coordinate services to meet enrollee's social needs

Colenda et al. (1998) identified potential disadvantages to participation in managed care plans by older adults with mental illness to include:

- Limiting providers to only participating mental health specialists, obscuring access to other community mental health professionals
- Precertification for psychiatric inpatient admissions could be disputed on the grounds of less-than-clearly defined medical necessity
- Authorization restrictions may limit outpatient services to basic psychopharmacology without adequate psychotherapy services
- Newer, safer, better tolerated but more expensive psychoactive medications may be excluded from drug formularies

Senior Centers

Social issues as well as physical and mental health problems affect the overall health of older adults. Senior centers, through positive social interaction, play a vital role in promoting healthy and successful aging and, along with Meals-On-Wheels, adult day care, transportation, and companion services, help to improve the quality of life of older adults. In the current climate of economic downturn, many state and local municipalities are confronting increased caseloads and shrinking budgets. Services most commonly provided at senior centers include: routine health screening, physical fitness programs, health promotion activities, nutritional screening and educational services, health risk assessments, and mental health screening, education, and referral (under the Administration on Aging State and Community Programs). Studies have shown that participation in senior centers may decrease the inappropriate use of health care providers, emergency rooms, and hospitals. The centrality of social ties to the health and well-being of older adults cannot be over-emphasized.

Substance Abuse and Mental Health Services Administration

This is the U.S. Department of Health and Human Services government division that specializes in producing publications, resources, and referrals for individuals including low-income and uninsured clients seeking health care, and those seeking alcohol treatment (information available at: www.find-treatment.samhsa.gov). This site allows the geropsychiatric nurse to enter his or her practice site Zip code to generate a list of treatment facilities, including those with free or sliding-scale alcohol-abuse services (telephone [888]ASK-HRSA).

▮▮▮ REIMBURSEMENT ISSUES FOR THE GEROPSYCHIATRIC NURSE

It is incumbent upon geropsychiatric nurses to understand reimbursement of mental health care services to older adults. This is important not only as clinicians, but for advocacy, case management, and health policy researcher and analyst role functions. Unless the client is paying out-of-pocket for his or her own health care, every encounter between a health care provider and an older adult client for psychiatric or mental health care will have a third-party participant, i.e., a payer (Buppert, 1998). There are three primary categories of third party payers that reimburse health care providers for mental health services including: federally funded programs (Medicare, Medicaid), managed care organizations (MCOs), and indemnity insurance companies.

Federally Funded Programs (Medicare, Medicaid) and APNs

The Balanced Budget Act of 1997 made direct Medicare reimbursement for Advanced Practice Nurses (APNs) possible. In order to receive reimbursement from Medicare, an APN must work collaboratively with a physician, meet state APN requirements, and be certified by a nationally recognized certifying body. There are two possible arrangements by which an APN may be reimbursed for services provided to a Medicare enrollee. The first is when Medicare reimburses the APN directly on a fee-for-service (FFS) basis through a local Medicare carrier agency. Self-employed APNs may bill directly for their services under their own Medicare provider number and receive 85% of the physician fee schedule for the billed procedure (MCNP, 2003). Alternatively, when employed by a physician or a practice, an APN may bill Medicare under the physician provider number and receive 100% of the physician charge subject to "incident to" provisions. The second reimbursement arrangement is when the Medicare beneficiary is enrolled in a capitated Medicare program such as a Health Maintenance Organization

(HMO) or a Managed Care Organization (MCO). In this scenario, Medicare pays the organization a lump sum for the health care services of the beneficiary and the HMO or MCO, in turn, pays the provider a predetermined capitated fee per member per month, regardless of how many times the client is seen (MCNP, 2003). To succeed in this type of arrangement, the APN must maximize cost-effective utilization of services.

APNs, like other providers, can decide annually whether they want to participate in Medicare in a given year. In 2003, almost 90% of Medicare providers enrolled to treat Medicare beneficiaries chose participating status and nearly 95% of Medicare claims were submitted by participating providers. Participating providers are paid using a higher fee schedule than used for nonparticipating providers, but agree to accept assignment and to bill beneficiaries only for the 20% copayment. The year 2004 started out on a positive note in relation to Medicare reimbursement for APNs. The CMS issued a final rule as part of the Medicare Prescription Drug, Improvement and Modernization Act of 2003 that increased payments to more than 875,000 health care providers for services under the Medicare Physician Fee Schedule by an average of more than 1.5% for calendar year 2004. All Medicare providers, including APNs, were scheduled to have a 4.5% fee reduction starting on January 1, 2004. Instead, legislators included a provision in the newly passed Medicare bill to include a 1.5% increase in reimbursement fees. These changes were implemented to provide health care professionals with higher payments to create incentives for APNs and other providers to continue to treat Medicare beneficiaries.

As with clients covered by Medicare, some Medicaid clients are enrolled in managed care plans and others are not (Buppert, 1998). The same two reimbursement arrangements apply to Medicaid reimbursement. In order to receive reimbursement under Medicaid,

an APN must apply and be accepted as a Medicaid provider by the state Medicaid agency. In the state of Massachusetts, for example, APNs may enroll as Medicaid (MassHealth) providers if the APN is a member of a private practice group, not salaried by a hospital, and compensated by the group practice in the same manner as the physicians and other APNs in the practice; or if the APN is a member of a group practice that solely comprises APNs; or the APN is in a solo APN private practice (MCNP, 2003). Medicaid then pays 70% of the fee-for-service (FFS) rates set for physicians and these rates vary from state to state. To provide care to a Medicaid client enrolled in an HMO, an APN must apply and be admitted to the provider panel of the HMO within which the client is enrolled (Buppert, 1998). Some states have Medicaid waivers from the federal government that allow the states to enroll all Medicaid patients in managed care organizations (MCOs).

One of the biggest challenges to APNs is ensuring that Medicaid regulations are applied correctly. While Medicare tends to be consistent and homogeneous, Medicaid may have heterogeneous influences based on variability in state government views or perspectives. In addition, public policy is subjected to various orientations such as those concerned with cure and rehabilitation versus those concerned with chronic care or palliative care. The National Heritage Insurance Company's Education and Outreach Unit has developed a guide to provide APNs with Medicare Part B non-physician reimbursement and billing information (National Heritage Insurance Company, 2004).

Managed Care Organizations

When an APN gains admission to a managed care organization provider panel, the designation Primary Care Provider (PCP) is awarded as well as a contract for providing care, credentialing, directory listing, and reimbursement (Buppert, 1998). MCOs sell a priced package of health services to their clients, who may be employers, individuals, or government agencies, such as the state Medicaid agency or Medicare. A client signs up for a particular plan and offers that plan to "members" who often share the cost of the plan (Buppert, 1998).

Indemnity Insurance Companies

An indemnity insurance company pays for the health care of its beneficiaries but does not deliver the care directly (e.g., Blue Cross, Blue Shield). Indemnity insurance companies privately credential individual providers, including APNs, as they deem necessary to meet the needs of their clientele. These companies pay APNs claims on a per-visit or per-procedure basis. The APN submits a bill to the insurance company and is reimbursed via a fee schedule based on "usual and customary" charges. Some companies reimburse at higher rates than others. The APN has the option of billing a predetermined price and is able to charge or balance bill the patient for the difference.

▮▮▮ CREATING A MENTAL HEALTH POLICY AGENDA FOR OLDER ADULTS

Mental illness in older adults can contribute to considerable morbidity and diminished quality of life (Colenda et al., 1998). Treatment is available for depression, dementia, and other geropsychiatric conditions but barriers including access to care, the social stigma of mental illness, a shortage of trained mental health professionals, underdiagnosis of mental disorders by health providers, and financial disincentives to provide quality care must be overcome (Colenda et al.). The nation's mental health care system is in need of a fundamental transformation—one that prizes

recovery instead of simply managing daily symptoms (Krisberg, 2003). The reality is that recovery is necessary to achieve cost-effectiveness. The New Freedom Commission on Mental Health, which was created by President George W. Bush in April 2002, was charged with examining the country's mental health delivery system. The final report of the Commission (2003) addressed six overarching goals:

1. To help Americans understand that mental health is essential to overall health

2. To make mental health consumer driven and family driven

3. To eliminate racial and ethnic disparity in mental health

4. To achieve early mental health screening, assessment, and referral

5. To assure that excellent mental health care is delivered and that research is expedited

6. To promote the use of technology to access mental health care as well as information on mental health

The achievement of these goals would improve the lives of millions of citizens now living with mental illnesses. Professional nurses have key positions in influencing health policy, advocacy, and research. Influence begins with awareness, creating networks, developing partnerships, and getting involved. The challenge for geropsychiatric nurses is to tailor these goals into policy reform initiatives that benefit a historically underserved population: older Americans.

It is encouraging that the mental health of aging Americans has been receiving increased attention in the legislature. The Positive Aging Act, for example, introduced in 2003, was designed to enhance vital mental health services for older adults by promoting models of care that integrate mental health services and medical care within primary care settings and to improve access to mental health services in community-based settings by:

- Offering competitive grants to reward projects that integrate multidisciplinary mental health programs into primary-care settings to create a collaborative health model for older adults

- Establishing competitive grants to reward public or private, nonprofit, community-based providers of multidisciplinary mental health services for older adults that deliver services where older adults reside, such as senior centers and assisted living communities

- Designating a Deputy Director for Older Adult Mental Health Services within the Center for Mental Health Services in the Substance Abuse and Mental Health Services Administration (SAMHSA) responsible for the development and implementation of initiatives to address the mental health service needs of older adults

- Reserving positions on the Advisory Council of the Center for Mental Health Services for representatives of older Americans, their families, and mental health specialists with appropriate training and experience in the treatment of older adults (American Association for Geriatric Psychiatry, 2003).

Although not enacted in 2003, this legislation was reintroduced in 2004 by Senators Hillary Rodham Clinton (D-New York) and Susan Collins (R-Maine), and others in the House of Representatives. The collaborative care model at the heart of the Positive Aging Act will undoubtedly help meet the mental health needs of our nation's growing population of older adults.

The mental health issues of older adults have not been adequately addressed, which has had an adverse effect on quality of life. Geropsychiatric nurses should assume a leadership role in defining and mobilizing practices for quality mental health care. Focusing views on health policy for older adults may reshape current thinking and decision making related to this important issue. Table 20-2 includes policy agenda considerations in planning holistic mental health care for an aging society. Reform begins with interventions to identify and optimally treat mental illness with individual clients in clinical practice. In turn, change evolves at the local and regional levels with awareness of the needs of those afflicted with mental illness at the community level. This must involve all constituencies with a stake in mental health care—clients, families, health care professionals, institutions, policymakers, and society. Targeting outreach and proactive interventions toward high-intensity, high-cost users of Medicare expenditures may enhance both quality of care and cost effectiveness.

Geropsychiatric and mental health nurses can support older adults in getting the best possible care by delineating the issues, exploring options, and promoting quality mental health care to policymakers. Quality of life in older adults with mental illness, and outcomes associated with the implementation of social, health, and long-term care programs for older adults need systematic evaluation. Partnerships between nurse researchers and health care policy analysts, as well as interdisciplinary efforts in practice and research related to mental illness and aging, are needed as we move into the 21st century. Geropsychiatric and mental health nurses in advanced practice roles are in key positions to facilitate positive changes in mental health policy for older adults through advocacy in policy issues at the local, state, and national levels.

TABLE 20-2   Mental Health Policy Agenda Considerations

Clinical
- Establishing centers of excellence for geriatric mental health care
- Identifying best practice models for depression, dementia, substance abuse, and schizophrenia in older adults
- Implementing and evaluating clinical practice guidelines
- Establishing methods to improve care coordination/case management
- Designing staffing models to optimize the provision of mental health care
- Defining unique interdisciplinary collaboration strategies in geriatric mental health care
- Exploring collaborative practice models and opportunities for the geriatric advanced practice nurse (APN)
- Improving/increasing benefits (pharmacy, psychotherapy, and social support services)

Academic
- Designing clinical faculty practice models in mental health care to older adults
- Promoting blended advanced practice nurse (APN) role development
- Facilitating caregiver and consumer education and opportunity
- Establishing municipal, regional, and national mental health care consortia
- Establishment of funding incentives for mental health professional education across disciplines

Research
- Developing quality indicators for treatment of mental illness in long-term care settings
- Designing and conducting outcomes research in geriatric mental health care
- Planning, implementing, and evaluating mental health service delivery programs
- Preventing mental illness in the elderly
- Testing creative financing and service delivery models for mental health care
- Improving quality of mental health care in nursing homes

Policy
- Assessing utilization patterns of acute and long-term care services
- Exploring integrated service delivery models in LTC (community versus institutional care)
- Designing local, regional, statewide, and national initiatives
- Enhancing access to mental health care
- Linking health care and social programs to help professionals and organizations cope with mental illness
- Eliminating disparities in the delivery of quality mental health care
- Developing national strategies for suicide prevention and alcohol dependence elimination
- Screening for mental illness and for medical comorbidities in all primary care and mental health settings
- Testing financing reform initiatives in the provision of mental health care

REFERENCES

Administration on Aging. (2003). *Older Americans Act.* Retrieved May 1, 2004, from http://www.aoa.gov

American Association for Geriatric Psychiatry. (2003). *The Positive Aging Act.* Retrieved May 1, 2004, from http://www.aagpgpa.org/advocacy/facts_posaging.asp

American Nurses Association. (1996). *Scope and standards of advanced practice registered nursing.* [Brochure]. Washington, DC: Author.

American Nurses Association. (2001). *Scope and standards of gerontological nursing practice.* [Brochure]. Washington, DC: Author.

Buppert, C. (1998). Reimbursement for nurse practitioner services. *The Nurse Practitioner, 23*(1), 67–81.

Centers for Medicare and Medicaid Services. (2004). *Medicaid information for states and territories.* Retrieved May 1, 2004, from http://www.cns.hhs.gov/medicaid

Centers for Medicare and Medicaid Services. (2003). *Medicare and your mental health benefits.* Retrieved August 18, 2003, from www.cms.hhs.gov

Centers for Medicare and Medicaid Services. (2004). *The Chronic Care Improvement Program.* Retrieved May 1, 2004, from http://www.cns.hhs.gov/medicarereform/ccip

Colenda, C. C., Banazak, D., & Mickus, M. (1998). Mental health services in managed care: Quality questions remain. *Geriatrics, 53*(8), 49–63.

Cubanski, J., Frank, R. G., & Epstein, A. M. (2004). Savings from drug discount cards: Relief for Medicare beneficiaries? [Electronic version]. *Health Affairs, W4*(10), 198–209. Retrieved May 1, 2004, from http://content.health affairs.org/cgi/content/abstract/hlthaff.w4.198

Department of Veterans Affairs. (2003). *VA fact sheets.* Retrieved May 1, 2004, from http://www1.va.gov/opa/fact/docs/vafacts.htm

Edmunds, M. (2003). Medicaid patients bear brunt of budget cuts. *The Nurse Practitioner, 28*(12), 11.

Hebert, L. E., Scherr, P. A., Bienias, J. L., Bennett, D. A., & Evans, D. A. (2003). Alzheimer's disease in the US population. *Archives of Neurology, 60*(8), 1119–1122.

HMO Workgroup on Care Management (1998). Essential components of geriatric care provided through health maintenance organizations. *Journal of the American Geriatrics Society, 46*(3), 303–308.

Krisberg, K. (2003). Presidential commission calls for U.S. mental health care reform. *The Nation's Health, 33*(7), 1–6.

Lantz, M. S. (2002). Depression in the elderly: Recognition and treatment. *Clinical Geriatrics, 10*(10), 18–24.

Lin, E. H. B, Katon, W., Von Korff, M., Tang, L., Williams, J. W., Kroenke, K., et al. (2003). Effect of improving depression care on pain and functional outcomes among older adults with arthritis: A randomized controlled trial. *Journal of the American Medical Association, 290*(8), 2428–2434.

Massachusetts Coalition of Nurse Practitioners. (2003). *Guide to nurse practitioner practice in Massachusetts.* Littleton, MA: Author.

Medicare: The official U.S. Government site for people with Medicare. Retrieved May 1, 2004, from http://www.medicare.gov

Melillo, K. D. (1996). Medicare and Medicaid: Similarities and differences. *Journal of Gerontological Nursing, 22*(7), 12–21.

National Heritage Insurance Company. (2004). *Physician assistant, nurse practitioner & clinical nurse specialist billing guide.* Retrieved September 12, 2004, from www.medicarenhic.com/providers/billing/nonphygd_mar04.pdf

National Institute of Aging (1993). *Discoveries in health for aging Americans. Special report on aging 1993.* Washington, DC: U.S. Department of Health and Human Services.

President's New Freedom Commission on Mental Health (2003). *Major federal programs supporting and financing mental health care.* Retrieved December 1, 2003, from http://www.mental-healthcommission.gov/reports/reports.htm

Rosenbach, M., & Ammering, C. (1997). Trends in Part B mental health utilization and expenditures for psychiatric services: 1995. *Health Care Financing Review, 18*(3), 19–42.

Satcher, D. S. (2000). Executive summary: A report of the Surgeon General on mental health. *Public Health Reports, 115*(1), 89–101.

Smoyak, S. (2000). The history, economics, and financing of mental health care. Part 3: The present. *Journal of Psychosocial Nursing*, *38*(11), 32–38.

U.S. Surgeon General (1999). *Mental health: A Report of the Surgeon General*. Rockville, MD: U.S. Department of Health and Human Services, Substance Abuse and Mental Health Services Administration, Center for Mental Health Services, National Institutes of Health, National Institutes of Mental Health.

CHAPTER 21

Future of Geropsychiatric and Mental Health Nursing in Addressing Older Adult Health Care Needs

As a fitting conclusion to this text, several nursing leaders were asked to address their vision of the future for geropsychiatric and mental health nursing. This specialty is rapidly evolving within nursing, and has advanced over the past several decades as more and more nurses have become involved in developing the scientific base for evidence-based practice in the area of geropsychiatric and mental health nursing. The nursing leaders who have contributed to this chapter have played an important role in this advancement of the specialty area through their involvement in education, research, dissemination of scholarly work, and technology development. The contributors speak to the optimistic future of geropsychiatric and mental health nursing and the need for more nurses to become adept at addressing the needs of a changing and aging adult population. The need for an increased number of nurses to become involved in research and technology related to mental health and psychiatric issues of older adults is also identified as an important aspect of the continued evolution of geropsychiatric and mental health nursing.

THE FUTURE OF GEROPSYCHIATRIC AND MENTAL HEALTH NURSING

Priscilla Ebersole, PhD, RN, FAAN

Priscilla Ebersole is a Professor Emerita from San Francisco State University and has been the editor of Geriatric Nursing *for 13 years. Her interest in geropsychiatric nursing has been sustained for 30 years, initially cultivated by Irene Burnside. She served for three years as field director of a geriatric nurse practitioner recruitment and training grant from the W. K. Kellogg Foundation and has held the Florence Cellar Chair of Gerontological Nursing at Frances Payne Bolton School of Nursing, Case Western Reserve University. She and Patricia Hess have written seven textbooks about healthy aging, and she is presently writing one about the history and progress of geriatric nursing, to be published by Springer Publications in 2005.*

Projecting the future of mental health and psychiatric care is greatly dependent upon the political climate. Another issue that must be considered is the population being addressed.

Speculation about the care of a circumscribed population holds some common denominators, not so with the aged. We are attempting to address a population that spans 50 years in age that encompasses numerous ethnic and cultural origins, gender differences, and evolving family constructs. In addition, the ready availability of mass information and as yet undiscovered technologic advancements adds uncertainty to the task. Based upon variations in social, cohort, and cultural origins, older adults do not all speak the same language or even understand the concepts of mental health and psychiatric aberrations in the same way. Given these cautions, with great audacity and presumption we will attempt to concoct the future mental health and geropsychiatric care of a widely variable and polyglot population.

Cohort Effects

Examining the cohort commonalities is one way to address these complex issues. The very old, from 85 to 95 years, and the oldest-old, from 95 to 110 years old, have seldom grown up in the lap of luxury and are generally a hardy lot. They often define mental health, if they think of it at all, as stoic acceptance and endurance of whatever situation they are in. Psychiatric therapies have rarely been their mode of problem solving. Those who are physically impaired often suffer an ongoing and subclinical depression. Their major concern may be how and when they will die. The end-of-life (EOL) movement offers more options than ever before and many more elders may opt for ending their life voluntarily or dying at home with hospice supports. There are many, however, that are vital, contributing citizens and will remain so until some brief condition strikes them down. These wise old elders are presently, and will continue to be, highly valued for their perspectives and survival skills.

Elders from 75 to 85 years old have always been on the cusp of change. They are the group that has lived through major shifts in social and political events that have impacted their lives and opportunities markedly. They are inured to political upheaval, have survived major social and psychological trends, and evolving concepts of mental health. They are extremely adaptable. They value education highly and have often sacrificed to secure a future and education for their children. The sophisticates of this group smoked and drank a lot in their youth and some still do. They are the prime targets for dementia research and it is hoped that they will be able to benefit from the numerous discoveries that will prolong healthy aging and mental competence. Advanced mental health interventions and evolving management skills will ensure a higher quality of life for the demented, as well as a more hopeful future.

Those individuals 65–75 years of age have been medicated and indoctrinated in an era of reliance on medical interventions though they are also the beneficiaries of health information technology. They are more likely to welcome psychiatric intervention and expect recognition of mental health issues and interventions when needed. They are also the group tending to transfer large amounts of assets to their younger generations. They are politically astute, and this political awareness and influence will continue to be crucial to the future of all elders.

The baby boomers, born between 1946–1964, are the subject of much present speculation among gerontologists. There are numerous predictions about their future that range from annihilation of social benefits and supports to a utopian old age. They are extremely aware of healthy life styles, proactively involved in maintaining health, and welcome the nontraditional and holistic therapies. Many have grown accustomed to a relatively affluent and comfortable life and have inherited substantial assets from their elders. These young-old people tend to be accepting of wide variations in lifestyle, culture, ethnicity, and alternative lifestyles. Yet the tendency toward uncritical acceptance and maintaining politically correct attitudes may result in some homogenization. Their ready acceptance of diversity will increasingly welcome and accommodate situations that in the past were considered mentally unhealthy. Their expectations are high and they will use their energies to develop a satisfying old age.

Defining Standards

The American Psychiatric Association published the Diagnostic and Statistical Manual of Mental Disorders (DSM-IV) in 1994 and in 2000 amended it with the DSM-IV TR to clarify some diagnostic criteria that had been misused or misunderstood. The purpose of the manual is to provide clear diagnostic criteria and to codify conditions for national statistical purposes. Changes incorporated into the DSM-IV TR of interest to geropsychiatric nurses include the abandonment of the subtypes of dementia of the Alzheimer's type (i.e., with delusions, with depression, with delirium). There is now a discrimination to indicate comorbid psychiatric symptoms arising from Alzheimer's disease. The code now indicates specific mental disorders due to a general medical condition on Axis I alongside dementia. These secondary conditions that can occur as part of dementia include psychotic disorders due to Alzheimer's disease, mood disorders due to Alzheimer's disease, anxiety disorders due to Alzheimer's disease, personality changes due to Alzheimer's disease, and sleep disorders due to Alzheimer's disease (DSM-IV-TR.org). This allows for much more specificity in coding.

The specifics of the DSM-IV-TR are available on the Web site (www.DSM-IV-TR). The next DSM is scheduled for 2011 or later. The criteria for describing and diagnosing mental disorders have changed markedly over the years reflecting many sociocultural changes. Other sources of interest are an outline of psychiatric practice (www.psych.org/psych_

pract/) and future research into psychopathology and psychiatric diagnosis (www.psych.org/research/). Updates on the research planning efforts for the DSM-V can be viewed on (www.dsm5.org). They will be of interest to all mental health professionals and input from professionals in the field is encouraged. Nurses are most likely to see the changing patterns of disorders and can provide important feedback related to future diagnostic formulations.

Encouraging trends from the American Psychiatric Association (APA) include a strong position statement on the needs of diverse populations, defined as issues of race, gender, age, country of origin, sexuality, religious and spiritual beliefs, social class, and physical disability. Indeed, almost any older person would fit into one of these categories and will benefit by increased awareness of diversity as it influences mental wellness. In addition the APA has developed an Association of Gay and Lesbian Psychiatrists (www.aglp.org) that addresses the special needs of these persons.

Depression, Anxiety, Psychoses, Substance Abuse, Chronicity, Delirium, and Dementia

It is impossible to determine the future magnitude of these various disorders among older persons, but we are currently aware of increases in substance abuse, anxiety, and depression. Chronicity of mental health disorders tend to ameliorate in the later years unless accompanied by dementia. We expect that with advances in the recognition and management of the complexity of these disorders the aged will be greatly benefited.

Where are the Elders?

In the states where the elderly reside in large proportions, we anticipate more attention to their mental health needs in order to maintain the benefits and environmental conditions that now attract them, as they are major contributors to economic and political activism.

Who are the Nurses?

At present we are well aware of the aging nurse phenomenon and concerns about the associated effects on care when these nurses retire. We see that the growing body of Advanced Practice Nurses (APNs) will definitely have an important role in the future care of the aged. Their holistic approach to care portends an erosion of segmented approaches with less emphasis on the present division of the mind and the body and stronger interpersonal alliances with the client. The American Psychiatric Nurses Association (APNA) in alliance with the APA, National Association of Psychiatric Health Systems (NAPHS) and the American Hospital Association (AHA), has created a compendium of strategies intended to develop an organizational culture that maximizes patient dignity and safety (www.apna.org/releases.html). A major issue is reducing the use of restraints and abusive situations.

Managed care is definitely the wave of the future. Though the early years of the movement were fraught with numerous problems, it is presently growing in strength and viability. The APNA position paper notes that managed care is based in health rather than illness, increases access to appropriate mental health care, and supports the meaningful participation of consumers and families (www.apna.org/resources/positionpapers.html). Shore and Beigel (1996) predicted that within 10 years, 90% of health care would be in a managed care environment. This will drive massive changes in professional practice and the definition of mental disorders.

The roles of psychiatric nurses in managed care are legion. Some the roles APNA have identified include:

- *Psychiatric-mental health nurses* with various levels of preparation are serving as direct care providers in facilities, psychiatric home health, and community settings. Advanced practice nurses now have prescriptive privileges in most states and can thus provide comprehensive primary care.

- *Care managers* are involved in developing treatment plans, coordinating resources, and managing psychiatric rehabilitation.

- *Assessment, evaluation, triage, and referral nurses* will direct patients to the appropriate levels of care and referrals when needed.

- *Utilization review nurses* serve as gatekeepers to mental health services.

- *Risk managers* are nurses who assess risk, implement strategies to reduce risk, and decrease the probability of adverse outcomes.

Other roles will doubtlessly develop as the managed care systems recognize the effectiveness and numerous abilities of nurses with mental health and psychiatric nursing skills.

Changing Situations

Long-Term Care We believe most elders will spend some time in long term care and the trend will be toward smaller facilities with a home-like atmosphere and opportunities to commune with the natural environment. The Eden model and others similar are developing momentum across the United States and are welcomed by families who now decry the effects of institutions on the mental health of residents. Subacute facilities that care for individuals needing extensive nursing care, though no longer appropriate for acute care, will need mental health and psychiatric nurses as residents cope with recovery and the possibility of increasing limitations as a result of serious illness. These individuals and families are becoming more vociferous and will advocate for much needed changes in the present care delivery systems. Continuing Care Retirement Communities (CCRCs), now limited to the affluent, could with efficiency be brought more predominantly into the long-term care arena and made available to those with fewer assets. Greater tax advantages for endowments to quality long-term care facilities would encourage investments into one's own future.

Caregiving

The recent California Family Paid Leave Law provides six weeks of partial pay when leaving work to care for a seriously ill family member, as well as for care of a new baby, foster, or adopted child (www.paidfamilyleave. org/) or (www.edd.ca.gov). This heralds an increasing awareness of the need to give additional supports to caregivers. There are presently a number of efforts to give more tax advantages and respite services to caregivers. A recent large grant from NIH to the Family Caregiver Alliance provides support for the development of interventions to enhance the mental health of family caregivers of persons with dementia and other chronic health conditions. The outcomes of this study are expected to assist in the design of support services to alleviate caregiver stress and enhance mental well-being (www.caregiver.org).

With the evolution of family structures and alternative types of families, the traditional family of one female mother, one male father, and some biologic children is rapidly becoming the exception rather than the rule. For the aged, and those not yet old, there are many questions about the availability of caregivers for those needing care. We expect many more local and regional supports will be necessary to avoid premature institutionalization of impaired elders.

Effects of Prolongevity

The future of human longevity and increased life expectancy is receiving a lot of attention from gerontologists and researchers in the antiaging movement. Some scientists are searching for the longevity gene. There is great debate about the ethics and reality of some of the research into prolongation of life. The mission of the International Longevity Center-USA is to help individuals and societies address longevity in positive and productive ways (ilcusa.org). CEO and President Robert Butler, says, "The average baby boomer consumer is the one being targeted by the anti-aging movement. A well informed consumer is the best defense." An e-mail newsletter, compiled by HR Moody, *Human Values in Aging,* is available for those interested in periodic updates (hrmoody@ yahoo.com).

As theorists and researchers continue to address the issues of life prolongation and antiaging, the major concern is extending the quality of life and wellness as long as possible. Some believe the primary purpose of life extension is to nurture and cultivate a society that is able to use the wisdom and experience of elders to enhance the lives of the young. At present there is disagreement about the possibility of surviving beyond the 120 years predicted by the Hayflick limit on cell division.

Gender

Feminist theorists of old age charge that feminists have largely ignored the issue of aging. However, Betty Friedan is on the Board of Directors of the International Longevity Center-USA, and her influence will be felt. As the boomers age, they will have a major influence on perceptions of old women. A Web site used to promote the wise stories, poetic songs, and essays of energetic elders is available at www.cronesunlimited.com.

Little attention has been given to the needs and mental health of males as they age. We know they are becoming increasingly involved in the caregiving process. They are seldom as vigorous or live as long as old women but those who survive the years between 75 and 85 are often more lively than females. More research is needed into this phenomenon.

Self-Care

The awareness among elders of informed self-care is burgeoning. The availability of information and elders' expanding use of Internet information provide great impetus for managing one's own care. And, it is becoming more apparent that one must be his or her own best advocate. Unfortunately, the information available is sometimes not well-founded and elders are prime targets for many scams and misinformation. Alternative and complementary strategies are becoming the refuge of many elders attempting to assuage the discomforts they are experiencing. The American Holistic Nursing Association is a reliable source of good information (www.ahna.org). Consumer-directed health care is a response to the increasing demand for self-care.

Presumptuous Projecting for a Decade

Given all the above factors and those we are yet unaware of, I would predict that in the near future we are unlikely to see sufficient federal support of mental health and just as unlikely to see a national health care system emerge, but managed care may function as a viable alternative. Nurse practitioners will provide most of the primary care in this system. Given their holistic perspective, the traditional mind–body separation will diminish. Their nursing roles will expand and change the face of mental health.

The 47 million individuals with no insurance of any kind must seek their own resources, often unaffordable. They will increasingly demand attention. The amount of funds used for the bureaucratic functions of Medicare, Medicaid, and insurance companies could be reduced and the savings diverted into personal health accounts and perhaps health care vouchers that would build a self-serving system.

Clinics for culturally indigenous groups, such as On Lok in San Francisco, will increase. We must always be aware, however, that cultural patterns and perceptions are never static and that mental wellness is integral to coping with everyday living for many individuals. (Lai, 2004). Mental health practitioners must avoid looking for simple models. The great variations in diverse groups will engender new philosophies of mental illness and mental health.

Rosowky (2004) observes that in the absence of frank pathology, people cope differently with various life stages. She believes that flexibility and the capacity for change, attitudinal adaptability, attunement to the reduction of physical and mental energy, and the capacity for self-transcendence through leaving something behind to extend beyond one's mortal end are all factors that lead to mental wellness. Given our changing society, politics, and population, we may look forward to an increased understanding of and attention to the complexities of mental health in an aging population that includes individuals from diverse groups, and an ever-increasing reliance on the skills of nurses with backgrounds and expertise in mental health, psychiatric nursing, and geriatric nursing advanced practice.

References

Lai, D. (2004). Cultural diversity and mental wellness for older adults. *Newsletter of Mental Health and Aging Network, 11*(1), 5.

Rosowsky, E. (2004). Dimensions. *Newsletter of Mental Health and Aging Network. 11*(1), 4.

Shore, M., & Beigel, A. (1996). The challenges posed by managed behavioral health care. *New England Journal of Medicine, 334*(2), 116–118.

THE FUTURE OF TECHNOLOGY IN MENTAL HEALTH NURSING—A NURSE GEROPSYCHTECHNOLOGIST?

Diane Feeney Mahoney, PhD, APRN, BC

Diane Feeney Mahoney is director of Gerontechnology and Enhancing Family Caregiving at the Research and Training Institute at the Hebrew Rehabilitation Center for Aged in Boston. She is a member of the faculty at the Division on Aging at Harvard Medical School, adjunct associate professor at the Boston University School of Public Health, and a fellow of the Gerontological Society of America. She is a social scientist, geriatric nurse practitioner, and for over a decade a gerontechnologist who has been developing and testing innovative ways to use telecommunication-based technologies with frail and cognitively impaired older adults and their family caregivers. Mahoney has authored numerous research publications and serves as a grant reviewer for NIH and foundation grant programs.

Under the aegis of the Department of Commerce Technology Opportunity Program, she tested remote wireless computational sensor technology designed to help working caregivers monitor frail elders residing alone at home. She received the first Alzheimer's Association/Intel Co. technology grant to adapt her sensor program for use in assisted living facilities. She has conducted a randomized clinical study of a computer-mediated automated telephone interactive voice response (IVR) system designed to support family caregivers of people with Alzheimer's disease as part of the NIA-funded national REACH project. In 1995 she conducted the first longitudinal qualitative analysis of an Internet-based virtual support group for family members of persons with Alzheimer's disease. In addition, through the aegis of an Alzheimer's Association grant, she and her team developed a computer-based interactive multimedia program that successfully taught older adults to recognize the differences between normal forgetfulness and more serious memory loss associated with Alzheimer's disease. Mahoney specializes in customizing technologies to make them personally relevant and tailored to the end user's needs and wants, as well as having policy and practice relevance.

Technology is revolutionizing the way professionals deliver and monitor health care. Medicine has embraced technology to develop a new field of telemedicine with specialty subgroups such as teleradiology, teledermatology, and telepathology. Home care nurses are increasingly conducting remote video visits to monitor high-risk patients. Advances in technology also influence the way consumers use the health care system. Patients now use the Internet to learn about conditions and treatment options. Computer-based programs have been developed to aid decision making when patients face choices between care strategies with differential risks. Internet-based support groups have enlisted numerous consumers and patients who seek alternative ways to gain disease-related information and counseling. As technologies advance, so too will patient and provider applications.

How will geropsychiatric nurses use these emerging technologies? I would like to address that question by sharing insights from the last decade of conducting technology-based interventions for elders with Alzheimer's disease and their family caregivers. By conducting prototype and implementation studies, one gains considerable knowledge about those who participate, the end users, those targeted to actually use the technology, the barriers and facilitators to technology adoption and its clinical potential. From my perspective, the future will certainly involve components from today's promising prototypes. And, we open the door for a new specialization—*a nurse geropsychtechnologist,* one who integrates geropsychiatric nursing and technology expertise to innovate and develop new mental health services.

Regardless of whether a formal role specialization evolves, all nurses have the potential to adopt technologies that offer increased access to mental health care for vulnerable elders and their caregivers. The following examples will offer nurses ideas and suggestions on how they may consider using technology in their clinical practice.

While now considered "low tech," the telephone is and always will be a very important form of technology. It doesn't matter if it changes form into a cell phone, wrist phone, or other microphone technology, it provides a means for us to send and receive messages from where and when we choose. The telephone offers several unique advantages. It is one of the most universally available forms of technology, ubiquitous, affordable, and familiar to everyone, including those with moderate levels of cognitive impairment. When one considers interventions to help primary family caregivers manage stress related to caregiving, the telephone needs to be considered. In the NIH-sponsored Resources to Enhance Alzheimer's Caregivers' Health (REACH) initiative, 1222 primary family caregivers and their respective elderly care recipients with Alzheimer's-related behavioral disorders were randomly assigned at six sites to one of 15 intervention or control groups (Schulz et al., 2003). Caregivers' interventions included traditional cognitive behavioral counseling sessions using an intensive series of individual and group counseling sessions, in-home environmental assessments and individualized counseling, ethnicity- or female-specific counseling sessions, family therapist-mediated group telephone call sessions, and totally automated interactive voice response (IVR) telephone sessions. Contrary to prevailing assumptions that intensive personal counseling results in better outcomes, findings from a meta-analysis at the 6-month point revealed that the automated telephone performed as well as the in-person interventions. Moreover, the family therapist-mediated group tele-

phone call program was the only intervention to target and demonstrate a statistically significant reduction in caregiver depression (Gitlin et al., 2003).

I developed the automated IVR telephone program to maximize the power of the computer to integrate baseline data into a personalized telephone conversation that assessed the caregivers' level of stress and, when desired, automatically relayed strategies to manage the identified behaviors evoking concern. Considered both innovative and "high tech," it also provided an individualized patient conversation for the caregiver to employ at any time when the person with Alzheimer's disease started to become agitated and needed to be distracted or the caregiver needed a safe activity to engage the elder and provide a short respite or break. It also offered voice mail connections to geriatric experts in medicine, nutrition, pharmacology, and other therapies, all triaged by an online gerontological nurse practitioner (Mahoney, 2000). I designed this program based on a nursing model of consumer empowerment, giving the caregiver the control and choice of components that could be tailored to match changing needs across the 12-month intervention period. As expected, we found differential patterns of usage among the caregivers, but overall they highly valued having an around-the-clock support program available and access to a credible source of information (Mahoney, Tarlow, Jones, Tennstedt, & Kasten, 2001). Our site-specific outcome analyses revealed that this intervention was most effective for those with low mastery, especially caregiving wives with low mastery and high anxiety (Mahoney, Tarlow, & Jones, 2003). From the clinical perspective, nurses can mimic the respite call by using the "talking" frames and albums now readily accessible in gift and gadget specialty shops. A loved one can tape a positive message to accompany the photo, or the family could do short clips for an album to be shown to divert an elder's attention onto more pleasant memories. In formal counseling sessions, consider using a speakerphone with call-in capability for multiple family members thereby enabling group sessions and the capacity to include distant family members.

Videophones are moving into their third generation and soon will overcome the speech delay, visual distortion, small screen, and number keypads that make it difficult for a frail elder to use independently. These too could become a tool for the nurse therapist, one that enables remote one-on-one counseling or links to others for family sessions or a support group. At-risk patients could be checked via videophone to assess their affect and mental health status. Socially isolated elders who today receive phone calls from elder volunteers could use the video component to increase personal engagement. The videophones do, however, offer the option of blocking images for those who do not want to be seen in their pajamas or without makeup. Alternatively, some have found that the screen image is an inducement to "dressing up," and in those situations it could be used as a motivational aid for personal grooming (Nakamura, Takehito, & Chiemi, 1999) and as a social presence in telepsychiatry (Cukor et al., 1998).

In 1997, I conducted a year-long content analysis of one of the first Internet-based Alzheimer's family caregivers support groups (Mahoney, 1998). At the time there were only a handful of patient support groups, and these were focused on specific types of cancer. Today, a similar search of Alzheimer's or patient support groups identifies too many to count. Clearly, the public has embraced this form of technology support. My analysis found that the postings online generally fell into three categories: information seeking, information sharing, and comments. From these data, a model of caregiver transitions emerged from the early stage of normalizing events through the middle stage of managing issues and into the advanced stage of surviving through the end-of-life period for the person with Alzheimer's disease. Each stage was mediated by caregiver vigilance and their need to "be there" for their loved one. Each stage brought new questions and issues and a quest by caregivers for assistance. Caregivers preferred advice from other caregivers, mainly those who had experiences similar to themselves and could offer practical tips and feedback related to their problem solving attempts. Professional input was valued when it added credibility to information such as new drugs, or exposed "cures" that were really quackery. Caregivers frequently expressed positive feelings about participating in an electronic caregivers group. They valued having a convenient alternative to traditional support groups. A minority also participated in traditional groups because they started there and had made friendships they wished to maintain. The majority, however, commented that they were not comfortable in face-to-face groups, did not have the time or desire to travel to meetings, had no elder sitter, or had conflicts with the scheduling. Consequently, therapists should consider that online groups work particularly well for people who are uncomfortable in group settings, "don't want to look into other people's eyes," have difficulty revealing themselves to strangers, enjoy asynchronous, around-the-clock communications, want to remain anonymous, or have sensitive information they don't want to personally share in public.

Technology can also be used as a means to reach out to patients with personally threatening, stigmatizing, or embarrassing conditions. When the Alzheimer's Association sought ways to better reach out to the public and educate them about the early signs of Alzheimer's disease, we developed a multimedia interactive computer program entitled: "Forgetfulness—What's Normal and What's Not." In a randomized controlled study of 113 elders recruited via the press, we found very large program effect sizes (Mahoney, Tarlow, Jones, & Sandaire, 2002). Viewers scored significantly higher in knowledge about the differences between normal forgetting and serious memory loss than the controls who were given the same information in traditional handout form. Besides the robust findings, this project was notable because we had an overwhelming response from the public and had to turn people away because of our resource constraints. We found that participants were worried about memory loss in a family member or themselves but did not wish to express their fear of Alzheimer's disease to a physician and be dismissed as silly or considered confused. Participants highly valued having a confidential, credible source of information, accessed in the privacy of their homes, one that offered a basic memory loss screening to affirm or allay an emotionally charged concern.

Other researchers have reported that many people are less embarrassed and more self-disclosing of sensitive topic areas when they interact with a computer rather than a person. Baer and his colleagues have numerous applications supporting this premise in the field of psychiatry. He tested the feasibility of using IVR technology as a means to administer the Zung Depression Index and found of the 1812 callers, 606 met the depression criteria, and the majority of these callers had received no previous treatment for depression (Baer et al., 1995). Baer and Greist (1997) also piloted studies using an IVR-administered self-assessment and self-help program for behavior therapy, as well as IVR technology comparisons with clinicians and controls (Greist et al., 2002). Zarate et al. (1997) tested the reliability of using videoconferencing to conduct psychiatric assessments in patients with schizophrenia and found it reliable and offering promise for providing psychiatric consultation to underserved remote populations. In Europe, the field of cybertherapy using the Internet and virtual reality programs is quickly evolv-

ing and currently has applications for panic disorders and agoraphobia (Riva, Botella, Légeron, & Optale, 2004).

Some may question whether problems with self-awareness might limit the usefulness of developing self-assessment applications for patients, especially those with depression and memory impairment. Mundt and colleagues demonstrated the feasibility of conducting either informant or self-assessment for dementia using IVR telephone screening (2000, 2001). Osgood-Hynes et al. (1998) demonstrated the feasibility of self-administered psychotherapy for depression using multiple IVR-based sessions coupled with a workbook to use at home.

Currently, "smart home" technologies are being developed and tested at several university and commercial sites across the country. It is postulated the home of the future will offer fully integrated technologies that not only control the environment but also monitor the residents' activities, provide activity reminders, and even communicate biometric monitoring results to residents and their clinical providers. How will this technology be received by elders and their caregivers? Will it improve their well-being or negatively affect personal privacy and clinical confidentiality? To prepare for the future, we have started to address those questions. We are nearing completion of a study using a wireless remote home monitoring system designed to help working caregivers with their oversight responsibilities for community-dwelling older adults with memory loss or physical frailty. Known as the WIN project (Worker Interactive Networking), an Internet-based program was developed to promote workplace intergroup support and links to a home-based wireless sensor monitoring system that informs and alerts workers about their elder caregiving concerns. As the system developer, my approach differed from the traditional home surveillance system approach that seeks to provide global safety monitoring by designing the WIN system to meet the specific needs of the working caregiver and their elderly family member (Mahoney, in press). We uniquely provide tailored information in real time with secured access limited to the worker. Primary control is given to the caregiving dyad as to when and how the monitoring will occur. From our early adopters—that is, those who readily embraced a new technology—we have learned that the system is viewed as an enabler, facilitating the elders' capacity to remain at home alone amid family concerns (Mahoney, 2004). One son has reported that now his telephone calls to his father are much more adultlike because he is not calling to nag him but to talk about more pleasant things such as baseball. Through this feasibility and implementation study, we are learning critical information about the ways caregivers and their family members view technology and the needs they express that technology may help address. I can envision Internet-based monitoring partnerships being developed to give caregivers respite breaks by widening the circle of care to include long-distance family caregivers or even contracted monitoring from formal caregivers. At a clinical level, the geropsychiatric nurse could be alerted when clients fail to take their psychiatric medications or take too many, or when their activity levels or sleeping patterns markedly change, possibly indicating depression.

Many opportunities will arise to integrate new technologies into health care applications (Steffen, Mahoney, & Kelly, 2003). According to DeJesus (2000), "In health care, unfortunately, about 80% of users are in the risk-averse category and only 1% are early adopters" (p. 50). My research on adoption of technology has documented that there are those working within a culture of personal relationships who strongly believe that the use of technology depersonalizes care and will result in worse outcomes. Our data does demonstrate that technology cannot com-

pletely substitute for in-person case assessment of frail elders. But technology can enhance care by providing real-time monitoring of vulnerable elders who otherwise would only receive intermittent case manager home visits, and it can send alerts about important changes in status to trigger more timely reassessment (Mahoney, Tennstedt, Friedman, & Heeren, 1999). Privacy concerns are another frequently stated major barrier to adoption that can be managed through secured Web sites, data encryptions, and clear consent acquisition for *all* involved parties (Mahoney, 2004). Should everyone then become an early adopter? Some words of wisdom: The first generation of new technologies translates ideas into reality, but their full potential is still promised. They also tend to have reliability and stability problems. Participation in feasibility trials to test utility and influence design will help to better meet caregiver needs. A champion is necessary in health care agencies, who is able to weather the inevitable frustrations of brand new applications. Otherwise, there is a risk of demoralizing the staff and turning them off to technology adoption.

It may be wise to defer major purchases of new technologies until their third generation, when they have become debugged, made easier to use, and more compact, but offer more capacity and features at lower costs. Other words of advice include considering leasing and subcontracting options. You reduce the risk of costly investments in systems that don't work as expected or desired. Mature systems offer better integration and flexibility. Avoid single system designs that depend on a sole source company for updates, enhancements, and repairs. "Off-the-shelf components," "universal elements," and "meets industry standards" are words to embrace to ensure timely fixing, easy modifications, and less cost. But don't fall into mediocrity or become outdated because you wait too long to embrace new technology. Partner with developers and participate in studies to ensure your needs are met and the technology translates well into geropsychiatric mental health nursing practice!

New practice possibilities will arise. Technology opens the door for flexible practice opportunities heretofore missing in nursing, such as telecommuting and scheduling at-home work hours. The nurse therapist can conduct remote home visits and group counseling sessions over the Internet from anywhere, including home. This flexibility may help attract and retain nurses longer, especially in rural, hard to travel areas. The need to develop new models of nursing care and to reinvent the work environment are recommendations made to address the nursing shortage (Robert Wood Johnson Foundation, 2002) that can be enabled through advanced technologies. It's time to reconceptualize the geropsychiatric nurse–patient relationship to include technology!

References

Baer, L., Jacobs, D., Cukor, P., O'Laughlen, J., Coyle, J., & Magruder, K. (1995). Automated telephone screening survey for depression. *Journal of the American Medical Association, 273*(24), 1943–1944.

Baer, L., Elford, D., & Cukor, P. (1997). Telepsychiatry at forty: What have we learned? *Harvard Review of Psychiatry, 5*(1), 7–17.

Baer, L., & Greist, J. H. (1997). An interactive computer-administered self-assessment and self-help program for behavior therapy. *Journal of Clinical Psychiatry, 58*(12), 23–28.

Cukor, P., Baer, L., Willis, B. S., Leahy, L., O'Laughlen, J., Murphy, M., et al. (1998). Use of videophones and low-cost standard telephone lines to provide a social presence in telepsychiatry. *Telemedicine Journal, 4*(4), 313–321.

DeJesus, E. (2000). Moving healthcare transactions online can improve efficiencies but barriers include technology—and a culture change. *Healthcare Informatics, 17*(6), 45–50.

Gitlin, L. N., Belle, S. H., Burgio, L. D., Czaja, S. J., Mahoney, D., Gallagher-Thompson, D., et al. (2003). Effect of multicomponent interventions on caregiver burden and depression: The REACH multisite initiative at six month follow-up. *Psychology and Aging, 18*(3), 361–374.

Greist, J. H., Marks, I. M., Baer, L., Kobak, K. A., Wenzel, K. W., Hirsch, M. J., et al. (2002). Behavior therapy for obsessive-compulsive disorder guided by a computer or by a clinician compared with relaxation as a control. *Journal of Clinical Psychiatry, 63*(2), 138–145.

Mahoney, D. (2000). Developing technology applications for intervention research: A case study. *Computers in Nursing, 18*(6), 260–264.

Mahoney, D., Tarlow, B., Jones, R., Tennstedt, S., & Kasten, L. (2001). Factors affecting the use of a telephone-based computerized intervention for caregivers of people with Alzheimer's disease. *Journal of Telemedicine and Telecare, 7,* 139–148.

Mahoney, D., Tarlow, B., & Jones, R. (2003). Effects of an automated telephone support system on caregiver burden and anxiety: Findings from the REACH for Telephone-Linked Care intervention study. *The Gerontologist, 43*(4), 556–567.

Mahoney, D. (1998). A content analysis of an Alzheimer family caregivers virtual focus group. *American Journal of Alzheimer's Disease, 13*(6), 306–316.

Mahoney, D., Tarlow, B., Jones, R., & Sandaire, K. (2002). An interactive CD-ROM program that increases user's knowledge about the differences between normal forgetfulness and serious memory loss. *Journal of the American Medical Informatics Association, 9*(4), 383–394.

Mahoney, D. F. (in press). Linking home care and the workplace through innovative wireless technology: The Worker Interactive Networking (WIN) project. *Home Health Care Management & Practice.*

Mahoney, D. F. (2004). Workplace response to virtual caregiver support and sensor home monitoring of elders: The WIN project. Working paper.

Mahoney, D., Tennstedt, S., Friedman, R., & Heeren, T. (1999). An automated telephone system for monitoring the functional status of community-residing elders. *The Gerontologist, 39*(2), 229–234.

Mundt, J. C., Freed, D. M. & Greist, J. H. (2000). Lay person-based screening for early detection of Alzheimer's disease: Development and validation of an instrument. *Journal of Gerontology, 55*(3), P163–P170.

Mundt, J. C., Ferber, K. L., Rizzo, M., & Greist, J. H. (2001). Computer-automated dementia screening using a touch-tome telephone. *Archives of Internal Medicine, 161*(20), 2481–2487.

Nakamura, K., Takehito, T., & Chiemi, A. (1999). The effectiveness of videophones in home health care for the elderly. *Medical Care, 37*(2), 117–125.

Osgood-Hynes, D. J., Greist, J. H., Marks, I. M., Bear, L., Heneman, S. W., Wenzel, K. W., et al. (1998). Self-administered psychotherapy for depression using a telephone-accessed computer system plus booklets: An open U.S.–U.K. study. *Journal of Clinical Psychiatry, 59*(7), 358–365.

Riva, G., Botella, C., Légeron, P., & Optale, D. (Eds.). (2004). *Cybertherapy: Internet and virtual reality as assessment and rehabilitation tools for clinical psychology and neuroscience*, Amsterdam: Ios Press. Retrieved July 15, 2004, from www.cybertherapy.info

Robert Wood Johnson Foundation. (2002). *Health care's human crisis: The American nursing shortage.* Retrieved May 15, 2003, from www.rwjf.org/special/nursingshortage

Schulz, R., Burgio, L., Burns, R., Eisodorfer, C., Gallagher-Thompson, D., Gitlin, L., et al. (2003). Resources for Enhancing Alzheimer's Caregiver Health (REACH): Overview, site-specific outcomes, future directions. *The Gerontologist, 43*(4), 514–520.

Steffen, A., Mahoney, D., & Kelly, K. (2003). Capitalizing on technological advances. In D. Coon, D. Gallagher-Thompson, & L. Thompson (Eds.), *Innovative interventions to reduce dementia caregiver distress—A clinical guide* (pp. 189–209). New York: Springer.

Zarate, C., Weinstock, L., Cukor, P., Moravito, C., Leahy, L., Burns, C., et al. (1997). Applicability of telemedicine for assessing patients with schizophrenia: Acceptance and reliability. *Journal of Clinical Psychiatry, 58*(1), 22–25.

ENVISIONING THE FUTURE OF GEROPSYCHIATRIC NURSING

Kathleen Coen Buckwalter, PhD, RN, FAAN

Dr. Kathleen Buckwalter, University of Iowa Foundation Distinguished Professor of Nursing, was named Associate Provost for Health Sciences in August 1997. In addition to her primary academic appointment as professor of nursing, she is Co-Director of the University's Center on Aging, Co-Director of the Hartford Center for Geriatric Nursing Excellence, Associate Director of the Gerontological Nursing Interventions Research Center, and has secondary appointments in the College of Medicine Departments of Psychiatry and Internal Medicine. Buckwalter is recognized internationally for her research in psychiatric nursing, aging, and long-term care, and has a sustained record of private and federal support related to the evaluation of clinical nursing interventions for geropsychiatric populations. Her particular interest is in behavioral management strategies for rural caregivers of persons with dementia and the effectiveness of community programs to prevent, minimize, and treat psychiatric problems in the rural elderly. With support from the NIMH and Administration on Aging, Buckwalter headed the Mental Health of the Rural Elderly Outreach Project. She also served as principal investigator of the PLST Model: Effectiveness for Rural ADRD Caregivers funded by NINR.

In 1999, Dr. Buckwalter received the Distinguished Contribution to Research Award from the Midwest Nursing Research Society and was elected to the National Academy of Sciences Institute of Medicine. In 2001 she was the recipient of the American Psychiatric Nurses Association Excellence in Research Award, and the first recipient of the National Gerontological

Nursing Association Board of Directors Award. Dr. Buckwalter serves on numerous review committees, editorial boards, and advisory groups. She has authored over 280 articles, over 90 book chapters, and co-edited eight books on topics such as geriatric mental health, memory, aging, and dementia.

Many changes have taken place since the term "geropsychiatric nursing" first appeared in the Cumulative Index to Nursing and Allied Health Literature in 1977 (Beck, 1988, p. 841). As I wrote nearly a decade ago, I remain very optimistic about the future of geropsychiatric nursing, but there is still much work to be done. "Nurses must work to create the professional and political will to avoid a crisis in long-term care. We must work to create models of care that are appropriate for the elderly and their families; pursue adequate funding and reimbursement for programming and services; support the preparation and retention of adequate numbers of qualified nursing providers; increase our research to assess the effectiveness of care strategies; increase our emphasis on health promotion, community-based services, and continuity of care; and strengthen the gerontological and professional ethics content of our curricula." (Maas & Buckwalter, 1996, pg. 247). As above, I envision changes and innovations in geropsychiatric nursing education, research, and practice in order to meet the "broad-based psychosocial, psychiatric, neurobiologic, and medical knowledge necessary to address the mental health needs of the elderly" (Wakefield, Buckwalter, & Gerdner, 1998, p. 914). Space limitations prohibit an exhaustive review of these changes, so I have limited my discussion to the following areas: new service delivery models or settings for care; needed research; emphasis on translation of research into practice; need to prepare more geropsychiatric nurse practitioners; health promotion; and disease prevention.

New Service Delivery Models/ Settings for Care

Nursing Homes Approximately 80% of persons who reside in nursing homes (NHs) have a diagnosable psychiatric disorder, with dementia being the most prevalent. Indeed, the prevalence of mental illnesses among NH residents is growing so dramatically that the Office of the Inspector General dubbed these nursing facilities, "de facto psychiatric hospitals" (Vickery, 2003). And yet, despite this high prevalence, and the associated behavioral problems, the majority of residents who need mental health services do not receive them (Tariot, Podgorski, Blazina, & Leibovici, 1993). Further, 50% of NHs report inadequate access to psychiatric consultation and 75% are unable to obtain the consultation and educational services they need to provide effective behavioral interventions for residents (Reichman et al., 1998). Currently, three primary models of mental health service delivery in nursing homes have been identified (Bartels, Moak, & Dums, 2002): psychiatrist-centered, multidisciplinary team, and nurse-centered models. The nurse-centered models emphasize consultation to NH personnel and the education of direct care staff to provide mental health interventions within the home. A "train-the-trainer" approach is used, in which geropsychiatric nurses outside of the NH provide ongoing training and consultation to staff who then become internal "experts" responsible for the training of others in the facility (Smith, Mitchell, Buckwalter & Garand, 1994; Smith, Mitchell, Buckwalter, 1995). In order to address current unmet needs for the delivery of mental health services to nursing homes, I foresee the emergence of more nurse-centered models of care, and an enhanced role for geropsychiatric nurses as members of multidisciplinary teams.

Assisted Living Facilities (ALFs) Common tenets of assisted living's philosophical model include autonomy, dignity, and service flexibility that facilitate maximum independence and aging-in-place. Over 500,000 older adults resided in 11,459 ALFs in 1998, and the number of persons entering assisted living is expected to double over the next decade. Of note, an estimated 34% to 50% of older people living in ALFs have dementia, and an estimated 30% of all facilities have dedicated dementia units, with growth in the number of dementia-specific facilities expected in the future (Hawes, Rose, & Phillips, 1999). The acuity levels of many ALF residents rival those of nursing homes a decade ago, without the same level of staffing and staff preparation. Thus, the rapid expansion of ALFs nationwide, including those that target the care of older adults with dementia, makes this environment an increasing focus of interest and concern for geropsychiatric nurses.

Geropsychiatric Inpatient Units To better accommodate the unique problems and mental health needs of older adults, changes are occurring in health care delivery systems. Once such adaptation is the development of specialized geriatric psychiatric inpatient units and services. Although these specialized units are increasingly common, little is known about how many, or what type of, services have developed nationwide—information that is essential for establishing best practices for these inpatient units, providing a foundation of knowledge upon which staff can build, and promoting networking among nurses who share common goals and needs. Thus, geropsychiatric nurses need to: (1) determine the current state of the art for inpatient geropsychiatric units, (2) develop specialized staff orientation and training that addresses both geriatric and psychiatric care needs, and (3) acknowledge the importance of interdisciplinary care in treating these complex patients, many of whom present with physical co-morbidities.

Regrettably, posthospitalization success is often limited, suggesting that improved understanding and communication between nurses working in nursing homes and hospital inpatient units is needed in order to solve the "revolving door" syndrome associated with transfer trauma for geropsychiatric patients. More joint conferences and other means of information sharing, problem solving, and networking between geriatric and psychiatric nurses are warranted (Smith, Buckwalter, & Maxson, 2002).

Co-located/Integrated Primary Care and Mental Health Services The lack of adequately trained geriatric mental health professionals is compounded by the fact that older adults seldom acknowledge their mental health problems or self-refer to psychiatric service settings because of barriers such as stigma, geographic access, limited funding and resources, and workforce issues. Even when mental health services are available, older adults do not use them. Less than 3% of elders report seeing a mental health professional for treatment, and only half of those who acknowledge mental health problems receive any kind of psychiatric treatment. Indeed, the primary care system has been called the "de facto mental health delivery system" (Peek & Heinrich, 2000), in that it manages, either directly or indirectly, about 30% of all patients with mental disorders. Undiagnosed and untreated mental disorders such as depression and anxiety can lead to increased disability, premature death, increased morbidity, increased risk of institutionalization, and a significant decrease in an elder's quality of life (Morris, 2001). Therefore, better integration of mental health and primary care for older people with mental illness is needed. Geropsychiatric nurses can play a pivotal role in promoting collaborative, cooperative approaches among health, mental health, primary care, and community and institutional care service providers, consumers, and family members, so that the system as a whole can deliver more effective and consistent services to mentally ill elders that support their functional status and quality of life (Cotroneo, Kurlowizc, Outlaw, Burgess, & Evans, 2001).

Expanded Roles

Geropsychiatric nurses are likely to be called upon to enact more of a clinical leadership and case management role in the future, to act as "bridge builders" of understanding across specialties, and as advocates for integration of mental health into a primary care framework to enhance the overall health and functioning of vulnerable elders (Cotroneo et al., 2001), and during end-of-life care. Care of the mentally ill elderly requires a systems orientation that involves coordination across medical, insurance, social support, and family systems, as well as among representatives of various disciplines such as medicine, pharmacy, social work, and so on (McBride, 2000). Geropsychiatric nurses will also be increasingly called upon to use telehealth and other techonology-based approaches and delivery methods to provide education and care for patients and their families in distant and underserved communities (Buckwalter, Davis, Wakefield, Kienzle, & Murray, 2002). In the future, geropsychiatric nurses will serve in a variety of independent practice roles, as well as collaborative and consultative roles. They will be active in determining cost-containment strategies while preserving quality care in our cost-driven health care reform process, and will serve as advocates for the most vulnerable special care elder populations such as minorities, the homeless, rural elders, developmentally disabled elders, those living alone, and the oldest-old.

Needed Research

Geropsychiatric nurses must conduct well-designed intervention and health service research in order to determine which treatments are most effective in a variety of institutional and community-based settings in which they practice, to ascertain the competencies that are essential for providers of mental health care to the elderly, and to evaluate the cost-effectiveness of interventions. For example, in spite of the increasing role played by ALFs in dementia care, little is known about important environmental variables that likely impinge on resident abilities. There has also been very little systematic study of psychiatric illnesses characteristic of residents in this setting. Intervention studies are sorely needed to ease distressing behavioral symptoms and to help ALF residents to maintain more active and independent social activities.

It is incumbent upon geropsychiatric nurses to then use their findings to change regulatory and reimbursement policies and to support improved mental health services to elders (Bartels et al., 2002). This is essential in an era of cost-driven health care reform, and because at present Medicare only reimburses about 50% of mental health care costs and fails to reimburse some services and diagnoses altogether. To achieve this goal, geropsychiatric nurses will need to undertake more translation of research findings into the development of evidence-based protocols to guide their clinical practice.

■ EMPHASIS ON TRANSLATION OF RESEARCH INTO PRACTICE

Three decades ago the need for greater use of research findings in practice was identified as one of the 15 priorities in clinical nursing research (Lindeman, 1975). Since that time, the emphasis on evidence-based practice (EBP) has generated a greater demand for nurses to use research to guide practice (Janken & Dufault, 2002). Despite regulatory and professional standards that address EBP, use of research in practice remains sporadic at best. Evidence-based practice is defined as the conscientious and judicious use of current best evidence, in conjunction with patient values and clinical expertise, to guide health care decisions (Sackett, Straus, Richardson, Rosenberg, & Haynes 2000). It encompasses dissemination of scientific knowledge and other types of evidence, critique, and synthesis of the evidence, determining applicability of the evidence in practice, developing an evidence-based practice standard, implementing the evidence-based practice, and evaluating changes in practice. Important roles for geropsychiatric nurses are facilitating the testing of selected EBP protocols in clinical sites, taking an active role with providers to promote adoption of EBPs, and creating EBP centers of excellence in acute and long-term care settings that can serve as exemplars for the provision of evidence-based care for mentally ill older adults.

Need to Prepare More Geropsychiatric Nurses

Nurses are still struggling with the issue of what it means to be a geropsychiatric nurse, and what qualifications and educational background are needed to best care for older adults with complex psychiatric and comorbid medical problems. Indeed, the number of currently practicing geropsychiatric nurses is unknown, in part because there is no certification procedure. However, one thing is certain: The demand for specialists in care of mentally ill and cognitively impaired elders will only increase in the coming years as the baby boom generation cares for their aging parents, begins to think about their own retirement and old age, and places financial demands on the health and mental health systems. The expectations and demands of "boomers" for rational and responsive systems of care will be enormous, and our current systems of elder care are unlikely to meet those demands, in large part because of the inadequate numbers of nurses prepared to care for the elderly,

especially those suffering from mental and neurological disorders. In that approximately 20% of older adults experience specific mental disorders that cannot be considered part of the normal aging process, these nurses will require a greater understanding of the behavioral science of aging to function as effective practitioners (McBride, 2000). Knowledge is necessary, not only of the unique presentation of psychiatric disorders in later life, but also about aspects of normal aging, disease, and disabilities associated with aging; psychopharmacology, genetics, and pharmacogenetics; a more integrated view of wellness and illness; and cultural differences among minority aged (Morris, 2001). Traditional geriatric nursing programs contain inadequate content related to the assessment and management of psychosocial needs of older adults. Nor do they prepare nurses to intervene using successful individual, group, family, and pharmacologic strategies. Similarly, most psychiatric nursing programs fail to provide adequate information on the unique needs of the older adult. Thus, more geropsychiatric nursing programs are needed, and happily, the number of such high-quality programs is expanding, thanks in large part to initiatives sponsored by the John A. Hartford Foundation under their Geriatric Nursing Education Project. For example, the Case Western Reserve University Frances Payne Bolton School of Nursing has incorporated more geriatric mental health content into the GNP curriculum, and the University of Arkansas for Medical Sciences College of Nursing has implemented a geropsychiatric initiative that includes a 4-semester program plus summer session and prepares practitioners to address a comprehensive array of mental and physical health needs of older adults. Similarly, the University of Michigan School of Nursing has developed a specialized concentration in geropsychiatric nursing that augments existing programs and uses distance-learning strategies, and the University of Nebraska

Medical Center College of Nursing has five courses in its advanced geropsychiatric nursing practice focus area. A number of other excellent courses, programs and post-baccalaureate and post-master's certificate programs have recently been implemented or are under development. As the specialty of geropsychiatric nursing further develops and continues to define itself, I expect the ANCC will develop an exam that will allow clinicians who care for the mentally ill elderly to be certified as such.

Health Promotion and Disease Prevention

Geropsychiatric nurses are concerned with both the prevention of health problems in elders and with care of those who have emotional, behavioral and mental disorders in a variety of community-based and institutional settings (Wakefield et al., 1998). However, much of our specialty focus to date has been on the care of frail and cognitively impaired elders. With increases in active life expectancy, and growing ethnic diversity among the elderly population, this focus may change to a greater emphasis on maintaining vitality/health and restorative models of care in well older adults; those who have the physical, mental, social, and spiritual function or resources to meet the needs of everyday living (Belza & Baker, 2000). This could entail greater attention to the mental health needs and education of well elders, development and evaluation of innovative mental health wellness centers and services, and assurance that adequate support systems (e.g. transportation, recreation, nutrition) and trained providers are available so that older adults can attain and maintain optimal mental health, remain actively engaged in their communities, feel a sense of personal control over their lives, and enjoy lifelong good interpersonal relationships (Belza & Baker). As functional status is strongly impacted by coping styles, social sup-

port, and affective status, it seems likely that geropsychiatric nurses could play a key role in optimizing the mental health of well elders. For example, they might provide pre-retirement counseling services, conduct mental health screening, lead problem solving and assertiveness groups, and train peer counselors at community centers.

Conclusion

I am confident, as I meet with new graduates who are choosing a career in geropsychiatric nursing, talk with nursing leaders at conferences, read the improved quality of the literature addressing geropsychiatric nursing issues, review innovative proposals submitted by nurses for private and federal funding to support their research related to care of mentally ill elders, and see the improvements that are slowly taking place in health care environments for elders, that geriatric nursing will not only survive, but will thrive in years to come. It's truly an exciting time to be a geropsychiatric nurse, and I feel so lucky to have gotten in on the ground floor of geropsychiatric nursing more than twenty years ago.

References

Bartels, S. J., Moak, G. S., & Dums, A. R. (2002). Models of mental health services in nursing homes: A review of the literature. *Psychiatric Services, 53*(22), 1390–1396.

Belza, B., & Baker, M. W. (2000). Maintaining health in well older adults: Initiatives for schools of nursing and the John A. Hartford Foundation for the 21st century. *Journal of Gerontological Nursing, 26*(7), 8–17.

Beck, C. K. (1988). The aged adult. In C. K. Beck, R. P. Rawlins, & S. R. Williams (Eds.), *Mental health-psychiatric nursing* (pp. 840–864, 2nd ed.). St. Louis, MO: C.V. Mosby.

Buckwalter, K. C., Davis, L. L., Wakefield, B. J., Kienzle, M. G., & Murray, M. A. (2002). Telehealth for elders and their caregivers in rural communities. *Family & Community Health, 25*(3), 31–40.

Cotroneo, M., Kurlowicz, L. H., Outlaw, F. H., Burgess, A. W., & Evans, L. K. (2001). Psychiatric-mental health nursing at the interface: Revisioning education for the specialty. *Issues in Mental Health Nursing, 22*(5), 549–569.

Hawes, C., Rose, M., & Phillips, C. (1999). *A national study of assisted living for the frail elderly: Results from a national survey of facilities.* Unpublished manuscript.

Janken, J. K., & Dufault, M. A. (2002, January 24). Improving the quality of pain assessment through research utilization. *The Online Journal of Knowledge Synthesis for Nursing, 2C,* Article OJ0011. Retrieved May 22, 2004, from http://www.stti.iupui.edu/library/ojksn/case_study/cc_doc2c.html

Lindeman, C. (1975). Priorities in clinical nursing research. *Nursing Outlook, 23*(11), 693–698.

Maas, M. L., & Buckwalter, K. C. (1996). Epilogue— gazing through the crystal ball: Gerontological nursing issues and challenges for the 21st century. In E. A. Swanson & T. Tripp-Reimer (Eds.), *Advances in gerontological nursing: Issues for the 21st century* (pp. 237–249). New York Springer.

McBride, A. B. (2000). Nursing and gerontology. *Journal of Gerontological Nursing, 26*(7), 18–27.

Morris, D. L. (2001). Geriatric mental health: An overview. *Journal of the American Psychiatric Nurses Association, 7*(6), S2–S7.

Peek, C. J., & Heinrich, R. L. (2000). Integrating behavioral health and primary care. In M. E. Maruish (Ed.), *Handbook of psychological assessment in primary care* (pp. 43–91). Mahwah, NJ: Lawrence Erlbaum.

Reichman, W. E., Coyne, A. C., Borson, S., Negron, A. E., Rovner, B. W., Pelchat, R. J., et al. (1998). Psychiatric consultation in the nursing home: A survey of six states. *American Journal of Geriatric Psychiatry, 6*(4), 320–327.

Sackett, D. L., Straus, S. E., Richardson, W. S., Rosenberg, W., & Haynes, R. B. (2000). *Evidence-based medicine: How to practice and teach EBM.* London: Churchill Livingstone.

Smith, M., Buckwalter K. C., & Maxson, E. (2002). Psychiatric and geriatric nurses together at the table: Evaluation of a combined conference. *Journal of the American Psychiatric Nurses Association, 8*(1), 3–8.

Smith, M., Mitchell, S., Buckwalter, K. C., & Garand, L. (1994). Geropsychiatric nursing consultation: A valuable resource in rural long-term care. *Archives of Psychiatric Nursing, 8*(4), 272–279.

Smith, M., Mitchell, S., & Buckwalter, K. C. (1995). Nurses helping nurses: Development of internal specialists in long-term care. *Journal of Gerontological Nursing, 21*(3), 25–33. Reprinted in: *Journal of Psychosocial Nursing, 33*(4), 38–42.

Tariot, P. N., Podgorski, C. A., Blazina, L., & Leibovici, A. (1993). Mental disorders in the nursing home: Another perspective. *American Journal of Psychiatry, 150*(7), 1063–1069.

Vickery, K. (2003). The complex path to managing mental illness. *Provider, 29*(5), 18–22.

Wakefield, B. J., Buckwalter, K. C., & Gerdner, L. A. (1998). Biopsychosocial care of the elderly mentally ill. In M. A. Boyd & M. A. Nilhart (Eds.), *Psychiatric mental health nursing* (pp. 912–939). Philadelphia: Lippincott.

INDEX